Basic and New Aspects of

# GASTROINTESTINAL ULTRASONOGRAPHY

**ADVANCED SERIES IN BIOMECHANICS**

Editor: Y C Fung *(University of California, San Diego)*

---

Vol. 1: Selected Works on Biomechanics and Aeroelasticity
Parts A & B
*by Y C Fung*

Vol. 2: Introduction to Bioengineering
*Ed. Y C Fung*

Vol. 3: Basic and New Aspects of Gastrointestinal Ultrasonography
*Eds. S Ødegaard, O H Gilja & H Gregersen*

Advanced Series in Biomechanics – Vol. 3

# Basic and New Aspects of GASTROINTESTINAL ULTRASONOGRAPHY

Editors

**Svein Ødegaard**
**Odd Helge Gilja**

*Haukeland University Hospital, and University of Bergen, Norway*

**Hans Gregersen**

*Aalborg Hospital, Denmark, and Aalborg University, Denmark*

World Scientific

NEW JERSEY • LONDON • SINGAPORE • BEIJING • SHANGHAI • HONG KONG • TAIPEI • CHENNAI

*Published by*

World Scientific Publishing Co. Pte. Ltd.
5 Toh Tuck Link, Singapore 596224
*USA office:* 27 Warren Street, Suite 401–402, Hackensack, NJ 07601
*UK office:* 57 Shelton Street, Covent Garden, London WC2H 9HE

**British Library Cataloguing-in-Publication Data**
A catalogue record for this book is available from the British Library.

*Cover design:* This 3D ultrasound reconstruction shows a pancreatic tumour and its surrounding structures. The tumour is depicted in grey, the liver in yellow, the gallbladder in light blue, the hepatic duct in pink, the aorta in green, and the superior mesenteric vein in red. The reconstruction is made in EchoPac3D, a software program dedicated for 3D ultrasound image analysis. The acquisition was performed by Dr. Odd Helge Gilja using the Bird System interfaced to a GE Vingmed System Five scanner with a 3.5 MHz curvilinear transducer.

**BASIC AND NEW ASPECTS OF GASTROINTESTINAL ULTRASONOGRAPHY**
**Advanced Series in Biomechanics — Vol. 3**



ISBN 981-238-845-1

Printed by Fulsland Offset Printing (S) Pte Ltd, Singapore

# PREFACE

Ultrasound nowadays is a well established diagnostic and therapeutic tool in diseases within several medical specialities. Furthermore, technical improvement of ultrasound equipment and continuous basic and clinical ultrasound research have increased the use of ultrasound within new fields.

In gastroenterology, ultrasound has been used for several decades to perform $B$-mode imaging of the abdominal organs. However, the development of new techniques, e.g. endoscopic ultrasonography, has made it possible to obtain detailed images of very small structures and to study pathophysiology of the gut. Ultrasound in gastroenterology is no longer limited to scanning of abdominal organs which, in many countries, is usually performed by radiologists. However, in gastroenterology, as in cardiology, gynaecology and obstetrics, basic and clinical education in this specific field is necessary to fully exploit the potential of ultrasound. Thus, external and endosonographic ultrasound has been used by our group to study gastrointestinal motility, allergy and inflammatory diseases using different ultrasound modes.

At the Division of Gastroenterology, Haukeland University Hospital, abdominal ultrasound was regarded as a promising investigation technique already in 1976. However, education and training within this field was necessary. To achieve this, we needed education abroad. Professor Harald Lutz, MD, Bayreuth, Professor Gerhard Rettenmaier, MD and Priv. Doz. Karlheinz Seitz, MD, Böblingen were pioneers within abdominal ultrasound and provided the help. We want to thank them and their coworkers for including members of our group in their training programmes and for their effort in continuous education within the field of abdominal ultrasound.

In 1987, we started to use endoscopic ultrasound in the Department of Gastroenterology. Within this field, the close collaboration with Professor Michael B. Kimmey, MD at the University of Washington in Seattle was of great importance. Furthermore, Professors Roy W. Martin, PhD, Fred E. Silverstein, MD, Alan Cheung, MD, Kirk Beach, MD and their research groups have been important coworkers within basic and clinical ultrasound.

The use of real-time $B$-mode ultrasound and Doppler-technology for studying gastrointestinal motility has become another major research field for our group and the clinical use of these techniques have, to some extent, replaced more stressful and expensive methods. Our group has developed original methods to study transpyloric flow, accommodation of the proximal stomach, intragastric distribution of meals, detailed strain estimation of the gastric muscle layers and endosonographic examination of the duodenal mucosa in patients with gastrointestinal allergy.

Three-dimensional ultrasound imaging has been an important part of our work for the last ten years. Basic research became possible in close cooperation with VingMed Sound and Christian Michelsen Research, Norway. Technical equipment and software development led to clinical applications both within external ultrasound and endosonography.

Education in ultrasound has been important for our group. For almost 20 years, we have offered ultrasound courses for doctors. Over the last 10 years, ultrasound was also included in the education of medical students. Clinical training of national and international colleagues has been an inspiration. Our network has extended to several new groups abroad, like the universities of Utrecht, Adelaide, Gothenburg, Aalborg and the University of Washington, Seattle.

In 2001, the Department of Medicine at Haukeland University Hospital was appointed National Centre for Ultrasound in Gastroenterology by the Norwegian National Health Authorities. Members of the centre are involved in several national and international ultrasound organisations, research and education programmes.

We are indepted to Professor Harald Lutz, MD, past president and Professor Sören Hancke, MD, Secretary, the World Federation for Ultrasound in Medicine and Biology and to Professor Michael B. Kimmey, MD, past president of the American Society for Gastrointestinal Endoscopy, for their written evaluation of our ultrasound activity. Furthermore, we wish to acknowledge Professor Jarle Ofstad, MD, Bergen, who has given us encouraging support. Their help was important for the decision of the Norwegian Authorities when deciding to give us the status as National Centre for Ultrasound in Gastroenterology.

We also want to thank the Health Authorities of Western Norway, the Administration of Haukeland University Hospital, the University of Bergen and Innovest Strategic Research Program for their enduring support. Hans Gregersen, now professor both in Bergen and Aalborg, has been supported by the Norwegian and Danish Research Councils. On the occasion of publishing this book, he wishes to acknowledge the mentorship in biomechanics by Professor Emeritus Yuan Cheng Fung, University of California, San Diego and in gastrointestinal physiology by Professor Emeritus James Christensen, University of Iowa Hospitals and Clinics. Finally, we wish to thank our loving families for their patience and support during the work with this book.

This book discusses basic and newer ultrasound applications in gastroenterology, partly based on the work from members of our Centre and from close collaborators. The book is intended both as an introduction to gastrointestinal ultrasonography for beginners as well as a presentation of new and advanced methods for experienced ultrasound colleagues.

Bergen, Norway, June 2004

Svein Ødegaard
Odd Helge Gilja
Hans Gregersen

# CONTENTS

## ABOUT THE EDITORS

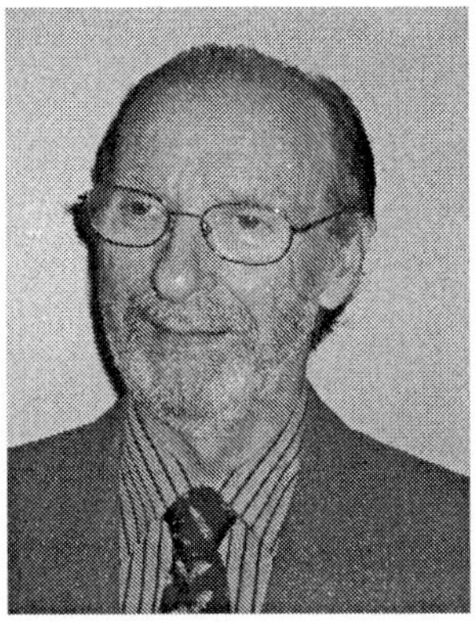

**Svein Ødegaard, Professor, University of Bergen, and Director, National Centre for Ultrasound in Gastroenterology, Haukeland University Hospital.**
Email: svein.odegaard@med.uib.no

M.D., Rheinische Friedrich Wilhelms Universitaet, Bonn, Germany, 1970. Specialist in Internal Medicine and Gastroenterology, Dr.med, University of Bergen, 1988. Professor, University of Bergen, 1995. Director Department of Medicine, Haukeland University Hospital from 1999–2004. President of the Norwegian Society for Diagnostic Ultrasound in Medicine 1989–1993. Board member European Federation for Ultrasound in Medicine and Biology 1993–2002. Visiting Professor, University of Washington, Seattle, USA, 1988, 1990, 1994. Senior member, American Institute of Ultrasound in Medicine. Advisory board member for European Journal of Ultrasound. Founder and Chairman, National Centre for Ultrasound in Gastroenterology, 2001. Three research awards.

**Research Interests:** Ultrasound in medicine. Imaging and signal conditioning. Three-dimensional ultrasound. Endoluminal ultrasound. Characterization of GI mucosa biopsies with flow cytometry and enzyme technology.

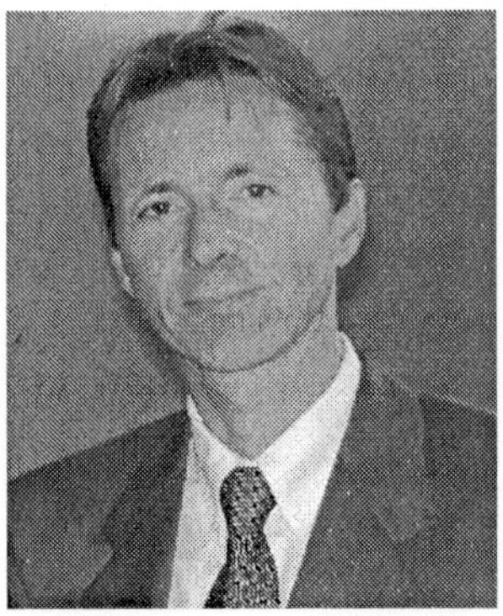

**Odd Helge Gilja, Professor, University of Bergen, and Consultant, National Centre for Ultrasound in Gastroenterology.**
Email: Odd.Gilja@med.uib.no

M.D., University of Bergen, 1990. Ph.D., University of Bergen, 1997. Consultant, Department of Medicine, Haukeland Hospital 2001 →. Associate Professor at Institute of Medicine, University of Bergen from 2001 and Professor from 2002. Secretary, National Centre of Ultrasound in Gastroenterology from 2001, consultant from 2003. President of Norwegian Society for Diagnostic Ultrasound in Medicine from 2001. Board member Scandinavian Association for Gastrointestinal Motility 1995–2001. Board member European Federation for Ultrasound in Medicine and Biology from 2002. Editorial Board of Neurogastroenterology and Motility from 2001. Editrial Board of Ultraschall in der Medizin from 2004. Vice-president of EUROSON congress 2003. Three international awards.

**Research Interests:** Ultrasonography. Functional dyspepsia, Gastric accommodation. Strain Rate Imaging. 3D imaging and reconstruction. Image analysis. Gastrointestinal motility. Biomechanics of the GI tract.

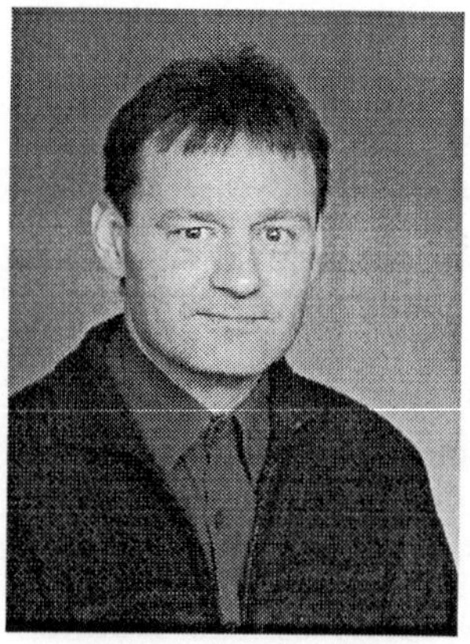

**Hans Gregersen, Professor of Bioengineering, Aalborg University, Denmark; Director of Research, Aalborg Hospital, Denmark.**
Email: hag@smi.auc.dk

M.D., Aarhus University 1988. Dr.M.Sci, Aarhus University, 1994. Master of Public Management, Odense University, 1999. Guest Professor, Institute of Mechanics and Materials and Department of Bioengineering, University of California, San Diego, 1994–1996. Editor on the book Essentials of Experimental Surgery 1996. Professor, Aalborg University from 1999, Advisory Professor, Chongqing University from 1999, Advisory Professor, Beijing Polytechnic University from 1999. Chairman of the Board, Accip Biotechnology from 1999. Guest Professor, Bergen University and Haukeland Hospital from 2001. Director of Research and Chairman of the Research Council, Aalborg Hospital from 2001. Three international research awards. Published the book Biomechanics of the Gastrointestinal Tract in 2002.

**Research Interests:** Gastrointestinal biomechanics and gastrointestinal tissue engineering. Development of equipment and imaging methods for studying soft tissue mechanical behavior. Development of a mathematical model for balloon distension studies. Modeling of the mechanical properties of multi-layered models of the GI tract. Non-cardiac chest pain and functional dyspepsia. Morphometric and biomechanical GI remodeling in neuromuscular diseases.

## ABOUT THE AUTHORS

**Arnold Berstad,** M.D., Ph.D.
Professor and Chairman
Division of Gastroenterology
Department of Medicine
Haukeland University Hospital
Institute of Medicine
University of Bergen
NO-5021 Bergen, Norway
E-mail: arnold.berstad@helse-bergen.no

**Peter Hans Dahl,** Ph.D.
Principal Engineer
Applied Physics Laboratory
Research Associate Professor
Department of Mechanical Engineering
University of Washington
Seattle, Washington 98105-6698, USA
E-mail: dahl@apl.washington.edu.

**Geir Folvik,** M.D.
Consultant
Division of Gastroenterology
Medical Department
Haukeland University Hospital
NO-5021 Bergen, Norway
Email: geir.folvik@helse-bergen.

**Odd Helge Gilja,** M.D., Ph.D.
Professor, Consultant
National Centre for Ultrasound in Gastroenterology
Department of Medicine
Haukeland University Hospital
Division of Gastroenterology
Institute of Medicine
University of Bergen
NO-5021 Bergen, Norway
E-mail: odd.gilja@uib.no

**Hans Gregersen, M.D., Dr.M.Sc., M.P.M.**
Professor of Bioengineering (SMI, Aalborg University)
guest professor, University of Bergen
Director of Research, Center of Excellence in Visceral Biomechanics and Pain
Aalborg Hospital, DK-9100 Aalborg, Denmark
Email: hag@aas.nja.dk

**Jan Hatlebakk, M.D., Ph.D.**
Associate Professor, Consultant
Division of Gastroenterology
Department of Medicine
Haukeland University Hospital
Institute of Medicine
University of Bergen
NO-5021 Bergen, Norway
E-mail: jan.hatlebakk@helse-bergen.no

**Trygve Hausken, M.D., Ph.D.**
Professor, Consultant
National Centre for Ultrasound in Gastroenterology
Division of Gastroenterology
Department of Medicine
Haukeland University Hospital
Institute of Medicine
University of Bergen
NO-5021 Bergen, Norway
E-mail: trygve.hausken@helse-bergen.no

**Andreas Heimdal, M.Sc., Ph.D.**
Senior Research Engineer
GE Vingmed Ultrasound
Forskningsparken, Gaustadalléen 21
NO-0349 Oslo, NORWAY
E-mail: Andreas.Heimdal@med.ge.com

**Kristian Hveem, M.D., Ph.D.**
Associate Professor, Consultant
Innherred Hospital
NO-7600 Levanger
Norway
Email: kristian.hveem@hnt.no

**Joo Ha Hwang, M.D.**
Department of Medicine
Division of Gastroenterology,
University of Washington
Seattle, Washington 98195 USA
Email: jooha@u.washington.edu

**Thomas Andersen, M.D.**
The Sam Laboratory
Institute of Experimental Clinical Research
Skejby Hospital
DK-8200 Aarhus N, Denmark
Email: ta@iekf.au.dk

**Michael B. Kimmey, M.D.**
Professor of Medicine
University of Washington
Seattle, Washington 98195, USA
Email: kimmey@u.washington.edu

**Ditlef Martens, M.Sc.**
Senior Development Engineer
GE Vingmed Ultrasound AS
Ibsensgt 104
NO-5052 Bergen, Norway
E-mail: Ditlef.Martens@med.ge.com

**Roy W. Martin, Ph.D.**
Research Professor
Departments of Anesthesiology and Bioengineering
Associate Director of Basic Research
Center for Medical and Industrial Ultrasound
Applied Physics Laboratory
University of Washington, Seattle WA 98195, USA
Email: rmartin@apl.washington.edu

**Knut Matre, M.Sc., Ph.D.**
Professor of Bioengineering and Biophysics
Institute of Medicine
University of Bergen
NO-5021 Bergen, Norway
knut.matre@med.uib.no

**Lars Birger Nesje, M.D, Ph.D.**
Director
Department of Medicine
Haukeland University Hospital
NO-5021 Bergen, Norway
lars.birger.nesje@helse-bergen.no

**Ole Martin Pedersen M.D., Ph.D.**
Consultant
Department of Heart Disease
Haukeland University Hospital
NO-5021 Bergen, Norway
Email: ole.pedersen@helse-bergen.no

**Solomon Tefera M.D., Ph.D., M.H.A.**
Consultant, Vice Chairman
Division of Gastroenterology
Medical Department
Diaconess University Hospital Haraldsplass
NO-5009 Bergen, Norway
Email: stef@haraldsplass.no

**Svein Ødegaard, M.D, Ph.D.**
Professor and Chairman
National Centre for Ultrasound in Gastroenterology
Department of Medicine
Haukeland University Hospital
Institute of Medicine
University of Bergen
N-5021 Bergen, Norway
E-mail: svein.odegaard@med.uib.no

CHAPTER 1

# BASIC TECHNOLOGIES IN ULTRASOUND

KNUT MATRE AND PETER HANS DAHL

## 1. Nature of Sound Waves

### 1.1. *Longitudinal waves and sound speed*

Biological tissues behave more like a fluid than a solid, insofar as being a medium through which sound waves propagate. This means that the elasticity of biological tissues is primarily in the form of compressibility, and that sound waves used in diagnostic ultrasound are primarily longitudinal waves for which a parcel of fluid under the influence of the sound wave moves back and forth with velocity, $\mathbf{u}$, in a direction parallel to that of the propagating sound wave. An important exception is solid bone tissue, which possess both compressive and shear elasticity, and thus both longitudinal and transverse sound waves, or shear waves, propagate within the bone. For transverse waves, motion of the medium is perpendicular to the direction of the propagating sound wave.

The displacement of a parcel of fluid, or tissue material, moving with velocity $\mathbf{u}$ (called the particle velocity) is exceedingly small, being much less than a nanometer. However, the passage of a longitudinal wave (Fig. 1) through the tissue causes parcels to be alternately compressed together to produce a high-pressure region and spread apart to produce a low-pressure region, also called rarefaction. The speed that this alternating pressure field propagates through the medium is the sound speed, $c$.

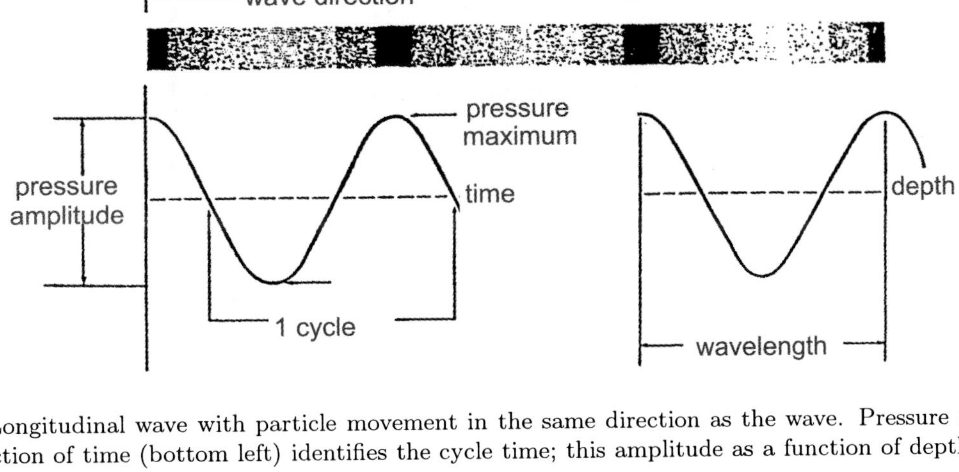


Fig. 1. Longitudinal wave with particle movement in the same direction as the wave. Pressure amplitude as a function of time (bottom left) identifies the cycle time; this amplitude as a function of depth (bottom right) identifies the wavelength.

The speed of sound in biological tissue depends on the density $\rho$ and the compressibility of the tissue according to

$$c = (K/\rho)^{1/2} \tag{1}$$

where $K$ is the bulk modulus of the material; this quantity is inversely related to compressibility, which is a measure of tissue stiffness. The sound speed for longitudinal waves is thus faster in relatively stiff material such as bone and slower in more compressible material such as soft tissue. A typical sound speed for soft tissue is 1550 m/s, with the relation between sound speed and particle velocity being such that $|\mathbf{u}|/c \ll 1$.

## 1.2. *Frequency and wavelength of ultrasound*

In addition to sound speed, sound waves are characterized by their frequency $f$, and wavelength $\lambda$; these three quantities are fundamentally related by

$$c = f\lambda \tag{2}$$

Sound wavelength is the spatial separation between regions of peak compression or peak rarefaction (Fig. 1). Diagnostic ultrasound uses sound frequencies well beyond the range of normal human hearing (approximately 20,000 Hz). Such high frequencies are used because the resulting short wavelengths are necessary to obtain high spatial resolution. In general, non-invasive medical ultrasound uses frequencies in the range 1–10 MHz (1 MHz = 1,000,000 Hz), while invasive methods use frequencies up to 40 MHz. Given a nominal soft tissue sound speed of 1550 m/s puts $\lambda$ in the range of 1.5 mm to 150 $\mu$m for frequencies between 1 and 10 MHz.

## 1.3. *Characteristic impedance and sound intensity*

The ratio of the sound wave pressure to particle velocity is defined as the characteristic acoustic impedance $Z$ of a material; $Z$ is also simply related to sound speed and density as follows:

$$Z = c\rho \tag{3}$$

and can also be thought of as a measure of the resistance to sound passing through the tissue. A typical $Z$ value for internal organ tissue is $1.62 \cdot 10^6$ kgm$^{-2}$s$^{-1}$ (the physical unit of $Z$ is the Rayl). Reflection of ultrasound at smooth tissue interfaces associated with changes in impedance is one of the primary mechanisms for ultrasound imaging. The other mechanism is diffuse scattering from rough tissue interfaces and tissue internal structures.

The strength of a sound wave is given by its intensity $I$ which is related to the pressure $P$ and acoustic impedance by

$$I = \frac{1}{2}\frac{P^2}{Z} \tag{4}$$

If the sound waveform is sinusoidal (often a good approximation) then the intensity is given by

$$I = \frac{1}{2}P_o u_o \tag{5}$$

where $P_o$ and $u_o$ are, respectively, the peak pressure and particle velocity for one cycle of the sine wave. A typical sound field intensity for a diagnostic ultrasonic waveform is 1–50 mWcm$^{-2}$.

## 1.4. *Specular reflection, refraction and scattering*

If the interface between the tissues is sufficiently smooth compared to the ultrasonic wavelength, a reflection process occurs at the interface (Fig. 2). For an angle of incidence close to 0° (called normal incidence) a fraction of the ultrasonic energy is reflected back towards the transducer and the remaining energy is transmitted into the second tissue with no change in the propagation angle. In general, $\theta_1$ will not be exactly 0°; in this case the reflected angle is the same magnitude as $\theta_1$ but of opposite sign. The relation between $\theta_1$ and the transmitted angle, $\theta_2$, is governed by Snell's Law for refraction:

$$\frac{\sin\theta_1}{c_1} = \frac{\sin\theta_2}{c_2} \tag{6}$$

where $c_1$ is the sound speed in the first tissue containing the incoming waveform, and $c_2$ is the sound speed in the second tissue.

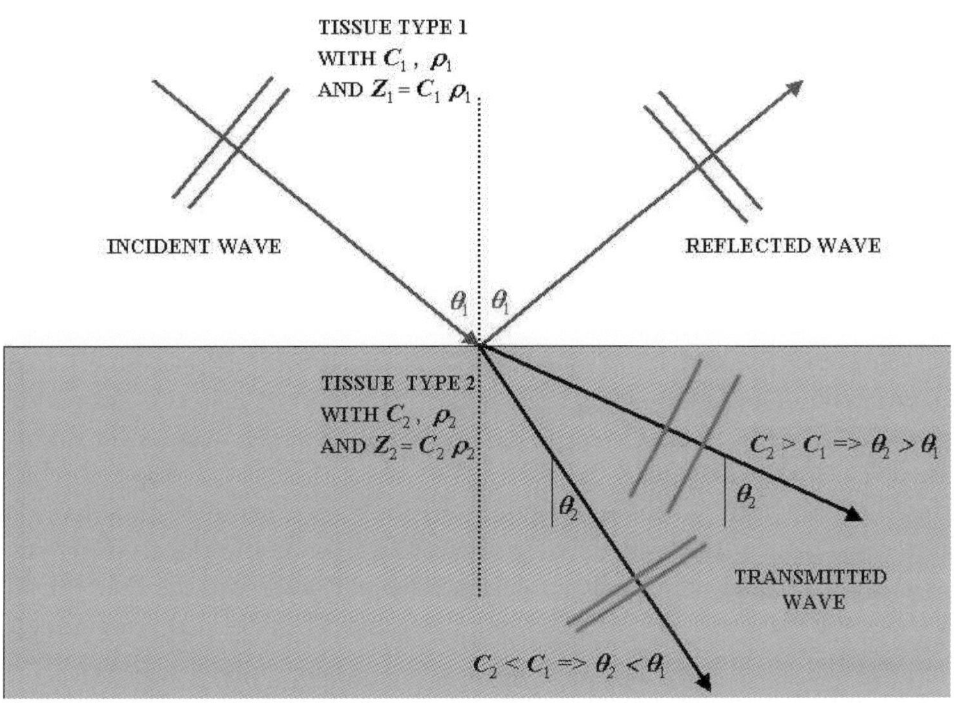


Fig. 2. Reflection, refraction and transmission at smooth interface between two tissues characterized by sound speed and density $c_1$, $\rho_1$ and $c_2$, $\rho_2$. Two different relations between $c_1$ and $c_2$ are shown. The incident waveform is symbolized by an arrow encountering the tissue interface at an angle of incidence, $\theta_1$. The two lines parallel to each arrow represents ultrasonic wave (or phase) fronts separated by distance $\lambda$; an increase or decrease in sound speed changes $\lambda$ accordingly.

The fraction of ultrasonic energy that is reflected at the interface is given by the intensity reflection coefficient $R$ which ranges from 0 to 1, and is given by

$$R = \left[\frac{(Z_2/Z_1 - \cos\theta_2/\cos\theta_1)}{(Z_2/Z_1 + \cos\theta_2/\cos\theta_1)}\right]^2 \tag{7}$$

where $Z_1$ is the characteristic acoustic impedance of the first tissue and $Z_2$ is that of the second tissue. This relation reduces to

$$R = \left[\frac{(Z_2/Z_1 - 1)}{(Z_2/Z_1 + 1)}\right]^2 \tag{8}$$

for normal incidence.

Thus, *refraction*, or the degree to which the direction an ultrasonic beam has changed within the second tissue, depends on the ratio of sound speeds for the two tissues, whereas *reflection* depends on the ratio of the characteristic acoustic impedances. For example, normal incidence reflection between two soft tissues, say fat ($Z_1 \approx 1.40 \cdot 10^6$ Rayls) and kidney tissue ($Z_2 \approx 1.62 \cdot 10^6$ Rayls), gives an $R \approx 0.005$, meaning that about 1/2% of the ultrasonic energy is reflected back from such an interface. On the other hand, the muscle-bone interface results in a much higher reflection coefficient ($R \approx 0.4$) because the characteristic acoustic impedance of bone is much higher than that for muscle. Another high reflection case is the abdomen, wherein the impedance of abdominal gas ($Z_2$) is much less than the impedance of the surrounding tissue ($Z_1$). For $Z_2 \ll Z_1$, then $R$ will be approximately 1, indicating the strongest of reflection, and ultrasonic transmission into the gas-filled abdominal areas is weak. Note that these relations apply for the case of small angles of incidence that are typical for medical imaging applications. However, if the angle of incidence $\theta_1$ is sufficiently large such that it exceeds the *critical angle*, then total reflection, and no transmission, occurs between the two tissue interfaces. The critical angle $\theta_c$ (also governed by Snell's Law) is given by:

$$\sin\theta_c = \frac{c_1}{c_2} \tag{9}$$

Finally, the above relation for $R$ describes only the reflection process for longitudinal waves. A conversion of acoustic energy originally in the form of longitudinal waves to shear waves (transverse waves) can occur at certain angles of incidence when solid tissues such as bone are involved in the reflection.

If the interface between tissues is irregular and rough compared to the ultrasonic wavelength, scattering, rather than reflection, occurs at the tissue interface. Here the incident energy is partitioned into a now smaller fraction reflected back towards the transducer; the remaining energy is scattered into a broad angular range of directions, including a fraction transmitted into the second tissue.

Another form of scattering, called diffuse scattering, is caused by tissue internal structures, such as blood vessels, tubules, etc, that are small in comparison with the ultrasonic wavelength. Again, sound is scattered into a broad angular range of directions, with the degree to which sound is scattered in a particular direction determined by the material properties of the tissue structure and the ultrasonic wavelength. An important form of diffuse scattering is known as *Rayleigh scattering*. This occurs if the characteristic dimension of the tissue structure $L$ is such that $L \ll \lambda$. When Rayleigh scattering applies, the scattered echo amplitude varies as the fourth power of ultrasonic frequency. Because diffuse scattering produces echoes that are much weaker than specular reflection, it is often necessary in grayscale ultrasonograhic processing that echo amplitudes be compressed in a non-linear manner in order to display both diffusely scattered and reflected echoes within the same image.

### 1.5. *Attenuation and TGC*

The ultrasound wave will be attenuated when it travels into the body. This attenuation is caused by several mechanisms including absorption (frictional losses), scattering from small objects and irregularities, and refraction and reflections at tissue interfaces. The most important factor is the absorption due to frictional losses for which sound energy is converted to heat. The attenuation is approximately proportional to the square of the transmitted frequency and varies for different types of tissue. Because the ultrasound wave is attenuated the echoes gradually become weaker. A compensation is made by a method called TGC (time gain compensation), giving the later-arriving echoes artificially higher amplification. Thus, a constant "grayscale" throughout all depths can be achieved for the ultrasound image.

## 2. Display Methods. Amplitude Imaging

### 2.1. *Ultrasound transducers*

Ultrasound waves are produced by transducers made of ceramic material having piezo-electric properties, meaning that a transducer (also called a crystal) will deform slightly when a voltage is applied across attached electrodes. The deforming vibrations produce an ultrasonic pressure waveform in the media to which the transducer is in contact with. Transducers are reciprocal devices, and carry out the reverse task of sound-to-electronic conversion associated with the pressure waves from echoes. A small (impedance-matching) layer of thickness $\lambda/4$ separates the tissue from the transducer face to increase the efficiency of this two-way conversion.

### 2.2. *A, B and M-modes*

The received (reflected) pulse or echo can be displayed by different methods summarized in Fig. 3. The first display method in clinical use was the $A$-mode ($A$ amplitude). Here the amplitude of the received pulse is displayed as a deflection of an oscilloscope beam in the $y$-direction and the $x$-direction is time $t$ which translates to penetration depth into the tissue $d$ using $t = 2d/c$ (e.g. $c = 1.55$ mm/$\mu$sec). In $B$-mode ($B$ brightness) the amplitude is presented as points with brightness proportional to the amplitude of the echoes. The transducer is stepped along an axis at a fixed rate to form a 2D image. An $M$-mode ($M$ motion) image displays the echoes as in $B$-mode but the time axis is constantly running, giving a display of position or movement of the echoes with time.

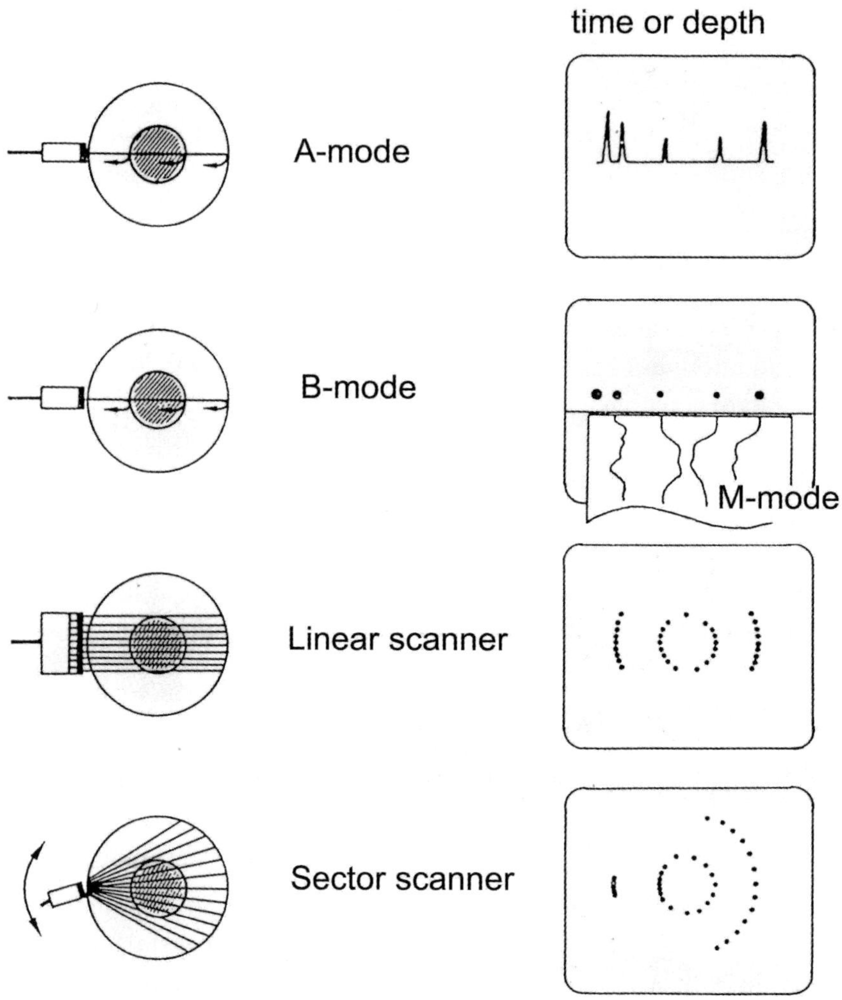


Fig. 3. Display methods. From the top, $A$-mode ($A$ = amplitude), $B$-mode ($B$ = Brightness), $M$-mode ($M$ = Motion) and the principle behind a linear scanner and a sector scanner. See text for additional details.

## 2.3. *Linear real-time scanning*

Real-time scanners produce a moving picture that is made possible by manipulating the ultrasound beam direction mechanically or electronically. The linear scanner has several crystals in a line and activates one or a small number of crystals at a time. This gives a square or rectangular ultrasound image and linear real-time scanning gives the same line density throughout all depths.

## 2.4. *Sector real-time scanning*

Sector scanning is obtained by changing the beam direction either mechanically or electronically. This technique was originally developed to image the heart, where access is restricted to an intercostal space, and thus the size (footprint) of the transducer must be small. The sector scanner is also used in abdominal scanning. The mechanical sector scanner may be either the rotational or oscillating type. All sector scanners are disadvantaged by a varying line density throughout the 2D image. The electronic sector scanner, called the phased array steers the beam without any mechanical components (Fig. 4). The probe has typically 18–64 crystals and transmits pulses with a time delay; the resulting beam from all separate crystals is steered in different directions by electronically varying the delay (phase) between the pulses.

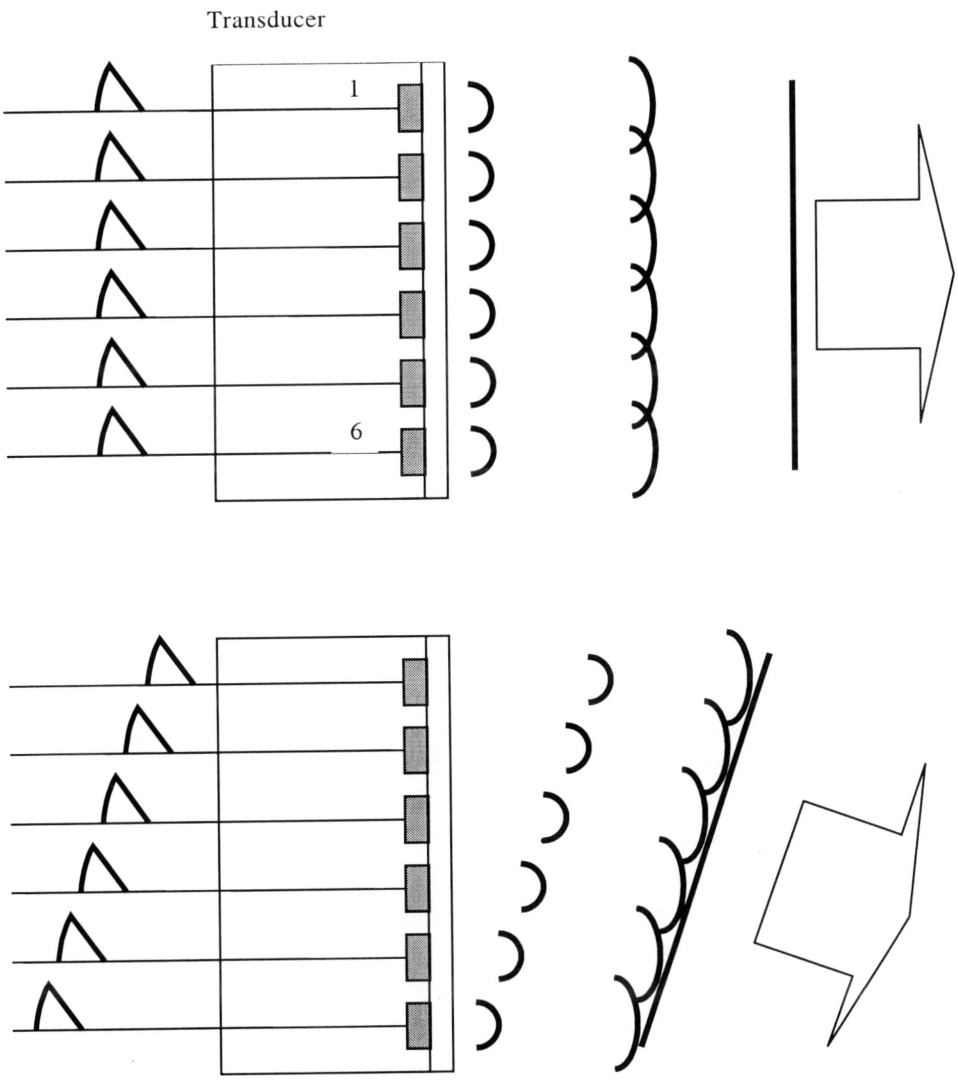


Fig. 4. Phased array for steering an ultrasound beam off axis by using different time delays for individual crystals. (Typical number of crystals in such an array is 18–64, and only 6 are shown here for clarity) Top panel: all 6 crystals are activated at the same time (no delays) with resulting beam tranmitted straight forward. Bottom panel: a time delay that depends on crystal position produces a beam steered in desired direction. Steering angle (arrow) is determined by the line perpendicular to the tangent to all six circular wave fronts.

## 2.5. *Curvilinear real-time scanning*

The surface of a linear probe can be made slightly convex. Such a curvilinear probe has both a good field of view close to the transducer and an extended field of view at increasing depth. The latter property makes the curvilinear probe less bulky for abdominal use compared to the linear probe.

## 2.6. *Improving quality factors for 2D tissue imaging*

The two most important factors governing image quality in ultrasound amplitude imaging are (1) spatial resolution and (2) contrast resolution. Methods to improve these are discussed below.

Resolution is the ability to display distinct echoes from two objects close to each other, and for an ultrasound image, resolution is defined in three orthogonal directions. The resolution along the beam axis is termed axial resolution. Resolution in the two directions perpendicular to the axial direction are known as lateral resolution and slice thickness (to distinguish these, imagine a 2D image possessing a certain axial and lateral resolution, or pixel size. Slice resolution is the distance between successive layers of such an image to form a 3D image). For a single circular crystal, slice thickness and lateral resolution are the same, but for non-circular crystals, or more complex imaging systems involving combinations crystals, these parameters differ. In general, axial resolution is better than lateral resolution and the first method used to improve the image resolution is to focus the beam in the lateral direction.

### 2.6.1. *Dynamic focusing*

Within a region close to the transducer, called the near field or Fresnel zone, the ultrasonic beam remains collimated and confined to within a region of approximately the same diameter as that of transducer. Further away from the transducer, in the far field or Fraunhofer zone, the ultrasonic beam begins to spread or diverge. The transition between these two regions occurs at a range equal to approximately $d^2/\lambda$, where $d$ is the diameter of a circular transducer (for transducers of any shape, this region begins at approximately $A/\lambda$, where $A$ is the transducer's area). Static focusing within the Fresnel zone is possible by placing a lens in front of the transducer, but at the cost of having the beam diverge in the Fraunhofer zone more than an unfocused beam. Electronic focus on transmission can also be achieved without a lens by transmitting on an array of crystals, with a transmit delay applied to crystals in the array's centre. Dynamic focusing represented a great improvement when it was introduced around 1980. (Fig. 5). With dynamic focusing, signals from an echo received by several crystals are summed with a time delay applied to the contribution from each crystal that increases for those positioned towards the centre crystal. The set of time delays that define a focal zone is called a focal function. When receiving echoes from tissue interfaces deeper in the patient the focal function can be altered, thus giving a different focal zone (1). The sweeping of the focus on receive, or dynamic focusing, improves resolution particularly for visualising abdominal regions (see Fig. 6).

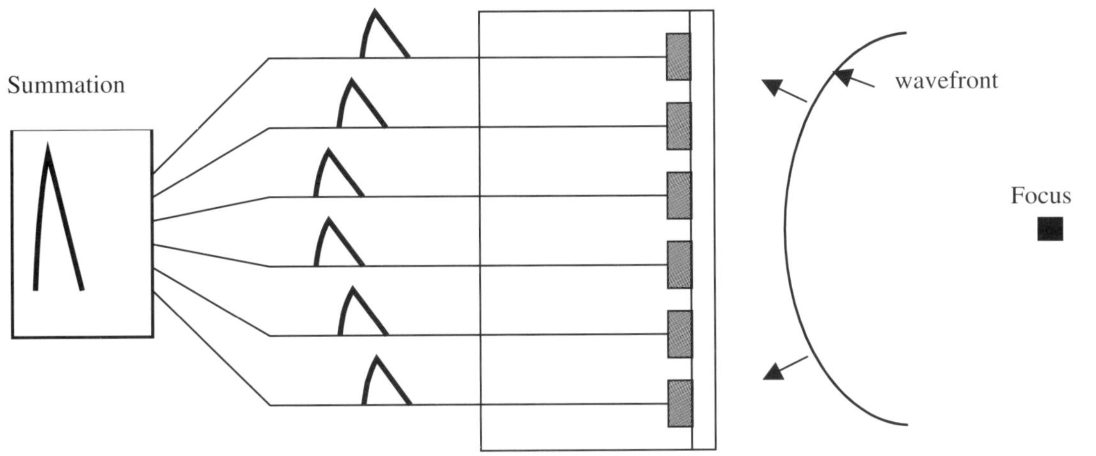


Fig. 5. Principle behind dynamic focusing. A non-planar wave front is sensed by multiple crystals used for receiving the reflected and scattered ultrasound. Signals from centrally located crystals receive a delay prior to summing the signals, which is equivalent to focusing at the position identified by the small square. The delays can be changed to change the focus position.

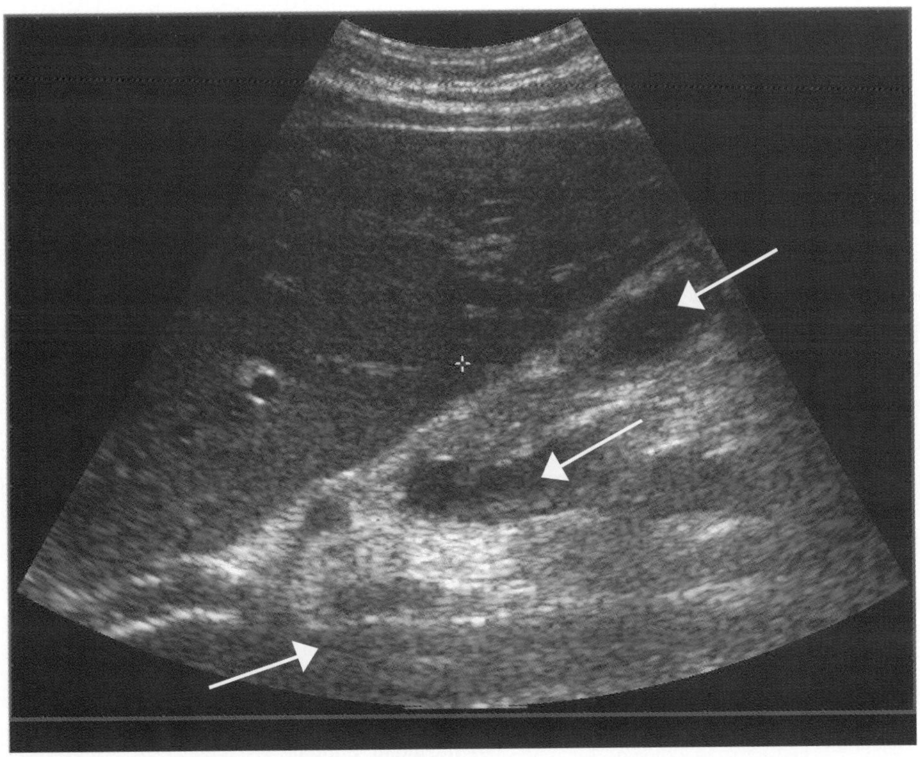

Fig. 6. An abdominal ultrasound *B*-mode image recorded with a curvilinear probe. To the left is shown the liver. Fluid filled lumens are shown black, top arrow the gastric antrum in cross-section, middle arrow the mesenteric vein and bottom arrow the aorta.

### 2.6.2. *Harmonic imaging*

The image quality of routine abdominal ultrasound scans can be reduced in some patients due to obesity or some post-operative states. Harmonic imaging represents a major improvement when examining such patients. The method was first developed for contrast microbubbles. When ultrasound waves encounter microbubbles they radiate overtones (harmonics) at twice the original transmit frequency. The receiver can be tuned to the second harmonic frequency and thus enhance the reflections from the microbubbles while suppressing signals from surrounding tissue structures.

Tissue harmonic imaging (THI) exploits the gradual generation of harmonic energy as ultrasound travels through tissue. This occurs because sound propagation through tissue is a nonlinear process resulting in a small amplitude distortion in the waveform, and with subsequent generation of higher harmonic frequencies, the farther the waveform propagates into the tissue. There are no harmonic frequencies present at the transducer face, thus the near field artefacts are suppressed when using detection of harmonic frequencies. (An artefact is any display of incorrect anatomy or velocity, for which such a display depends on the physical assumptions in medical ultrasound usage concerning ultrasound propagation, scattering, reflection and refraction. Artefacts are discussed further in Section 5.) Near field artifact is associated with echoes that originate from a region near the transducer face and out of the focal zone, producing image clutter that is difficult to interpret. It can also include echoes associated with side lobes of the main ultrasound beam, which are small portions of ultrasound leaving the probe surface in a direction different from that of the main beam. As well as reducing this image clutter, THI reduces the noise and thereby improves the image signal to noise ratio (2).

Also, since the majority of the harmonic energy is generated close to the beam centre, the result is that lateral resolution of the image is improved. It was first believed that harmonic components were too weak to be detected, but system improvement has made it possible. Harmonic imaging requires a receiver system with excellent sensitivity and dynamic range, and a sharp filter to remove energy close to the fundamental frequency. Images based on harmonic imaging will show a much cleaner picture, especially in patients with poor images obtained using fundamental frequencies.

The operator is able to adjust resolution, penetration, and artefact rejection (Table 1) to optimize image quality. There is a compromise between resolution and penetration,

Table 1. Quality factors for 2D ultrasound tissue amplitude imaging.

| Factor | Increased by |
|---|---|
| Resolution | - higher frequency<br>- dynamic focus<br>- harmonic imaging |
| Penetration | - lower frequency<br>- higher intensity |
| Dynamic range | - larger gray scale<br>- lower noise level |
| Artefact rejection | - smaller sidelobe |

resulting in the use of several frequencies for the same clinical procedure depending on the echogenicity of the patient. Modern ultrasound probes transmit a range of frequencies, e.g. 2.5–5.0 MHz for a probe with 3.5 MHz centre frequency. The sensitivity is, however, usually highest at the probe's resonance frequency. Dynamic range is the ability to simultaneously record both strong and weak echoes which is important because sometimes the pathology is characterized by strong echoes (e.g. calcified processes) and sometimes by weak echoes (e.g. small tumors).

## 3. Ultrasound Doppler Methods

The ultrasound Doppler methods originally developed for the heart and peripheral vessels are now used in most medical ultrasound applications, including abdominal scanning.

### 3.1. *The Doppler effect*

All Doppler methods are based on the estimation of velocity from a Doppler shift, which is the difference between the transmitted and received ultrasound frequency. When either the source, reflector or receiver or a combination of these are moving, a change in frequency results and the frequency difference (Doppler shift) is proportional to the relative velocity. Figure 7 shows the effect on a stationary receiver when the sound source is moving. If the

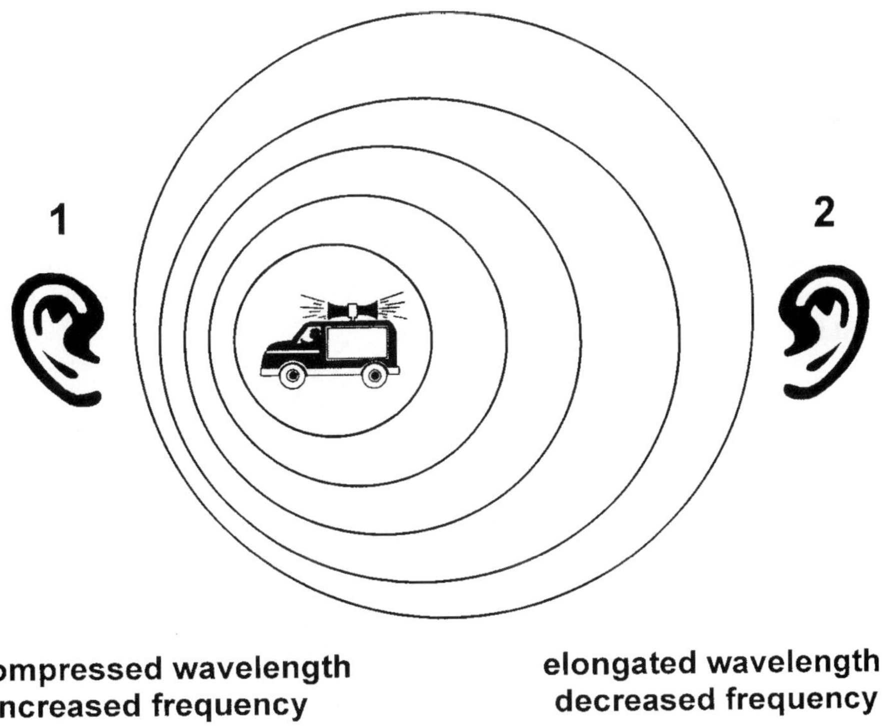


Fig. 7. The Doppler effect. Observer 1 experiences an increased frequency (compressed wavelength, positive Doppler shift) from the ambulance moving towards him, while observer 2 experiences a decreased frequency (elongated wavelength, negative Doppler shift).

source is moving towards the receiver a compressed wavelength results and the frequency of the source appears increased. The opposite effect is experienced if the source is moving away from the receiver. In medical ultrasound Doppler methods, it is the reflector that is moving (e.g. as in blood flow) and both the receiver and source are stationary.

### 3.2. *CW and PW Doppler methods*

The two primary Doppler methods are known as continuous wave (CW) and pulse wave (PW), both of which are illustrated in Fig. 8. A CW Doppler transmits a continuous wave train on one crystal, while the other crystal acts as a receiver. The transmitted ultrasound is reflected from tissue interfaces and these reflections have the same frequency. If the ultrasound hits moving blood, the reflection from blood will experience a shift in frequency ($f_D$) given by the Doppler equation

$$f_D = 2f_0(|\mathbf{v}|/c)\cos\theta \tag{10}$$

where $f_0$ is the transmitted frequency, $|\mathbf{v}|$ is the magnitude of the velocity of blood flow, $\theta$ is the angle between the ultrasound beam and the blood vessel, and $c$ is the speed of sound in blood, approximately 1,570 m/s. The Doppler shift is typically 20–10,000 Hz, and thus with signal conditioning this Doppler signal from blood flow can be made audible. The factor 2 arises because during transmission blood is a moving receiver and experiences a Doppler shift. During reflection the blood acts as a moving transmitter, and receiving crystal experiences both Doppler shifts. Note that the velocity $v$ cannot be recorded without

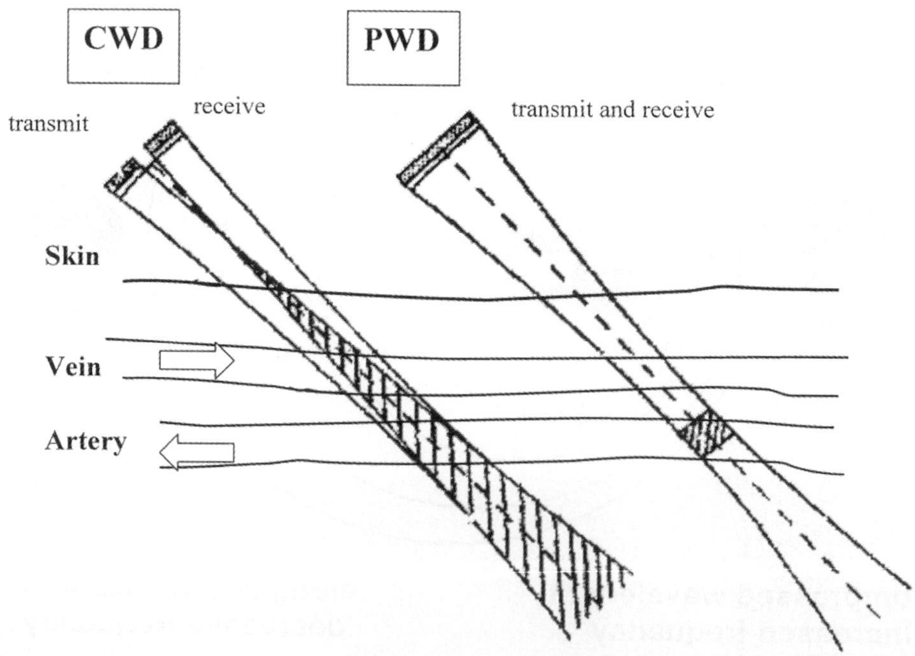


Fig. 8. Continuous Wave (CWD) and Pulsed Wave (PWD) Doppler methods. With CWD, Doppler shifts are registered from both the vein and artery. With PWD, depth resolution allows the sample volume to be placed in either vessel, shown here in the artery.

knowing the angle $\theta$. Only the component of this velocity along the ultrasound beam is measured; thus if $\theta = 90°$ no Doppler shift is recorded as in this case $\cos\theta = 0$.

For the PW Doppler method, a short ultrasound pulse is transmitted from the crystal and the same crystal then acts as the receiver, similar to $B$-mode imaging. Depth resolution is obtained by ignoring Doppler-shifted signals returning to the transducer until a pre-selected time interval after transmission. The duration of this time interval determines the length of the collecting region, called a range gate or sample volume. An effect known as aliasing can occur in PW Doppler devices (including the methods that use color Doppler display), which limits the maximum measurable velocity. In PW Doppler systems, the Doppler frequency is sampled once every transmitted pulse and the sampling frequency is equal to the pulse repetition frequency (PRF), which is typically 5 kHz. The Doppler frequency can be no greater than half the sampling frequency to be correctly reconstructed. This is also called the Nyquist frequency, and it will vary if the PRF changes. This limit in measurable velocity does not apply for CW Doppler. One method of increasing the Nyquist frequency is to increase the PRF until the next pulse is transmitted before all reflected ultrasound is received, called high pulse repetition frequency (HPRF). Thus, when high velocity is present, an alternative of using CW Doppler is to use HPRF Doppler (Fig. 9). This will, however, introduce two or more sample volumes along the same beam and depth resolution is degraded. Using only one sample volume is often called Low Pulse Repetition

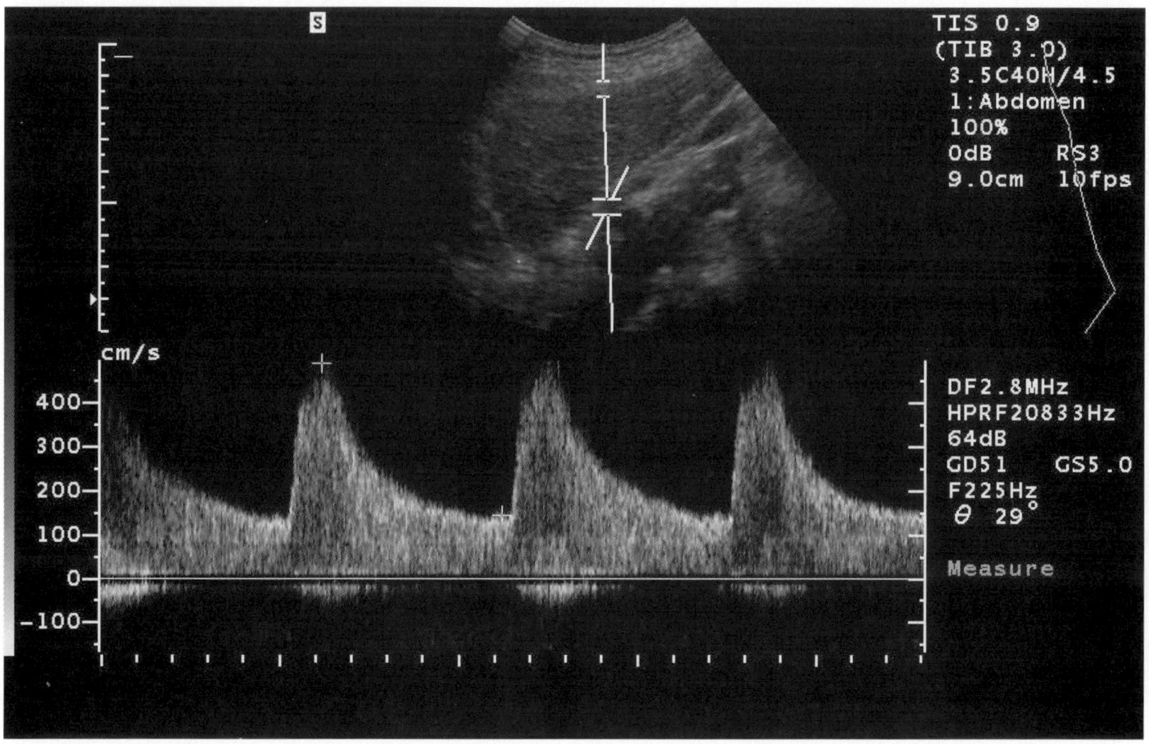


Fig. 9. A display of HPRF Doppler showing a peak systolic velocity of more than 4 $ms^{-1}$ in the mesenteric artery with stenosis in a patient with postprandial abdominal pain. Two sample volumes along the Doppler beam can be seen in the upper display.

Table 2. Doppler method properties.

| CWD | PWD | PWD (HPRF) |
|---|---|---|
| No depth resolution | Depth resolution | Ambiguous depth resolution |
| All velocities | Limited velocities | Extended velocity range |
| Poor sensitivity | Good sensitivity | Good sensitivity |

Frequency (LPRF). Properties of CW and PW Doppler methods are compared in Table 2, including the trade-offs of using the higher PRF (HPRF) with PW methods.

Because the reflected ultrasound energy originates from a distribution of velocities associated with blood cell flow, the result will be a distribution of Doppler shifts. Spectrum analysis is one method for displaying this distribution and a spectrum display of the velocities in the common carotid artery is shown in Fig. 10. From this spectral display of velocities several important parameters are obtained. The width of the spectrum (spectral broadening) is a measure of the amount of disturbed flow present; if velocities in both

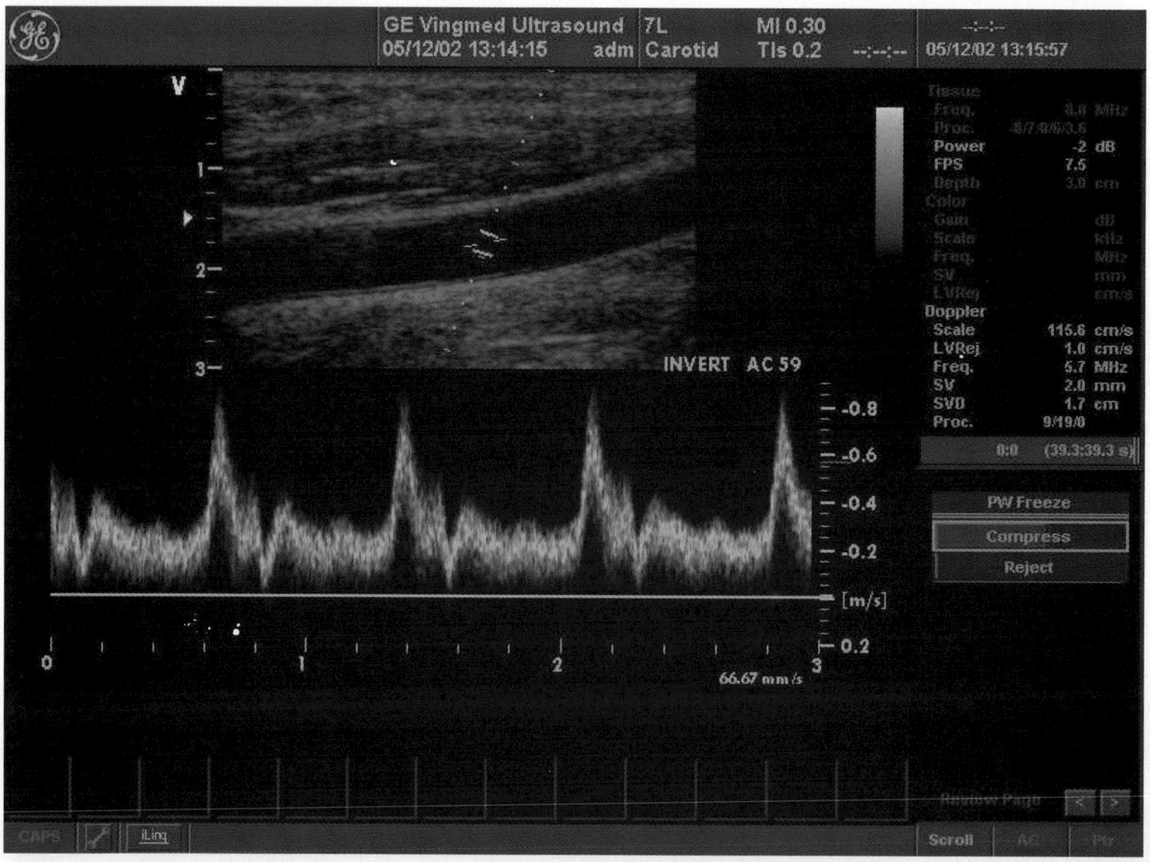


Fig. 10. Duplex scanning that combines a *B*-mode image (upper plot) and spectral Doppler recordings (lower plot) from the common carotid artery. For the Doppler data, horizontal axes is time (here showing 3 s of data) and vertical axes shows the blood velocity. The grayscale is proportional to the amplitude of the spectrum.

direction at the same time are recorded, turbulence is present. If the angle $\theta$ is small or known the velocity can be recorded either as the maximum velocity at any time (tracing envelope of velocity spectrum) or the mean velocity within the sample volume.

### 3.3. *Duplex scanning*

Using the Doppler alone (often called Doppler stand alone systems) is difficult and time-consuming because there is no image to guide the direction of the Doppler beam. When Doppler methods were combined with the $B$-mode image (often called Duplex scanning, Figs. 9 and 10), this combination became widespread within most specialities using ultrasound imaging. Used in this manner, the Doppler signal becomes particularly useful in examining tissue regions expressing otherwise low echogenicity in the $B$-mode image, such as venous or arterial blood flow.

In the $B$-mode image, a cursor placed along the center axis of the vessel gives an angle correction of the velocity scale, thus enabling the velocity along the vessel axes to be measured (see sample volume Figs. 9 and 10). The combination of a $B$-mode image and Doppler allows measurement of both blood flow and blood velocity. Blood flow ($Q$) is estimated from

$$Q = \bar{v}A \tag{11}$$

where $\bar{v}$ is the velocity averaged over the vessel lumen and time, and $A$ is the cross-sectional area. Accuracy of flow measurement depends on several criteria to be fulfilled. If a single diameter is measured it must be verified that the lumen is circular. The internal luminal cross-sectional area should be used, which is not always easily obtainable. Velocity must be the velocity averaged over the whole lumen, normally obtained with a large sample volume. Care must be taken in adjusting the filters used to remove the Doppler signal associated with wall motion, to avoid unwanted filtering of the Doppler signal from slow-moving blood. The angle $\theta$ must be known and the average (spatial average) velocity must be computed over several heart cycles to remove variation due to respiration. With these criteria fulfilled flow can be measured with good accuracy.

### 3.4. *Color Doppler*

The forerunner of color Doppler methods were instruments based on multiple range gates. Here, the backscattered Doppler-shifted ultrasound from a large number of range gates or sample volumes was recorded simultaneously. The velocity profile of a blood vessel could thus be measured. Using the multi-range gated method (typically 128 sample volumes) while sweeping the beam gave velocity information in a 2D area. Color coding of the velocities produces a color flow map (CFM) of velocities that are superimposed on a $B$-mode image (Fig. 11). The most common color coding is red towards the probe, blue away from the probe, and yellow or green for high velocities. Combining $B$-mode imaging, spectral Doppler (as shown in Fig. 9), and CFM is often called a Triplex display. Since CFM Dopplers utilize a PW Doppler method, aliasing can occur. This, in addition to the fact that the frame rate of the CFM real-time recording is often low, makes color Doppler the primary method for visualization of blood flow. By reducing the length and width of the color area, modern scanners have an improved frame rate of typically 25–50 frames per second (FPS).

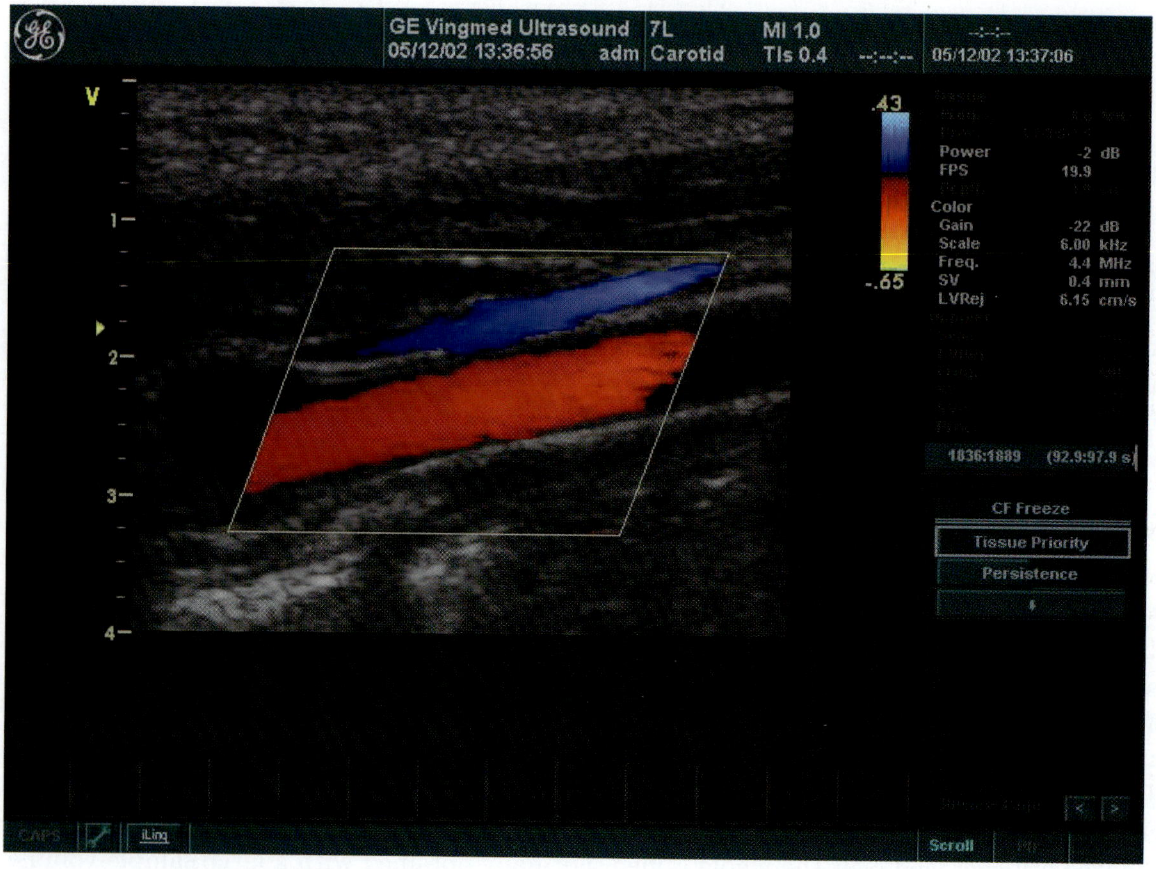


Fig. 11. Color flow mapping (CFM). In this case, red shows arteriel velocities (away from probe) and blue shows venous velocities (towards probe).

### 3.5. *Power Doppler*

The color flow image changes for an artery with every heart cycle and a complex vessel matrix of both arteries and veins produces a color image that may be difficult to interpret. Power Doppler (also called amplitude Doppler or Doppler angio) was developed to easily visualize complex vessel structures. Here all velocities (high or low velocities in both directions) are displayed in yellow, or orange if the Doppler-shifted ultrasound is of high amplitude. A filter with a time constant of several seconds is used to display the velocities in a manner similar to an angiographic X-ray contrast picture. The use of power Doppler has been limited, but there are advantages with this method, especially, for example, when the internal diameter of a vessel should be measured, and blood flow in the kidney is imaged showing low flow areas.

### 3.6. *Tissue velocity imaging*

Removing the Doppler shifted ultrasound from moving blood leaves the Doppler shifts associated with moving tissue, and displaying these Doppler shifts as color or spectral displays are called tissue velocity imaging (TVI). This can be used to detect the velocity of

Table 3. Use of different Doppler methods on the abdomen.

| Problem | Method |
|---|---|
| Identify echo-free region | CFM, PWD, PD |
| Velocity through stenosis | PWD (HPRF), CWD |
| Diameter | $B$-mode, PD |
| Flow | $B$-mode, PD + PWD |

different segments of the myocardium (3). From the velocity of two points along the one beam, the strain rate and strain of one region can be estimated and displayed as a color strain rate map (SRI — strain rate imaging) (4). TVI and SRI have only recently been introduced as methods suitable for evaluating the function of the gastrointestinal tract (5).

### 3.7. *Elastography*

The elastic behavior of tissue can be evaluated by a method called elastography. This method is based on the recording of $B$-mode images during small external tissue compressions using a mechanical device. By comparing the pre and post-compression signals in the 2D images, and employing the cross-correlation function, the displacement and the strain can be estimated (6, 7).

## 4. Special Techniques

### 4.1. *Endoscopic ultrasound*

Endoscopic imaging typically utilizes frequencies of 5–30 MHz and is performed from the gastrointestinal tract lumen. It is most often performed with radial mechanical ultrasound endoscopes. With this type of transducer a balloon facilitates acoustic contact between the transducer and the gastrointestinal tract wall, and 360° radial scans are obtained. It takes time to perform the 360° movement, thus the endoscopic scanner has a lower frame rate than transcutanous real-time scanners, typically 5–20 frames per second. Alternatively, linear or curvilinear electronic probes are available for endoscopic ultrasound. They provide axial scans, giving a reduced image size but having the advantage of higher frame rates. The higher frame rates facilities Doppler methods which are difficult with the slow moving 360° mechanical scanners.

An alternative method is to use transendoscopic miniature probes which can be introduced through the biopsy channel (internal diameter typically 2.8 mm). The first of these transducers was designed for static scanning where the operator performed the scanning movement: later rotational 360° probes have been applied. Special Doppler probes can also be introduced through the biopsy channel, but these cannot so far be combined with $B$-mode imaging (8, 9).

Using a higher frequency compared to transcutaneous applications, endoscopic ultrasound methods give much better axial resolution (along the ultrasound beam). Lateral resolution is not affected in the same way due to the lack of focusing of the beam and the limited line density for the 360° scan. Most endoscopic ultrasound methods are capable of

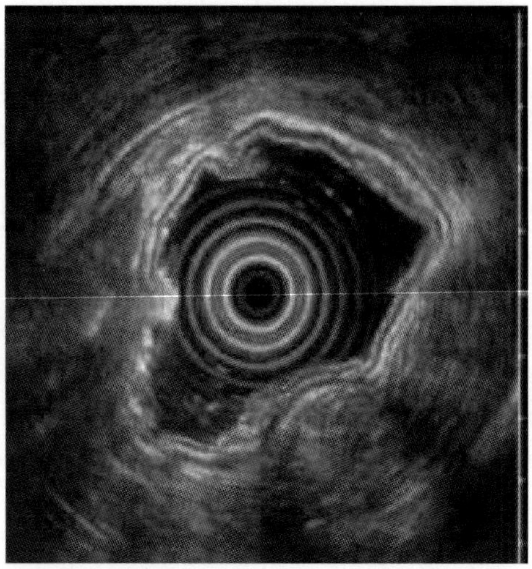

Fig. 12. Endoscopic ultrasound image of the stomach obtained with a 7.5 MHz intraluminal transducer showing the 5-layer wall structure. Note the circular artefacts produced by reverberation from the transducer capsule.

imaging the separate layers of the gastrointestinal tract wall (Fig. 12); the interpretation of the multiple echo layers is a major challenge for the operator of endoscopic ultrasound methods (10).

## 4.2. *3D imaging*

A large number of systems have been designed to obtain 3D ultrasound images. Both rotational and translational probe adaptors are commercially available as well as position sensors mostly based on magnetic sensing. The latter method is frequently used on the abdomen, because of the freedom in probe angling and manipulation (11, 12). Also 3D imaging of the gastrointestinal tract has been reported using endoscopic ultrasound (13). Recently, the first commercially real-time electronic scanner for the heart was introduced. It uses a 2D crystal array and will likely be the future system for 3D imaging. It has several advantages over the electronic/mechanical probes, most notably its increased frame-rate.

## 4.3. *Ultrasound guided biopsy*

Fine needle biopsies are today almost exclusively performed under ultrasound guidance. An open channel in a specially designed linear or curvilinear probe can accommodate the biopsy needle. By cutting the tip of the needle at an oblique angle, the tip can be seen in the $B$-mode image for improved control. When used in tandem with a mechanical or electronic sector probe the biopsy needle is introduced via an attachment outside the probe head.

## 5. Artefacts

Artefacts are echoes appearing in the $B$-mode image that do not correspond to actual interfaces in the patient. Similarly Doppler artefacts are velocities that appear in regions (color Doppler) where there is no flow, as well as lack of detected velocities where flow is present. The most common ultrasound artefact in $B$-mode imaging is reverberation. This artefact results from the ultrasound pulse being reflected back into the patient either by the transducer surface or the patient's skin. On the $B$-mode screen this artefact appears as another interface deeper in the image. In endoscopic ultrasound the water-filled balloon used as coupling between the transducer and the gastrointestinal tract wall often produces reverberation artefacts. A similar artefact can appear for echoes from the acoustic window in the transducer casing, which often filled with oil.

A mirror artefact is similar to the reverberation artefact but the extra reflection comes from within the body itself and is often reflected off an angle to another interface. On screen, the artefact appears as a virtual object, as in a mirror. Interfaces that can produce mirror artefacts are strong tissue/fluid transitions and the diaphragm.

Refraction, the bending of the ultrasound beam when passing through an interface at an oblique angle, can cause the image of the next interface to be displaced. This sometimes occurs when the beam passes through fluid.

Side lobes are present in any acoustic beam, and although much effort has been done to design transducers with small side lobes, they can still produce artefacts. The primary side lobes artefact are echoes from strongly reflective structures that can originate from positions outside the main beam.

Doppler artefacts are commonly due to range ambiguity and side-lobes, in addition to those linked with aliasing in PW Dopplers. Range ambiguity might occur with HPRF Dopplers where two sample volumes are present at the same time and the Doppler shifts from, for example, a vein and an artery can be mixed and difficult to interpret. Side-lobes can hit a strong blood jet, as in heart valves, and the resulting image can be misleading. A Doppler beam can be affected also by reverberation and mirror effects, which can result in a color image appearing where there is no flow.

Despite the improvement in signal transmission and processing in modern ultrasound devices, artefacts control remains a real challenge for the operator. Understanding the physics of ultrasound is the basis for recognizing and understanding these artefacts.

## 6. Biological Effects of Ultrasound and Potential Risks

Much attention has been given to the study of the potential hazards of diagnostic ultrasound, with considerable research effort directed towards studies on ultrasound exposure of macromolecules, cells and laboratory animals, in addition to follow-up studies of patients. There is particular interest in whether ultrasound exposure of fetuses affects a child's performance later in life. To date, such studies have not confirmed any significant biological effect after exposure to diagnostic ultrasound, although some have sparked debate both in the press and in the scientific community.

In clinical practice, the range of ultrasound exposure is large, including both pulsed and continuous ultrasound at frequencies 1–40 MHz. In general, higher intensities are used in conjunction with Doppler applications than for $B$-mode tissue imaging. Beam focusing increases the peak intensity (in space) compared with unfocused systems. The typical range intensities use for $B$-mode imaging is 1–50 $mWcm^{-2}$ and is 10–100 $mWcm^{-2}$ for Doppler applications, compared to typical intensities used in physiotherapy 500–2,000 $mWcm^{-2}$ (spatial peak, temporal average intensities).

High intensity ultrasound has well known biological effects associated with absorption (leading to heat production), cavitation (the dynamic behavior of gas nuclei and bubbles in an ultrasound field), streaming of intracellular material, and pressure forces acting over several wave cycles. These are in addition to the primary particle displacement and resulting particle pressure.

One alarming result leading to debate was the experiments by Machintosh and Davey in the 70s. They performed *in vitro* experiments on lymphocytes in solution with a fetal heart detector and reported chromosome changes (14). Other workers in this field failed to reproduce the results and the authors withdrew their findings in 1972 (15), concluding that the findings in their first study "must be due to some unknown artefact". Also experiments with ultrasound exposure of small rodents have shown effects at 500 $mWcm^{-2}$. Most of the reported effects in small animals are due to temperature effects and the findings are difficult to extrapolate to humans.

Clinical studies have followed both adults and children who had been examined by ultrasound in utero. One study (16) showed a higher incidence of dyslexia in school children who had been examined by ultrasound in utero; however, this incidence was not statistically significant. A recent study has found a weak but significant association between ultrasound and left handiness in boys (17). The careful interpretation of these results reveals no contraindication to perform routine ultrasound examinations in pregnant women.

The American Institute of Ultrasound in Medicine provided guidelines for ultrasound exposure as early as 1976; there is no significant biological effect shown for exposures under 100 $mWcm^{-2}$. This limit was based mainly on the observation that in most biological tissues, intensities under 100 $mWcm^{-2}$ do not produce a significant temperature rise. This limit continues to be the guideline standard.

Ultrasound safety in clinical practice must continue to be monitored as new ultrasound instrumentation is often based on significantly different transmitted pulse and ultrasonic field. As for all medical diagnosis where the patient is subjected to a form of energy, a monitoring program is essential.

## References

1. Selbie, R. D., Hutchison, J. M. S. and Mallard, J. R., The Aberdeen phased array: A real-time ultrasonic scanner with dynamic focus. Med Biol Eng Comput 1980; 18: 335–343.
2. Tranquart, F., Grenier, N., Eder, V. and Pourcelot, L., Clinical use of ultrasound tissue harmonic imaging. Ultrasound Med Biol 1999; 25: 889–894.
3. McDicken, W. M., Sutherland, G. R., Moran, C. M. and Gordon, L. N., Colour Doppler velocity imaging of the myocardium. Ultrasound Med Biol 1992; 18: 651–654.

4. Heimdal, A., Stoylen, A., Torp, H. and Skjaerpe, T., Real-time strain rate imaging of the left ventricle by ultrasound. J Am Soc Echocardiogr 1998; 33: 822–27.
5. Gilja, O. H., Heimdal, A., Hausken, T., *et al.*, Strain during gastric contractions can be measured using Doppler ultrasonography. Ultrasound Med Biol 2002; 28: 1457–1465.
6. Ophir, J., Cespedes, I., Ponnekanti, H., Yazdi, Y. and Li, X., Elastography: A quantitative method for imaging the elasticity of biological tissues. Ultrason Imaging 1991; 13: 111–134.
7. Ophir, J., Garra, B., Kallel, F., Konofagou, E., Krouskop, T., Righetti, R. and Varghese, T., Elastographic imaging. Ultrasound Med Biol 2000; 26(Suppl 1): S23–S29.
8. Martin, R. W., Gilbert, D. A., Silverstein, F. E., Deltenre, M., Tytgat, G., Gange, R. K. and Myers, J., An endoscopic Doppler probe for assessing intestinal vasculature. Ultrasound Med Biol 1985; 11: 61–9.
9. Matre, K., Ødegaard, S. and Hausken, T., Endoscopic ultrasound Doppler probes for velocity measurements in vessels in the upper gastrointestinal tract using a multifrequency pulsed Doppler meter. Endoscopy 1990; 22: 268–270.
10. Kimmey, M. B., Martin, R. W., Haggitt, R. C., Wang, K. Y., Franklin, D. W. and Silverstein, F. E., Histologic correlates of gastrointestinal ultrasound images. Gastroenterology 1989; 96: 433–441.
11. Gilja, O. H., Smievoll, A. I., Thune, N., Matre, K., Hausken, T., Ødegaard, S. and Berstad, A., *In vivo* comparison of 3D ultrasonography and magnetic resonance imaging in volume estimation of human kidneys. Ultrasound Med Biol 1995; 21: 25–32.
12. Matre, K., Stokke, E. M., Martens, D. and Gilja, O. H., *In vitro* volume estimation of kidneys using three-dimensional ultrasonography and a position sensor. Eur J Ultrasound 1999; 10: 65–73.
13. Molin, S. O., Nesje, L. B., Gilja, O. H., Hausken, T., Martens, D. and Odegaard, S., 3D-endosonography in gastroenterology: Methodological clinical applications. Eur J Ultrasound 1999; 10: 171–177.
14. Machintosh, I. J. and Davey, D. A., Chromosome aberrations induced by an ultrasonic fetal pulse detector. Br Med J 1970; 4: 92–3.
15. Machintosh, I. J. and Davey, D. A., Relationship between intensity of ultrasound and induction of chromosome aberrations. Br J Radiol 1972; 45: 320–7.
16. Stark, C. R., Orleans, M., Haverkamp, A. D. and Murphy, J., Short and long term risks after exposure to diagnostic ultrasound in utero. Obstet Gynecol 1984; 63: 194–200.
17. Salvesen, K. Å., Ultrasound and left-handedness: A sinister association? Ultrasound Obstet Gynecol 2002; 19: 217–221.

CHAPTER 2

# THE USE OF ULTRASOUND IN BIOMECHANICS

HANS GREGERSEN AND KNUT MATRE

## 1. Introduction

Mechanics is the study of the motion of matter and the forces that cause such motion. The analysis of the stress, deformation and stability of thin-walled tubes is a classical subject in physics and engineering. This chapter serves to give an introduction to the mechanics of the gastrointestinal tract and to show how ultrasonography can greatly contribute to this field. The chapter first introduces basic principles of mechanics. Then it gives a review of the ultrasound techniques that are useful for obtaining the geometric preliminaries for biomechanical analysis or for directly providing mechanical data.

Biomechanics requires an understanding of biology in addition to mathematics, mechanics and statistics. Biomechanics seeks to explain the mechanical behavior of living organisms. When applied to gastrointestinal biology, it requires a thorough understanding of gastrointestinal structure, anatomy, function, pathophysiology and symptomatology. The complexity of the gastrointestinal tract demands a multidisciplinary effort through the use of experimental, analytical and numerical methods. Although the gastrointestinal tract can be viewed as a complex mechanical device, the scientific study of its mechanics has only begun. Physiology and medicine have long disregarded the mechanics of the gut as a matter for serious consideration, despite the prominence of disordered mechanics in clinical gastroenterology. A degree of disorder in motor function characterizes many if not most patients with gastrointestinal complaints. Nearly all patients with esophageal disease, for example, exhibit some abnormality in mechanical function in that organ, and mechanical dysfunction often complicates the connective tissue diseases, diabetes and neurological disorders.

Biomechanical principles can be applied to almost any problem related to gastrointestinal function and pathophysiology. The term, gastrointestinal motility, is defined as the quality of the gut to generate motions. It encompasses a very wide area, comprising the movements of the walls, the controls of those motions, and the movement of the luminal contents induced by those motions. Hence, biomechanics is central in the study of gastrointestinal motility, being required both to describe the way in which the intent of the neural control system is expressed and the way in which the flow of the gastrointestinal contents is produced. A mechanical analysis of the operation of the gastrointestinal tract can be important to advance our understanding of such a wide-ranging set of matters as

- the passive viscoelastic properties of the wall
- the responses of the wall to mechanoreceptor stimulation such as the peristaltic reflexes

- the mechanics of bolus transport and the development of smooth muscle tone
- the origin of perceptions or sensations from the gut
- the growth and development of the gut
- geometric and biomechanical remodeling in the gut
- the origin of gastrointestinal diseases characterized by mechanical dysfunction
- the development of new clinical tests for mechanical dysfunction in the gut.

The mechanics of solids is different from that of fluids. A constant force transmitted to a solid material generally elicits a discrete, finite, time-independent deformation, whereas the same force transmitted to a fluid causes a continuous and time-dependent response called flow. In other words, a fluid is a material continuum that is unable to withstand a static shear stress. Unlike an elastic solid which responds to a shear stress with a recoverable deformation, a fluid responds with an irrecoverable flow. An intermediate response characterizes the fluid-solid state, which constitutes viscoelastic material behavior. In solid mechanics, the analysis of the basic relations between stress and strain is fundamental. In fluid mechanics, variables needed to define a fluid and its environment are pressure, velocity, density, viscosity, body force and time. Examples of fluids include gases and liquids. Typically, liquids are considered to be incompressible, whereas gases are considered to be compressible. Fluid flow can be either laminar or turbulent.

Many solid materials express simple stress-strain relations because the material is homogenous, behaves in an isotropic manner and show infinitesimal deformation even at large stresses. Such materials often obey Hooke's law, where Young's modulus is the constant of proportionality between stress and strain. However, biological tissues such as the wall of the gastrointestinal tract differ in several ways from the usual engineering materials that exhibit such behavior. Specifically, the gastrointestinal wall exhibits:

- heterogeneous materials
- complex geometry with layered structure and tissue buckling
- viscoelastic behavior, in that the tissue has the mechanical properties of both solids and fluids
- anisotropic mechanical behavior (behavior that differs in one direction or dimension from another)
- behaviors in which large deformations produce non-linear stress-strain curves
- the intrinsic active properties of muscle cells and their associated nerves.

The gastrointestinal tract consists of a series of organs that exhibit somewhat different behaviors. The mechanical characteristics of the wall of esophagus differ from those of the stomach wall, for example. There are differences even between one region of a single organ and another, for example between the gastric fundus and the gastric antrum. This complexity makes the mechanical analysis of the gut wall much more difficult than that of structures made of the usual engineering materials. The study of gastrointestinal mechanics has suffered greatly from the inaccessibility of the gut, which requires the development of special methods if the gastrointestinal tract is to be examined *in vivo*. Recently, balloon distension techniques and non-invasive imaging with ultrasound, MR-scanning and multi-slice

CT-scanning for biomechanical analysis *in vivo* are becoming established in gastrointestinal physiology.

## 2. Basic Mechanics

One principal objective in tissue biomechanics is to determine the stresses and strains in biological tissues when forces are acting on them. The determination of these quantities over a range of loads, from a stage that approximates the unloaded state up to loads that cause failure, gives a complete picture of the biomechanical behavior. The fact that forces applied to solids deform them demands a study of the force-deformation relationship. Soft biological tissues such as the gastrointestinal tract express mechanical properties that are intermediate between solid and fluid properties; that is to say, anisotropy prevails due to the heterogeneous laminated structure, the finite deformation, the non-linear stress-strain relation, and the pronounced viscoelastic behavior. The mechanical properties are time-dependent in that the stress-strain response does not occur instantly.

One must consider the structure and geometry of gastrointestinal tissues when dealing with the mechanical properties of the gastrointestinal tract. For simplicity, the basic geometry of the gastrointestinal tract may be considered cylindrical. Three principal directions, longitudinal ($z$), radial ($r$) and circumferential ($\theta$) can be defined. The pressure $P$ from a bolus or a distending balloon will induce a normal stress that will stretch the tube in circumferential directions and probably also cause longitudinal extension and radial compression, meaning that the wall becomes thinner. Assuming that the pressure is generated by a moving bolus, forces will also occur in longitudinal direction, causing a shear stress in the mucosa (Fig. 1). The normal stresses and shear stresses together with corresponding strains will be dealt with below and mechanical definitions are given in Table 1.

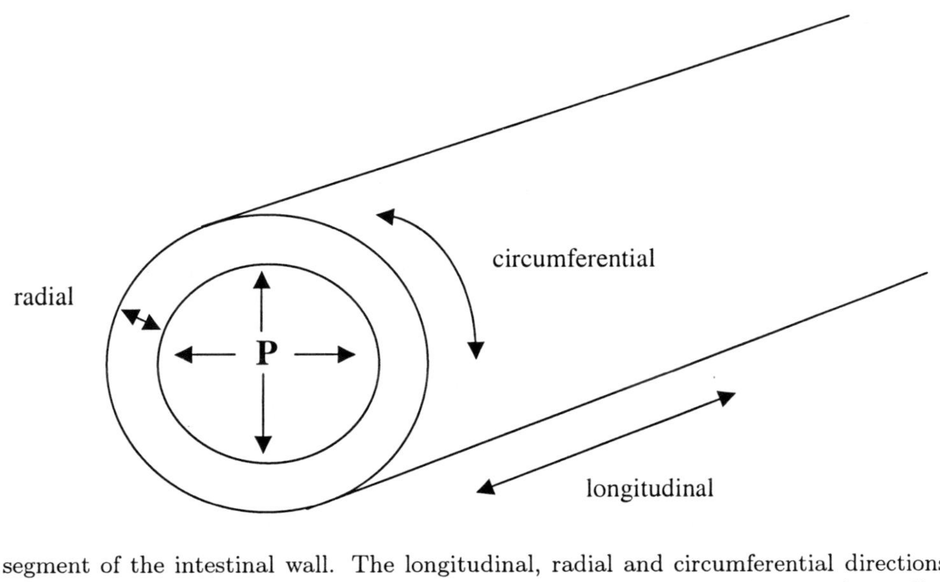


Fig. 1. A segment of the intestinal wall. The longitudinal, radial and circumferential directions are illustrated. The pressure $P$ from a bolus or a distending balloon induces a normal stress that will stretch the tube in circumferential directions and radial compression (a thinner wall). Longitudinal extension may also occur. A moving bolus will also cause shear stresses in the mucosa.

Table 1. Common terms used in solid and fluid mechanics.

| | |
|---|---|
| Composite materials | A structural composite is a material system consisting of two of more phases on a macroscopic scale. Many types of composites exist, e.g. laminated structures or fibers embedded in a matrix. |
| Constitutive equation | In mechanics a constitutive equation describes the mechanical properties of a material (the stress-strain relation). |
| Deformation | Forces applied to solids cause deformation or strain. If the deformation is elastic, the material returns to its initial state when the stress is removed. If it does not return to the initial state, the deformation is plastic. |
| Density | The mass of fluid per unit volume. |
| Elastic modulus | The proportionality constant between stress and strain. Hooke's law applies for a homogenous linearly elastic material. |
| Incompressible | An incompressible fluid is one whose density is constant everywhere. |
| Isotropy | A material is isotropic when its properties are the same in all directions or are independent of the orientation of the reference axis. Materials whose mechanical properties depend on directions are said to be anisotropic. Biological tissues are usually anisotropic, mainly because of their heterogeneous, layered structure. |
| Laminar flow | An organized flow field that can be described with streamlines. In order for laminar flow to be permissible, the viscous stresses must dominate over the fluid inertia stresses. |
| Membrane tension | Multiplying the uniform stress with wall thickness gives the membrane tension, expressed as force per unit length. In place of "membrane tension", some authors use "stress resultants" or "membrane stress resultants" to recognize the fact that they are the integrals of stresses throughout the thickness of the membrane wall. |
| Newtonian fluid | A Newtonian fluid is a viscous fluid whose shear stresses are a linear function of the fluid strain rate. Most fluids do not behave as Newtonian fluids. |
| Preconditioning | In mechanical testing of living tissues *in vitro*, loading and unloading are repeated for a number of cycles until the stress-strain relation becomes stabilized so that repeatable results are obtained. |
| Pressure | A measure of the force per unit area exerted, for example by a fluid. The SI unit is $Nm^{-2}$ or Pascal. |
| Reynolds number | The factor that determines whether laminar or turbulent flow is present is the ratio of inertia forces to viscous forces within the fluid, expressed by the non-dimensional Reynolds number. |
| Rotational | A rotational fluid flow can contain streamlines that loop back on themselves. Fluid particles following such streamlines will travel along closed paths. Bounded viscous fluids exhibit rotational flow, typically within their boundary layers. All real fluids exhibit a level of rotational flow somewhere in their domain. |
| Strain | Forces applied to solids cause deformation or strain. Consider a string with initial length $L_O$ and stretched length $L$. It is useful to describe the change by dimensionless ratios such as $L/L_O$ or $(L - L_O)/L_O$ since it eliminates the absolute length from consideration. Elongation causes tensile (positive) strain while shortening causes compressive (negative) strain. Strain is a tensor quantity. |
| Streamline | A path in a steady flow field along which a given fluid particle travels. |
| Stress | The force per unit surface area that the part lying on the positive side of a surface element (the side on the positive side of the outer normal) exerts on the part lying on the negative side. Stress is a tensor quantity. A normal stress is perpendicular to the surface while shear stress is parallel to the surface. |
| Turbulent flow | A flow field that cannot be described with streamlines in the absolute sense. In turbulent flow, the inertia stresses dominate over the viscous stresses, leading to small-scale chaotic behavior in the fluid motion. |
| Viscoelasticity | Time dependence of the response to stress or strain. Stress relaxation, creep and hysteresis are features of viscoelasticity. |
| Viscosity | The property of resisting deformation of a fluid. A fluid property that relates the magnitude of fluid shear stresses to the fluid strain rate, or more simply, to the spatial rate of change in the fluid velocity field. |

## 3. Stress

A large specimen can sustain a large force where the small specimen can sustain a much smaller force. Therefore, the force relative to the size is important. Stress is defined as force per unit cross-sectional area ($\sigma = \frac{F}{A}$) with units of Pa or $\mathrm{Nm}^{-2}$ (the SI unit for force is Newton, being the force required to give a mass of one kilogram an acceleration of 1 $\mathrm{ms}^{-2}$). On any surface, the force may be applied perpendicular to the surface, such as the bolus pressure (normal stress) exerted on the wall, or parallel to the surface, such as the force exerted by the fluid flow (shear stress) on the wall. Normal stresses may be either compressive or tensile. A force may be applied in any direction and can induce stresses and strains in various directions. At any given point in the body, the state of stress is described by a stress tensor that consists of three normal stresses and six shear stresses, three of which are independent.

To understand the concepts of tensors it is useful first to consider a vector. A vector is a quantity having both magnitude and direction such as velocity, force and acceleration. Tensor analysis can be regarded as a generalization of vector analysis to certain entities known as tensors that require more than three components for their complete specification. Tensor analysis is used as a mathematical tool to make physical laws independent of any particular coordinate system. A vector is a first-order tensor with three components. In the example of stress an elastic body that deforms can be considered. At any particular point within the body nine components ($\tau_{ij}$ where $i, j = 1, 2, 3$) are sufficient for fully specifying the state of stress. This means that stress is a second-order tensor. Similar considerations can be made for strain, i.e. strain also consists of nine components. Since both stress and strain are second-order tensor quantities, the stress-strain relation will be of fourth order, i.e. contain 81 components. Thus, in general, it would require 81 elastic constants to characterize a material fully. Assumptions such as the isotropy assumption can reduce the number of components considerably. For example, if the stress and strain tensors are symmetric, the number of constants is reduced to 36.

It is not the intention to use tensor analysis in this chapter but it is important to keep the concept in mind. This following is primarily based on derivation of equations for simple geometric structures based on equilibrium equations. La Place's law is such an example. Ultrasonography is useful for obtaining such geometric data.

In the following, we will assume that the gastrointestinal tract is a thin-walled cylindrical pressure vessel and that the weight of the pressure vessel and its contents can be neglected. In a cylindrical tube, we deal with radial, circumferential and longitudinal components of stress in the respective directions. These are the normal components of stress in the wall of the cylinder (Fig. 2). In the following, we shall consider the circumferential stress, also called the hoop stress, and the longitudinal stress, also called the axial stress.

### 3.1. *Circumferential stress in a thin-walled cylinder*

In tubular organs the major tensile stress induced by distension is in the circumferential direction (1, 2). During luminal pressure loading, the equilibrium condition requires that the force in the intestinal wall in the circumferential direction to be balanced by the force in the

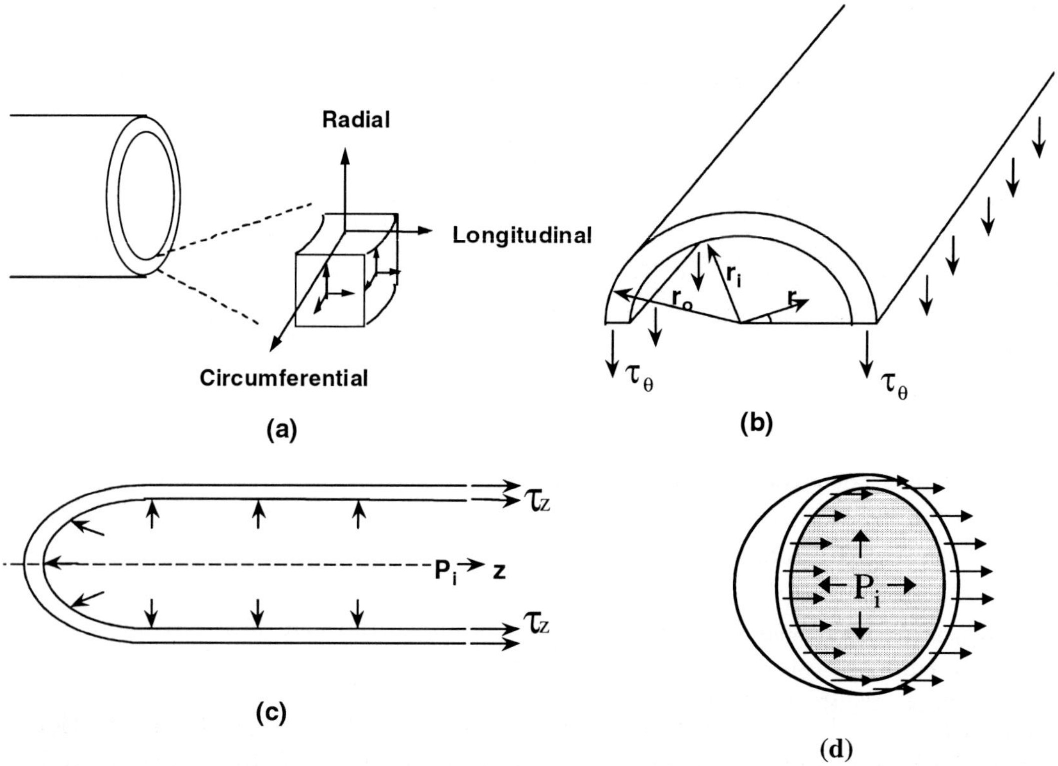


Fig. 2. A pressurized cylindrical tube and sphere. (a) An infinitesimal element of the cylindrical tube showing the radial, longitudinal and circumferential directions. (b) A free-body diagram of half of the tube cut parallel to the central axis. (c) A free-body diagram of the tube cut perpendicular to the central axis. (d) A free-body diagram of the pressurized spherical shell. See the text for explanation of symbols.

intestinal lumen contributed by the inflation pressure. Consider a section of a circular cylindrical intestine subjected to an internal pressure $P_i$, as shown in Fig. 2(a). The pressure in the intestine induces stress in the intestinal wall. Under equilibrium conditions, the force in the intestinal wall in the circumferential direction $2\tau_\theta(r_o - r_i)L$, is balanced by the force in the intestinal lumen contributed by the pressure $2Lr_iP_i$, as shown in Fig. 2(b). Hence, under equilibrium conditions $2\tau_\theta(r_o - r_i)L = 2Lr_iP_i$ and the equilibrium equation in the circumferential direction can be expressed as

$$\tau_\theta = \frac{Pr_i}{r_o - r_i} \tag{1}$$

where $\tau_\theta$ is the average circumferential stress, $r_i$ is the internal radius and $r_o$ is the outer radius. Because $r_o - r_i = h$, then Eq. (1) is simplified to Eq. (2).

$$\tau_\theta = \frac{Pr_i}{h} \tag{2}$$

where $P$, $r_i$, and $h$ are the pressure, internal radius, and wall thickness, respectively.

It should be noted that the stress in Eq. (2) is averaged over the thickness of the segment and does not describe any regional distribution of stress across the wall thickness. Furthermore, the Laplace stress may refer to either the wall thickness in the undeformed state ($h_0$) (named the engineering stress) or to the thickness in the deformed state (true stress).

If the segment geometry is conical, the circumferential stress is given as (3)

$$\tau_\theta = \frac{Pr_i}{h\cos\alpha} \tag{3}$$

where $\alpha$ is the angle between the wall of the cone and the centre line axis. If $\alpha$ is small, Eq. (3) reduces to Eq. (2). If the deformation is expressed in terms of Green strain (large deformation theory with reference to the initial state (Lagrangian description, see later)), the stress must be expressed as a commensurate measure and should in that case be expressed in the sense of Kirchhoff stress

$$S_{\theta\theta} = \frac{Pr_i}{h\lambda_\theta^2} \tag{4}$$

where $\lambda$ is the average circumferential stretch ratio.

The Kirchhoff stress is especially useful in bi-axial strain energy functions with uniform $S_{\theta\theta}$ *and* $S_{zz}$. Stress in radial direction is ignored.

### 3.2. *Longitudinal stress in a thin-walled cylinder*

The longitudinal stress in an intestinal wall can be determined in a similar way as the circumferential stress based on the equilibrium of forces in the longitudinal direction. The product of the longitudinal stress and the cross-sectional area of the intestinal wall is the force that balances the total longitudinal force acting on the intestine as shown in Fig. 2(c). The longitudinal force in the intestinal wall $\tau_z\pi(r_o^2 - r_i^2)$ is balanced only by the pressure component $P_i\pi {r_i}^2$ since the external pressure is assumed to be zero. Thus, $\tau_z\pi(r_o^2 - r_i^2) = Pi\pi r_i^2$ and the longitudinal stress $\tau_z$ can be expressed as:

$$\tau_z = \frac{Pr_i^2}{r_o^2 - r_i^2} \tag{5}$$

If the wall thickness-to-radius ratio is small, so that $r_o = r_i = r$ and $r_o - r_i = h$, then the equation for longitudinal stress is simplified to

$$\tau_z = \frac{Pr_i}{2h} \tag{6}$$

### 3.3. *Stress in a thin-walled spherical shell*

The free-body diagram for the geometry is shown in Fig. 2(d). Similarly to the longitudinal direction of a pressurized pressure vessel, it can be shown that the force in the wall of a sphere $\tau_z\pi(r_o^2 - r_i^2)$ is balanced only by the pressure component $P_i\pi r_i^2$. With the same assumptions as above, Eq. (6) also account for the thin-walled pressurized spherical shell.

### 3.4. *Laplace's law*

The law of Laplace [Eqs. (2) and (6)] has been used extensively in gastroenterology and the cardiovascular field due to its simplicity to explain why rupture occurs when segments are excessively distended. An important implication of the law is that the wall stress is related to pressure and radius-to-wall thickness ratio. Hence, the conventional comparison of wall properties such as the distensibility and tone at the same pressure and threshold for mechanoreceptor response regardless of the radius-to-wall thickness ratio is often misleading.

Using Laplace's law, it is important to recognize the assumptions it is based upon. In fact it was probably never meant to be used in physiology. The following assumptions apply: the geometry of the segment must be circular cylindrical with equal thickness along the circumference, the material properties must be isotropic and a static equilibrium of forces is required, i.e. acceleration must not occur. The question arises whether the gastrointestinal tract can be regarded as being thin-walled or thick-walled. This is important because the stress cannot be assumed uniformly distributed through the wall thickness in a thick-walled cylinder. The limit is often said to be at a thickness-to-radius ratio of 10% (if so, there is less than a 5% difference in the stress distribution from the inner to outer surface of the wall). The heart, arteries and arterioles have thickness-to-radius ratios of 0.25, 0.20 and 1.0 and must be modeled as thick-walled shells. The corresponding value for veins is 0.03. Hence, only veins can be strictly regarded as being thin-walled. However, theory for thin-walled structures has often been employed for other parts of the cardiovascular system and justified by the fact that the average stress is a good approximation. Considering the gastrointestinal tract, only few data on the thickness-to-radius ratio appear in the literature. The esophagus is thick-walled, especially at low pressures where the lumen is small. Even the duodenum and jejunum must be considered as thick-walled organs whereas the ileum approximates the thin-walled structure. Gao and Gregersen (4) provided data that the large intestine can be considered a thin-walled organ.

Perhaps the following formulas are more known to the readers as Laplace's law. In this case the organ is considered to be very thin-walled. Hence, membrane theory must be considered rather than the shell theory presented above and tension is computed rather than stress. This approach is often used in physiology when the wall thickness is inmeasurable.

Laplace's law originally refers to the relationship between the pressure difference, the wall tension, and the curvature of the membrane surface. Consider a thin-walled membrane surface and assume that the wall tension is constant everywhere, then the law of Laplace reads:

$$T = \Delta P \left( \frac{1}{r_1} + \frac{1}{r_2} \right)^{-1} \tag{7}$$

where $r_1$ and $r_2$ are the principal radii of curvature of the surface, $T$ is the total tension per unit length of the mid-surface of the membrane, and $\Delta P$ is the transmural pressure difference. $\Delta P$ is often assumed equal to the pressure inside the membrane due to the assumption that the external pressure is zero. The equation reduces to $T = \Delta P r$ in the case of a cylinder since one of the radii tends to infinity, and to $T = \Delta P \frac{r}{2}$ for a sphere since the two radii in this case are equal.

Equation (7) is valid as long as the membrane is so thin that bending rigidity can be neglected. Furthermore, there are several underlying assumptions: Firstly, a cylindrical lumen must be assumed. Secondly, the material property is assumed to be isotropic. Although the isotropy assumption is not valid for many biological tissues, the parameter is still useful. Finally, the analysis requires a static equilibrium of forces and consequently zero inertial forces. The circumferential tension is equal to the product of the average circumferential stress [Eq. (2)] and wall thickness.

### 3.5. *The thick-walled cylinder*

If the organ is thick-walled it is erroneous to average the stress over the thickness. In that case, the circumferential distribution of stress across the circular cylinder can be computed according to Fung (5) as

$$\sigma_\theta = -\frac{r_o^2 r_i^2 (P_o - P_i)}{r^2 (r_o^2 - r_i^2)} + \frac{P_i r_i^2 - P_o r_o^2}{r_o^2 - r_i^2} \tag{8}$$

where $r_o$ and $r_i$ are outer and inner radii whereas $r$ is the radial location of a point in the wall. $P_o$ and $P_i$ are the outside and inside pressures. In a similar fashion, it is possible to compute the radial stress distribution (5). The thick-walled approach is better than the thin-walled one if we want to determine the stress in the vicinity of the mechanoreceptors located in the wall of the gastrointestinal tract, especially in the thick-walled esophagus. However, one important consideration must be done. The gastrointestinal tract is a layered structure where the mechanical properties differ between the layers. This fact greatly complicates mechanical studies and puts emphasis on development of composite models.

### 3.6. *Strain and strain rate*

The term deformation refers to a change in the shape of a continuum (a continuous distribution of matter in space) between some initial (undeformed) configuration and a subsequent (deformed) configuration. A force may be applied in any direction and can induce strains in various directions. On any surface, the strain may be perpendicular to the surface (normal strain), or parallel to the surface such as the strain exerted by the fluid flow (shear strain) on the wall. At any given point in the body, the state of strain is described by a strain tensor that consists of three normal strains and six shear strains.

Deformation can take many forms, e.g. if we pull a tissue strip, it stretches, and if we inflate a tubular organ, it distends. To be able to describe such deformations quantitatively, the *strain* measures must be introduced. For a continuum subjected to deformation, strains can be defined in several different ways in relation to the deformation gradient. For simplicity, consider a tissue strip of initial length $L_0$ [Fig. 3(a)]. If we stretch it to length $L$, the change in length can be described by several dimensionless ratios such as

$$\text{Stretch ratio } \lambda = \frac{L}{L_0}, \quad \text{Cauchy strain } \varepsilon = \frac{L - L_0}{L_0}, \quad \text{Green's strain } E = \frac{L^2 - L_0^2}{2L_0^2}. \tag{9}$$

Thus, for a continuum subjected to finite deformation, strains can be defined in several different ways in relation to the deformation gradient (6). The selection of proper strain measures is dictated primarily by the stress-strain relationship. The strains can be computed for all surfaces or interfaces between layers where the geometric data can be obtained. The measures are dimensionless. This is advantageous since it eliminates the absolute length and any system of units from consideration. This makes comparison possible between specimens of various sizes. In Eq. (9), the strain measures are expressed as a fraction of the initial length (Lagrangian strains). However, they may also be expressed as a fraction of the

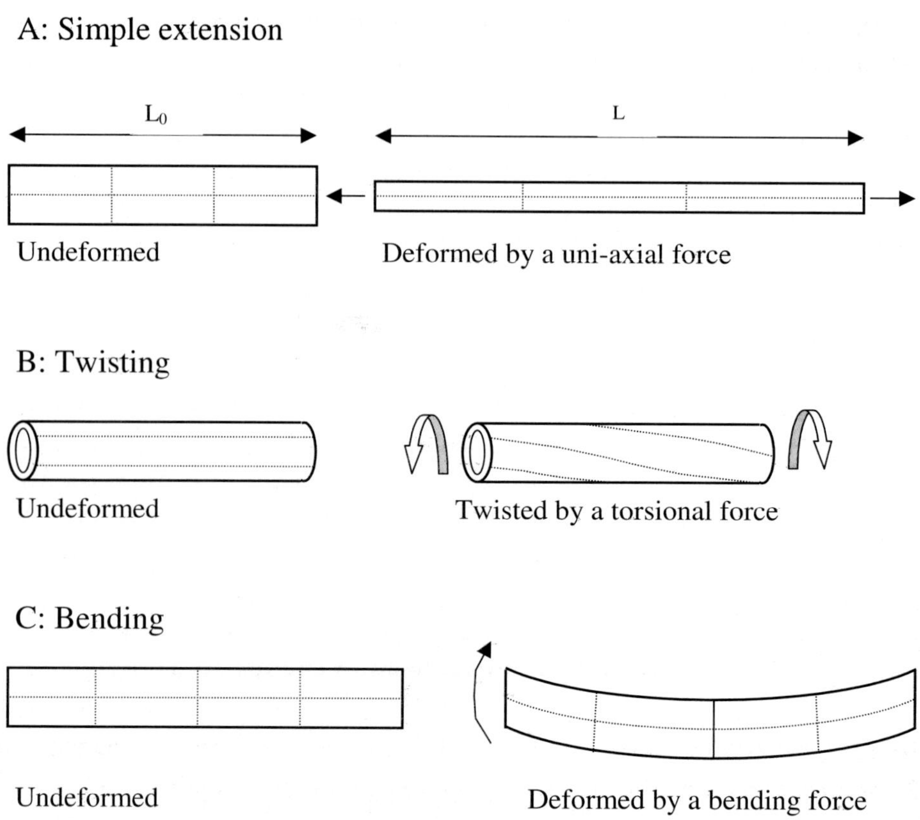


Fig. 3. (A) extension of a bar with undeformed length ($L_0$) at resting state and length $L$ at deformed state caused by a uni-axial force. The force induced a positive (tensile) strain. A force in the opposite direction will induce a negative (compressive) strain, (B) the effect of twisting a tissue strip, (C) the effect of bending a specimen. No strain occurs at the horizontal dotted line. Therefore, this line is called the neutral axis. On the convex side the tissue is in tension, on the concave side the tissue is in compression.

final length (Eulerian strains). Either of these strain measures are useful. In infinitesimal elongations, the strain measures are equal. However, in finite elongations, they are different which easily can be shown by examples. The Cauchy strain is especially useful in linearized theory of elasticity, which is valid when $\varepsilon$ is infinitesimal. Hence, it is usually called the "infinitesimal strain" or "engineering strain". For finite deformations, strain defined by Green is more conveniently related to stress. One strain measure can readily be transformed into another as shown below:

$$\varepsilon = \lambda - 1 \quad \text{and} \quad E = \frac{(\varepsilon + 1)^2 - 1}{2}. \tag{10}$$

Due to the incompressible nature of tissue, stretching a tissue strip causes a lateral contraction (radial narrowing). The ratio of lateral strain to longitudinal strain in a body under tensile or compressive forces is called Poisson's ratio. For biological materials which is regarded as incompressible in the physiological range the Poisson's ratio is often regarded as 0.5. Thus, deformation in one direction causes deformation in other directions.

In some cases, one strain measure may have advantages over others. As stated before, Green strain and Kirchhoff stress are commensurate measures useful in strain energy functions. On the other hand, the stretch ratio is a convenient measure when the tissue can be considered incompressible. In case of incompressibility the product of the stretch ratios in the three principal directions equals 1. Thus, if two stretch ratios are known it is possible to compute the last one. The proof for this relation is simple. Consider a rectangular block of tissue with length $L$, width W and height $H$. In the undeformed state we use the subscript 0. In the undeformed state, the volume $V_0 = L_0W_0H_0$ and in the deformed state $V = LWH$. If the tissue is incompressible $V = V_0$. Therefore, $L_0W_0H_0 = LWH$ or

$$\frac{LWH}{L_0W_0H_0} = 1 \quad \text{or} \quad \lambda_L\lambda_W\lambda_H = 1\,. \tag{11}$$

It is characteristic for soft biological tissue that they can undergo large deformations with a very low degree of compressibility. Thus, these tissues resist volume changes much more that shape changes. For the majority of practical applications within the physiological range, soft tissues can be considered incompressible. This has been verified for arterial tissue but is yet an assumption in gastroenterology.

In this chapter, focus is primarily on deformations caused by applying luminal forces (pressure) in tubular organs such as the esophagus and the intestines. This approach obviously is more physiological than tissue strips specimens. The strain measures can readily be used for studying organs of complex configuration as long as the geometric data can be obtained. In the case of the gastrointestinal tract let us for simplicity consider a straight circular cylindrical tube of homogenous material. We may refer to radial, circumferential and longitudinal components of strain in the respective directions as defined before. These are the normal components of strain in the wall of the cylinder. During luminal pressure loading (distension) the circumferential length usually increases (tensile circumferential strain), the wall thickness decreases (compressive radial strain) and compression or elongation may occur in the longitudinal direction (dependent on the material properties).

One issue that has not been touched yet is the determination of the initial (reference) length. It is apparent from Eq. (9) that the strain measure depends on the correct determination of the initial length. This is a difficult task for several reasons. First, it may be difficult to suppress smooth muscle activity. Secondly, strain may vary throughout the intestinal wall. Finally, the *in vivo* state may not reflect the true unstressed (zero stress) state.

There are several ways to obtain strain measures. *In vitro*, strains are often computed from measurements of changes in the total length of a strip, because of the change in distance between markers located on the surface or embedded in the tissue, or from the measurement of changes in diameter in intact specimens. *In vitro*, it will also often be possible to determine the zero-stress state as the reference. *In vivo*, we often rely on balloon distension techniques with measurement of volume or cross-sectional area along with the balloon pressure. Jørgensen *et al.* (7) made a promising development by combining impedance planimetry with high-frequency endoluminal ultrasonography. Hereby, it is possible to correct for variation in wall thickness to obtain a measure of stress-strain distributions *in vivo*. These methods are treated in the next chapter. Several ultrasound techniques also seem promising. When comparing *in vivo* experiments with *in vitro* experiments, it is important to notice that the segments are often free to lengthen *in vitro*, but they may be tethered to the surrounding structures *in vivo*. An important observation is that esophagus is always under considerable longitudinal stress *in vivo*. When removed from the body, it shortens by up to 50% as observed in guinea-pigs with a corresponding increase in the diameter. This large residual longitudinal strain may have important physiological implications during bolus transport in the esophagus.

The *strain rate* is the temporal derivative of the strain:

$$\dot{\varepsilon} = \frac{d\varepsilon}{dt} . \tag{12}$$

This means that while the strain indicates the amount of deformation, strain rate indicates the *rate* of the deformation. The relation between strain rate and strain can be compared to the relation between velocity and displacement. Assuming the velocity is constant, displacement equals time multiplied with velocity. Similarly, assuming the strain rate is constant, strain equals time multiplied with strain rate. A positive strain rate means that the length of the object is increasing, while a negative strain rate means that the length is decreasing. If the length is constant, the strain rate is zero.

The unit of the strain rate is normally $s^{-1}$ (per second). In other applications, the unit Hertz (Hz) is used for $s^{-1}$, but this is not recommended for strain rate. Hertz means number of cycles per second, while for strain rate it is more correct to speak of amount of deformation per second. A strain rate of $-2\ s^{-1}$ applied over one second would result in a relative strain of $-2$.

## 4. The Stress-Strain Relation (Constitutive Equation)

The properties of materials are specified by constitutive equations. A constitutive equation in solid mechanics relates stress and strain through a set of material constants. The proportionality constant between stress and strain is called the *elastic modulus* and for a linear Hookean material it is called Young's modulus. For such material, the mechanical properties are elastic and the constitutive equation is simplified to Hooke's law. In biological tissues, however, the relation between stress and strain is non-linear and the strain is usually large (finite deformation). Examples of non-linear stress-strain curves for gastrointestinal tissue are found elsewhere in this book. The non-linear (usually exponential-like) mechanical behavior, which likely reflects the mechanical properties of collagen, facilitates stretch in the physiological pressure range and prevents overstretch and damage to the tissue at higher stress levels. Overstretch can induce a plastic deformation in which the tissue can no longer return to its original state when unstressed. Due to the non-linearity, it is necessary to compute an incremental elastic modulus. The gastrointestinal wall resembles other biological tissues in that it possesses complex three-dimensional structures that have different material properties in different directions. This important feature, anisotropy, implies that a large set of material constants have to be specified in order to completely describe the mechanical behavior.

The constitutive equations of a solid that consists of a homogeneous, isotropic, linearly elastic material contain only two material constants

$$\varepsilon_{ij} = \frac{1}{2\mu}\left[\frac{-\lambda}{3\lambda + 2\mu}\tau_{\alpha\alpha}\delta_{ij} + \tau_{ij}\right] \tag{13}$$

where $\mu$ and $\delta$ are Poissons ratio and stress and $i$ and $j$ are indices ranging from integers 1 to 3. The $i$th index denotes the component in the $i$th direction whereas the $j$th index denotes the surface perpendicular to the $j$th direction. The repetition of an index in a term denotes a summation with respect to that index over its range.

Material constants are often derived with the use of exponential or polynomial laws. The stress-strain data are plotted and then fitted using a least-square method with an exponential stress-strain relationship such as of the form

$$\sigma = \beta[\exp(\alpha\varepsilon) - 1] \tag{14}$$

for the circumferential and longitudinal directions, respectively. Since the strain is referred to the zero-stress state, we must have $\sigma = 0$ when $\varepsilon = 0$, as satisfied by Eq. (14). A least square fit is used to determine the values of $\alpha$ and $\beta$ for the circumferential and longitudinal directions at the various times. The tangent modulus, $E$, is the slope of the stress-strain relationship (a measure of tissue stiffness) and can be computed analytically from Eq. (14) as

$$E = \frac{d\sigma}{d\varepsilon} = \alpha[\sigma + \beta]\,. \tag{15}$$

In the linear stress-strain range, the tangent modulus is equivalent to Young's modulus. Normally, a linear relation will be found between the tangent modulus and the stress as a result of the exponential nature of the stress-strain relation. This equation was originally proposed for uni-axial experiments, but it can be used independently for circumferential and longitudinal data obtained from gastrointestinal distension experiments. A bi-axial approach is given below.

Since the behavior is non-linear, incremental elastic moduli can also be computed. In order to compare these moduli, they must be measured under conditions of constant strain.

### 4.1. *Biaxial constitutive equation for determination of material constants in the GI Wall*

In order to quantify wall stresses, it is necessary to have an accurate measurement of the strain field to which the gastrointestinal tract is subjected and a reliable constitutive equation that relates those strains to stresses. Based on previous data, the wall is assumed an incompressible, non-linearly elastic orthotropic material subjected to finite deformation. This implies the use of a strain energy function for which the strains must be given with reference to the zero-stress state. The strain energy function represents stored energy per unit volume of the gastrointestinal wall. One of the forms for the strain energy function in a two-dimensional analysis is expressed as follows (5)

$$\rho_o W = \frac{C}{2} e^Q \tag{16}$$

$$Q = a_1(E_{\theta\theta}^2 - E_{\theta\theta}^{*2}) + a_2(E_{zz}^2 - E_{zz}^{*2}) + 2a_4(E_{\theta\theta}E_{zz} - E_{\theta\theta}^{*}E_{zz}^{*})] \tag{17}$$

where $\rho_o$ is the material density of the artery (mass per unit volume). $W$ is the strain energy per unit mass, $\rho_o W$ is the strain energy per unit volume, $E_{\theta\theta}$ and $E_{zz}$ are the circumferential and longitudinal Green's strains, respectively. $E_{\theta\theta}^*$ and $E_{zz}^*$ are reference strains measured at a physiological pressure, and $C$, $a_1$, $a_2$, and $a_4$ are material coefficients. Under assumptions that materials in a wall are homogeneous and pseudoelastic (i.e. the loading and unloading curves of the stress-strain relation are considered to represent properties of two materials with different elasticity), the strain energy function can be applied to loading and unloading processes separately and stress components expressed as

$$S_{ij} = \frac{\delta(\rho_o W)}{\delta(E_{ij})} \tag{18}$$

where $S_{ij}$ and $E_{ij}$ are components of Kirchhoff's stress and Green's strain, respectively. The assumption on homogeneity in the wall can in part be tested in the case of esophagus by separating the layers of the esophagus and testing the layers separately. By combining Eqs. (16) and (18) with the radial component and all shear components neglected, the stress-strain relations of a gastrointestinal segment in both circumferential and longitudinal directions can be obtained. The stress and strain components can be determined experimentally and the coefficients of the strain energy function, $C$, $a_1$, $a_2$, and $a_4$ can be determined by using a non-linear curve-fitting method (6).

The circumferential length of the inner and outer walls of the segment must be measured at the unstressed state with the aid of an image analysis system. The mid-wall circumferential length of the segment can then be computed as Cauchy strains [Eq. (9)]

The mid-wall strain and average stress of the segment (or its sub-layers after separation) can be determined under assumptions that the materials in the wall are homogenous and the shape is cylindrical. The mid-wall circumferential strain can be calculated on the basis of experimentally measured outer diameters at varying inflation and deflation pressures and reference mid-wall circumferential length at zero-stress state. With an assumption that materials in the wall are incompressible, the middle wall circumferential length of the segment at a given inflation or (deflation) pressure can be computed based on the outer diameter and longitudinal length of the pressurised segment, and the inner- and outer-wall circumferential and longitudinal lengths at zero-stress state. The middle-wall circumferential stretch ratio of the segment, $\lambda_\theta$, at a given pressure can be computed with respect to zero-stress state as the ratio between the mid-wall circumferential length at a given pressure and the middle-wall circumferential length at zero-stress state. Similarly, the longitudinal stretch ratio, $\lambda_z$, at a given pressure can be computed with respect to the zero-stress state as the ratio between the longitudinal length of the segment at a given pressure and the longitudinal length at zero-stress state. The circumferential and longitudinal strains of the segment at a given pressure can be computed with the following equations

$$E_{\theta\theta} = \frac{\lambda_\theta^2 - 1}{2} \quad \text{and} \quad E_{zz} = \frac{\lambda_z^2 - 1}{2} \tag{19}$$

where $E_{\theta\theta}$ and $E_{zz}$ are circumferential and longitudinal Green's strains, respectively. At an equilibrium condition, the average circumferential and longitudinal stresses in the wall at a given pressure can be computed with an assumption that the shape is cylindrical

$$S_{\theta\theta} = \frac{Pr_i}{h\lambda_\theta^2}, \quad S_{zz} = \frac{Pr_i^2}{h\lambda_z^2(r_o + r_i)} \tag{20}$$

where $S_{\theta\theta}$ and $S_{zz}$ are the circumferential and longitudinal Kirchhoff's stress, $P$ is the inflation pressure, $r_i$ is the inner radius, $r_o$ is outer radius at a given pressure, and $h$ is the wall thickness at the given pressure. These parameters can be determined experimentally as detailed earlier. With a similar approach, average longitudinal stress in the wall at a given pressure can be computed using the following equation:

By substituting Eq. (16) into Eq. (18), the following stress-strain relations for the gastrointestinal segment in both the circumferential ($\theta$) and longitudinal ($z$) directions can be obtained

$$S_{\theta\theta} = C(a_1 E_{\theta\theta} + a_4 E_{zz})e^Q \quad \text{and} \quad S_{zz} = C(a_2 E_{zz} + a_4 E_{\theta\theta})e^Q \,. \tag{21}$$

Reference strains $E^*_{\theta\theta}$ and $E^*_{zz}$ are selected as the strain components at physiological pressures in the circumferential and longitudinal directions, respectively. A Marquardt's nonlinear least-squares algorithm (6) can be used to fit the experimental data, and the coefficients $C$, $a_1$, $a_2$, and $a_4$, can be determined by minimizing the sum of the squares of the differences between experimental and theoretical data.

## 5. Viscoelasticity

Biological tissues reveal properties of both elastic solid and viscous fluid. Thus, the stress depends not only on the applied strain as in a solid, but also on the rate of strain as in a viscous fluid. In other words, the response is time-dependent in that the stress-strain response does not occur instantly. When the material is suddenly strained and the strain is maintained constant, the corresponding stresses induced in the wall decrease with time. This phenomenon is called stress relaxation (Fig. 4). If the material is suddenly stressed and

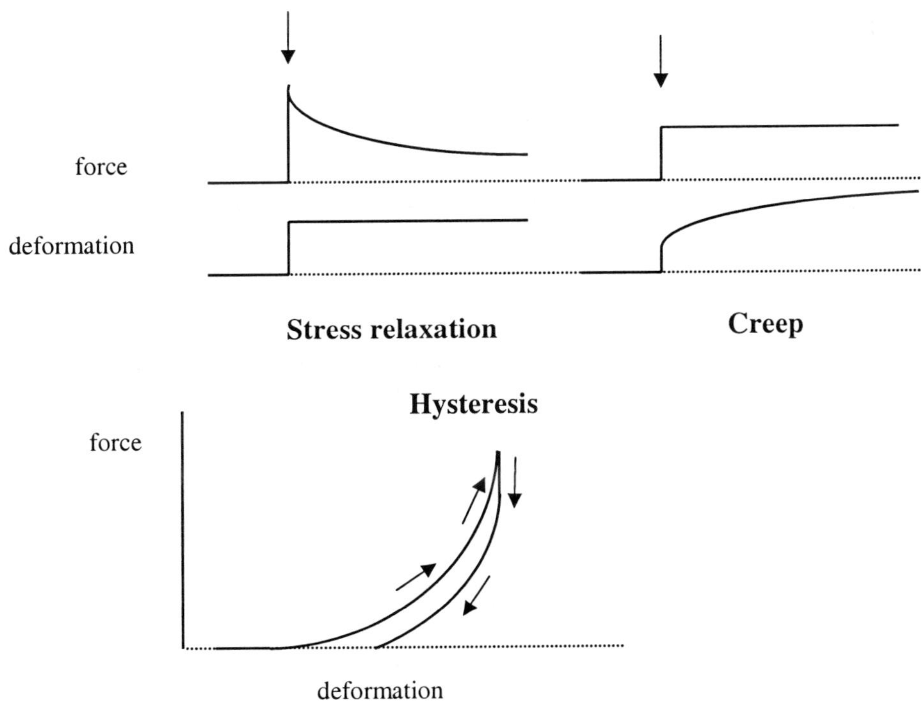


Fig. 4. Illustration of stress relaxation, creep and hysteresis.

the stress is maintained constant, the material will continue to deform. This phenomenon is called creep. If the material is subjected to a cyclic loading, the stress-strain relationship in the loading process is somewhat different from that in the unloading process (Fig. 4) and the phenomenon is called hysteresis (1, 2, 5, 8). Stress relaxation, creep, and hysteresis are features of viscoelasticity.

Viscoelastic properties in terms of pressure relaxation curves have been described for the normal and diseased human rectum (9). Often, the viscoelastic behavior is described in terms of models. Three simple models are often used, the Maxwell model, the Voigt model and the Kelvin model (standard linear solid). The models combine linear springs (constant $\mu$) and dashpots with coefficient of viscosity ($\eta$). The spring is supposed to produce an instant deformation proportional to the load whereas the dashpot produces a velocity proportional to the load at any instant. The relationship $F = \mu u$, where $F$ is a force acting on the spring and $u$ is the extension of the spring describes the spring. For the dashpot we have the relationship $F = \eta\dot{u}$ where $\dot{u}$ is the velocity of deflection. The Maxwell body is the combination of a spring and dashpot in series. The Voigt body is the spring and dashpot in parallel whereas the Kelvin model has a Maxwell body in parallel with a dashpot. On basis of the equations for the dashpot and spring, creep functions and relaxation functions can be derived for these models (10). Figure 5 illustrates the creep behavior for the three models. More complex functions exist. However, viscoelastic models does not account for all history-dependent mechanical behavior (11).

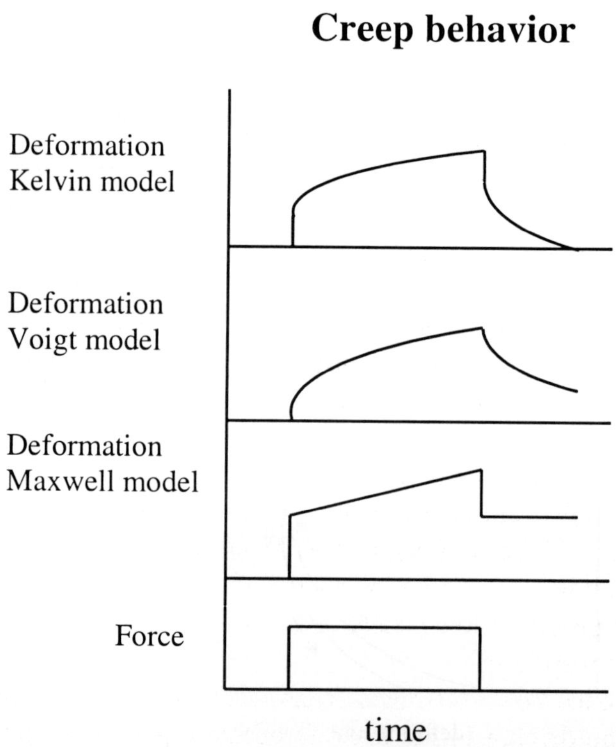


Fig. 5. Illustration of the creep behavior in the three viscoelastic models.

## 6. Fluid Mechanics

This chapter does not intend to provide a detailed analysis of gastrointestinal fluid mechanics, despite the fact that flow is the main result of the motion of the gastrointestinal tract. The reason for this is that relatively few data and valid models are available for gastrointestinal flow. The GI tract has received very little attention from the point of view of fluid mechanics. Furthermore, the fact that the geometry of the tract is complex and the fluids are non-Newtonian complicates matters greatly. A Newtonian fluid is a viscous fluid for which the shear stress is linearly proportional to the rate of deformation (air and water can be treated as nonviscous in many engineering problems, in relation to gastrointestinal function they probably cannot).

In this chapter, we merely wish to point out the most important concepts for the study of fluids in motion. Three significant concepts in fluid flow are:

- the principle of conservation of mass
- the principle of kinetic energy
- the principle of momentum

from which the equations of continuity, flow equations and equations evaluating dynamic forces exerted by flowing fluids are developed.

Fluid mechanics in the gastrointestinal tract encompasses many processes. The gross mass transport of contents from the proximal to the distal tract is just one aspect of these processes and perhaps the easiest to measure. However, secondary and retrograde flows, the addition of volume by secretion, the reduction of volume by absorption, physical changes in the fluid as it flows, the mixing of heterogeneous fluids, gas production by microorganisms, etc produce a complex flow system that challenges the most advanced methods of contemporary fluid mechanics. An analysis, however, is necessary for those who wish to truly understand gastrointestinal physiology. It is just as inappropriate to ignore flow in the gastrointestinal tract as it would be to ignore blood flow in the cardiovascular system.

Compared to the work on visceral muscle contractility, the work on gastrointestinal flow seems much more scattered, probably because of the difficulties involved in its study from and the complexity of the geometry, the unfamiliar composition and properties of the fluids, and the kinds of flows that seem to occur. Several studies, more or less theoretical by nature, have been published on flow in the gastrointestinal tract and the consequences of various types of contractions. Brasseur and coworkers applied bioengineering principles in their extensive work on bolus flow in the esophagus (see for example Refs. 12 and 13). In addition, the reader should consult the work by Bertuzzi (14), Denli (15), Stavitsky (16), Macagno (17), Fung (18), Tözeren (19), and Miftakhov (20, 21). Though the complexity is enormous *in vivo*, fluid flow *in vitro* can be controlled in experimental set-ups. For example, it is possible to impose predetermined shear stresses and shear rates to cells grown in culture in order to study their responses.

Many factors influence flow and bolus transport in distensible organs such as the gastrointestinal tract. The driving forces are the pressure generated by the contractile peristaltic forces and, to a lesser extent, the hydrostatic force of gravity. Biomechanical models indicate that the important determinants of flow include such factors as the shape and size of the luminal cross-section, the size and viscosity of the bolus, and the viscoelastic properties of the tissue (the elastic modulus, strain rate and shear properties of the wall). The gastrointestinal tract may be stretched in the vicinity of a bolus. That is, the contents propelled in front of a peristaltic contraction may tend to bulge out the wall. This is the source of the idea that intestinal reflexes initiated by local stretch are important in the generation of antegrade flow. Although the degree to which such reflexes actually regulate flow in normal conditions is debatable, distension studies might help us to understand the complex fluid mechanical behavior of the gastrointestinal tract.

Esophageal flow properties have been studied by Brasseur and coworkers while gastric emptying, antroduodenal mechanics, and intestinal flow properties were described primarily by Macagno, Christensen, Meyer, Schulze-Delrieu and their coworkers. Weems reviewed the literature on flow properties in the gastrointestinal tract. Mathematical modeling of peristaltic transport in distensible tubes has also been attempted by Stavitsky, Srivastava, Fung, Li, Brasseur and Miftakhov. The mathematical modeling of peristaltic transport is based on the premise that the interaction between gastrointestinal elasticity and bolus transport is best understood by examining the fluid dynamics equations (equations describing bolus transport) and equations describing gastrointestinal deformation (the constitutive equations). The interaction between these equations is governed by the boundary conditions.

## 7. Ultrasound Approaches

The speed of sound in biological tissue depends on the density, $\rho$, and the compressibility of the tissue according to

$$c = (K/\rho)^{1/2} \tag{22}$$

where $K$ is the bulk modulus of the material; a quantity inversely related to compressibility which is a measure of tissue stiffness. The sound speed for longitudinal waves is rather low in materials which are compressible such as soft tissue. A typical sound speed for soft tissue is 1550 $\mathrm{ms}^{-1}$, with the relation between sound speed and particle velocity being such that $|\mathbf{u}|/c \ll 1$.

### 7.1. *Transabdominal B-mode ultrasonography*

In $B$-mode (Brightness-mode) ultrasonography the received echoes from tissue interfaces are displayed as points on the screen with brightness proportional to the amplitude of the echo. This is different from the $A$-mode (Amplitude-mode) where the echos are displayed as the amplitude of the deflection in the $y$-axis when the beam is running along the $x$-axis. Both static and real-time $B$-mode ultrasonography can be used to visualize areas of the gastrointestinal tract such as the stomach, pylorus and duodenum. Usually, a 3–7.5 MHz ultrasound probe is used, providing a fairly good resolution and a sufficient penetration range. Short pulses of ultrasound will pass through a liquid but are partially reflected by interfaces where one or both media are tissue, producing echoes. The depth of the reflecting interface determines the time taken for an echo to return to the ultrasound transducer. In real-time ultrasonography a continuous, moving, two-dimensional $B$-mode image is obtained. The technique is useful for the study of gastric emptying and antroduodenal motility and antral size. Some problems may, however, arise from individual anatomic variations that may prevent visualization in a single plane. Furthermore, subcutaneous fat and bowel gas may blur the images.

Several scanning techniques have been developed. These include:

- **Linear real-time scanning** where a moving picture is made possible by mechanically or electronically manipulating the ultrasound beam direction. The linear electronic scanner is characterized by having several crystals in a line, activating one or a small number of crystals at a time. This type of real-time scanning gives the same line density throughout all depths.
- **Curvilinear real-time scanning** where the surface is made slightly convex. This provides a good field of view close to the transducer and an extended field of view at increasing depth. The latter property makes the curvilinear probe less bulky for abdominal use compared to the linear probe.
- **Sector real-time scanning** where the image is obtained by changing the beam direction mechanically or electronically. The mechanical sector scanner can be of the rotational or the oscillating type. All sector scanners have a varying line density throughout the 2D image. The electronic sector scanner, called the phased array, uses Huygen's principle to steer the beam without any mechanical components.

$B$-mode ultrasonography is useful for obtaining geometric measures in the parts of the gastrointestinal tract where scanning is possible. Hence, it is useful for measuring luminal dimensions, wall thickness and layer thicknesses at various conditions such as during contractile activity. However, to compute stresses (according to the equations provided previously in this chapter) the pressure must also be measured. Therefore, ultrasonography must be combined with intraluminal manometry. Furthermore, a balloon may be added to the manometry probe in order to actively distend the gastrointestinal tract. In some regions of the gastrointestinal tract such as in the antrum, it is possible to obtain good images using transabdominal ultrasonography. If combined with balloon distension where the pressure is measured and can be controlled, it is possible to compute stress-strain relations *in vivo*. This has in fact been used for studying the geometry during balloon distension (Fig. 6) and the stress-strain relationship of the gastric antrum (22). Healthy volunteers underwent stepwise inflation of a bag located in the antrum with volumes up to 60 ml. The stretch ratio and Cauchy stress and strain were calculated from measurements of pressure, diameter, and wall thickness in periods without and with administration of relaxant drugs. The strain was positive in circumferential direction, negative in the radial direction, and no strain in the longitudinal direction. The stress-strain relation was exponential. Furthermore, the wall stress was decomposed into its active and passive components, i.e. the well-known length-tension diagram from *in vitro* studies of smooth muscle strips could be reproduced. The maximum active tension appeared at a stretch ratio of 1.5.

### 7.2. *Endoscopic ultrasonography (EUS)*

Performing the scan from the gastrointestinal tract lumen enables higher frequencies to be used. Endoscopic imaging typically utilizes frequencies of 5–30 MHz and is most often performed with radial mechanical ultrasound endoscopes. With this type of transducer 360°

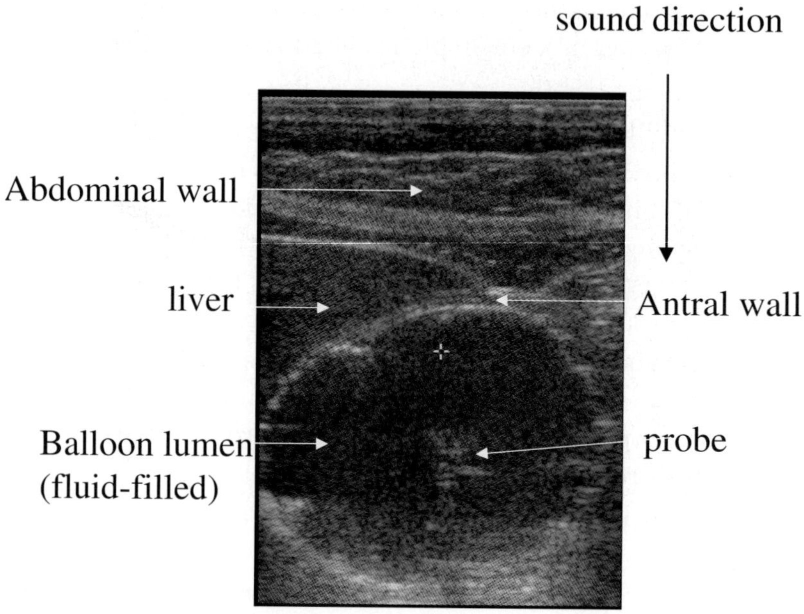


Fig. 6. *B*-mode ultrasonographic image of the antrum (cross-section) during balloon distension. The image is obtained with an 8 Mhz scanner. The probe on which the balloon is mounted is visible in the centre of the balloon. Several layers can be identified in the antrum wall. This is especially evident in the part of the antrum closest to the transducer.

radial scans are obtained and a balloon facilitates acoustic contact between the transducer and the gastrointestinal tract wall. The endoscopic scanner has a lower frame rate than transcutanous real-time scanners, typically 5–20 frames per second. Alternatively, linear or curvilinear electronic probes are available for endoscopic ultrasound. They provide axial scans, giving less image view but having the advantage of higher frame rates and also facilities for Doppler methods, something which is difficult with the slow moving 360° mechanical scanners.

An alternative method is also available — using a standard gastroscope miniature probes can be introduced via the biopsi channel (internal diameter typically 2.5 cm). The first of these transducers were designed for static scanning where the operator performed the scanning movement.

The increased frequency in EUS compared with transcutaneous applications gives a much better resolution, especially the axial resolution (along the ultrasound beam). The lateral resolution is not affected in the same way due to the lack of focusing of the beam (mechanical transducers) and the limited line density for the 360° scan. Most endoscopic ultrasound methods are capable of imaging the separate layers of the gastrointestinal tract wall. The interpretation of the multiple echoes from these layers is a major challenge for the operator of endoscopic ultrasound methods.

By now, endoscopic ultrasonography has been used for several biomechanical studies of the esophagus. Figure 7 shows an EUS view of the human esophagus using a 15 MHz probe.

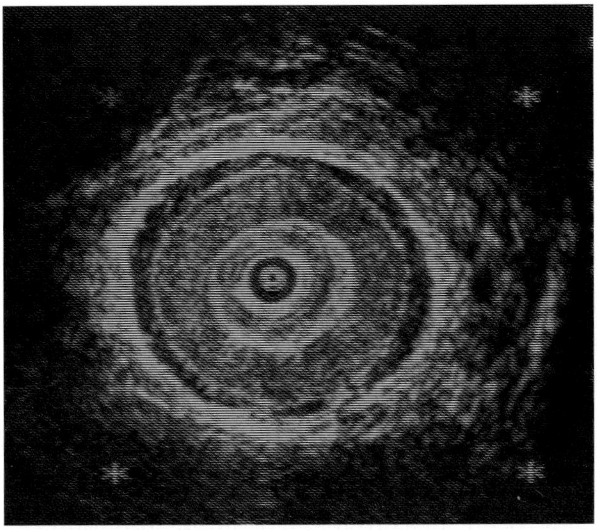

Fig. 7. Ultrasonographic image of esophageal wall during a contraction (primary peristalsis). The image is obtained using a 15 MHz endoscopic ultrasound probe in a young volunteer at Haukeland Hospital in Bergen, Norway. Several layers and their interfaces are visible.

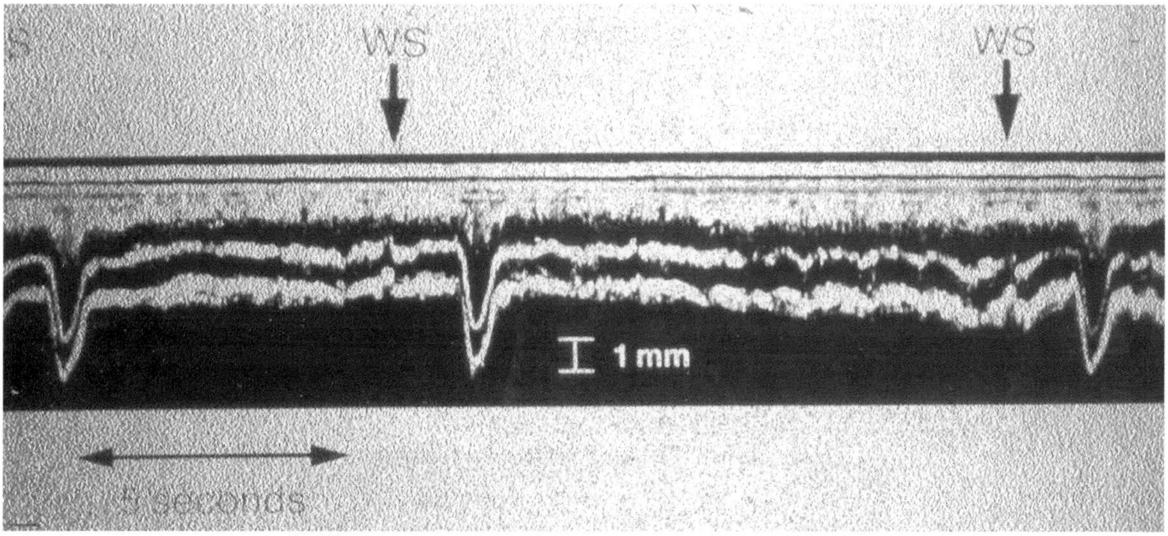


Fig. 8. $M$-mode representation of esophageal contractions (courtesy of R. Martin).

## 7.3. *M-mode*

Displaying the echoes in $B$-mode but with the time axis constantly running, it gives a display of position or movement of the echoes with time called $M$-mode (Motion-mode). An example is provided in Fig. 8. This application is especially useful in dynamic biological systems like the gastrointestinal tract for evaluating wall motions, giving a high time-resolution.

### 7.4. *3D-ultrasound*

Both rotational and translational probe adaptors for 3D ultrasound acquisition are commercially available as well as position sensors mostly based on magnetic sensing. The latter method is most frequently used on the abdomen, because of the freedom in probe angling and manipulation (23). An example of a reconstruction of the stomach geometry from 3D ultrasonography is shown in Fig. 9.

The method of recording dynamic 3D rendered images obtained by sequentially acquisition of 2D images has been available for some time. The method use a workstation to input 2D images for Cartesian coordinate conversion and volume rendering. Outside research settings, this rather time-consuming process proved cumbersome and has not been extensively used in clinical practice. Now these technical and practical issues have been addressed and real-time 3D sonography has recently been introduced with great potential to impact both patient care and throughput in a number of ways, including better pre- and post-surgical planning, improved measurement of organ function, and decreased examination times. With real-time 3D ultrasound images, clinicians will be able to better quantify size, shape and function of the gastrointestinal organ. However, the most important contribution of real-time 3D sonography in gastroenterology may be improvement in locating abnormalities for surgical planning.

## 8. Spectral Doppler

Spectral Doppler methods are based on the estimation of velocity from Doppler shifts which is the difference between the transmitted and received ultrasound frequency. When either the source, reflector or receiver or a combination of these are moving, a change in frequency results and the frequency difference (Doppler shift) is proportional to the relative velocity. If the source is moving towards the receiver, a compressed wavelength will be experienced and the frequency of the source will appeared increased. The opposite effect will be experienced if the source was moving away from the receiver. In medical ultrasound Doppler methods,

Fig. 9. 3D reconstruction of the human stomach.

it is the reflector that is moving (in our case gastric contents) and both receiver and source are stationary.

The two simplest methods are the continuous wave (CW) Doppler and pulsed wave (PW) Doppler. The CW Doppler transmits a continuous wave train on one crystal, while the other crystal acts as a receiver. The transmitted ultrasound is reflected from tissue interfaces and these reflections have the same frequency. If the ultrasound hits moving objects, the reflection will experience a shift in frequency ($f_d$). This signal is called the *Doppler shift*. The frequency of the Doppler signal is related to the velocity of the moving fluid in the sample region through the Doppler equation

$$f_d = \frac{2f_0 v}{c}. \tag{23}$$

In this equation, $f_0$ is the central frequency of the transmitted ultrasound pulse, $c$ is the speed of sound, and $v$ is the velocity component of the fluid in the ultrasound beam direction. The Doppler shift is in the audible range typically 20–10,000 Hz, and is often called the Doppler signal. The factor 2 arises from the fact that during transmission the moving medium is a moving receiver and experiences a Doppler shift. During reflection, the moving medium acts as a moving transmitter and the receiving crystal experiences both Doppler shifts.

In the PW Doppler method a short ultrasound pulse is transmitted from the crystal and the same crystal then acts as the receiver similar to $B$-mode imaging. Ignoring Doppler shifted signals returning to the transducer until a preselected time interval after transmission, depth resolution is obtained. The duration of this time interval determines the length of the collecting region called range gate or sample volume.

The distribution of Doppler shifts can be displayed as a spectrum where time is running along the $x$-axis, velocity on the $y$-axis and the amplitude of the different velocities given as a grey scale.

### 8.1. *Duplex scanning*

Application of the stand-alone Doppler was restricted to the heart and peripheral vessels. When these Doppler methods were combined with the $B$-mode image (often called Duplex scanning), their use became widespread within most specialities using ultrasound imaging. Quick verification of areas with no or little echoes in the $B$-mode image for venous or arterial blood flow or no blood flow gave important information about these structures.

In the $B$-mode image, a cursor placed along the center axis of the vessel gave an angle correction of the velocity scale, thus enabling the velocity along the vessel axes to be measured. In addition, the combination of $B$-mode image and Doppler gave the opportunity to measure blood flow and not only the blood velocity. Blood flow ($Q$) are estimated from

$$Q = \bar{v}A \tag{24}$$

where $\bar{v}$ is the velocity averaged over the vessel lumen and time, and $A$ is the cross-sectional area. Although a simple relationship, the accuracy of such flow measurement depends on several criteria to be fulfilled. If the diameter of the vessel is measured, it must be verified that the lumen is circular and it is the internal luminal cross-sectional area that should be used which is not always easily obtainable. The velocity must be the velocity averaged over the whole lumen, normally obtained with a large sample volume. The wall motion filters must be at a minimum removing only wall motion Doppler shifts and not Doppler shifts from slow moving blood. The angle $\theta$ must be known and the average (spatial average) velocity must also be the mean over several heart cycles to remove variation due to respiration. With these criteria fulfilled flow can be measured with good accuracy.

Movements of luminal contents across the pylorus has been studied by duplex sonography (24). The relationship between motility and transpyloric movements of luminal contents have been studied after ingestion of 500 ml meat soup in healthy subjects. Accurate timing of antegrade and retrograde flow were recorded using bidirectional velocity curves. The quantification of velocity depends on the knowledge of ultrasound velocity $c$ of the administrated fluid.

### 8.2. *Color Doppler*

In the multirange gated Doppler, the backscattered Doppler-shifted ultrasound from a large number of range gates or sample volumes was recorded simultaneously. The velocity profile of a blood vessel could thus be measured with this instrument. Using the multi-range gated method (typically 128 sample volumes) and in addition sweeping the beam gave velocity information in a 2D area (picture). Color coding the velocities gives a color flow map (CFM) of velocities that could be superimposed on the $B$-mode image. Color Doppler has been used to estimate gastric emtying and duodenogastric reflux in volunteers (25).

## 9. Tissue Doppler and Strain Rate Imaging

Strain rate imaging (SRI) is a novel technique to measure deformations in biological tissue. The technique is based on tissue velocity imaging, which is an ultrasound technique that provides quantitative information on the velocity of the tissue. By color-coded tissue velocity imaging, velocity samples from the whole field of view are available simultaneously. This allows for extraction of parameters such as strain and strain rate through spatial and temporal processing of the velocity data. The methods have primarily been used in echocardiography but measurements of gastric motor function have also been done recently.

### 9.1. *Tissue velocity imaging*

Tissue velocity imaging (TVI) is a technique where the velocity of the moving tissue towards or away from the transducer is measured and displayed. The velocities can be calculated and displayed as a PW spectrogram or as a color-coding of the image. The two methods both calculate the velocity based on the echoes of several ultrasound pulses fired in the same direction. Each echo is sampled at a fixed depth, and the samples are collected into a new signal representing a certain position in the image, called the *Doppler signal.* The frequency of the Doppler signal is related to the velocity of the tissue in the sample region through the Doppler equation stated in the section on spectral Doppler.

In PW TVI, the Doppler signal from only one sample region is collected. In the basic type of processing, the signal is first split into overlapping segments, and the frequency content of each signal segment is next calculated using the Fourier transform. Other, more advanced processing methods involving data from several sample regions may also be used. The result is a signal spectrum for each segment, representing the frequency content at a certain time. The signal spectra are collected in a spectrogram, with Doppler frequency on the vertical axis and time or velocity on the horizontal axis.

In color TVI, a Doppler signal is collected for each depth and each ultrasound beam. This normally requires more time, so each Doppler signal consists of fewer samples per time unit than in the PW case. This normally limits the ability to calculate full signal spectra for each position in the image. Instead, only the mean Doppler frequency is estimated for each position.

The most common way to estimate this mean frequency is to calculate the phase shift relative to the transmitted ultrasound pulse for each sample in the Doppler signals. The difference in phase shift from sample to sample in the Doppler signal can thus be used to calculate the mean velocity.

When the mean velocity has been estimated for all parts of the ultrasound image, each pixel is color coded according to the velocity. As mentioned earlier, the Doppler acquisition is usually separate from the image acquisition, so for each grey scale image there is at least one corresponding velocity image. The velocity image may have a lower resolution than the grey scale image, but is normally interpolated to match the resolution of the grey scale image. This means that neighboring pixels in the color-coded image may represent identical velocity values.

### 9.2. *Strain, strain rate and velocity gradients*

Strain and strain rate are characteristics of changes in shape, i.e. deformations. The strain and strain rate can be defined and measured in various ways as stated previously in this chapter. For example, the Lagrangian (Cauchy) strain and the natural strain are defined as

$$\varepsilon = \frac{L - L_0}{L_0} \quad \text{and} \quad \varepsilon' = \ln\left(\frac{L}{L_0}\right) \tag{25}$$

The strain rate is the temporal derivative of the strain. The relation between strain rate and strain can be compared to the relation between velocity and displacement. Assuming the velocity is constant, displacement equals time multiplied with velocity. A positive strain rate means that the length of the object is increasing, while a negative strain rate means that the length is decreasing. Since there are several definitions of strain, there are a corresponding number of similar definitions for strain rate. For example, the natural strain rate is defined as

$$\dot{\varepsilon}' = \frac{d\varepsilon'}{dt} = \frac{1}{L}\frac{dL}{dt} \tag{26}$$

Under certain assumptions and since the temporal derivative of spatial position is velocity, the natural strain rate of the object can be written

$$\dot{\varepsilon}' = \frac{1}{L}\frac{dL}{dt} = \frac{1}{L}\left(\frac{dx_b}{dt} - \frac{dx_a}{dt}\right) = \frac{v_b - v_a}{L} = \frac{dv}{dx} \tag{27}$$

where $v_a$ and $v_b$ are the instantaneous velocities of the end-points of the segment. The equation is correct if the spatial velocity distribution within the segment is assumed to be linear. In practice, it is rarely feasible to accurately track the end-points of such a segment, and a fixed "strain length" or "strain sample size" $\Delta x$ may be used instead. As long as the velocities are linearly increasing or decreasing within the region, this method will give the same answer.

The velocity gradient may be estimated using only the two velocity estimates $v_1$ and $v_2$ from the end-points of the estimation area as

$$\dot{\varepsilon}' = \frac{v_2 - v_1}{\Delta x} \tag{28}$$

or a linear regression of all the velocity samples within the area may be performed.

### 9.3. *Integrating strain rate to get strain*

The strain can be found as the temporal integral of the strain rate, calculated for each time point during the deformation

$$\varepsilon' = \int_{T_0}^{T} \dot{\varepsilon}'(t)dt \tag{29}$$

where $T_0$ and $T$ are the time points of the start and end of the deformation. Note that it is the natural strain that is found through this integral.

One of the major advantages of TVI and strain rate imaging is that it allows quantitative analysis of the motion pattern of the tissue. In pulsed wave TVI, accurate timing and velocity measurements may be performed from the spectrogram. In the color modes, each pixel in the image represents a measurement, and the quantitative value can be presented in various ways, as described in the following sections.

Strain rate imaging has thus far only been used in one gastrointestinal study (26). Healthy fasting subjects were studied with both grey-scale and Doppler US data acquired with a 5- to 8-MHz linear transducer in cineloops of 97 to 256 frames. Rapid stepwise inflation (5 to 60 mL) of an intragastric bag was carried out and bag pressure and SRI were measured simultaneously. The balloon distension gave values of strain on passive deformation of −20 to −40% in the antrum in the circumferential direction and 0 to 160% in the radial direction. Great variations in strain distribution of the muscle layers were found. Radial strain was much higher in the circular than in the longitudinal muscle layer. Strains derived from SRI correlated well with strains obtained with $B$-mode measurements ($r = 0.98$) and an inverse correlation was found between pressure and radial strain ($r = -0.87$). Intraobserver correlation of strain estimation was $r = 0.98$) and the intraobserver agreement was 0.2%. Hence, it was concluded that SRI enables detailed mapping of radial strain distribution of the gastric wall and correlates well with $B$-mode measurements.

The above data are in accordance with yet unpublished bench studies showing good agreement for the SRI method with both $B$-mode and calculated values for strain. However, the examination preferably should be undertaken with a speed at least corresponding to a tissue velocity 0.5 mm/s to give accurate strain estimates with the SRI method, and averaging over several ultrasound beams increase the accuracy.

## 10. Elastography

An alternative method to estimate the elastic behavior of biological tissue has been published (27, 28). This method, called elastography, utilizes the recording of the radio frequency signals in a $B$-mode registration and has been applied to the GI tract, kidney, muscle, breast and the heart (29–31). The underlying principle is that the deformation of tissue by a mechanical excitation is a function of its mechanical properties. The deformation of the tissue is determined using ultrasound. For gastrointestinal purposes, the intraluminal pressure may be used as the excitation force. The radial strain in the tissue is obtained by cross-correlation techniques on the radio frequency signal. The strain is color-coded and plotted as a complimentary image to the IVUS echogram.

## 11. Ultrasound Microscopy

Data relating microscale biomechanical properties and gastrointestinal histology are sparse although tissue components for force transmission, i.e. smooth muscles and collagen have been identified. Scanning acoustic microscopy (SAM) can provide such data *in vitro* by means of ultrasound in the GHz-range and use of elementary theory of elasticity. The following shows how advanced high-frequency ultrasound and elementary theory of elasticity can be utilized to quantify the intestinal properties on the micrometer scale (32).

### 11.1. *SAM microscope*

The SAM microscope utilizes ultrasound signal frequencies ($f$) in the GHz-range to image and measures elastic properties in sectioned tissue specimens. In both imaging and measurement mode, operation is by way of a focused acoustic lens with a piezo-electric transducer transmitting and receiving ultrasound to and from the tissue. The microscope may be operated at $f = 500$ MHz using a lens with a numerical aperture (NA) of 0.98 to yield a resolution ($w$) of approximately 1.8 $\mu$m.

In image mode, the lens $x$–$y$-scans fields of interest, magnifying between 125$\times$ and 600$\times$. In this mode, the reflected ultrasound is converted to 512 by 512 pixels 8-bit grey scale images. Once an image is obtained, the microscope is switched to the time-resolved measurement mode where it scans the lens along a programmed scan-line while digitizing and recording individual reflected ultrasound waves.

Elementary elasticity theory can be applied to SAM measurements for the calculation of $c_{11}$ which expresses the elastic stiffness. In acoustics, the speed $C$ and acoustic impedance $Z$, where the latter is the ratio of stress or pressure to particle displacement velocity, are the parameters necessary to calculate $c_{11}$. The recorded ultrasound waves contain echoes in the form of voltage amplitude signals originating from the upper tissue surface and the tissue-substrate interface. The method of detecting the relevant echoes by way of computer-based signal deconvolution and waveform recognition is described in detail by Briggs *et al.* (33). For the determination of $C$ and $Z$, we need

(1) individual wave amplitudes ($A_1$ and $A_2$) and timings ($t_1$ and $t_2$)

(2) reference amplitude and timing of an echo in a wave received from a substrate without tissue ($A_0$ and $t_0$)

(3) standard $C$ and $Z$ values of the couplant (1,532.9 ms$^{-1}$ and 1.53 MPa sm$^{-1}$, respectively) into:

$$C = C_{\text{couplant}} \frac{t_0 - t_1}{t_2 - t_1} (\text{ms}^{-1}) \tag{30}$$

and

$$Z = Z_{\text{couplant}} \frac{A_0 + A_1}{A_0 - A_1} (\text{Pa sm}^{-1}) \tag{31}$$

In the analysis, we neglect absorption in the thickness of the sample, and take the variables in Eq. (31) to be real-valued.

$c_{11}$ is computed from

$$c_{11} = CZ \text{ (Pa)} \tag{32}$$

According to Briggs (34), $c_{11}$ is related to Young's modulus ($E$) by the relationship

$$c_{11} = \frac{(1-\sigma)E}{(1+\sigma)(1-2\sigma)} \tag{33}$$

where $\sigma$ is the Poisson's ratio. Because $\sigma$ is only slightly less than 0.5 for soft tissue, $c_{11}$ may be considerably higher than $E$.

### 11.2. *Scanning Laser Acoustic Microscopy (SLAM) for determination of the propagation speed of sound*

The SLAM is a transmission mode instrument that creates real-time acoustic images of a sample throughout its entire thickness. A collimated continuous-wave ultrasound beam at frequencies from 10 to 500 MHz is produced by a piezoelectric transducer located beneath the sample. When the ultrasound wave propagates through the sample, the wave is affected by mechanical inhomogeneities in the material. A scanned laser beam is used as the ultrasound detector. The ability of the SLAM to produce simultaneously optical and acoustic images from which the acoustic properties of the specimen can be calculated facilitates its use in this field of biology. The ultrasonic attenuation and propagation speed can be estimated from the obtained information. Conventional tissue fixation and staining are not required for the SLAM imaging. Living cells and tissues can be studied.

Three SLAM modes produce three different images. For all modes, the sample is located between the SLAM stage and plastic coverslip. The coverslip is coated with a partially reflecting optical layer. In the *optical mode*, a focused laser beam scans the specimen from above, and is transmitted through the coverslip and specimen to a photodiode at the base of the stage. The received photodiode signal is electronically processed and displayed to a TV-monitor; the SLAM's optical image is comparable to that of conventional optical microscopy at a magnification of 100X, but is not comparable in that the light source is that of a laser. In the *acoustic mode*, the specimen is insonified with an ultrasonic wave generated by a piezoelectric transducer located below the specimen. The sound wave traverses the specimen and is incident on the lower surface of the coverslip, the surface with the coating. The acoustic generated deflections on this surface of the coverslip are scanned by the laser beam that in turn is reflected to a photodiode. The laser signal is then processed into an acoustic-mode image and displayed in real time on the TV monitor. The ultrasonic attenuation of the specimen can be calculated from this acoustic image (35, 36). In the *interference mode*, the laser beam is detected by the same photodiode as in the acoustic mode and it is then mixed with a reference signal to produce an interference image displayed on the TV-monitor. From the interference image, the acoustic propagation speed is calculated from the lateral (horizontal) shift of the vertical interference lines. The lines shift to the right when the sound waves enter an object having a higher speed relative to the coupling reference medium. Quantitative speed profiles can be obtained from several image regions in different loci. The propagation speed of the specimen is calculated in relation to that of the reference medium according to the following expression

$$C_x = \frac{C_o}{\sin\theta_o}\left[\tan^{-1}\left(\frac{1}{\frac{1}{\tan\theta_o} - \frac{\lambda_o N}{T\sin\theta_o}}\right)\right] \text{ms}^{-1} \tag{34}$$

where $C_x$ is the propagation speed in the specimen of interest, $C_o$ is the propagation speed in the reference medium, $\lambda_o$ is the wavelength of sound in the reference medium, $T$ is the specimen thickness, $N$ is the measured normalized lateral fringe shift, $\theta_o$ is the angle between the direction of sound propagation in the reference medium and the normal to the stage surface, and is determined from Snell's Law:

$$\theta_o = \sin^{-1}\left[\frac{C_o}{C_s}\sin\theta_s\right] \tag{35}$$

where $C_s$ is the propagation speed in the fused silica stage (5968 $\text{ms}^{-1}$), and $\theta_s$ is the angle the sound wave travels through the stage (45°). Measurements of the propagation speed can be done along the vertical line in each layer of the wall to yield a speed profile. Preliminary data obtained in the guinea pig esophagus are given by Assentoft and coworkers (37).

In summary, ultrasound is very useful in biomechanical studies where it is used primarily for measurement of geometric data such as wall thickness and diameters. Techniques are evolving for the future where strain rate imaging and 3D geometry likely will be important tools of investigation.

## References


1. Gregersen, H., Biomechanics of the gastrointestinal tract. Springer-Verlag. 2002.
2. Gregersen, H. and Kassab, G. S., Biomechanics of the gastrointestinal tract. Neurogastroenterol Motility 1996; 8: 277–297.
3. Nash, W., Theory and problems of strength of materials. 3rd. edition. McGraw-Hill Inc., USA. 1994.
4. Gao, C. and Gregersen, H., Biomechanical and morphological properties in the rat large intestine. J Biomech 2000; 33: 1089–1097.
5. Fung, Y. C., A first course in continuum mechanics. Prentice Hall, Englewood Cliffs. 1994.

6. Fung, Y. C., Biomechanics: Motion, flow, stress and growth. Springer-Verlag, New York. 1990.
7. Jørgensen, C. J., Dall, F. H., Jensen, S. L. and Gregersen, H., A new combined ultrasound-impedance planimetry measuring system for quantification of organ wall biomechanics *in vivo*. J Biomech 1995; 28: 863–867.
8. Fung, Y. C., Biomechanics. Its scope, history, and some problems of continuum mechanics in physiology. Applied Mechanics Reviews 1968; 21: 1–20.
9. Arhan, P., Faverdin, C., Persoz, B., *et al.*, Relationship between viscoelastic properties of the rectum and anal pressure in man. J Appl Phys 1976; 41: 677–82.
10. Fung, Y. C., Biomechanics. Mechanical properties of living tissues. Springer-Verlag, New York. 1993.
11. Gregersen, H., Emery, J. and McCulloch, A. D., History-dependent mechanical behavior of the guinea-pig small intestine. Annals Biomed Eng 1998; 26: 1–9.
12. Brasseur, J. G., A fluid mechanical perspective on esophageal bolus transport. Dysphagia 1987; 2: 32–39.
13. Brasseur, J. G., Mechanical studies of the esophageal function. Dysphagia 1993; 8: 384–386.
14. Bertuzzi, A., Salinari, S., Mancinelli, R. and Pescatori, M., Peristaltic transport of a solid bolus. J Biomechanics 1983; 16: 459–464.
15. Denli, N., An analytical model of flow induced by longitudinal contractions in the small intestine. Thesis. University of Iowa. 1975.
16. Stavitsky, D., Flow and mixing in a contracting channel with applications to the human intestine. Thesis. University of Iowa. 1979.
17. Macagno, E. O. and Christensen, J., Fluid mechanics of gastrointestinal flow. In: Physiology of the gastrointestinal tract. Eds. Johnson LR *et al.* Raven Press; New York. 1981; Chapter 10.
18. Fung, Y. C. and Yih, C. S., Peristaltic transport. J Applied Mechanics 1968; 669–675.
19. Tözeren, A., Özkaya, N. and Tözeren, H., Flow of particles along a deformable tube. J Biomechanics 1982; 15: 517–527.
20. Miftakhov, R. N., Abdusheva, G. R. and Christensen, J., Numerical simulation of motility patterns of the small bowel. Part I-formulation of a mathematical model. J Theoretical Biology 1999; 197: 89–112.
21. Miftakhov, R. N. and Wingate, D. L., Numerical simulation of the peristaltic reflex of the small bowel. J Biorheology 1994; 31: 309–325.
22. Gregersen, H., Gilja, O. H., Hausken, T., Heimdal, A., Gao, C., Matre, K., Ødegaard, S. and Berstad, A., Biomechanical wall properties in the human gastric antrum using B-mode ultrasonography and volume-controlled antral distension. Am J Physiol 2002; 283: G368–G375.
23. Matre, K., Stokke, E. M., Martens, D. and Gilja, O. H., *In vitro* volume estimation of kidneys using three-dimensional ultrasonography and a position detector. Eur J Ultrasound 1999; 10: 65–73.
24. Hausken, T., Odegaard, S., Matre, K. and Berstad, A., Antroduodenal motility and movements of luminal contents studied by duplex sonography. Gastroenterology 1992; 102: 1583–1590.
25. Hausken, T., Li, X. N., Goldman, B., Leotta, D., Ødegaard, S. and Martin, R. W., Quantification of gastric emptying and duodenogastric reflux stroke volumes using three-dimensional guided digital color Doppler imaging. Eur J Ultrasound 2001; 13: 2050–213.
26. Gilja, O. H., Heimdal, A., Hausken, T., *et al.*, Strain during gastric contractions can be measured using Doppler ultrasonography. Ultrasound Med Biol 2002; 28: 1457–1465.
27. Ophir, J., Cespedes, I., Ponnekanti, H., Yazdi, Y. and Li, X., Elastography: A quantitative method for imaging the elasticity of biological tissues. Ultrason Imaging 1991; 13: 111–134.

28. Ophir, J., Garra, B., Kallel, F., Konofagou, E., Krouskop, T., Righetti, R. and Varghese, T., Elastographic imaging. Ultrasound Med Biol 2000; 26(Suppl 1): S23–S29.
29. Cespedes, I., Ophir, J., Ponnekanti, H. and Maklad, N., Elastography: Elasticity imaging using ultrasound with application to muscle and breast *in vivo*. Ultrason Imaging 1993; 15: 73–88.
30. Hiltawsky, K. M., Krüger, M., Starke, C., *et al.*, Freehand ultrasound elastography of breast lesions: Clinical results. Ultrasound Med Biol 2001; 27: 1461–1469.
31. Konofagou, E. E., D'hooge, J. and Ophir, J., Myocardial elastography — a feasibility study *in vivo*. Ultrasound Med Biol 2002; 28: 475–482.
32. Assentoft, J. E., Gregersen, H. and OBrien, Jr., W. D., Propagation speed of sound assessment in the layers of the guinea-pig esophagus by means of acoustic microscopy. Ultrasonics 2001; 39: 263–268.
33. Briggs, G. A. D., Wang, J. and Gundle, R., Quantitative acoustic microscopy of individual living human cells. J Microsc 1993; 172: 3–12.
34. Briggs, G. A. D., A little elementary acoustics. In: Acoustic microscopy. Clarendon Press; Oxford. 1992; 78–101.
35. Tervola, K. M. U., Foster, S. G. and O'Brien, Jr., W. D., Attenuation coefficient measurement technique at 100 MHz with the scanning laser acoustic Microscope IEEE Transactions on Sonics and Ultrasonics 1985; 32: 259–265.
36. Tervola, K. M. U., Gummer, M. A., Erdman, Jr., J. W. and O'Brien, Jr., W. D., Ultrasound attenuation and velocities in rat liver as a function of fat concentration: A study at 100 MHz using a scanning laser acoustic microscope. J Acoust Soc Am 1985; 77: 307–313.
37. Assentoft, J. E., Jørgensen, C. S., Gregersen, H., Christensen, L. L., Djurhuus, J. C. and O'Brien, W. D., Scanning laser acoustic microscopy as a method for characterizing the acoustic properties of the individual layers of biological tissue. Engineering in Medicine and Biology 1996; 15: 42–45.

Published with permission

*Neurogastroenterol. Mot.* (1996) **8**, 277–297

REVIEW ARTICLE

# Biomechanics of the gastrointestinal tract

H. GREGERSEN[1] & G. KASSAB[2]

[1]Centre of Biomechanics and Motility, The Institute of Experimental Clinical Research, Skejby University Hospital, Denmark
[2]Department of Bioengineering, University of California, San Diego, La Jolla, CA, USA

***Abstract*** *As the function of the gastrointestinal tract is to a large degree mechanical, it has become increasingly popular to acquire distensibility data in motility research based on various parameters. Hence it is important to know on which geometrical and mechanical assumptions the various parameters are based. Currently, compliance and tone derived from pressure-volume curves are by far the most often used parameters. However, pressure-volume relations obtained in tubular organs must be carefully interpreted as they provide no direct measure of luminal cross-sectional area and other variables useful in plane stress and strain analysis. Thus, erroneous conclusions concerning tissue distensibility may be deduced. Other parameters, such as wall tension, stress and strain, give more useful information about mechanical behaviour. Distensibility data procure significance in fluid mechanics and in the study of tone, peristaltic reflexes, and mechanoreceptor kinematics. Such data are needed for the determination of the interaction between stimulus, electrical responses in neurons and the mechanical behaviour of the gut. Furthermore, from a clinical perspective, investigation of viscoelastic properties is important because GI diseases are associated with growth and remodelling. For example, prestenotic dilatation, increased collagen synthesis, dysmotility and altered distensibility are common features of obstructive diseases. The purpose of this review is to discuss the physiological and clinical importance of acquiring biomechanical data, distensibility parameters and interpretation of these results and their associated errors. We will also discuss some aspects of the relationship between morphology, growth and biomechanics. Finally, we will outline a number of techniques to study the mechanical properties of the GI tract.*

***Keywords*** *compliance, distensibility, mechanoreceptors, peristaltic reflex, strain, stress, tension, tone, viscoelasticity.*

## INTRODUCTION

The mechanical properties of the gastrointestinal (GI) tract are important for its function as a digestive organ. Hence, in the last decade it has become increasingly popular to acquire distensibility data in motility research by luminal balloon distension or bolus injection. This popularity stems from the many reasons that will be discussed in later sections. It is well known that phasic contractility and its co-ordination play an important role for flow in the GI tract. Unfortunately, we know very little about tone and distensibility and their effects on flow mainly owing to the lack of applicable methods for obtaining and interpreting quantitative data. Furthermore, it is difficult to obtain 'true' measures of viscoelasticity *in vivo* due to the very complex structure of the GI tract. Consequently, data interpretation of biomechanical parameters rely on geometric assumptions. Commonly, parameters such as compliance, pressure elastic modulus and tension-strain relations are used to describe the biomechanical properties *in vivo* and *in vitro*. It is, however, imperative to know the basic principles of biomechanics and its nomenclature (Table 1 is a reference guide to common terms). Knowing the basic principles facilitates the understanding of the parameters and their inherent assumptions. The compliance parameter and tone based on pressure-volume curves are by far the most used in motility research. Pressure-volume relations are, however, often misinterpreted which lead to erroneous conclusions.

Several techniques have been developed to study distensibility and tone in the GI tract. It is, however, outside the scope of this paper to describe and review

*Address for correspondence*
Hans Gregersen, M.D., Centre of Biomechanics and Motility, Institute of Experimental Clinical Research, Skejby University Hospital, DK-8200 Aarhus N, Denmark.
*Received*: 19 January 1996
*Accepted for publication*: 1 May 1996

Published with permission



**Table 1** Reference guide to some common mechanics terms

| Term | Definition |
|---|---|
| Stress | Force per unit surface area that the part lying on the positive side of a surface element (the side on the positive side of the outer normal) exerts on the part lying on the negative side. Stress is a tensor quantity with six independent components ($\tau_{11}$, $\tau_{22}$, $\tau_{33}$, $\tau_{12} = \tau_{21}$, $\tau_{13} = \tau_{31}$, and $\tau_{23} = \tau_{32}$). The components $\tau_{11}$, $\tau_{22}$, and $\tau_{33}$ are called normal stresses, and the remaining components are called shear stresses. A normal stress is perpendicular to the surface while a shear stress is parallel to the surface. |
| Strain | Forces applied to solids cause deformation or strain. Consider a string with initial length $L_0$ and stretched length $L$. It is useful to describe the change in length by dimensionless ratios such as $L/L_0$ or $(L - L_0)/L_0$ as this eliminates the absolute length from consideration. Elongation causes tensile (positive) strain while shortening causes compressive (negative) strain. |
| Elastic modulus | The proportionality constant between stress and strain. Hooke's law applies for a homogenous, isotropic, linearly elastic material implying that a single elastic modulus describes the stiffness. As the mechanical behaviour in biological tissues is non-linear, an incremental approach must be used. |
| Isotropy | Materials whose mechanical properties do not depend on directions are said to be isotropic. Biological tissues are usually anisotropic, mainly owing to their heterogeneous, layered structure. |
| Viscoelasticity | Time dependence of the response to stress or strain. Stress relaxation, creep and hysteresis are features of viscoelasticity. |
| Preconditioning | In mechanical testing of living tissues *in vitro*, the loading and unloading processes are repeated for a number of cycles until the stress–strain relation becomes stabilised and repeatable results are obtained. |
| Constitutive equation | A constitutive equation describes the material properties of a material, e.g. the stress–strain relation. |
| Zero-stress state | The tissue configuration where no stress is present. For a tubular organ, the zero-stress state is obtained by making radial cuts in a ring of tissue so that it springs open into a sector. The difference in strain between the zero-stress state and the no-load state where all external forces are absent is called residual strain. |
| Plastic deformation | Deformation that does not return to its initial state when the stress is removed. |

these methods; instead some guidelines are suggested as to which measures are useful when studying intact segments of the GI tract *in vivo* and *in vitro*. This review outlines a basic overview of biomechanics as it pertains to motility research in the GI tract with minimal use of complicated equations (some theoretical aspects are described in appendices). Furthermore, the physiological and clinical importance of biomechanical data (in particular; distensibility and tone), definitions of some important biomechanical terms as well as some aspects of the relationship between morphology, biomechanics and growth/remodelling will be discussed. The reader is referred to other articles for more detailed information on gastrointestinal flow properties and phasic motility patterns (see critical reviews in ref. 1). Finally, several promising methods are proposed for the study of GI anatomy and mechanical properties.

## THE CONCEPT OF STRESS AND STRAIN

Biomechanics is mechanics applied to biology. Mechanics is the study of motion of matter and the forces that cause such motion. Forces applied to solids cause deformation while forces applied to fluids cause flow. When external forces are applied to a GI segment, it deforms resisting the forces. It is common practice to use distensibility and stiffness to describe the deformation and the resistance to deformation, respectively. However, definition of these parameters for the GI tract can be difficult since no single parameter can describe the complex mechanical behaviour of the GI system. To arrive at useful approximations, it is important to understand the basic relations between stress and strain.

 

Published with permission

Volume 8, Number 4, December 1996 GI mechanics

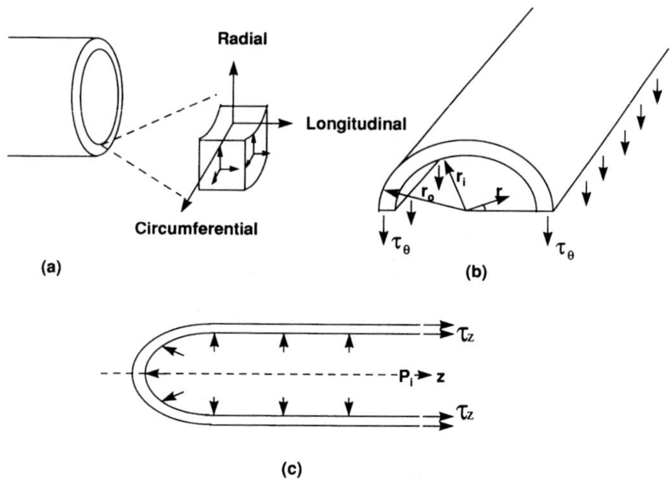


**Figure 1** A pressurized cylindrical tube. (a) An infinitesimal element of the cylindrical tube showing the radial, longitudinal and circumferential directions. (b) A free-body diagram of half of the tube cut parallel to the central axis. (c) A free-body diagram of the tube cut perpendicular to the central axis.

*Stress* is force per unit cross-sectional area. On any surface, the force may be applied perpendicular to the surface, such as the bolus pressure (normal stress) exerted on the wall, or parallel to the surface, such as the force exerted by the fluid flow (shear stress) on the wall. Normal stresses may be either compressive or tensile. A force may be applied in any direction and can induce stresses and strains in various directions. At any given point in the body, the state of stress is described by a stress tensor that consists of three normal stresses and six shear stresses, three of which are independent. In a cylindrical tube, we may refer to radial, circumferential and longitudinal components of stress in the respective directions. These are the normal components of stress in the wall of the cylinder (Fig. 1). There are also three additional shear components. In tubular organs the major tensile stress induced by distension is in the circumferential direction[2] and hence we shall focus mainly on the circumferential stress and strain. During luminal pressure loading, the equilibrium condition requires that the force in the intestinal wall in the circumferential direction to be balanced by the force in the intestinal lumen contributed by the inflation pressure. Under the assumption that the geometry is cylindrical, it can be shown that the average circumferential wall stress is

$$\tau_\theta = \frac{Pr}{h} \tag{1}$$

where $P$, $r$ and $h$ are the pressure, internal radius and wall thickness, respectively. This formula is commonly known as Laplace's law and its derivation appears in Appendix A. This law explains why rupture occurs when segments are excessively distended. Another important implication of the law is that the wall stress is related to pressure and radius-to-wall thickness ratio. Hence, the conventional comparison of wall properties such as the distensibility and tone at the same pressure and threshold for mechanoreceptor response regardless of the radius-to-wall thickness ratio is often misleading.[3–7] It should also be noted that the stress in eqn (1) is averaged over the thickness of the segment and does not describe any possible regional distribution of stress across the wall thickness. Furthermore, residual strain (prestress) is often found in biological tissues as shown by a vessel segment opening into a sector when cut radially.[8] A cylinder that is not prestressed will bear the highest tensile stress at the inner edge which will further increase during loading as the radius-wall thickness ratio increases. However, the residual strain in biological tissues may serve as a mechanism of reducing the stress gradient from the inner to the outer wall under homeostatic conditions (Gregersen *et al.* unpublished results). Thus, residual strain may prevent damage to the mucosa in the GI tract during large bolus transport.

*Strain* refers to deformation of a material and is usually expressed as a fraction of the initial length (Lagrangian strain). It may also be defined in terms of stretch ratio (length divided by initial length) which is useful if the material is incompressible since the product of the stretch ratios in the three principal directions is equal to 1. Hence knowing the stretch ratios in two directions allows us to compute the third stretch ratio. The relation between Lagrangian strain ($\varepsilon$)

Published with permission



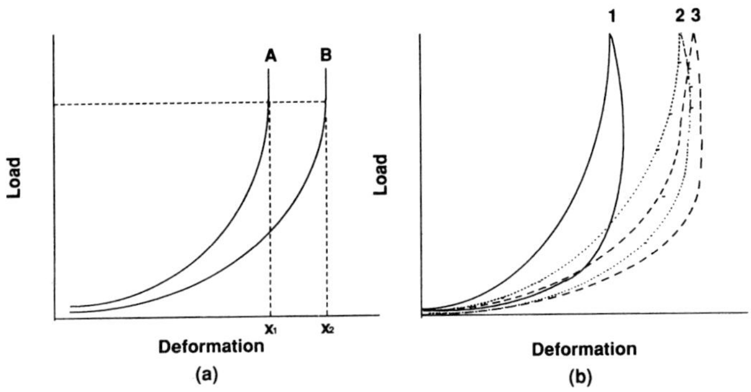


**Figure 2** Graphs showing (a) the load–deformation plot typical of pressure–volume, pressure–cross-sectional area, tension–strain, or stress–strain relations. Curve A is shifted to the left when compared to curve B which implies, in case of a stress–strain relation, that curve A represents a stiffer material. Hysteresis and preconditioning are demonstrated in graph (b). Curves 1, 2, and 3 refer to the first, second, and third loading cycle, respectively.

and stretch ratio ($\lambda$) is $\varepsilon = \lambda - 1$. In contrast to stress, strain is dimensionless and the gradient in circumferential strain is more uniform across the wall in tubular organs. The dimensionless property of strain facilitates comparison of various experiments. However, the strain is dependent on the determination of the correct initial length as will be discussed later. This is a difficult task because in some tissues, e.g. taenia coli smooth muscle preparations, the resting length is not unique since it depends on the method of suppression of smooth muscle contractile activity.[9]

A tensile stress imposed on a material leads to elongation (positive strain) while a compressive stress leads to shortening (negative strains). Like stress, strain is a tensor with corresponding components. For example, in the wall of a cylinder, we describe radial, circumferential and longitudinal strains in the respective directions as well as six additional shear strains, three of which are independent. *In vitro*, strains are often computed from measurements of changes in distance between markers located on the surface or embedded in the tissue. In intact organs, the change in radius or circumference can be used as a measure of strain as will be discussed later. In *in vitro* experiments, the segments are often free to lengthen, but *in vivo* the organs may be tethered to the surroundings. An important observation is that the oesophagus is always under considerable longitudinal stress *in vivo*. When removed from the body, it shortens by up to 50% (unpublished observations in guinea-pigs) with a corresponding increase in the diameter. This large residual longitudinal strain may have important physiological implications during bolus transport in the oesophagus.

The proportionality constant between stress and strain is called the *elastic modulus* and for a linear, Hookean material it is called Young's modulus. For such a material the mechanical properties are elastic and the constitutive equation can be simplified to Hooke's law (see Appendix B). However, in biological tissues the relation between stress and strain is non-linear and the strain is usually large (finite deformation). Figure 2(a) illustrates a typical stress–strain curve. The non-linear (usually exponential-like) mechanical behaviour facilitates stretch in the physiological pressure range and prevents overstretch and damage to the tissue at higher stress levels. Overstretch can induce a plastic deformation whereby the tissue can no longer return to its original state when unstressed. Owing to the non-linearity of the material it is necessary to compute an incremental elastic modulus. The gastrointestinal wall is similar to other biological tissues in that it has complex three-dimensional structures that have different material properties in different directions. This important feature is called anisotropy and it implies that a large set of material constants have to be specified in order to completely describe the mechanical behaviour. The so-called constitutive equation relates stress and strain through a set of material constants. Appendix B illustrates the constitutive equation for an isotropic, Hookean, elastic solid. Recently, Jørgensen *et al.*[10] made a promising development by combining impedance planimetry with high-frequency endoluminal ultrasonography. Hereby, it is possible to correct for variation in wall thickness to obtain a measure of stress–strain distributions *in vivo*.

## VISCOELASTICITY

Biological tissues reveal properties of both elastic solid and viscous fluid. Thus, the stress depends not only on the applied strain as in a solid, but also on the rate of strain as in a viscous fluid. In other words, the response is time-dependent in that the stress–strain response does not occur instantly. When the material is suddenly strained and the strain is maintained constant, the corresponding stresses induced in the wall decrease with time. This phenomenon is called stress relaxation. If the material is suddenly stressed and the stress is

Published with permission

Volume 8, Number 4, December 1996 

maintained constant, the material will continue to deform. This phenomenon is called creep. If the material is subjected to a cyclic loading, the stress–strain relationship in the loading process is somewhat different from that in the unloading process (Fig. 2b) and the phenomenon is called hysteresis.[2,9,11] Stress relaxation, creep, and hysteresis are features of viscoelasticity. Viscoelastic properties in terms of pressure relaxation curves have been described for the normal and diseased human rectum.[12,13] Often, the viscoelastic behaviour is described in terms of models, e.g. the Maxwell model describes the mechanical behaviour using a spring and a dashpot in series.[9]

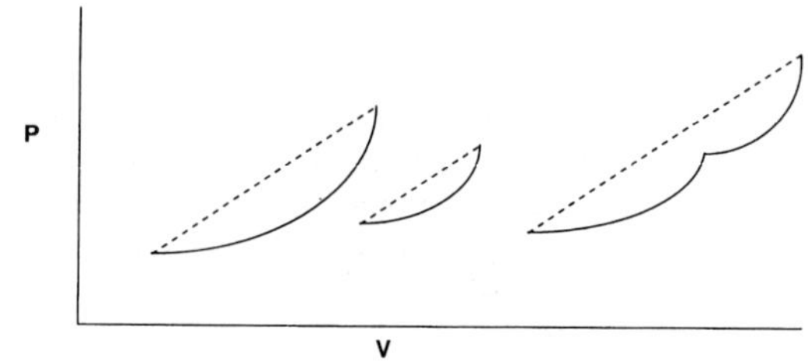


**Figure 3** Example of pressure–volume curves. Curves A, B and C have the same compliance according to the definition ($C$=d$V$/d$P$) even though they behave differently. The linear approach as illustrated in this figure does not consider the non-linear variation of the curves.

## DEFINITION AND MEASUREMENT OF STIFFNESS AND DISTENSIBILITY

It is clear that such complexities of the gastrointestinal wall as anisotropy, non-linear behaviour, finite deformation, and viscoelasticity make simple estimates of stiffness unsound. In fact, even techniques with far better resolution than those currently available would not permit complete characterization of the three-dimensional mechanical behaviour of the gastrointestinal tract *in vivo*. However, some general expression of the overall stiffness is useful. Several commonly used elasticity parameters are defined and discussed below.

### Compliance

Compliance is defined as the change in luminal dimension (volume or cross-sectional area) divided by the corresponding change in pressure

$$C = \frac{\Delta V}{\Delta P}, \quad \text{or} \quad C = \frac{\Delta CSA}{\Delta P} \tag{2}$$

where $V$, $CSA$ and $P$ are volume, cross-sectional area and pressure, respectively. In this respect, compliance is the reciprocal of stiffness. Usually, it is given either as a single averaged value or as a function of pressure. The compliance parameter merely expresses the differences in luminal dimensions between pressure steps. Hence, the parameter does not take into account the actual degree of stretch that occurs under luminal pressure loading, the variations in the unstressed basal luminal diameter, or the wall thickness. Consequently, compliance should in general, be avoided. Figure 3 shows examples of compliance derived from pressure-volume curves.

### Pressure elastic modulus and cross-sectional area distensibility

The pressure elastic modulus is a measure of stiffness and is defined as follows

$$E_p = \frac{\Delta P}{\left(\frac{\Delta r}{r}\right)} \tag{3}$$

where $\Delta P$ and $\Delta r$ denote changes in internal pressure and radius. This parameter can be used to compare segments with different pressures. It is more advantageous than compliance because it considers the degree of stretch but still does not account for the wall thickness. Although this variable has units of *pressure* similar to an elastic modulus, it is different from the elastic modulus of the wall because the pressure in the lumen is not the same as the tensile stress in the wall. It is often advantageous to express the distensibility rather than stiffness in terms of cross-sectional area and transmural pressure. Thus, the distensibility is defined as the ratio of fractional change of cross-sectional area (CSA) to the change in transmural pressure ($P_{tm}$)

$$D = \left(\frac{1}{CSA_0}\frac{\Delta CSA}{\Delta P_{tm}}\right) \tag{4}$$

where $CSA_0$ is the reference cross-sectional area. This parameter can be directly computed from a $P$–$CSA$ curve. Despite this, it is useful to convert such a measurement into an incremental Young's modulus for circumferential extensions of the whole intestinal wall, modelled as a uniform cylinder with homogenous, isotropic walls. The use of an incremental Young's modulus is made necessary by the non-linearity of the relation between circumferential stress and cross-sec-

 

Published with permission



tional area. Hence, a single elastic parameter can be defined by considering small departures from a mean, prestressed, *in vivo* state, and linearizing the stress–strain curves. This may be useful if the amplitude of the pressure is small. For an increase in pressure within a thin-walled isotropic intestinal segment whose length is held constant, Young's modulus is related to the distensibility $D$ by

$$D^{-1} = \frac{E}{1-\alpha^2}\frac{h}{d} \tag{5}$$

where $h$ is the wall thickness, $d$ is intestinal diameter and $\alpha$ is Poisson's ratio (equal to 0.5 if the material is incompressible, see Appendix B). This result follows from the classical elasticity of shells and is referenced by Bergel[14] in a more general form for thick-walled tubes.

## Circumferential wall tension: the law of Laplace

Laplace's law refers to the relationship between the pressure difference, the wall tension and the curvature of membrane surface. Consider a thin-walled membrane surface and assume that the wall tension is constant everywhere, then the law of Laplace reads

$$T = \Delta P\left[\frac{1}{r_1} + \frac{1}{r_2}\right]^{-1} \tag{6}$$

where $r_1$ and $r_2$ are the principal radii of curvature of the surface, $T$ is the total tension per unit length of the midsurface of the membrane, and $\Delta P$ is the transmural pressure difference. $\Delta P$ is often assumed equal to the pressure inside the membrane owing to the assumption that the external pressure is zero. The equation reduces to $T = \Delta P\, r$ in the case of a cylinder as one of the radii tends to infinity, and to $T = \Delta P(r/2)$ for a sphere as the two radii become equal. Laplace's law is often used for balloon distension studies in tubular organs when the balloon is long compared to its radius. More general equations have to be considered if the luminal cross-sectional area is elliptical rather than circular.

Equation 6 is valid as long as the membrane is so thin that bending rigidity can be neglected. Furthermore, there are several underlying assumptions. Firstly, a cylindrical lumen must be assumed. Pressurising the balloon achieves a cylindrical configuration during distension as has been confirmed in human studies by means of radiography.[15] Secondly, the material property is assumed to be isotropic. Although the isotropy assumption is not valid for many biological tissues, the parameter is still useful.[16,17] Finally, the analysis requires a static equilibrium of forces and consequently zero inertial forces. The tension given by eqn 6 is equal to the product of the average circumferential stress (given in Appendix A) and wall thickness.

## Circumferential strain

Lagrangian strain or stretch ratio in the form of

$$\varepsilon = \frac{r - r_0}{r_0}, \quad \text{and} \quad \lambda = \frac{r}{r_0} \tag{7}$$

can be computed, where $r$ is the midwall radius determined at various inflation pressures and $r_0$ is the midwall radius at zero pressure. As it is difficult to determine the wall thickness *in vivo*, strain is computed at the inner wall using the luminal radius. For comparison of strains (and tension–strain relations) between different segments or before and after intervention, it is best to determine $r_0$ at the same level of tension rather than at the same pressure level in accordance with Laplace's law. Thus, a plot of tension *vs* radius for each set of data can be extrapolated to give the lowest tension value. At this specific tension, it is easy to determine $r_0$ graphically for the different specimens. For ease of measurements, $r$ and $r_0$ can be replaced by $c$ and $c_0$ which are the corresponding circumferences. Ideally, $c_0$ should be the midwall circumference at the zero-stress state. The strain measure is very useful in biomechanics as it expresses a dimensionless fractional change in dimensions and is related to stress.

The slope of the tension–strain and stress–strain relation is a better measure of tissue distensibility than compliance.[16,17] Several methods are used to analyse stiffness from tension-strain and stress–strain curves.[9] Using an exponential approach, the data can be curve-fitted to the function

$$T = \alpha e^{\beta \cdot \lambda} \tag{8}$$

using a least-square fit method. In this context $\alpha$ represents the $y$-intercept and $\beta$ is the slope of the curve. As the slope is a measure of wall stiffness, the derivative of tension with respect to stretch ratio yields the stiffness function

$$\frac{dT}{d\lambda} = \beta T. \tag{9}$$

As the behaviour is non-linear, incremental elastic moduli must be computed. In order to compare these

Published with permission



moduli, they must be measured under conditions of constant length and expressed as function of strain. Bergel[14] and Dobrin[18] provide examples of the error introduced in expressing the modulus as a function of pressure and different length settings in the cardiovascular system.

## WHAT DETERMINES THE SHAPE OF THE DISTENSIBILITY CURVES?

Smooth muscle cells contribute to the distensibility passively through the synthesis of extracellular collagen and actively through contraction. We shall primarily consider the passive state that can be studied *in vitro*[17] and to some extend *in vivo* when appropriate smooth muscle relaxants are administered.[16]

It is well known that the passive elastic behaviour of biological tissues is non-linear.[9,16,17,19] This mechanical feature protects the tissue against overdistension and damage at high luminal pressure loads while distending easily and facilitating flow in the physiological pressure range. In arteries, it has been demonstrated that collagen bears circumferential loads at high stress levels.[2,20] As gastrointestinal tissue is rich in collagen,[21] it is likely that collagen is a major determinant of the curve shapes. There is very little data, however, concerning the relation between elastic properties and morphology in the GI tract. Previously, Fackler *et al.*[23] and Orberg *et al.*[24] showed the biaxial orientation of collagen fibres in submucosa and demonstrated how the fibres uncrimp to low levels of stress rather than being directly stretched. Recently, our studies have shown a correlation between the total collagen content and the biomechanical properties in obstruction models[22] (and unpublished data).

Parameters such as wall tension, stress, and strain at equilibrium are likely to depend mainly on the elastic properties of tissue or the pseudo-elastic properties[9] as the stress–strain curve shows a high degree of non-linearity. The parameters are likely to reflect properties of the parallel elastic component according to the Hill-Maxwell model. The parallel elastic component seems to be anatomically located in the connective tissue as the contractile element of smooth muscle by itself does not contribute significantly to the passive tension.[25,26] Using this model the parallel elastic component determines the shape of the curve.

The distensibility *in vivo* depends not only on the passive properties but also on the physiological state of the muscle. Smooth muscle cells are orientated both circumferentially and longitudinally and their contractile state may change the geometry of the lumen and the wall stiffness considerably. For example, it is well known that longitudinal contraction increases the diameter of the intestine[27] which may affect its distensibility. Furthermore, the circular layer of the GI tract contracts at the site of distension.[28,29] Such contractions seem to be nerve-mediated via cholinergic pathways rather than being a direct smooth muscle response to distension.[30,31] These contractions arise proximal to the distension site and propagate anally. As discussed earlier, this implies that the measured distensibility depends not only on the degree of phasic contractility but also on the dynamic properties of the instruments used for the measurements. Although it is more difficult to study the passive *properties in vivo* due to contractility and difficulties in quantitating the transmural pressure, phasic contractions can, to a variable degree, be eliminated by administration of drugs such as Buscopan. Lowering the contractile activity to a level within the frequency range of the measuring equipment facilitates differentiation between passive and active properties. The passive tension can be evaluated in between the contractions where inertial forces are negligible under the assumptions of Laplace's law. However, active properties in the form of specific tone may still be present. This may cause a shift at the lower end of the tension–strain curves which may be difficult to differentiate from the pure passive properties. Animal studies are needed to evaluate the possible contribution of tone and to validate the baseline pressure determination and to elucidate the contribution of tethering to the transmural pressure in the organ wall during distension.

## THE IMPORTANCE OF DISTENSIBILITY DATA

Mechanical properties are important for cardiovascular[2,32] and urogenital function.[19,33] These organs are similar to the GI tract in that they are subjected to changes in wall stresses and strains. In the GI tract, distensibility data are important for an understanding of passive viscoelastic properties, peristaltic reflexes, perception, mechanoreceptor responses, tone, bolus transport mechanics, growth, and remodelling in experimental and clinical studies. These fields of investigation are in many ways related.

### Mechanoreceptors, peristaltic reflex activity and sensory function testing

Distension of the gastrointestinal tract elicits reflex-mediated inhibition and stimulation of motility via intrinsic or extrinsic neural circuits. Many studies have focused on the stimulus-response function and

Published with permission



the mechanisms involved in distension; for instance, in the oesophagus, the effect of distension has been studied in animal models, and in humans with normal oesophagus and with oesophageal chest pain.[3,4,6,7,34–36] Much of the basic work in the GI tract was done in the late 1950s.[37–40] The sensing elements are afferent neurons with the mechanoreceptors located in the GI wall. For example, those receptors involved in the peristaltic reflex pathway are located in the muscularis externa, the myenteric plexus and mucosa.[37,41–43] The variability in location may be important for the sensitivity to different mechanical stimuli. The mechanoreceptors have also been classified on the basis of their pressure or volume thresholds to balloon distension which in turn relates to whether the afferents project to the vagal nerve or to the spinal cord.[4] Furthermore, multimodal receptors reacting both to chemical and mechanical stimuli exist in the mucosa. Grundy[44] has recently reviewed the mechanoreceptors in the GI tract. Some of the work done in the upper human small intestine is referenced by Edelbroek *et al.*[45]

It is a common mistake to believe that mechanoreceptors are sensitive to variations, in pressure or volume. A large variation in the pressure and volume thresholds needed to trigger the peristaltic reflex and perception have been found in various studies and species[30,31,35,46–48] suggesting that pressure is not the direct stimulus. Instead, the receptors are stimulated by forces and deformations acting in the intestinal wall due to changes in transmural pressure.[49] The same mechanism accounts for the baroreceptors in the cardiovascular system. Despite the name (baro = pressure), the baroreceptor nerve activity is associated with wall deformation, because restricting wall distension abolishes baroreceptor-mediated reflexes.[50] In a similar fashion, it was demonstrated that stretch is a potent stimulus for gastrointestinal mechanoreceptors rather than increased transmural pressure.[49,51] The fact that the receptors are also stimulated by visceral tension and deformation developed actively during contractions in the small intestine[37] further suggests that they are sensitive to deformation. However, it is important to recognize that different mechanoreceptors respond to different kinds of mechanical stimuli, e.g. mucosal receptors respond to distortion and pinching but are relatively insensitive to contraction and distension.[52]

As pressure is not the direct stimulus, a large variation arises when expressing the receptor response as a function of pressure making it difficult to draw conclusions. Gregersen *et al.*[31] studied the ascending peristaltic reflex response as function of circumferential wall tension in the isolated perfused porcine duodenum (Fig. 4). Although this approach was important in that it quantified the stimulus in terms of wall tension rather than pressure or volume, more detailed analysis is needed in future studies. Despite the vast number of studies in this area, the essential stimulus has not yet been defined. Further analysis must consider the fact that mechanical forces imposed on the tissue induce stresses and strains in various directions. Thus, distension will, in addition to circumferential tensile stress and strain, cause longitudinal tensile stress and strain and radial compressive stress and strain. For the study of mechanoreceptor kinematics, it is therefore important to express the stimulus in terms of magnitude and direction of stress, strain, and strain rate. Unfortunately, it is impossible to measure stresses and strains exactly at the receptor sites. Theoretical solutions based on experimentally determined mechanical properties in different layers of the GI wall may therefore be necessary. A numerical solution to the peristaltic reflex of the small bowel is provided by Miftakhov and Wingate.[53] By determining the nature of these mechanical stimuli we may learn more about the mechanoreceptors and how they adapt to the physical environment. This will allow us to establish the relation between the activity in the neurons, electrical responses in neurons, and the mechanical behaviour of the gut. On the other hand, if the appropriate mechanical stimulus is not known, the data are merely qualitative. Models that preserve the structural integrity of the tissue to the *in vivo* condition are most useful in this respect.

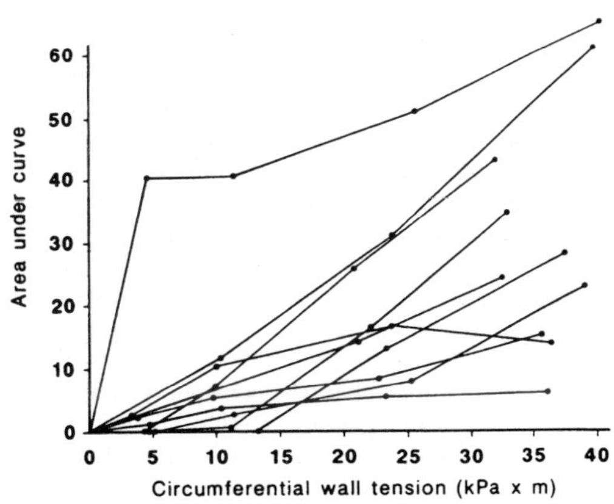


**Figure 4** Relation between area under the pressure curve of the peristaltic reflex response and the wall tension from isolated perfused porcine duodenum. Adapted with permission from *J Gastrointest Mot* 1992; **4**:125–35.

Published with permission



## Tone

Tone is not yet defined clearly in gastroenterology because it is difficult to measure and because phasic activity often interferes with the measurements. This review considers specific tone (sustained muscle contraction) with the terminology adapted from Mandrek and Golenhofen[54,55] rather than tetanic tone caused by fused phasic contractions. For many years it was believed that only the smooth muscles in sphincter regions are capable of developing tonic contractions. During the last decades several reports have indicated that smooth muscle cells outside sphincters are capable of developing tonic contractions, e.g. the small intestine became dilated during administration of smooth muscle relaxants such as glucagon.[56–58] Furthermore, animal studies using serosal strain gauges (force transducers) and videofluoroscopy have indicated that tonic contractions of the smooth muscle cells in the small intestine may occur during the fasted state.[59,60] Indications of specific tone during phase I of the migrating motility complex have been proposed from impedance planimetric studies in the human duodenum.[46,61] Long-lasting tonic contractions occur in the colon and may be important for its function.[62] Data suggestive of tone have been obtained by use of the barostat in different species in the oesophagus,[63] gastric fundus,[64–68] duodenum and jejunum,[46,61,69,70] colon,[71,72] and in the rectum.[73] Tonic contractions often do not occlude the lumen but merely change the cross-sectional area of the lumen which in turn changes the flow properties or the storage capacity of the organ. Hence, tonic contractions cannot be measured by means of conventional manometry.

It is a common misconception to define tone of the oesophagus and the intestines as the slope of the volume-pressure relation or as the change in volume at a constant pressure.[63,66,69,72,74,75] Tone refers to a sustained reduction in luminal cross-sectional area and circumference due to activation of the smooth muscle cells in accordance with urological and cardiovascular studies.[76] Analogously, tone in globular organs refers to a sustained reduction in surface area. Since surface area cannot be measured directly *in vivo*, methods such as the barostat have been developed to measure volume. However, the notion that 'the barostat system, which maintains a constant gastric wall tension by applying a constant pressure, records gastric tone by measuring changes in tissue length (variations in volume)' [65] is fundamentally wrong from a biomechanical point of view. This stems from the fact that the stomach is not spherical and the tension induced in the stomach wall is not uniformly distributed when applying a constant pressure. Furthermore, propagating phasic contractions recorded in distal parts of the stomach will influence the measurement of volume if part of the balloon is located in that area (for further details see Table 2 and the section Balloon Techniques: Consideration of Geometrical Factors). Finally, balloons with lengths of up to 15 cm have been used in studying tone in the intestines[69,70,73] whereby recordings are obtained from a large area making it difficult to differentiate between phasic activity and specific tone.

## Bolus transport mechanics

Many factors influence flow and bolus transport in distensible organs such as the GI tract. The driving force is the pressure generated by the contractile peristaltic forces and to a lesser extend the hydrostatic force of gravity. Brasseur and co-workers[77] have demonstrated that bolus volume, viscosity and abdominal compression influence bolus pressure in the oesophagus. Biomechanical models predict that factors such as the shape and size of the luminal cross-section, tissue viscoelastic properties such as the elastic modulus and shear modulus of the wall are also important determinants of flow. Recent studies in pigs and guinea-pigs have revealed that differences in luminal cross-sectional area and passive elastic properties exist between proximal and distal regions of the oesophagus and small intestine.[16,17,78] These findings are associated with the existence of differences in flow properties and motility between these regions.[1,5] The gastrointestinal tract is stretched in the vicinity of a bolus,[79] i.e. the contents propelled in front of a peristaltic contraction bulge out the intestinal wall.[79,80] This supports the hypothesis that the intestinal reflexes initiated by localized stretch are of physiological significance for flow. Brasseur[81] have demonstrated that the bolus pressure in the human oesophagus can range up to 3–5 kPa. Hence, the bolus pressure corresponds to the most elastic part of the distensibility curves and serves to reduce resistance to flow while the wall is much stiffer at higher pressure, which may prevent overstretching.

Distensibility studies may help us understand the complex fluid mechanical behaviour of the GI tract. Thus far, oesophageal flow properties have been studied in detail by Brasseur and coworkers[77,81,82] while gastric emptying, antroduodenal mechanics, and intestinal flow properties were described primarily by Christensen's group,[27,83,84] Ehrlein's group,[59,79] Meyer and co-workers,[85] Schulze-Delrieu and co-workers,[5,86,87–89] as well as by other investigators.[90,91] A promising method based on impedance measurements for evaluation of

 

Published with permission



**Table 2** Differences between the barostat and impedance planimetry

| | Barostat | Impedance planimetry |
|---|---|---|
| Variable measured | Volume | Cross-sectional area |
| Organs | Oesophagus, stomach, gall bladder, small intestines, large intestines | Oesophagus, small intestine, rectum, urogenital tract, cardiovascular system |
| Dynamic properties | Relatively fast | Relatively slow |
| Does the method provide a measure of the geometry? | No | No |
| Does longitudinal balloon distension affect the measured variable directly? | Yes | No |
| Is the boundary of the geometrically measured parameter in contact with the measurand? | No | Yes |
| Do phasic contractions affect results? | Yes | Only if contractions are very frequent in the mid-balloon area |
| Under assumption of known geometry, does the method provide a measure of specific tone? | Only if phasic contractions are not present along the entire balloon length | Yes |

bolus shape in the oesophagus was introduced in gastroenterology by Fisher *et al.*[92] and was later refined by Silny and co-workers.[93] A detailed review of the GI flow properties is given by Weems.[94] Mathematical modelling of peristaltic transport in distensible tubes have also been attempted.[95–98] The mathematical modelling of peristaltic transport is based on the premise that the interaction between GI elasticity and bolus transport is best understood by examining the fluid dynamics equations (equations describing bolus transport) and equations describing GI deformation (the constitutive equations). The interaction between these equations is governed by the boundary conditions.

## Mechanical forces, growth, remodelling, and morphology

Mechanical forces are a major determinant of tissue behaviour and are likely the single most important factor influencing growth and remodelling of tissue. An understanding of this relationship is important in deciphering how the gastrointestinal tract responds and adapts to changes in the physical environment. The passive elastic properties of the intact organ must be studied since these properties reflect the state of the structural components determining a specific function or malfunction, e.g. the wall tension is modulated by changes in the wall structure due to obstructive diseases.[22,99,100] Therefore, it is desirable to study the biomechanical and morphological properties of the tissue concurrently. The literature is relatively sparse in this regard. Gabella[21,101] has reviewed the structural apparatus for force transmission in smooth muscles, and Orberg *et al.*[24] described the biaxial orientation of the collagen fibrils and the pattern of uncrimping in response to stress. Gregersen *et al.*[22] found, in a partially obstructed model of the opossum oesophagus, a linear relation between the amount of collagen and the wall tension. It is likely that collagen synthesis was stimulated because of dilation and increased wall tension proximal to the site of obstruction in the oesophagus. Collagen may also be a major determinant of the biomechanical properties of the small intestine since large amounts are found in its wall[21]. Recently, our group found an increase in collagen content and wall thickening and a correlation between the elastic modulus and the collagen content proximal to the site of partial obstruction in the small intestine at stress levels of 10 kPa and 70 kPa (Storkholm *et al.*, unpublished data). Furthermore, the growth effect of epidermal growth factor on the biomechanical properties of the rat small intestine *in vitro* was studied recently.[102] Further studies are needed to clarify the relation between the biomechanical properties of the gut and its morphology. Such studies should also utilize molecular techniques. The advent of molecular techniques provide an opportunity to study the effect of mechanical stimuli on the gene expression of various structural proteins such as collagens, fibronectin and stress proteins on the transcriptional level. This approach is now widely used in cardiovascular research and will undoubtedly provide us with important new insights into the mechanisms of structural remodelling of tissue in health and disease.

## Clinical perspectives

The clinical aspects of gastrointestinal biomechanics are mainly related to bolus transport and remodelling. As distensibility is important for the physiologic function of the gut, it also plays an important role in diseases that affect wall structure and motility. There are several diseases that cause tissue remodelling that are closely related to changes in the mechanical properties. In obstructive diseases, proximal dilatation and wall thickening is a common phenomenon.[22,78,103] This is perhaps caused by the repeated stretch during passage of foods due to the increased resistance to flow and the repetitive high-pressure contractions proximal to the site of obstruction.[100] Increased wall stress due to progressive dilatation and strain are likely responsible for the development of collagenous infiltration[22,104]. Hirschsprung's disease, ulcerative colitis, diabetes, systemic sclerosis and sclerotherapy-induced damage are some examples of diseases and treatments associated with remodelled morphology and biomechanical properties.[12,15,105–107] Balloon distension tests are also relevant in studying dysmotility, non-cardiac chest pain, and perception.[3,34–36] Distensibility studies therefore have potentially diagnostic and prognostic value. High-frequency ultrasound systems for imaging the wall and its layers may also be useful in clinical studies.[108,109]

## BALLOON TECHNIQUES: CONSIDERATION OF GEOMETRICAL FACTORS

As the distensibility data available are based mainly on balloon distension methods, we will consider this method in greater detail. The most important aspects relate to the experimental design, the probe design, the method of measurement, the geometry and mechanical properties of the balloons, and the assumptions for the analysis, e.g. the analysis depends on the mode of filling (continuous or stepwise). In general, the boundary of a geometrically measurable parameter must be in complete contact with the measurand, i.e. when measuring the cross-sectional area of a tube or the volume of any organ, the whole circumference and surface area of the balloon must be in contact with the tissue. This is never completely attained in volume measurements in the intestines and the stomach (see Figs 1 and 2 in reference no. 65). It is important to ensure that the applied pressure is properly transmitted to the tissue, i.e. that the balloon is sufficiently large so that it does not contribute its own elastic properties to the results. Thus, the pressure drop must be confined to the wall itself (as long as the surrounding structures do not contribute, e.g. by tethering). Hysteresis of the balloon and infusion system and friction between the tissue and balloon wall are usually negligible. To avoid difficulties in interpretation of results in studies of the intestines and oesophagus, the balloon length should be short in order to provide a localized distension to imitate the size and shape of a bolus. Some studies use long balloons.[69,70,73] This has little physiological significance and data on tone and distensibility may be difficult to interpret since reflex stimulation and inhibition of phasic activity are likely to occur simultaneously at the proximal and distal end of the balloon. Consequently, volume measurements in a long balloon may show no change even though the shape changes are considerable and visa versa. Results will consequently depend on the phasic contractile properties of the segment under study. Therefore, the previous definition of specific tone does not apply for studies using the barostat since this technique provides a three-dimensional measure of tone that is difficult to differentiate from phasic contractility (tetanic tone is a summation of phasic contractions). The dynamical characteristics of the measurement system also make it difficult to compare results from different studies, e.g. short balloons encounter only a few contractions while long balloons sum up phasic contractions in a tetanic tone pattern. Consequently, the luminal cross-sectional area should be measured rather than volume and in any case, the balloon should be short. This is further exasperated by the fact that the balloon will tend to elongate rather than distend the organ wall due to resistance to deformation in the radial direction. The degree of elongation is obviously dependent on the balloon material but will inevitably occur with any balloon (Fig. 5). This has two very important implications. Firstly, parameters such as wall tension and compliance are over-estimated.[110] Furthermore, the large variation in rectal size between subjects gives rise to the large variation in pressure–volume relations and compliance found in the rectum.[110] Secondly, even a small error in volume in the low pressure range, as shown in Fig. 5, will affect the results of any tension-strain analysis as $r_0$ is determined in this range. Fortunately, impedance planimetric and endosonographic methods for measurement of luminal cross-sectional area exist.[31,111,112] Cross-sectional area as a

 

Published with permission



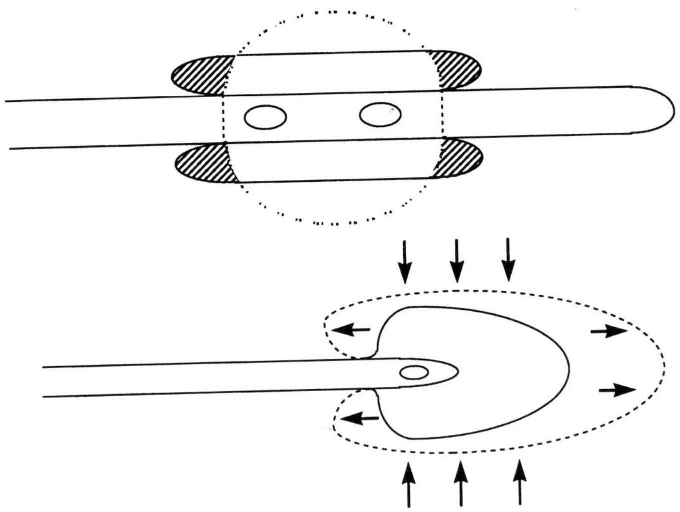

**Figure 5** A schematic illustration of two commonly used balloon types. Top: A rigid balloon showing elongation at low pressures (solid balloon line). The ends bulge out owing to the radial resistance to stretch. At high pressures, the balloon may conform to a spherical shape (dashed balloon line). The hatched area shows the volume in the elongated part of the balloon at low pressures. This type of balloon is often used in oesophageal and small intestinal studies. Bottom: A compliant end-mounted balloon at low pressures (solid balloon line) and at higher pressures (dashed balloon line), where the radial resistance to stretch causes the balloon to stretch in the longitudinal direction. This type of balloon is often used in rectal studies. In both cases, the volume measurements will cause large errors in the computation of compliance and other biomechanical parameters.

function of pressure provides important information on luminal dimensions during loading but gives little information about material properties without further mechanical analysis.

Biomechanical analysis is dependent on geometrical factors. Most of the equations used in biomechanics are derived under certain geometrical assumptions. As an example, the Laplace equation in Appendix A is valid for a circular tube. Appendix C and Fig. 6 demonstrate the magnitude of the error induced when an elliptical geometry is considered to be circular. In more complex geometries, the expressions for possible errors can be even more complex. Obviously this has important consequences for interpretation of data on tone and distensibility, but yet none of the studies published consider the proper geometry, i.e. tubular sections of the gastrointestinal tract are assumed circular and the stomach is assumed spherical. The current knowledge therefore is based on qualitative data and more sophisticated analysis is greatly needed.

## HOW DO MECHANICAL DATA OBTAINED *IN SITU* COMPARE WITH DATA OBTAINED BY CONVENTIONAL STRIP METHODS *IN VITRO*?

Mechanical data obtained from intact segments are not directly comparable to data obtained using isolated smooth muscle strips. This is due to the many differ-

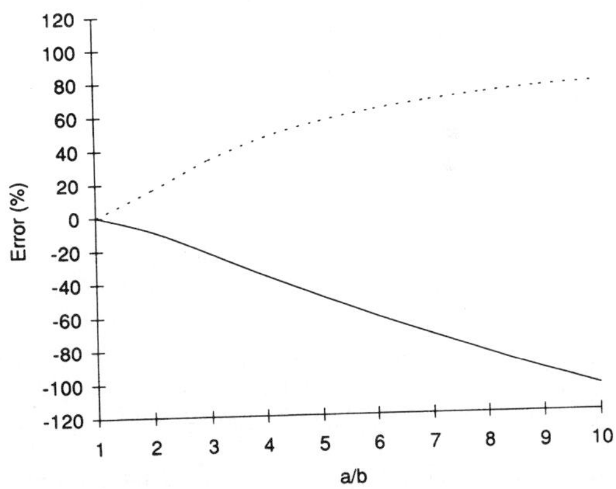


**Figure 6** The graph shows the resulting error when an elliptical cross-section is assumed to be circular as a function of the major-to-minor axis ratio ($a/b$). The dashed line shows the error in the CSA for a constant circumference while the solid line shows the error in the circumference at constant CSA. The curves are based on the equations given in Appendix C. When the $a/b$ ratio increases, the cross-section becomes more elliptical. This plot shows that without any change in circumference (tone), changes in geometry can cause the CSA or volume to vary considerably. The $a/b$ ratio is high in the intestines at low pressures because they are collapsed in the resting state. Thus, unless geometry is taken into account, the measurement of circumference (tone) is at best qualitative. Data on the geometry could potentially be measured using imaging techniques.

Published with permission



ences between the two techniques. In strip studies it is common to determine the active and passive length-tension relations, force-velocity relations, and stress relaxation.[113–116] Furthermore, it is possible to study the behaviour under either isotonic or isometric conditions in uni-axial isolated strip experiments. Unfortunately, in the isolated strip studies, the structural integrity of the organ wall is not preserved and the strip is not necessarily in its zero-stress state at resting conditions since large residual strains exist in the GI tract (unpublished data, see Fig. 7). This zero-stress state must be considered in the analysis of stress distribution in the organ and in the determination of the resting length. The isolated strip technique, however, is useful for studying the effect of pharmacological agents on smooth muscle and it may provide useful data on the mechanical properties of individual layers in the wall by studying circular and longitudinal strips. Also, Yamada has provided extensive data on the passive properties of GI tissues *in vitro*.[117] In contrast to strip investigations, it is more difficult to compute stress *in vivo* where the data cannot be obtained under purely isometric or isotonic conditions. On the other hand, the advantage of studying intact organs is that one can measure their biomechanical properties in conditions closer to the *in vivo* condition[9] with proper geometry and boundary conditions.

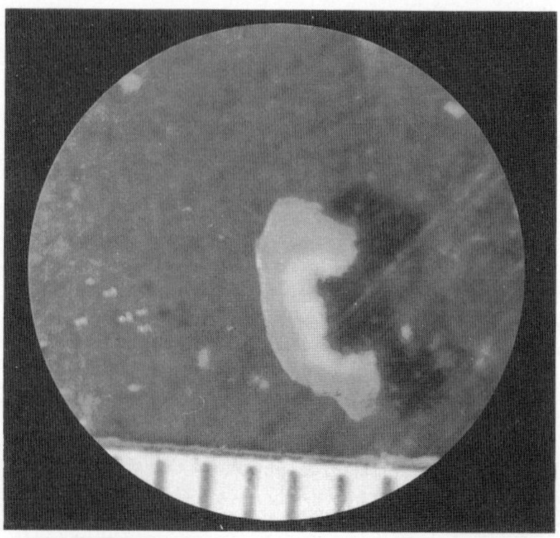

**Figure 7** Photograph showing an oesophageal specimen in its zero-stress state. A radial cut in the tissue ring caused it to spring open into a sector which can be characterized by an opening angle.

In mechanical testing of living tissues *in vitro*, preconditioning is necessary to obtain repeatable results. This means that after the test specimen is prepared and mounted on the testing machine, the loading and unloading processes are repeated for a number of cycles until the stress–strain relationship becomes reproducible. The number of cycles depends on the tissue and the method of preparation. Usually, preconditioning is not done in testing of GI tissue *in vivo*. The basic rationale for preconditioning is that tissues are disturbed in the process of preparation by cutting, changes in stress, strain, temperature, blood flow, chemical environment, ischaemia, hypoxia, contracture of muscle, etc., and need to be restored to a stable condition by preconditioning.[118]

## FUTURE INVESTIGATIONS

A biomechanical analysis of GI physiology requires a complete database on GI geometry and mechanical properties. The database can then be used in conjunction with the basic laws of physics to write down the governing equations and solve the appropriate boundary value problems. Today, a full set of data describing the geometric properties of the entire GI tract does not exist. Recently, Gregersen *et al.* (unpublished data) have reconstructed the geometry of the entire duodenum using an elastomer casting method.[119] Briefly, portions of the GI tract were cannulated and perfused with silicone elastomer at physiologic pressures. The elastomer hardened and render a cast of the internal geometry. Hence, both the external and the internal geometries were measured.

The question of mechanical properties, on the other hand, can be formulated in many different forms, varying in degree of generality and difficulty. We have thus far discussed pressure-volume measurements, balloon distensions and tension-strain relations. The mechanical properties can in part be determined in terms of pressure-diameter experiments, zero-stress state experiments, strain measurements, bending and torsion experiments. Although most of these experiments are *in vitro*, they may contribute significantly to our understanding of the complex behaviour of the GI tract in health and disease.

### Pressure–diameter experiments

The pressure–diameter relation has been extremely popular among cardiovascular physiologists as it plays an important role in the pressure–flow relationship of blood through an organ.[120] This approach can be used to understand the distensibility of the intestine. The compliance of an intestine as expressed by the percentage change in diameter *vs* change in transmural pressure can be shown to be a function of the ratio of the wall thickness to intestinal diameter and of the Young's modulus of the wall material. A simple estimation can be made based on the assumption of a thin-walled tube. According to Laplace's formula, the tensile stress in the wall of a tube of diameter $D$ is given by

$$\tau_\theta = \Delta P_{\text{tm}} \frac{D}{2h} \tag{10}$$

where $h$ is the wall thickness. The strain $\tau_\theta/E$, which is also the change in diameter divided by the diameter (see Appendix B), can be written as

$$\frac{\Delta D}{D_0} = \frac{D}{2hE} \Delta P_{\text{tm}}. \tag{11}$$

Hence, the compliance $D/2hE$ is proportional to the diameter–wall thickness ratio, $D/h$, and inversely proportional to the material constant, $E$.

The reference diameter $D_0$ cannot be taken as the diameter at zero-pressure as the cross-sectional area of the intestine is not circular at that pressure. Upon luminal pressure loading, the intestine becomes circular and hence it is useful to analyse the tendency for the cross-section to become circular as the pressure increases. The complex differential equations for a cylindrical shell[121,122] can be simplified considerably if the deformation is taken to be the same along each generator line, so that a cylinder deforms into another with a different cross-section. The following assumptions are necessary: (1) the wall thickness–diameter ratio is sufficiently small, (2) the material is isotropic and obeys Hooke's law with a Young's modulus $E$ and Poisson's ratio $v$ (see Appendix B for definitions), and (3) the cylinder has an elliptical cross-section in the no-load condition so that its curvature can be expressed by the equation

$$C_0 = \frac{1}{a} + \frac{\varepsilon}{a} \cos 2\theta \tag{12}$$

where $a$ is the mean initial radius, $\theta$ is the polar angle, and $\varepsilon$ is a measure of the ellipticity of the cross-section. It has been shown[123] that a simple solution can be analytically determined if the initial ellipticity is small ($\varepsilon \ll 1$). The solution can be expressed as the change of curvature $\Delta C$ as follows:

$$\Delta C = \frac{-\frac{\varepsilon}{a}\cos 2\theta}{1 + \frac{Eh^3}{3(1-v^2)a^3 \Delta P_{\text{tm}}}}. \tag{13}$$

This solution shows that when the transmural pressure $\Delta P_{\text{tm}}$ is zero, the denominator tends to infinity and $\Delta C = 0$, so that the original elliptical cross-section is obtained. When the transmural pressure tends to infinity, the solution becomes

$$\Delta C = \frac{-\varepsilon}{a} \cos 2\theta \tag{14}$$

which implies a circular cross-section.

The transmural pressure at which the ellipticity is reduced to 5% of its initial value can be obtained by setting the denominator of the fraction on the right-hand side of eqn 13 to 1.05:

$$\Delta P_{\text{tm}} = \frac{E}{0.15(1-v^2)} \left(\frac{h}{a}\right)^3. \tag{15}$$

Hence, assuming that the material is incompressible ($v = 0.5$), the value of the transmural pressure required to reduce the ellipticity to 5% of its initial value can be computed given the material's Young modulus and thickness to radius ratio.

## Zero-stress state experiments: determination of residual strain

To compute the stress and strain in the GI tract under physiological or pathophysiological conditions, one must know the zero-stress configuration. Recent studies have shown that the zero-stress state in blood vessels, heart and trachea is very different from the no-load state in which all external loads are removed.[8,124,125] For a tubular organ, two cuts transverse to the longitudinal axis of the tube will produce a ring which will open into a sector when cut radially. Figure 7 shows the zero-stress state of an oesophageal ring. The strain difference between the zero-stress state and the no-load state is called the residual strain. Any rigorous mechanical modelling must use the zero-stress configuration as the reference state. Cardiovascular studies have shown that the residual strain serves to reduce the stress at the inner wall.[126] The residual strain may have a similar effect in the GI tract. In the absence of residual strain, the mucosa would develop a larger stress during bolus transport. Residual strain in the GI tract may serve as a mechanism to relieve stress concentration at the mucosa during peristalsis (Gregersen *et al.*, unpublished results). The residual stress in the resting condition may also serve as a growth-regulating factor.[127]

### Strain measurements: determination of local strain distributions using implanted ultrasound crystals or surface markers

It is often more important to know local strain distributions rather than averaged midwall strains in the various directions. For example, a detailed strain analysis would yield more information about the mechanical behaviour during muscle contraction and deformation in the vicinity of mechanoreceptors. Several methods have been developed to determine strain fields. Surface strains can be computed from photomicrographs of ink dots, beads or other markers on the surface of the tissue[128] while intramural strains can be determined using implanted ultrasonic transducers.[129,130] Commonly, two-dimensional strains are computed from the change of coordinates of a triangle of markers when the tissue deforms.[128]

### Bending experiments: determination of the elastic properties in a two-layer model

Experimental results on gastrointestinal elasticity have thus far been analysed with the GI wall treated as a homogeneous material. As the structure of the wall in the GI tract is non-uniform, we must evaluate the stress–strain relations of different layers of the wall. Hence, important data on the force-deformation relation in the vicinity of mechanoreceptors at various locations can be obtained. Experiments involving pressurization and longitudinal stretching yield a single strain. Hence, non-axisymmetric deformation must be studied so that the different layers and locations along the wall deform to different degrees. Bending is one way of imposing a non-axisymmetric deformation on the wall of a tubular organ. In experiments based on bending theory, Yu *et al.*[128] showed a large difference between Young's modulus of the intima-media and the adventitia layers in the pig thoracic aorta. The method is applicable to the GI tract where differences in elasticity between individual layers would be expected due to the differences in the structure, e.g. the orientation and configuration of collagen fibres.

### Torsion experiments: determination of the shear modulus

We have thus far primarily considered normal stresses and strains in the circumferential and longitudinal directions. Shear components, however, are also important in the longitudinal–circumferential directions. Hence, the data on the shear modulus and its dependence on the circumferential and longitudinal stresses must be included in the constitutive equation. Recently, Deng *et al.*[118] presented an experimental method to determine the shear modulus of arteries. They applied torsion to an arterial segment *in vitro* and subsequently measured the torque and shear deformation to solve for the shear modulus $G$ from the equilibrium of forces equation:

$$T = GJ\frac{\theta}{L} \tag{16}$$

where $T$ is the torque, $J$ is the polar moment of inertia of the vessel cross-section and $\theta/L$ is the angle of twist per unit length. The method is equally applicable to the GI tract and may provide the necessary information for the determination of the proper stimulus for the mechanoreceptors. Data on the shear modulus of elasticity is also important for studying tissue growth and remodelling using molecular approaches since shear flow stimulates collagenase gene expression in smooth muscle cells from the human duodenum (Gregersen *et al.*, unpublished results).

### Biaxial experiments

Uni-axial loading experiments such as the conventional strip experiments and balloon distension cannot provide the full relationship between all the components of stress and strain. Biaxial and triaxial tests are required to provide further information for the constitutive equation of a material.[9] A biaxial test for a tubular organ consists of inflation and longitudinal distension.[131] In triaxial testing, torsion is added to inflation and longitudinal distension of a tubular organ.[118] In organs of more complex geometries, such as the heart, lung or stomach, a thin sheet of tissue is excised. After mounting the sheet in a biaxial testing machine, forces are applied in the two orthogonal directions of the plane and the corresponding strains measured.[9,132]

## CONCLUDING REMARKS

Organisms must contend with the physical characteristics of their environment as they carry out a wide

 

Published with permission



range of physiological and mechanical functions. Mechanical forces are a major determinant of tissue behaviour and are probably the single most important factor determining tissue remodelling. Biomechanics is the study of mechanical forces and their resulting deformations. Hence, the application of biomechanics to the gastrointestinal system is warranted. A rational approach to the study of the biomechanics of the GI tract consists of the following: study the morphology, anatomy and ultrastructure of the GI tract; determine the constitutive equations of the tissue; apply the basic laws of physics to write down the governing equations; specify appropriate initial and boundary conditions; solve the mathematical equations analytically or numerically; perform physiological experiments that will test the solutions of the mathematical equations; compare the experimental results with the corresponding theoretical results and seek applications of the theory and experiments in health and disease.[9] The application of the biomechanics approach to the study of the gastrointestinal structure and function, represents an important interdisciplinary approach that can add rigorous insight to our understanding of gastrointestinal design and function.

A basic outline of biomechanics and its application to distensibility data in the GI tract has been reviewed. This is important because in addition to considering phasic motility patterns, measurement of tone and distensibility is an important concept for GI physiologists. A review of the work done in this area has shown that the major criticisms of some of the previous studies are that the proper geometry is not considered; pressure-volume relations are not appropriate when studying tubular organs; the distension protocol, in pressure-volume measurements and the properties of the balloon and measurement system have not been evaluated in each case; and compliance measures have not considered the non-linear tissue properties and were expressed as functions of the luminal pressure only. Instead, when studying the tubular parts of the GI tract, it is important to use stress and strain models based on measurements of pressure, luminal cross-sectional area (luminal diameter or circumference) and wall thickness. Such data are greatly needed to enhance our understanding of mechanoreceptors, peristaltic reflexes, perception and pain, bolus transport mechanics, tissue growth and remodelling, and their relation to many GI diseases with altered structure and function. Finally, there were many issues such as the complex geometry, non-uniform material properties, layering and buckling of the GI tract which were not discussed in this review. However, these as well as other complex features of the GI tract may be tackled by a multidisciplinary effort through the use of experimental, analytical and numerical methods.

## REFERENCES

1 Johnson LR, Christensen J, Jackson MJ, Jacobson ED, Walsh JH, eds. *Physiology of the gastrointestinal tract* 3th edn. New York: Raven Press, 1994.

2 Dobrin PB. Mechanical properties of arteries. *Physiol Rev* 1978; **58**:397–460.

3 Paterson WG, Selucky M, Hynna-Liepert TT. Effect of intraesophageal location and muscarinic blockade on balloon distension-induced chest pain. *Dig Dis Sci* 1991; **36**:282–8.

4 Sengupta JN, Saha JK, Goyal RK. Differential sensitivity to bradykinin of esophageal distension-sensitive mechanoreceptors in vagal and sympathetic afferents of the opossum. *J Neurophysiol* 1992; **68**:1053–67.

5 Schulze-Delrieu K. Intrinsic differences in the filling response of the guinea pig duodenum and ileum. *J Lab Clin Med* 1991; **117**:44–50.

6 Sengupta JN, Saha JK, Goyal RK. Stimulus-response function studies of esophageal mechanosensitive nociceptors in sympathetic afferents of opossum. *J Neurophysiol* 1990; **64**:796–812.

7 Sengupta JN, Kauvar D, Goyal RK. Characteristics of vagal esophageal tension-sensitive afferent fibers in the opossum. *J Neurophysiol* 1989; **61**:1001–10.

8 Liu SQ, Fung YC. Zero-stress state of arteries. *J Biomech Eng* 1988; **110**:82–84.

9 Fung YC. *Biomechanics Mechanical properties of living tissues.* New York. Springer-Verlag, 1993.

10 Jørgensen CJ, Dall FH, Jensen SL, Gregersen H. A new combined ultrasound-impedance planimetry measuring system for quantification of organ wall biomechanics *in vivo*. *J Biomech* 1995; **28**:863–7.

11 Fung YC. Biomechanics. Its scope, history, and some problems of continuum mechanics in physiology. *Appl Mech Rev* 1968; **21**:1–20.

12 Arhan P, Devroede G, Danis K *et al.* Viscoelastic properties of the rectal wall in Hirschsprung's disease. *J Clin Invest* 1978; **62**:82–7.

13 Arhan P, Faverdin C, Persoz B *et al.* Relationship between viscoelastic properties of the rectum and anal pressure in man. *J Applied Physiol* 1976; **41**:677–82.

14 Bergel DH. The properties of blood vessels. In: Fung YC, Perrone N, Anliker M, eds. *Biomechanics: Its foundations and objectives.* Englewood Cliffs, New Jersey: Prentice-Hall, 1972: 105–138.

15 Villadsen GE, Petersen JAK, Vinter-Jensen L, Juhl CO, Gregersen H. Impedance planimetric characterisation of the normal and diseased oesophagus. *Surg Res Comm* 1995; **17**:225–42.

16 Gregersen H, Vinter-Jensen L, Juhl CO, Dajani EZ. Impedance planimetric characterization of the distal oesophagus in the Goettingen minipig. *J Biomech* 1996; **29**:63–8.

17 Storkholm JH, Villadsen GE, Jensen SL, Gregersen H. Passive elastic wall properties in the isolated guinea-pig small intestine. *Dig Dis Sci* 1995; **40**:976–82.

18 Dobrin PB. Vascular mechanics. In: *Handbook of Physiology – The Cardiovascular System.* Chapter 3, pp. 65–102.

Published with permission



19 van Duyl WA. A model for both the passive and active properties of urinary bladder tissue related to bladder function. *Neurourol Urodyn* 1985; **4**:275–83.

20 Roach MR, Burton AC. The reason for the shape of the distensibility curves of arteries. *Can J Biochem Physiol* 1957; **35**:681–90.

21 Gabella G. Structure of muscles and nerves in the gastrointestinal tract. In: Johnson LR, Christensen J, Jackson MJ, Jacobson ED, Walsh JH, eds. *Physiology of the gastrointestinal tract.* 2nd edn. New York: Raven Press, 1987: 335–382.

22 Gregersen H, Giversen IM, Rasmussen LM, Tøttrup A. Biomechanical wall properties and collagen content in the partially obstructed opossum esophagus. *Gastroenterology* 1992; **103**:1547–51.

23 Fackler K, Klein L, Hiltner A. Polarizing light microscopy of intestine and its relationship to mechanical behaviour. *J Microscopy* 1981; **124**:305–11.

24 Orberg J, Baer E, Hiltner J. Organization of collagen fibers in the intestine. *Connective Tissue Res* 1983; **11**:285–97.

25 Conklin J, Goyal RK. Gastrointestinal smooth muscle. In: Sleisenger MH, Fordtran JS, eds. *Gastrointestinal disease.* 4th edn. Philadelphia: W.B Saunders Company, 1989: chapter 3.

26 Murphy RA. Contractile system function in mammalian smooth muscle. *Blood vessels* 1976; **13**:1–23.

27 Melville J, Macagno E, Christensen J. Longitudinal contractions in the duodenum: their fluid-mechanical function. *Am J Physiol* 1975; **228**:1887–92.

28 Furness JB, Costa M. *The enteric nervous system.* New York: Churchill Livingstone, 1987: 207–238.

29 Hukuhara T, Masuda K, Kinose S. Über das Gesetz Des Darmes. *Pflügers Archives der Gesamte Physiologie* 1936; **237**:619–30.

30 Gregersen H, Jørgensen CS, Dall FH, Jensen SL. Spontaneous and evoked motility in the isolated perfused porcine duodenum. *J Appl Physiol* 1992; **73**:9–19.

31 Gregersen H, Jørgensen CS, Dall FH. Biomechanical wall properties in the isolated perfused porcine duodenum. An experimental study using impedance planimetry. *J Gastrointest Mot* 1992; **4**:125–35.

32 Mulvany MJ. Determinants of vascular hemodynamic characteristics. *Hypertension* 1984; **6** (Suppl. III): 13–17.

33 Coolsaet BLRA, van Duyl WA, van Mastrigt R, Van der Zwart A. Visco-elastic properties of the bladder wall. *Urol Int* 1975; **30**:16–26.

34 de Caestecker JS, Pryde A, Heading RC. Site and mechanism of pain perception with oesophageal balloon distension and intravenous edrophonium in patients with oesophageal chest pain. *Gut* 1992; **33**:580–6.

35 Williams D, Thompson DG, Heggie L, Bancewitz J. Responses of the human esophaus to experimental intraluminal distension. *Am J Physiol* 1993; **265**: G196–203.

36 Paterson WG. Neuromuscular mechanisms of esophageal responses at and proximal to a distending balloon. *Am J Physiol* 1991; **260**: G148–55.

37 Iggo A. Gastro-intestinal tension receptors with un-myelinated afferent fibres in the vagus of the cat. *Q J Exp Physiol* 1957; **42**:130–43.

38 Paintal AS. Responses from mucosal mechanoreceptors in the small intestine of the cat. *J Physiol* 1957; **139**:353–68.

39 Bülbring E, Lin RCY, Schofield G. An investigation of the peristaltic reflex in relation to anatomical observations. *Q J Exp Physiol* 1958; **43**:26–37.

40 Hukuhara T, Yamagami M, Nakayama S. On the intestinal intrinsic reflexes. *Jpn J Physiol* 1958; **8**:9–20.

41 Hukuhara T, Fukuda H. The motility of the isolated guinea pig small intestine. *Jpn J Physiol* 1965; **15**:125–39.

42 Yokoyama S, Ozaki T. Effects of gut distension on Auerbach's plexus and intestinal muscle. *Jpn J Physiol* 1980; **30**:143–60.

43 Hukuhara T, Nakayama S, Nanba R. Locality of receptors concerned with the intestino-intestinal extrinsic and intestinal muscular intrinsic reflexes. *Jpn J Physiol* 1960; **10**:420–6.

44 Grundy D. Mechanoreceptors in the gastrointestinal tract. *J Smooth Muscle Res* 1993; **29**:37–46.

45 Edelbroek M, Horowitz M, Dent J *et al.* Effects of duodenal distention on fasting and postprandial antroduodenal motility in humans. *Gastroenterology* 1994; **106**:583–92.

46 Gregersen H, Orvar K, Christensen J. Biomechanical wall properties and tone during phase I and phase II of the MMC. *Am J Physiol* 1992; **263**: G795–801.

47 Holzer P. Ascending enteric reflex: Multiple neurotransmitter systems and interactions. *Am J Physiol* 1989; **256**: G540–5.

48 Akervall S, Fasth S, Nordgren S, Oresland T, Hulten L. Rectal reservoir and sensory function studied by graded isobaric distension in normal man. *Gut* 1989; **30**:496–502.

49 Ginzel KH. Investigations concerning the initiation of the peristaltic reflex in the guinea-pig ileum. *J Physiol* 1959; **148**:75–76P.

50 Hauss WH, Kreuziger H, Asteroth H. Uber die reizung der pressorezeptoren im sinus caroticus beim hund. *Z Kreislaufforsch* 1949; **38**:28–33.

51 Kosterlitz HW, Robinson JA. Reflex contractions of the longitudinal muscle coat of the isolated guinea-pig ileum. *J Physiol* 1959; **146**:369–79.

52 Yuan SY, Furness JB, Bornstein JC, Smith TK. Mucosal distorsion by compression elicits polarized reflexes and enhances responses of the circular muscle to distension in the small intestine *J Autonom Nervous System* 1991; **35**:219–26.

53 Miftakhov R, Wingate D. Numerical simulation of the peristaltic reflex of the small bowel. *Biorheology* 1994; **31**:309–25.

54 Mandrek K, Golenhofen K. Tonic duodenal contractions – a process for regulation of duodenal transit. In: *Frontiers in smooth muscle research.* Alan R. Liss, Inc, 1990: 459–62.

55 Mandrek K, Golenhofen K. Phasic-rhythmical and tonic components in gastrointestinal motility. In: *Frontiers in smooth muscle research.* Alan R. Liss, Inc, 1990: 463–81.

56 Chernish SM, Miller RE, Rosenak BD, Scholz NE. Hypotonic duodenography with the use of glucagon. *Gastroenterology* 1972; **63**:392–8.

57 Diamant B, Picazo J. Spasmolytic action and clinical use of glucagon. In: Lefebre, ed. *Handbook of experimental pharmacology,* Berlin: Springer-Verlag, 1983: 614–43.

58 Summers RW, Karacic JJ, Anuras S. Pseudo–obstruction syndrome in multiple sclerosis *J Gastrointest Mot* 1991; **3**:144–50.

59 Ehrlein H-J, Scheemann M, Siegle M-L. Motor patterns of small intestine determined by closely spaced extra-

 

Published with permission




luminal transducers and videofluoroscopy. *Am J Physiol* 1987; **253**: G259–67.

60 Reinke DA. Patterns and parameters of dog gastrointestinal contractile activity monitored by extraluminal force transducers. Thesis, University of Michigan, 1964.

61 Gregersen H, Kraglund K, Djurhuus JC. Variations in duodenal cross-sectional area during the interdigestive motility complex. *Am J Physiol* 1990; **259**: G26–31.

62 Sarna SK. Cyclic motor activity: Migrating motor complex. *Gastroenterology* 1985; **89**:894–913.

63 Mayrand S, Diamant NE. Measurement of human esophageal tone *in vivo*. *Gastroenterology* 1993; **105**:1411–20.

64 Azpiroz F, Malagelada J-R. Intestinal control of gastric tone. *Am J Physiol* 1985; **249**: G501–9.

65 Azpiroz F, Malagelada J-R. Physiological variations in canine gastric tone measured by an electronic barostat. *Am J Physiol* 1985; **248**: G229–37.

66 Azpiroz F, Malagelada J-R. Isobaric intestinal distension in humans: sensorial relay and reflex gastric relaxation. *Am J Physiol* 1990; **258**: G202–7.

67 Azpiroz F, Malagelada J-R. Perception and reflex relaxation of the stomach in response to gut distension. *Gastroenterology* 1990; **98**:1193–8.

68 De Ponti F, Azpiroz F, Malagelada J-R. Reflex gastric relaxation in response to distension of the duodenum. *Am J Physiol* 1987; **252**: G595–601.

69 Rouillon J-M, Azpiroz F, Malagelada J-R. Reflex changes in intestinal tone: relationship to perception. *Am J Physiol* 1991; **261**: G280–86.

70 Rouillon J-M, Azpiroz F, Malagelada J-R. Sensorial and intestinointestinal reflex pathways in the human jejunum. *Gastroenterology* 1991; **101**:1606–12.

71 Steadman CJ, Phillips SF, Camilleri M, Haddad AC, Hanson RB. Variations of muscle tone in the human colon. *Gastroenterology* 1991; **101**:373–81.

72 Steadman CJ, Phillips SF, Camilleri M, Talley NJ, Haddad A, Hanson R. Control of muscle tone in the human colon. *Gut* 1992; **33**:541–6.

73 Bell AM, Pemberton JH, Hanson RB, Zinsmeister AR. Variations in muscle tone of the human rectum: recordings with an electromechanical barostat. *Am J Physiol* 1991; **260**: G17–25.

74 Premen AJ, Soika CY, Dabney JM, Dobbins DE. Effects of gastrointestinal hormones on ileal vascular and visceral smooth muscle. *Am J Physiol* 1984; **246**: G1–7.

75 Premen AJ, Dobbins DE, Soika CY, Dabney JM. Relationship between substance P, intestinal wall compliance and vascular resistance in the canine ileum. *Reg Peptides* 1984; **9**:119–27.

76 VanBavel E, Giezeman JMM, Mooij T, Spaan JAE. Influence of pressure alterations on tone and vasomotion of isolated mesenteric small arteries of the rat. *J Physiol* 1991; **436**:371–83.

77 Ren J, Massey BT, Dodds WJ *et al.* Determinants of the bolus pressure during esophageal peristaltic bolus transport. *Am J Physiol* 1993; **264**: G407–13.

78 Orloff Juhl C, Vinter-Jensen L, Djurhuus JC, Gregersen H, Zapher Dajani E. Biomechanical properties of the oesophagus damaged by endoscopic sclerotherapy. An impedance planimetric study in minipigs. *Scand J Gastroenterol* 1994; **29**:867–73.

79 Siegle M-L, Ehrlein H-J. Effects of various agents on ileal postprandial motor patterns and transit of chyme in dogs. *Am J Physiol* 1989; **257**: G698–703.

80 Bayliss VM, Starling EH. The movements and innervation of the small intestine. *J Physiol* 1901; **26**:125–38.

81 Brasseur JG. Mechanical studies of the esophageal function. *Dysphagia* 1993; **8**:384–6.

82 Li M, Brasseur JG, Kern MK *et al.* Viscosity measurements of barium sulfate mixtures for use in motility studies of the pharynx and esophagus. *Dysphagia* 1992; **7**:17–30.

83 Macagno E, Melville J, Christensen J. A model for longitudinal motility of the small intestine. *Biorheology* 1975; **12**:369–76.

84 Macagno EO, Christensen J. Fluid mechanics of the duodenum. *Ann Rev Fluid Mech* 1980; **12**:139–58.

85 Meyer JH, Gu Y, Elashoff J, Reedy T, Dressman J, Amidon G. Effects of viscosity and fluid outflow on postcibal gastric emptying of solids. *Am J Physiol* 1986; **250**: G161–4.

86 Schulze-Delrieu K. Clearance patterns of the isolated guinea pig duodenum. *Gastroenterology* 1992; **102**:849–56.

87 Schulze-Delrieu K, Ehrlein HJ, Blum AL. Mechanics of the pylorus. In: *Gastric and gastroduodenal motility*. Praeger Publishers, 1984: 87–101.

88 Schulze-Delrieu K, Brown BP, Custer-hagen T. Contraction and accomodation of guinea pig duodenum *in vitro*. *Am J Physiol* 1991; **261**: G364–72.

89 Schulze-Delrieu K, Wall JP. Determinants of flow across isolated gastroduodenal junctions of cats and rabbits. *Am J Physiol* 1983; **245**: G257–64.

90 Keane FB, DiMagno EP, Dozois RR, Go VLW. Relationships among canine interdigestive exocrine pancreatic and biliary flow, duodenal motor activity, plasma pancratic polypeptide, and motilin. *Gastroenterology* 1980; **78**:310–16.

91 Kerlin P, Zinsmeister A & Phillips S. Relationship of motility to flow of contents in the human small intestine. *Gastroenterology* 1982; **82**:701–6.

92 Fisher MA, Hendrix TR, Hunt JN, Murrils AJ. Relation between volume swallowed and velocity of the bolus ejected from the pharynx into the esophagus. *Gastroenterology* 1978; **74**:1238–40.

93 Nguyen HN, Silny J, Wuller S, Marschall HU, Rau G, Matern S. Chyme transport patterns in human duodenum determined by multiple intraluminal impedancometry. *Am J Physiol* 1995; **268**: G700–8.

94 Weems WA. Intestinal fluid flow: Its production and control. In: Johnson LR, Christensen J, Jackson MJ, Jacobson ED, Walsh JH, eds. *Physiology of the gastrointestinal tract*. New York: Raven Press, 1987: 571–93.

95 Stavitsky D, Macagno EO, Christensen J. Finite-element analysis of flow induced by contractions like those of the intestine. *J Biomechanics* 1981; **14**:183–93.

96 Srivastava LM, Srivastava VP, Sinha SN. Peristaltic transport of a physiological fluid. Part I. Flow in non-uniform geometry. *Biorheology* 1983; **20**:153–166.

97 Fung YC, Yih CS. Peristaltic transport. *J Applied Mechanics* 1968; 669–75.

98 Li M, Brasseur JG. Non-steady peristaltic transport in finite-length tubes. *J Fluid Mechanics* 1993; **248**:129–51.

Published with permission




99 Schulze-Delrieu K, Shirazi S, Sprunger K, Noel S, Tung H. Functional denervation of the esophagus from experimental obstruction. *Gastroenterology* 1988; **94**: A414 (abst.).

100 Ravinder KM, Ren J, McCallum RW, Shaffer HA, Sluss J. Modulation of feline oesophageal contractions by bolus volume and and outflor obstruction. *Am J Physiol* 1990; **258**: G208–15.

101 Gabella G. Structural apparatus for force transmission in smooth muscles. *Physiological Rev* 1984; **64**:455–77.

102 Vinter-jensen L, Duch BU, Pedersen JAK, Ryslev A, Gregersen H. Systemic treatment with epidermal growth factor in the rat. Biomechanical properties of the growing small intestine. *Regulatory Peptides* 1996; **61**:135–42.

103 Tung H-N, Schulze-Delrieu K, Shirazi S, Noel S, Xia Q, Cue K. Hypertrophic smooth muscle in the partially obstructed opossum esophagus. The model: histological and ultrastructural observations. *Gastroenterology* 1991; **100**:853–64.

104 Jensen LS, Laurberg S, Andreassen TT. Endoscopic sclerotherapy of oesophageal varices in rabbits. The long-term effect on oesophageal collagen content and mechanical strength. *Scand J Gastroenterol* 1989; **24**:613–16.

105 Denis Ph, Colin R, Galmiche JP, Geffroy Y, Hecketsweiler Ph, Lefrancois R, Pasquis P. Elastic properties of the rectal wall in normal adults and in patients with ulcerative colitis. *Gastroenterology* 1979; **77**:45–8.

106 Nowak TV, Harrington B, Weisbruch JP, Kalbfleish JH. Structural and functional characteristics of muscle from diabetic rodent small intestine. *Am J Physiol* 1990; **258**: G690–8.

107 Jensen LS, Laurberg S, Juhl CO, Andreassen TT. Esophageal collagen content and mechanical; strength after endoscopic sclerotherapy of esophageal varices. *Scand J Gastroenterol* 1987; **22**:743–9.

108 Kimmey MB, Martin RW, Haggitt RC, Wang KY, Franklin DW, Silverstein FE. Histolog correlates of gastrointestinal ultrasound images. *Gastroenterology* 1989; **96**:433–41.

109 Martin RW, Silverstein FE, Kimmey MB. A 20-MHZ ultrasound system for imaging the intestinal wall. *Ultrasound Med Biol* 1989; **15**:273–80.

110 Madoff RD, Orrom WJ, Rothenberger DA, Goldberg SM. Rectal compliance: a critical reappraisal. *Int J Colorect Dis* 1990; **5**:37–40.

111 Gregersen H, Andersen MB. Impedance measurement system for quantification of cross-sectional area in the gastrointestinal tract. *Med Biol Eng Comput* 1991; **29**:108–10.

112 Alstrup NI, Skjoldbye B, Rasmussen O, Christensen NEH, Christiansen J. Rectal compliance determined by rectal endosonography. *Dis Colon Rectum* 1995; **38**:32–6.

113 Meiss RA. Some mechanical properties of cat intestinal muscle. *Am J Physiol* 1971; **220**:2000–7.

114 Price JM, Patitucci P, Fung YC. Mechanical properties of taenia coli smooth muscle in spontaneous contraction. *Am J Physiol* 1977; **233**: C47–55.

115 Nowak TV, Harrington B. Effect of cholinergic agonists on muscle from rodent proximal and distal small intestine. *Gastroenterology* 1985; **88**:1118–25.

116 Tøttrup A, Forman A, Uldbjerg N, Funch-Jensen P, Andersson KE. Mechanical properties of isolated human esophageal smooth muscle. *Am J Physiol* 1990; **258**: G338–43.

117 Yamada H. *Strength of biological materials*. Baltimore: The Williams & Wilkins Company, 1970.

118 Deng SX, Tomioka J, Debes JC, Fung YC. New experiments on shear modulus of elasticity of arteries. *Am J Physiol* 1994; **266**: H1–10.

119 Kassab GS, Rider CA, Tang NJ, Fung YC. Morphometry of pig coronary arterial tree. *Am J Physiol* 1993: **265**: H350–65.

120 Fung YC. *Biodynamics Circulation*. New York: Springer-Verlag, 1984.

121 Flügge W. *Stresses in shells*. Berlin: Springer-Verlag, 1960.

122 Prescott J. *Applied elasticity*. New York: Dover Publications, 1946.

123 Yen RT, Fung YC, and Bingham N. Elasticity of small pulmonary arteries in the cat. *J Biomech Eng* 1980; **102**:170–7.

124 Han HC, Fung YC. Residual strains in porcine and canine trachea. *J Biomech* 1991; **24**:307–15.

125 Omens JH, Fung YC. Residual strain in the rat left ventricle. *Circulation Res* 1990; **66**:37–45.

126 Fung YC, Liu SQ. Strain distribution in small blood vessels with zero-stress state taken into consideration. *Am J Physiol* 1992; **262**: H544–52.

127 Fung YC, Liu SQ. Changes of zero-stress state of rat pulmonary arteries in hypoxic hypertension. *J Appl Physiol* 1991; **70**:2455–70.

128 Yu Q, Zhou J, Fung YC. Neutral axis location in bending and Young's modulus of different layers of arterial wall. *Am J Physiol* 1993; **265**: H52–60.

129 Omens JH, MacKenna DA, McCulloch AD. Measurement of strain and analysis of stress in resting rat left ventricular myocardium. *J Biomech* 1993; **26**:665–76.

130 Villarreal FJ, Waldman LK, Lew WYW. Technique for measuring regional two-dimensional finite strains in canine left ventricle. *Circulation Res* 1988; **62**:711–21.

131 Takamizawa K, Hayashi K, Matsuda T. Isometric biaxial tension of smooth muscle in isolated cylindrical segments of rabbits arteries. *Am J Physiol* 1992; **263:** H30–4.

132 Humphrey JD, Strumpf RK, Yin FCP. Biaxial mechanical behavior of excised ventricular epicardium. *Am J Physiol* 1990: **259**: H101–8.


## APPENDIX A

### Derivation of circumferential stress (Laplace's law) and longitudinal stress

Consider a cylindrical intestine subjected to an internal pressure $P_i$, as shown in Fig. 1(a). The pressure in the intestine induces stress in the intestinal wall. Under equilibrium conditions, the force in the intestinal wall in the circumferential direction $2\tau_\theta(r_o - r_i)L$, is balanced by the force in the intestinal lumen contributed by the pressure $2Lr_iP_i$, as shown in Fig. 1(b). Hence, the equilibrium equation in the circumferential direction is

$$\tau_\theta = P_i r_i/(r_o - r_i) \qquad \text{(A1)}$$

Published with permission



where $\tau_\theta$ is circumferential stress, $r_i$ is internal radius and $r_o$ is outer radius.

The longitudinal stress in an intestinal wall can be determined based on the equilibrium of forces in the longitudinal direction. The product of the longitudinal stress and the cross-sectional area of the intestinal wall is the force that balances the total longitudinal force acting on the intestine as shown in Fig. 1(c). The longitudinal force in the intestinal wall $\tau_z\pi(r_o^2 - r_i^2)$ is balanced only by the pressure component $P_i\pi r_i^2$ as the external pressure is assumed to be zero. Thus,

$$\tau_z = P_i r_i^2/(r_o^2 - r_i^2) \tag{A2}$$

where $\tau_z$ is the longitudinal stress. If the wall thickness-radius ratio is small, so that $r_o = r_i = r$ and $r_o - r_i = h$, then these equations are simplified to

$$\tau_\theta = P_i r/h, \qquad \tau_z = P_i r/2h. \tag{A3}$$

## APPENDIX B

### Constitutive equation of an elastic solid

The constitutive equations of a solid that consists of a homogeneous, isotropic, linearly elastic material contain only two material constants:

$$\varepsilon_{ij} = \frac{1}{2\mu}\left[\frac{-\lambda}{3\lambda + 2\mu}\tau_{ij}\delta_{ij} + \tau_{ij}\right] \tag{B1}$$

where $i$ and $j$ are indices ranging from integers 1–3. The $i$th index denotes the component in the $i$th direction whereas the $j$th index denotes the surface perpendicular to the $j$th direction. The repetition of an index in a term denotes a summation with respect to that index over its range.

Consider several special cases:

**1** a uni-axial state of stress with the non-zero stress-component $\tau_{11}$ corresponding to the $x_1$-direction. From eqn (B1) we obtain

$$\varepsilon_{11} = \frac{\lambda + \mu}{\mu(3\lambda + 2\mu)}\tau_{11}, \qquad \varepsilon_{22} = \varepsilon_{33} = \frac{-\lambda}{2\mu(3\lambda + 2\mu)}\tau_{11}. \tag{B2}$$

The coefficient

$$E = \mu\frac{(3\lambda + 2\mu)}{\lambda + \mu} \tag{B3}$$

is called the *elastic modulus* or *Young's modulus*, which can be readily measured in a uni-axial tension test. The ratio $-\varepsilon_{22}/\varepsilon_{11} = -\varepsilon_{33}/\varepsilon_{11}$ is given by

$$= \frac{\lambda}{2(\lambda + \mu)} \tag{B4}$$

which is known as Poisson's ratio. It is a measure of the lateral contraction (extension) produced by an axial tension (compression). The physical dimension of $E$ is force divided by squared length, while is a dimensionless quantity.

**2** Consider a state of plane stress in pure shear in which the only non-zero component of the stress tensor is $\tau_{12} = \tau_{21} \neq 0$. The corresponding non-zero strain component is given by

$$\varepsilon_{12} = \frac{1}{2\mu}\tau_{12}. \tag{B5}$$

The ratio of shearing stress $\tau_{12}$ and the corresponding change $2\varepsilon_{12}$ of an initially right material angle is known as the shear modulus. In the engineering literature, the symbol $G$ is widely used to describe the shear modulus.

**3** Finally, consider a hydrostatic state of stress, i.e.

$$\tau_{ij} = -p\delta_{ij}. \tag{B6}$$

Combining this result with eqn (B1) yields

$$\varepsilon_{ij} = \frac{-1}{3\lambda + 2\mu}p\delta_{ij}. \tag{B7}$$

Setting $i = j$, and summing on $j$, we obtain

$$-p = K\varepsilon_i \tag{B8}$$

where $\varepsilon_{ii} = \varepsilon_{11} + \varepsilon_{22} + \varepsilon_{33}$ and constant

$$K = \lambda + \frac{2}{3}\mu \tag{B9}$$

is known as the bulk modulus. It is a measure of the compressibility of the solid. For an incompressible material, $K$ and hence $\lambda$ are unbounded ($\rightarrow\infty$). If a hydrostatic pressure is to be accompanied by a volume decrease, then the bulk modulus $K$ must be positive. Moreover, we expect that the shearing should occur in the direction of the shearing stress. Therefore, form a purely physical consideration, we expect that

$$\infty \geq (\lambda + \frac{2}{3}\mu) > 0, \qquad \infty > \mu > 0.$$

Published with permission



The corresponding bounds on $E$ and are

$$0 < E \leq 3\mu, \qquad -1 < v \leq \frac{1}{2}. \tag{B10}$$

Hence, a simple tension is always accompanied by an extension. On the other hand, in a direction normal to the direction of this tension, a contraction may take place.

## APPENDIX C

### The resulting error when an elliptical cross-section is assumed to be circular

Consider a segment of a tubular GI organ with a fixed length. Next, consider two special cross-sectional geometries of the organ: a circle with radius $r$ and an ellipse with major and minor radii $a$ and $b$, respectively. The following equations relate the circumference and luminal cross-sectional area (or volume if the length is constant) to the radii for the two geometries:

**elliptic shape**

Cross-sectional area $= \pi \cdot a \cdot b$ (C1a)

Circumference $= \int_0^{2\pi} [a^2 \sin^2\theta + b^2 \cos^2\theta]^{1/2} d\theta$ (C1b)

**circular shape** (where $a = b = r$)

Cross-sectional area $= \pi \cdot r^2$ (C2a)

Circumference $= 2 \cdot \pi \cdot r$ (C2b)

Now, the resulting error in the area ($E_A$) when an elliptical cross-section is assumed to be circular is

$$E_A = \frac{\pi r^2 - \pi ab}{\pi r^2} = 1 - \left(\frac{ab}{r^2}\right). \tag{C3}$$

If we assume that the circumference is constant, then

$$2\pi r = \int_0^{2\pi} [a^2 \sin^2\theta + b^2 \cos^2\theta]^{1/2} d\theta,$$

or (C4)

$$r = \frac{1}{2\pi} \int_0^{2\pi} [a^2 \sin^2\theta + b^2 \cos^2\theta]^{1/2} d\theta.$$

Hence, substitution of $r$ from Eq. (C4) into Eq. (C3) yields

$$E_A = 1 - \frac{4\pi^2 ab}{\left[\int_0^{2\pi} [a^2 \sin^2\theta + b^2 \cos^2\theta]^{1/2} d\theta\right]^2} \tag{C5}$$

or

$$E_A = 1 - \frac{4\pi^2}{I^2} \tag{C6}$$

where

$$I = \int_0^{2\pi} \left[\left(\frac{a}{b}\right) \sin^2\theta + \left(\frac{a}{b}\right)^{-1} \cos^2\theta\right]^{1/2} d\theta.$$

The dashed curve in Fig. 6 illustrates the error in cross-sectional area as a function of the $a/b$ ratio when the geometry deviates from a circle. It can be seen that the error in the CSA or volume can be considerable at a constant circumference (equivalent to no variation in tone). Thus, the circular assumption may introduce large errors when the cross-section is elliptical. The $a/b$ ratio is high in the resting state because the intestines are collapsed and become more circular as the distension pressure is increased.

In a similar fashion, we can compute the resulting error in the circumference ($E_C$) when an elliptical section is assumed to be circular as follows:

$$\begin{aligned} E_C &= \frac{2\pi r - \int_0^{2\pi} [a^2 \sin^2\theta + b^2 \cos^2\theta]^{1/2} d\theta}{2\pi r} \\ &= 1 - \frac{1}{2\pi} \frac{\int_0^{2\pi} [a^2 \sin^2\theta + b^2 \cos^2\theta]^{1/2} d\theta}{r}. \end{aligned} \tag{C7}$$

If we assume a constant cross-sectional area so that

$$\pi r^2 = \pi ab, \quad \text{or} \quad r = \sqrt{ab}, \text{ then} \tag{C8}$$

$$E_C = 1 - \frac{I}{2\pi}. \tag{C9}$$

The solid line curve in Fig. 6 illustrates the error in circumference as a function of the $a/b$ ratio. Equations (5) and (9) can be used to relate the error in circumference to that in areas as follows:

$$E_C = 1 - \frac{1}{\sqrt{1 - E_A}}. \tag{C10}$$

It must be emphasized that these equations only consider the case when an elliptical cross-section is assumed to be circular. The evaluation of errors (in, for example, volume or surface area) is considerably more difficult for organs with more complex geometry, e.g. the stomach.

CHAPTER 3

# ULTRASONOGRAPHY OF THE LIVER, BILIARY SYSTEM AND PANCREAS

OLE MARTIN PEDERSEN AND SVEIN ODEGAARD

## 1. Liver

### 1.1. *Anatomy*

In the interpretation of ultrasound images, it is crucial to understand cross-sectional anatomy. The liver is the largest abdominal organ located predominantly on the right side under the dome of the right diaphragm. It varies considerably in size and shape. In some patients the bulk of the liver may be located mainly on the right, perhaps with a Riedel's lobe and a correspondingly small left lobe, while in others there is a small right lobe with a large left lobe extending across the mid-line.

#### 1.1.1. *Blood vessels*

The liver possesses a dual blood supply, with roughly 75% of the blood coming from the portal vein and 25% from the hepatic artery. Both arterial and portal venous vessels branch and divide until they reach the hepatic sinusoids. The portal vein is divided into a right and left branch. The right branch of the portal vein passes transversely within the liver substance for a few centimeters before dividing into anterior and posterior branches, while the left branch curves anteromedially, branching into the parts of the liver it traverses. The hepatic arterial branches follow the same pattern.

The hepatic veins (Fig. 1) include three main veins, the right, middle and left, which drain the hepatic sinusoids of the liver and empty into the upper part of the inferior vena cava. The right hepatic vein runs in the coronal plain and empties separately into the inferior vena cava (IVC). The middle hepatic vein passes from the position of the gallbladder fossa and joins the left hepatic vein to form a short common trunk of approximately one centimeter before entering the anterior aspect of the IVC just below the diaphragm.

The sonographic differentiation between hepatic and portal veins (Fig. 2) is usually not difficult. The hepatic veins come from the periphery of the liver and converge just below the diaphragm. They have anechoic walls and run a dominantly straight course with few bifurcations. In contrast, the portal veins diverge from the porta hepatis running towards the periphery of the liver. The portal veins bifurcate more often and their walls are usually highly echogenic as compared with the surrounding liver tissue. Because the portal veins bring blood to the periphery of the liver, the red cells move towards the transducer. This causes a positive Doppler shift which is coded red on color Doppler images. However, the liver veins, which bring blood from the periphery, cause a negative Doppler shift and thus appear blue on color Doppler images.

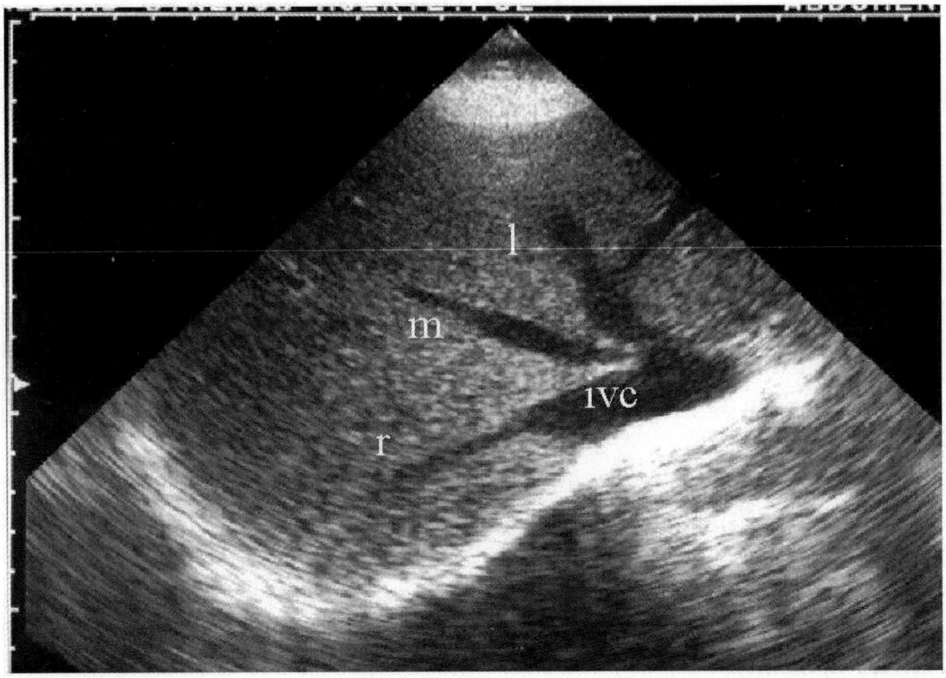


Fig. 1. Transverse sonogram of the three main hepatic veins, the right (r), middle (m) and left (l), which empty into the upper part of the inferior vena cava (ivc).

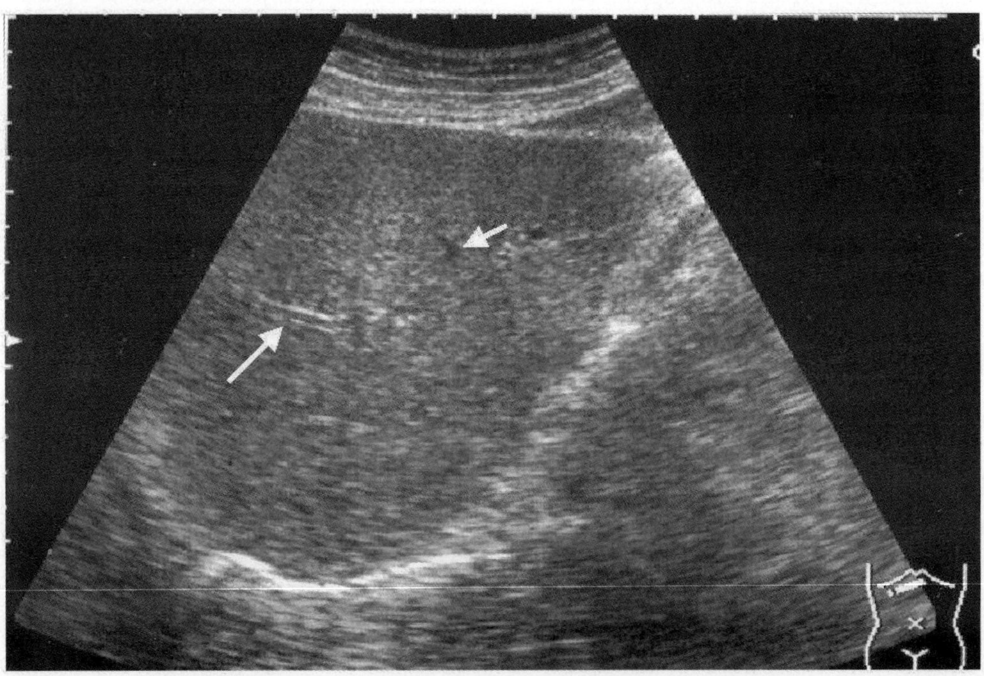

Fig. 2. Subcostal view of the right lobe of the liver. Long arrow — small branch of the portal vein. Short arrow — hepatic vein.

### 1.1.2. *Bile ducts*

The overall arrangement of the bile ducts is similar to that of the portal vein — the smaller hepatic ducts joining to form the right and left hepatic ducts. These generally lie anterior to the associated portal vein branches. Normally the intrahepatic bile ducts are not well differentiated from the portal vein radicle, but may sometimes be visualized as a separate vessel parallel to the portal vein. They are regarded as non-dilated as long as their internal diameter is less than 1.0 mm.

### 1.1.3. *Liver segments*

The liver is divided into right and left lobes along an imaginary plane extending from the gall bladder fossa to the anterior vena cava. The most commonly used system of classifying different liver segments, the Couinaud classification system (1, 2), divides the right lobe into anterior and posterior segments, each with a superior and inferior subsegment. The left lobe is divided into medial and lateral segments, each with an inferior and superior subsegment. Each subsegment is given a number from 1 to 8, proceeding in a clockwise direction (3).

Segment one is the retrocaval portion of the caudate lobe. The other segments are defined cranio-caudally by a transverse or axial section through the porta hepatis at the level where the main portal vein divides into right and left portal vein branches (on ultrasonography, this plane is best obtained subcostally in deep inspiration). Moving from right to left, this horizontal plane divides, segment 6 from 7, 5 from 8, 4a from 4b, 2 from 3. The liver is then divided by longitudinal planes radiating from the IVC in the plane of each of the three hepatic veins. The plane through the right hepatic vein and inferior vena cava divides the right lobe into the postero-lateral segments 6 and 7 and the antero-medial segments 5 and 8. The two medial segments of the left lobe, 4a and 4b, are divided from the left lateral segments, 2 and 3 by the left hepatic vein and falciform ligament. The segmental anatomy is thus defined by the major vascular tree and identifies clear surgical planes for resection. The localization of tumors according to this system is fully possible with ultrasound (4).

### 1.1.4. *Sonographic view of the porta hepatis*

The best view of the porta hepatis is often obtained through one of the right lateral intercostal spaces, either with the patient in a left lateral decubitus position or standing. With the patient in one of these positions the liver is shifted downwards and medially providing a better ultrasonic window for obtaining a view of the porta hepatis, gallbladder (GB) and pancreas. In this scanning plane, the portal vein (PV) is usually visualized in a longitudinal section. The common duct (CD) is also visualized in a longitudinal fashion where the common hepatic duct crosses the right branch of the PV (Fig. 3). More, distally it is seen running anterolaterally and parallel to the portal vein. When visualized, the hepatic artery appears in cross-section as it crosses in between the CD and PV. In a few patients, however, the hepatic artery may be found anterior to the CD. With this angle of interrogation, the IVC may be intersected as well and thereby constitutes a third tubular structure, running parallel to the CD and PV. When the CD is dilated the three parallel running tubular structures may look rather like a three-lane highway (Fig. 4).

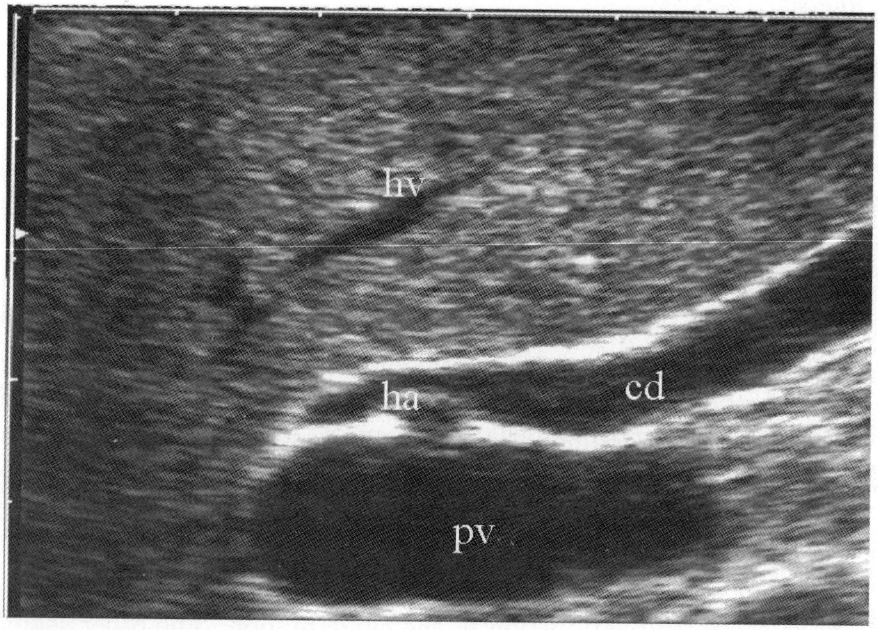


Fig. 3. Oblique view of the porta hepatis where the common duct (cd) crosses the right branch of the portal vein (pv) with the hepatic artery (ha) in between. hv — hepatic vein.

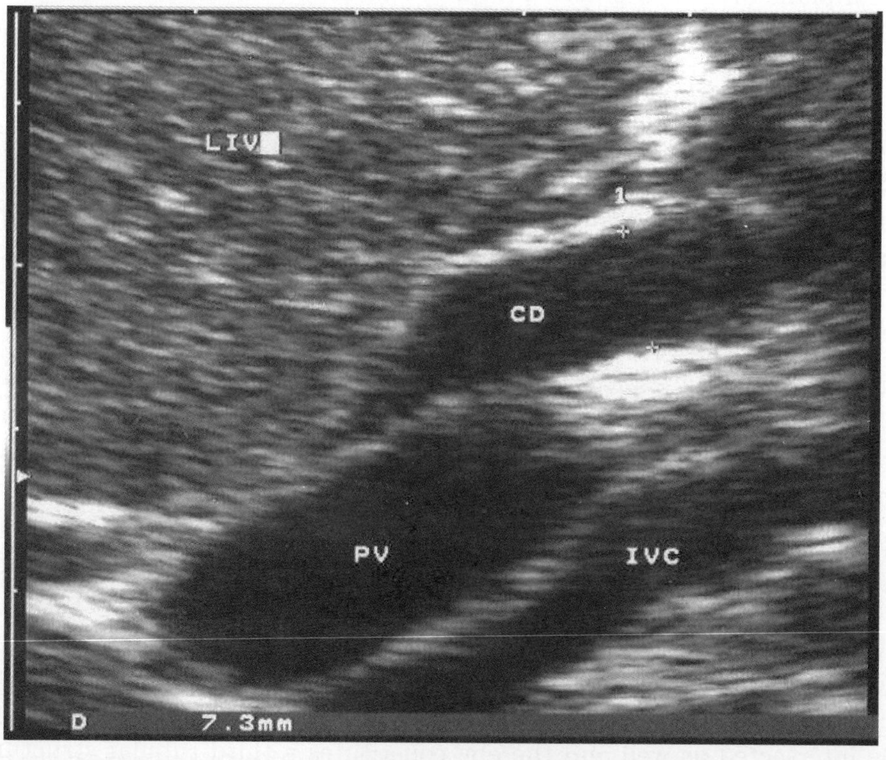


Fig. 4. Oblique section of the porta hepatis visualizing three parallel running tubular structures, the common duct (CD), portal vein (PV) and inferior vena cava (IVC). 1 — common duct diameter = 7.3 mm.

## 1.2. *Benign liver disease*

### 1.2.1. *General sonographic findings in diffuse liver disease*

The normal liver has a smooth surface and wedge shaped edges, which may become blunt in cirrhotic patients. The echoes of normal liver parenchyma are similar in size and shape and are a mid grey in signal intensity. Together they form a uniform sponge-like pattern interrupted by the vessels. According to the nature of the liver pathology, this pattern may change, becoming finer or coarser or irregular.

Various pathological processes may result in either an increase or a decrease in echo-amplitude, in disturbances in echo pattern and in alterations in the size and shape of the liver. It is difficult to visualize the entire liver with sonography even under the best circumstances. Difficult areas include the superficial liver above the costal margin, the left tip of the lateral segment of the left lobe, and the ventral subdiaphragmatic regions (5).

The liver is best visualized with the patient in the supine and left lateral decubitus positions, starting with 3–7 MHz curved linear array transducers. A subcostal acoustic window should be used first, supplemented with intercostal scans. Small sector transducers should be used to image areas inaccessible to the larger curved linear transducers. The anterior surface of the liver (usually the ventral left lobe or the right lobe through intercostal views) should be evaluated for nodularity with a 5–12 MHz linear array transducer. Surface characteristics are easier to appreciate in real-time and when there is ascites.

Liver size is difficult to measure due to its complex shape and the need for many different views, only obtained through a series of different ultrasonic windows and patient positions. The most reliable measurement is probably the sagittal dimension from the dome to the tip of the right lobe, measured at the midclavicular line. If the dome-tip measurement exceeds 15.5 cm, the liver is probably enlarged (5). In 95% of normal subjects, this measurement is less than 13 cm (6).

Loss in amplitude with depth is known as attenuation. Normal liver parenchyma attenuates the ultrasound beam at around 1 dB/MHz/cm of depth. Studies have shown that abnormal liver parenchyma tend to show either increased or decreased attenuation (7). Parenchymal echogenicity, inversely related to ultrasound attenuation, may be increased in diffuse liver disease, especially when there is fatty infiltration. The degree of increase in echo intensity, however, is difficult to establish because of the lack of an echo amplitude or echo intensity standard. Such standards have been worked out for computer tomography (CT), where the attenuation of X-rays is given as Hounsfield numbers (attenuation numbers). To overcome this problem, liver echogenicity is judged by comparison with adjacent organs (Fig. 5), most often the kidneys and spleen, which normally should be lower. The echo amplitudes of the parenchymal liver are slightly higher than those returned from the renal cortex at the same depth in the image.

In the normal liver, the portal venous radicals are visualized as clear white lines, more brilliant than the less echogenic parenchyma. Increased reflectivity of the liver parenchyma may therefore cause the portal veins to appear less distinct. Conversely, unduly prominent portal veins indicate reduced echogenicity of the liver parenchyma consistent with the "dark liver" seen in hepatitis.

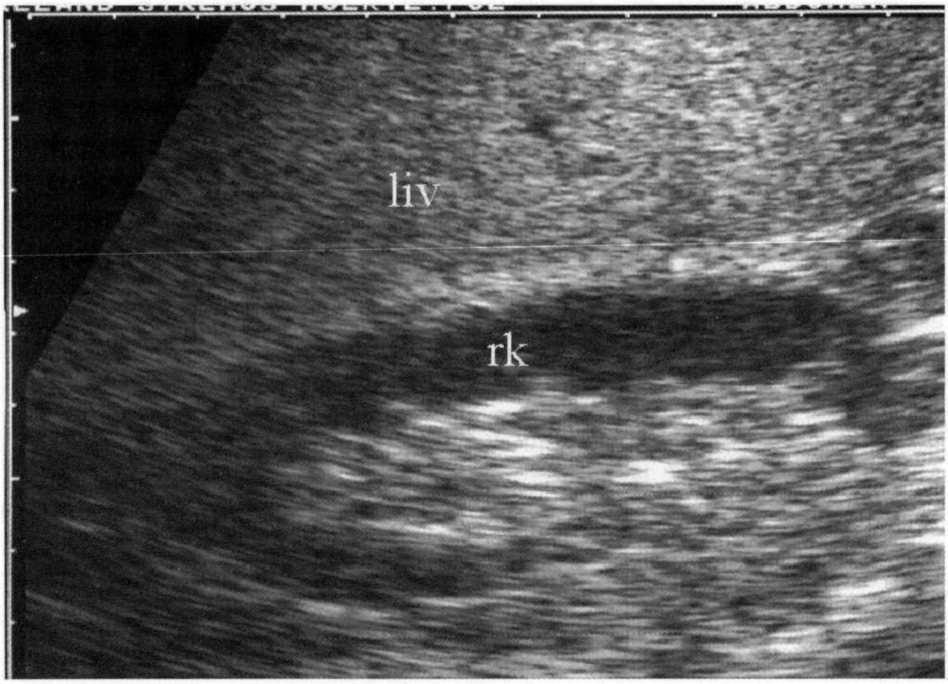


Fig. 5. Section through a hyper-echogenic, fatty infiltrated, right lobe of the liver (liv) as compared with the echo-poor cortex of the right kidney (rk).

### 1.2.2. *Hepatitis*

Acute hepatitis is not associated with any specific ultrasound findings. The most common sonographic finding is probably hepatomegaly. Infrequently (2.4%), the liver may appear darker than usual, "dark liver", and the portal vein echoes appear brighter than usual, *starry night liver* (5). The main value of ultrasound in acute viral hepatitis is usually to exclude obstructive jaundice. Another striking sonographic feature of acute hepatitis is the marked thickening of the gallbladder wall, sometimes reaching 20 mm (normal $< 3$ mm) due to direct inflammation and edema (5). Acute alcoholic hepatitis can vary from a mild anicteric illness to fulminant hepatic failure. The liver is almost always enlarged and there is increased reflectivity and attenuation (8, 9). Many patients with acute viral hepatitis, especially hepatitis $C$, have periportal adenopathy (10, 11).

Chronic hepatitis is usually associated with an inhomogeneous patchy or diffusely increased echogenicity depending on the amount of fatty infiltration and fibrosis. The liver surface is smooth unless cirrhosis is also present.

### 1.2.3. *Fatty liver*

The accumulation of fatty droplets within hepatocytes occurs in response to a variety of injuries to the liver including alcohol, diabetes mellitus, obesity, pregnancy, drugs (especially corticosteroids) and toxic substances, malnutrition, parenteral hyperalimentation and inborn errors of metabolism (12). Fatty infiltration is a dynamic process; its severity may alter rapidly, over weeks or even days, and is usually completely reversible (9, 13).

The liver is often enlarged (75%) and the ultrasound pattern is usually that of fine, closely packed echoes which in severe cases may make the liver appear *whitish* or *bright*, tending to make blood vessels and the diaphragm become less distinct (14). This sonographic appearance is helpful in distinguishing fatty infiltration from cirrhosis when the liver is normal in size or shrunken (15). In mild degrees of fatty infiltration, its presence may be made more evident by using higher ultrasound frequencies, 5 MHz or more, which increases the attenuation of ultrasound.

Although ultrasound is highly sensitive for the detection of fatty infiltration (sensitivity 86% for mild and almost 100% for moderate and severe degrees), the specificity is lower (14).

### 1.2.4. *Tissue harmonic imaging in conjunction with micro-bubble contrast agents*

Recently, tissue harmonic imaging (THI), especially when used in combination with new types of liver-specific ultrasound contrast agents, has greatly enhanced the ability of ultrasound to detect and differentiate focal liver lesions. Tissue harmonic imaging utilizes the non-linear ultrasound waves generated at each instant in the propagation of the transmitted pulse. The frequencies of these waves are twice that of the transmitted or fundamental frequency (second harmonic). The source pressure of the fundamental wave and the second harmonic wave has a non-linear relationship.

The second harmonic signals are separated from the fundamental echoes using filters or "phase inversion technology" based on the elimination of the fundamental pulse by transmitting a second pulse 180 degrees out of phase with the first pulse, down each ultrasound line. Upon receiving the paired echo, the signals are summed. Linear echoes at fundamental frequency cancel while the non-linear harmonic echoes are added and further processed. Since the harmonic signals are generated in the tissues during propagation of the fundamental pulse, they are not distorted by near field artifacts, where the weaker side-lobes and scatter play an important role. This greatly improves the lateral resolution and signal-to-noise ratio (16, 17). Further improvement of the image resolution is achieved by an increase in the axial resolution due to the higher frequency of the second harmonic waves. Together, these improvements have led to a significant increase in the detection rate of small focal liver lesions (18).

The full benefit of tissue harmonic imaging can only be exploited when this technology is used in conjunction with the new micro-bubble contrast agents. At low acoustic powers, micro-bubbles (<10 $\mu$m) behave as linear backscatterers, alternatively contracting and expanding according to the positive and negative pressures of the sinusoidal sound waves. As acoustic power increases, the gas-filled micro-bubbles start to resonate in a non-linear or asymmetric fashion called "stimulated acoustic emission". The emitted sound waves contain frequencies that are harmonics to the transmitted fundamental frequency.

The intensity of the ultrasound emitted by the bubbles is augmented by up to 25 dB (greater than 300-fold increase) due to resonant behavior (19). The production of harmonic frequencies is due to non-linearity in the oscillation of the bubbles. At higher ultrasound powers the bubbles resist compression more than expansion. At still higher powers, bubble disruption or destruction occurs (20). Micro-bubbles are fragile and easily disrupted by ultrasound, even at diagnostic energies (19). Newer contrast agents with lower solubility of micro-bubble gases, however, are less susceptible to bubble disruption. This enables continuous imaging at low mechanical index (acoustic power) without the need for time intervals between scans for the replenishment of contrast agents (21).

To make a complete characterization of different liver lesions, it is important to obtain images reflecting all the different vascular phases: (1) the arterial phase (15–25 s after the start of the injection); (2) portal in-flow phase (40–55 s); (3) the full portal phase (70–85 s); and (4) the delayed or late liver-specific phase (180–300 s) (21).

The newly developed liver-specific micro-bubble sonographic contrast agents such as Sonazoid (Nycomed Amersham), Sonovist (Shering), and BR 14 (Bracco), accumulate in normal liver parenchyma but not in malignant tissue (21). This is probably due to a lack of normally functioning reticuloendothelial cells in primary liver cancer and liver metastases as compared with benign focal lesions such as regenerative nodules and focal nodular hyperplasia (22). The "pulse-inversion technique", which eliminates fundamental echoes, causes areas of malignant tissue to appear anechoic in an otherwise bright contrast-enhanced liver. High spatial resolution due to the high frequency harmonic imaging causes even small sub-centimeter metastases to appear sharply limited (23). The late phase liver-specific sonographic contrast enhancement is analogous to sulfur colloid scintigraphy and MR imaging with liver-specific contrast agents (19).

### 1.2.5. *Focal fatty infiltration*

Fatty infiltration is commonly generalized, but may also be patchy or focal where it appears as an area of increased echogenicity. The distribution may be lobar, segmental or subsegmental. Both focal fat and spared areas have a tendency to be pyramidal, with flame-shaped, tapered margins. These areas are often seen dorsal to the gall bladder or may include the region of the porta hepatis, near the falciform ligament, the dorsal left lobe, and caudate lobe (5). The less affected *spared* areas in a fatty liver may be misinterpreted as echo-poor lesions (24). Regions of fatty infiltration differ from masses in that normal vessels can be seen to pass through the affected portions of liver without displacement (25). These features usually allow differentiation from highly reflective metastases, especially important when fatty infiltration appear as single or multiple discrete areas of increased reflectivity (26).

Thus, fatty infiltration may be defined as increased echogenicity of the liver parenchyma without obvious mass effect and slightly impaired or poor visualization of the intrahepatic vessels and diaphragm (27).

### 1.2.6. *Cirrhosis*

Liver cirrhosis is a progressive disease characterized by fibrosis and conversion of the normal liver architecture into structurally abnormal nodules. In the acute stage there is a mixture of cellular necrosis, degeneration and inflammatory response. Later in this destructive phase, regenerative nodules start to form. At first the nodules consist of local proliferation of hepatocytes surrounded by fibrous septa. In more advanced disease nodules may independently reflect the different phases of the cirrhotic process (28). In this process hepatocytes of regenerative nodules may become less and less differentiated, and ultimately develop into HCCs.

Cirrhotic nodules are classified morphologically by their size in "micronodular" cirrhosis where the nodules are <3 mm and in "macronodular" cirrhosis which is characterized by many nodules being >3 mm (29). Hepatocellular carcinoma more commonly arises in macronodular cirrhosis. The regenerative nodules, which consist of local hepatocyte proliferation surrounded by fibrous septa, develop as part of the repair process. Their blood supply is similar to that of normal liver, mainly from the portal vein with a small arterial contribution (29).

Surface nodularity is usually readily detected by US when ascites is present, but is much more difficult when it is absent. On ultrasound this nodularity of the liver may be looked for at the anterior or superficial surfaces, preferably using high resolution linear array transducers. However, in a recent study using standard sector- and curved-array transducers, the sensitivity of sonography for detecting surface nodularity was greater for deep surfaces that abut on the retroperitoneal ligamentous, or pericholecystic fat (86%), as compared with that (53%) of the superficial surfaces (28). The only other notable cause of surface nodularity is multiple subcapsular tumor nodules, usually from metastasis. Rarely, surface nodularity may be caused by involution from treated metastases or from liver necrosis with parenchymal collapse (5).

The essential ultrasonographic features of liver cirrhosis are increased parencymal echogenicity due to replacement by fibrous tissue and a concomitant loss of definition of portal vein wall (9, 30–32). In contrast to fatty infiltration, there is no significant increase in attenuation, which is useful in distinguishing fibrosis from fatty infiltration. This is especially important in alcoholic disease, where the two pathologies often co-exist (7, 33).

It is also important to look for redistribution of the liver volume toward the caudate and left lobe, especially the lateral segment, as well as splenomegaly, ascites and varices in the more advanced stages (28). The caudate and left lobes tend to be relatively less affected by cirrhosis than the right lobe, sometimes resulting in a small right lobe with left and caudate lobe hypertrophy, especially in hepatitis B (5).

In liver disease with few liver parenchymal changes and portal hypertension, color Doppler sonography may be useful in demonstrating portal vein flow reversal or portal collaterals, which indicate severe liver disease. Concomitantly, there may be conspicuously enlarged and tortuous hepatic arteries with increased flow. These arteries may appear together with portal thrombosis, portal vein flow reversal, and portosystemic shunts. The normal main portal vein measures slightly more than 1 cm in diameter. Although only marginally useful, an increase in size to a diameter of >13 mm may be used as a sign of possible portal hypertension. More valuable is the lack of respiratory variation in size (increase during inspiration and a decrease during expiration), which may sometimes be the sole indication of portal hypertension (5, 34). The most common collaterals occurring in portal hypertension are left gastric (coronary) and paraumbilical (recanalized umbilical) veins. Left gastric vein collaterals, although by far the most frequent porto-systemic collaterals, are often difficult to visualize because of their deep location in the lesser omentum. The tissue distortion associated with cirrhosis may also lead to the narrowing of the hepatic veins due to compression.

### 1.2.7. *Budd-Chiari syndrome*

This is caused by partial or complete obstruction of the hepatic venous outflow. The obstruction may be central or peripheral and is occasionally a result of an inferior vena caval web, but is more frequently associated with hypercoagulable states. If the venous obstruction is complete and of rapid onset, patients usually die of acute liver failure. Those who present for ultrasound examination usually have a disease of slow onset and with the sparing of one or more of the major hepatic veins. The ultrasound features in the acute phase are of hepatomegaly and ascites combined with relatively normal spleen size. Later thrombus may form within the major hepatic veins which may be difficult to detect by Doppler. This condition may also be associated with the reverse flow in the portal vein.

### 1.2.8. *Liver cysts*

Ultrasound is highly accurate in the demonstration of liver cysts including features like cyst smoothness and regularity, septa, fluid levels and possible internal echoes and posterior acoustic enhancement. Simple hepatic cysts may be primary or secondary. Primary liver cysts are congenital and arise from developmental defects in the formation of bile ducts. These cysts tend to be superficial and are lined with cuboidal epithelium. They have an average size of 3 cm and are rarely palpable and usually do not cause liver enlargement. Occasionally, simple cysts may present with pain and a right upper quadrant mass secondary to haemorrhage or infection (35).

Acquired cysts are usually secondary to trauma, inflammation or parasitic infection and are often indistinguishable from primary cysts on ultrasound. The diagnostic accuracy of ultrasound in the diagnosis of simple liver cysts approaches 100%. The differential diagnosis includes a necrotic metastasis, hydatid cyst, hepatic cystadenocarcinoma, haematoma or abscess. Currently, simple liver cysts that have become symptomatic are drained under sonographic guidance, followed by the introduction of a sclerosing agent such as 96% ethanol. Re-accumulation of fluid after this procedure is nearly always temporary (36).

Multiple cysts in the liver occasionally occur as an isolated phenomenon; however, they are most commonly seen in patients with underlying adult polycystic liver disease. The majority of patients with this disease also have renal cysts. Polycystic liver disease is more likely to be symptomatic than single cysts, the most common presentation being hepatomegaly. These may benefit the most by image guided drainage followed by sclerotherapy (36).

### 1.2.9. *Echinococcal cysts (hydatid disease)*

Hydatid disease is a parasitic disease caused by one of the two species of Echinococcus: Echinococcus granulosus (cystic hydatid disease) or Echinococcus multilocularis (alveolar hydatid disease). Infection with the eggs of the dog tapeworm occurs most commonly in persons who raise sheep or cattle, and who have contact with dogs. Echinococcus granulosus which causes unilocular hydatid disease, are typically ingested during play with dogs or through consumption of garden vegetables or water contaminated by dog feces. Cysts develop mostly in the liver where more than half of the cysts are found, and less frequently in the lung, but any internal organ or bone can be infected (37).

A solitary or single cyst may vary from 1 to 20 cm in size and may be indistinguishable from a simple congenital liver cyst. The liver tissue between the cysts appear normal. The following features indicate hydatid cysts: (1) wall calcification which hardly ever is found in simple cysts. Inactive lesions may have a complete rind of calcification (38); (2) debris consisting of sand or scolices which are best seen when the patient changes position during the ultrasound examination; (3) daughter cysts which develop from the lining germinal membrane, these may appear as cysts enclosed within a cyst (39). The hydatid cysts which are classified as noncomposite include simple (uniloculated) cysts, cysts with a daughter cyst, cysts containing coarse echoes, or cysts with a partially detached germinal layer. Composite cysts may have either a rosette or honeycomb pattern (large number of small daughter cysts leaving no space inside the mother cyst). In the absence of membrane separation or daughter cyst formation, the differentiation from other cystic lesions may be difficult (40).

Recent reports indicate that the PAIR (puncture, aspirate, injection of scolicidal agents into the cyst cavity, and reaspirate) technique combined with albendazole therapy is an effective and safe alternative to surgery for the treatment of uncomplicated hydatid cysts of the liver and requires a shorter hospital stay. Treatment of alveolar hydatid disease is based on radical surgical resection of parasitic lesion and many years of chemotherapy or in some cases of extensive hepatic disease, and liver transplantation (41, 42).

### 1.2.10. *Pyogenic abscess*

Pyogenic liver abscess is a condition with significant mobidity and mortality. Hematogenous spread from distant foci was common in the past. In more recent series, liver abscesses most frequently arise as a complication to biliary tract disease, mostly by portal venous spread to the liver (43, 44).

The causative organism is commonly Escherichia coli, Klebsiella and streptococcus milleri but anaerobic bacteria are also found. Fever and chills, leucocytosis and elevated alkaline phosphatase are the most common clinical and laboratory findings (43, 44).

Abdominal ultrasound may be diagnostic for liver abscesses in >90% of cases (43, 44). The abscesses tend to be visualized on ultrasound as sperical, oval or slightly irregular echo-poor lesions with distal attenuation in three-quaters of cases (45). A significant number of these may contain echogenic material including bubbles of gas and thus appear to be more echogenic than the surrounding liver parenchyma (46). The differential diagnosis of an abscess includes complicated hepatic cysts and necrotic tumors. A pyogenic or amoebic abscess, for example, can simulate a metastasis but the liver is usually locally tender and the history of fever is suggestive.

The treatment of choice is percutaneous abscess drainage (PAD) guided by ultrasound, CT, and fluoroscopy (47). In most centers, CT is the preferred modality for imaging abscesses due to its ability to visualize the entire abdomen and retroperitoneum despite distended bowel or overlying bandages. Once an abscess is identified by CT, US may be well suited to guide catheter insertion, especially for peripheral liver abscesses (48). Indications for PAD continue to expand, and currently almost all abscesses are considered amenable (47). Simple unilocular abscesses are cured almost uniformly by PAD while more complicated abscesses, such as those with enteric fistulas or pancreatic abscesses, have cure rates ranging from 65% to 90% (47).

### 1.2.11. *Amoebic abscess*

Amoebic liver abscess should be suspected in travelers returning from endemic areas or in immuno-compromised patients who present with fever, right upper quadrant pain, hepatomegaly, and a liver lesion on the US or CT scan. The disease is contracted by ingesting the entamoeba histolytica in contaminated food and water. The ingested trophozoites colonize and ulcerate the colon with subsequent spread of the amoebae through the portal venous system to the liver where abscess formation may occur in 25% of the infected patients (48).

An amoebic abscess can be indistinguishable from a pyogenic abscess, but ought to be suspected when appearing as punched-out lesions lacking significant wall echoes. The abscesses tend to be subcapsular, hypoechogenic, oval or round lesions with a homogenous pattern of internal echoes and increased sound transmission. (48).

Currently the primary mode of treatment of amoebic liver abscess is the administration of oral or intravenous metronidazole for approximately 14 days. The drug is effective against luminal cysts in only 50% of patients and another luminal antiamoebic agent may be needed to eradicate the parasite. Image-guided drainage of an amoebic liver abscess is indicated in patients who do not respond to antimicrobial therapy or who are at risk of abscess rupture (49).

### 1.2.12. *Lipomas*

Lipomas, which show the typical high reflectivity of fatty tumors, are rare primary benign tumors arising from mesenchymal elements (50). They are non-encapsulated and in continuity with the normal liver parenchyma.

### 1.2.13. *Hematoma*

The etiology of a liver hematoma may be blunt abdominal trauma or rupture of a neoplasm such as a hepatic adenoma or cavernous hemangioma. The hematoma may be centrally located, subcapsular or in the most severe cases rupture of both the liver and its capsule.

An acute central hematoma tends to be highly reflective because of fibrin and erythrocytes forming multiple acoustic interfaces. With time, the clot undergoes liquefaction, causing a reduction in echogenicity. The size of the lesion may increase due to osmotic absorption of fluid and eventually over a period of months the hematoma may become completely cystic with fibrous strands traversing the lumen. Eventually, the lesion resolves leaving a residual fibrous scar or a small cystic space.

### 1.2.14. *Cavernous hemangiomas*

Benign hepatic neoplasms are rare with the exception of the cavernous hemangioma, which is the most common benign tumor of the liver with a prevalence of 4% to 7% (51). They are usually congenital and are known for their lack of growth over time. The tumor is composed of a network of vascular endothelial-lined spaces filled with blood. In the majority of patients, this is asymptomatic and requires no treatment.

The commonest (60–70%) sonographic appearance of hemangiomas (Fig. 6) is a homogeneously strongly echogenic focal lesion less than 3 cm in diameter (52). They may or may not have small central areas of hypoechogenicity. Not infrequently, hemangiomas show posterior acoustic enhancement (52). The margins are well defined but irregular (53). Atypical features are more common in larger lesions. These include heterogeneous echogenicity areas due to necrosis, hemorrhage, partial thrombosis or scarring and sometimes calcification (19). These lack evidence of invasion and there is usually no mass effect, at least when the hemangiomas are small. In contrast to highly echogenic metastases, hemangionomas lack the echo-poor halo that may be seen around metastases. Hemangiomas are usually solitary and are mostly found in a subcapsular or perivascular position.

A number of other benign conditions and lesions including focal fatty changes, adenomas, focal nodular hyperplasia and, lipoma as well as malignant lesions, especially hepatocellular carcinomas, can mimic hemangiomas at ultrasonography (53).

In liver cirrhosis, however, the differential diagnosis of a hemangioma-like lesion may be somewhat more complicated. In a recent study of 1,982 patients with newly diagnosed liver cirrhosis, US depicted hemangioma-like lesions in 44 patients. These small hyperechogenic lesions consisted of 22 hemangiomas and 22 hepatocellular carcinomas. Alfa-fetoprotein

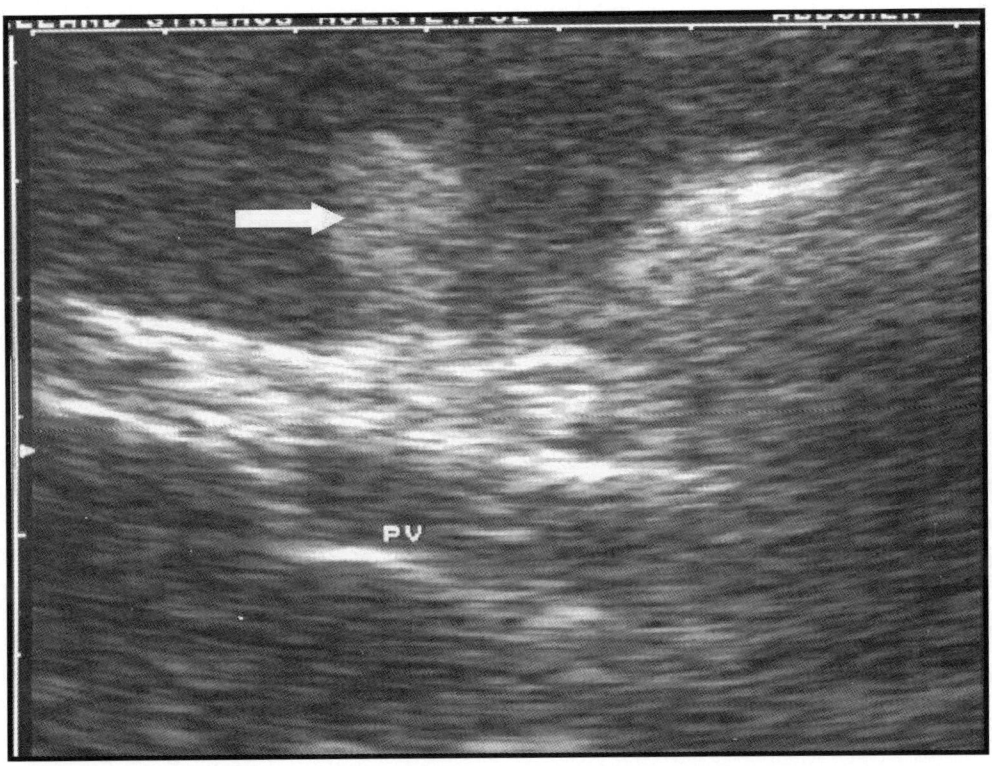


Fig. 6. View of the porta hepatis with an hemangioma (arrow) characteristically consisting of strong homogeneous echoes. PV — portal vein.

levels were of little use in the differentiation between the two lesions as only 22% of 383 patients with hepatocellular carcinoma in this series had $\alpha$-fetoprotein levels suggestive of the diagnosis (53).

In asymptomatic patients with no known history of malignancy or liver disease, however, a classical US pattern consistent with hemangioma may be regarded as diagnostic, obviating the need for further imaging (19). In patients with unusual ultrasound appearance, the diagnosis often needs to be confirmed by follow-up examination with US, CT, MR, or red cell scintigraphy. However, in some cases a reliable diagnosis of a hemangioma may be impossible without biopsy guided by US or CT (54). To confine possible bleeding associated with the biopsy, it is important that there is a long liver path.

Despite their vascular nature the blood flow within a hemangioma is too slow to be detected by conventional Doppler modes. Recently, micro-bubble contrast-enhanced power Doppler sonography has demonstrated peripheral nodular arterial enhancement with a pattern of solitary circular vascularity with no irregular intratumoral vessels followed by the classic delayed centripetal filling-in similar to that observed on contrast-enhanced CT or MR (19). The presence of this vascular pattern is particularly helpful in atypical hemangiomas with central hypoechogenicity and usually allows reliable diagnosis with no further imaging (19).

### 1.2.15. *Focal nodular hyperplasia*

Focal nodular hyperplasia (FNH) is the second most common solid benign liver tumor with an incidence of 1–3%. It is multiple in 20% and measures less than 5 cm in 65% (19). It is often discovered by chance and most typically found in a subcapsular location in women of 20–40 years of age (55). Most patients are asymptomatic but up to one-third may have pain or hepatomegaly.

The pathologic findings of FNH are usually distinctive and characteristic. Histologically, FNH is composed of normal hepatic constituents (hepatocytes, Kupffer cells and bile ducts) in an abnormal arrangement. Contrary to true adenomas, which are always cold on scintigraphy, focal nodular hyperplasia may take up colloid. Therefore, the combination of a lesion larger than 2 cm in diameter on ultrasound (or CT) without a cold area on the isotope scan is almost diagnostic of focal nodular hypeplasia (56, 57).

On ultrasonography the lesion is a non-encapsulated, well circumscribed, lobulated lesion with a central stellate scar in 45% (19). The differentiation from a hepatocellular carcinoma (HCC), however, may present a problem. A hypoechoic rim (halo) around an intrahepatic tumor, has usually been considered to be suggestive of malignancy (e.g. hepatocellular carcinoma or liver metastases) (58). Recent studies, however, have shown that this hypoechoic rim is also frequently detectable in benign liver lesions such as focal nodular hyperplasia (FNH), benign liver adenoma, liver abscess, or atypical hemangioma (59). On US images focal nodular hyperplasia is usually homogenously isoechoic, but may also be slightly hyper- or hypoechoic compared with normal liver parenchyma.

As mentioned earlier, micro-bubble contrast-enhanced ultrasonography with liver-specific agents such as Levovist and Sonozoid, which are taken up by normal liver, has been shown to be highly reliable in the diagnosis of FNH. The diagnosis is primarily based on characteristic FNH vascularity including typical centrifugal filling to the periphery at the arterial phase and a uniform or lobulated dense stain at the capillary phase (19, 60, 61). This vascular pattern is both sensitive (83%) and specific (98%) of FNH (62). Small FNHs often lack these typical features and may therefore be confused with metastases especially in young women with breast cancer.

### 1.2.16. *Liver cell adenoma*

Adenoma is a rare benign neoplasm found mainly in young women. It consists of normal or slightly atypical hepatocytes but unlike focal nodular hyperplasia they do not contain bile ducts or Kupffer cells. Adenoma is closely associated with the use of oral contraceptives and is much more common in women (63). Hepatic adenomas may regress following cessation of the contraceptive pill. The mass is usually symptomatic with presentations including a palpable mass, right upper quadrant pain and hemorrhage either into the tumor or from rupture into the peritoneum. Up to 60% of patients with hepatic adenoma have areas of hemorrhage and necrosis compared with 6% with focal hyperplasia (57). Adenomas usually measure 8–10 cm at presentation and have have a propensity to malignant transformation and recurrence following resection (19).

Differentiation from focal nodular hyperplasia is important as this lesion may be followed conservatively while surgery is the treatment of choice for hepatic adenoma. Liver cell adenomas usually manifest as smooth solitary masses that are well marginated and completely or partially encapsulated. However, there are no definite ultrasound features that distinguish hepatic adenoma from focal nodular hyperplasia on conventional B-scans (57). The ultrasound pattern is variable depending on the amount of bleeding and the time that has passed since the bleeding took place.

Color Doppler may show large peripheral subcapsular vessels and sometimes central vessels but these are not usually as prominent as in focal nodular hyperplasia. Ultrasound contrast enhances vascular imaging which is usually (68%) able to demonstrate enhancement in the arterial phase, but contrary to FNH, does not demonstrate enhancement in the post vascular or late liver-specific imaging phase (62).

## 1.3. *Malignant liver disease*

With the exception of cysts and typical haemangiomas, definitive characterization of a focal liver lesion is often not possible on conventional ultrasound. Primary liver cancer comprises two major histopathological types: hepatocellular carcinoma (HCC) and cholangiocarcinoma (64, 65). The liver is among the commonest sites of metastatic involvement and its assessment is an important part of the staging of patients with malignancy.

Ultrasound visualizes liver tumors, whether primary or secondary, by the demonstration of a mass which is characterized by an area where the echogenicity differs from that of the surrounding liver. Most malignant liver tumors have an hypoechoic rim in the periphery of a lesion (sonographic halo sign). The importance of this sign was illustrated in a study where the halo sign was present in 88% of malignant liver tumors and in 14% of benign tumors, the positive and negative predicted values of the halo sign being 86% and 88%, respectively (66). The sign was especially important in differentiating liver hemangiomas from metastases. A malignant tumor may also be characterized by expansion or invasive

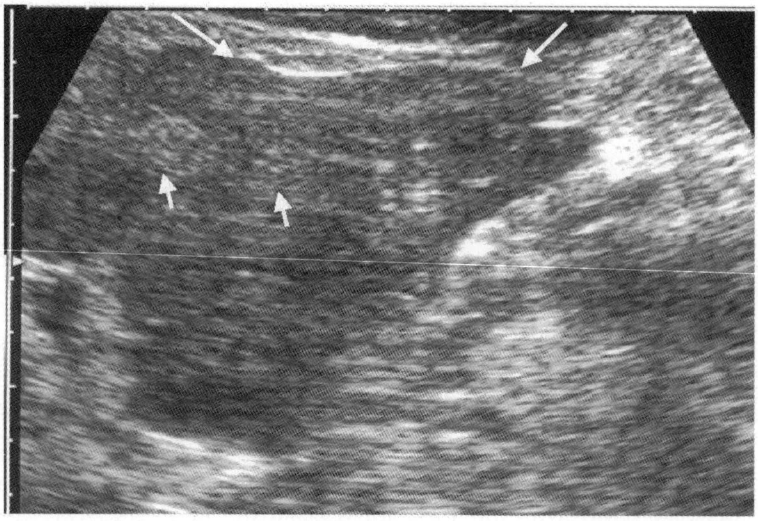

Fig. 7. Longitudinal section of the right lobe of the liver. Its bulgy contour (long arrows) is seen more easily than the individual liver metastases (short arrows).

growth. Differing echogenicity is especially important in the detection of small masses. In contrast, larger masses may be suspected even when they are iso-echoic due to the displacement of surrounding structures such as hepatic vessels. This is especially evident when the mass lesion causes deviation of the normal straight or gently curved course of the liver veins. Tumor expansion may also have effect on the liver surface (Fig. 7) where a tumor may be suspected due to development of a local hump.

In liver malignancies, tumor vessels characteristically penetrate the tumor from one or several sites. They are usually both tortuous and irregular in outline (67). Hepatocellular carcinomas tend to be well vascularized in comparison to metastases where vessels are few and usually much more difficult to detect with both color and power Doppler.

Any type of liver tumor may invade vessels, but invasion is observed more frequently with the more aggressive types and is especially common in hepatocellular carcinoma (HCC). Invasion may cause thrombosis and obstruction of both the portal and the hepatic veins. Contrary to intravascular clotting, invading tumors tend to be echogenic and may expand the vessel. Arterial Doppler signals from within the thrombus strongly suggest tumor invasion contrary to blood thrombus. Occlusion is best detected by color Doppler imaging.

Bile ducts may also be invaded and occluded and thus cause intrahepatic duct dilatation. This is a specific feature of the cholangiocarcinoma, which typically obstructs the main ducts at the porta. Bile duct dilatation, however, may also be caused by other primary or secondary tumors. Mostly, obstructive jaundice occurs only when the main ducts are involved due to the livers large reserve capacity for bile excretion.

### 1.3.1. *Hepatocellular carcinoma*

Hepatocellular carcinoma (HCC) remains widely prevalent in tropical Africa and Southeast Asia and is largely related to chronic hepatitis B and C virus infection. Hepatocellular carcinoma, which occurs in three forms, solitary, multiple nodules, and diffuse infiltrative, is strongly associated with cirrhosis (present in 80% of the patients) and viral hepatitis (19).

The pathogenesis of HCC in liver cirrhosis is a multistep de-differentiation process progressing from regenerative nodule via dysplastic or borderline nodule to HCC (68). Dysplastic nodules, which are present in 15–25% of cirrhotic livers at the time of transplantation, contain atypical cells without definite histologic features of malignancy. The nodules may be classified as low or high grade malignant depending on the degree of cellular atypia (68). They are typically hypovascular lesions (68).

Compared with regenerative nodules, the dysplastic nodules more frequently show signs of neoplastic angiogenesis (unpaired or isolated arteries not accompanied by bile ducts). The number of unpaired arteries increases as the dysplastic nodules progress from low to high grade dysplasia to HCC (68). The HCCs obtain their blood supply almost exclusively from the hepatic artery.

Hepatocellular carcinoma in cirrhosis may be solitary, multifocal or less frequently diffusely infiltrative. Small HCCs (<3 cm) tend to be well-differentiated and commonly have a capsule. In contrast, the less well-differentiated tumors are often larger at presentation and tend to be associated with vascular invasion and metastases. The diffusely infiltrating HCCs grow rapidly and frequently invade the main portal and hepatic veins.

In many patients the only cure is liver transplantation. The survival of cirrhotic patients undergoing transplantation with solitary HCCs <2 cm is similar to that of patients with non-malignant conditions. In patients with 1–3 lesions <3 cm or solitary lesion measuring 3–5 cm, the 4 year survival rate is 75% (68). In a patient with cirrhosis every solid nodule of the liver must be suspected of being a hepatocellular carcinoma until proved otherwise.

Liver transplantation is of little use in cases of hepatic vessel invasion, lymph node metastases or in the presence of distant metastatic disease (68). Current surveillance programs in Europe aimed at early detection of HCC, include measurements of serum levels of alpha-fetoprotein and ultrasound imaging every 6 months. This approach has been adopted due to reported mean doubling time of 4 months in lesions <5 cm (68).

The sonographic appearance of HCC range from highly echogenic tumors to apparently cystic masses. Some have a mixed echo pattern with areas of both increased and reduced reflectivity. Most HCC (77.4%) are small (<3 cm) and tend to be poorly reflective (69). These small HCC are often demarcated by an echo-poor rim or halo. Approximately 50% of large HCCs are echogenic which usually is due to the presence of haemorrhage, fibrosis and necrosis (19). However, some of the small HCCs may both have increased echogenicity and lack the echo-poor rim characteristic of most malignant lesions and may thus be impossible to differentiate from hemangiomas by ultrasound alone (53).

Ultrasonography with the aid of guided biopsy (aspiration cytology and cutting biopsy) which provides diagnostic material in more than 90% of the HCCs and 100% of the hemangiomas, has significantly improved detection of small, asymptomatic, hepatocellular carcinomas (69), which has opened up new therapeutic options including radiofrequency ablation, cryotherapy, and percutaneous ethanol injection. These forms of treatment may also be regarded as worthwhile palliative options for non-surgical candidates (68). Detection of small HCCs is especially evident in sonographic screening programs. Here, more than half (55–65%) of the HCCs were smaller than 2 cm (70, 71).

The importance of early detection of HCCs was demonstrated in a recent US screening study. Here the rate of operability and feasibility of treatment by transcatheter intra-arterial chemoembolization (TACE) was significantly higher in patients with small asymptomatic HCCs than in patients with symptomatic tumors (72). Although hepatocellular carcinoma (HCC) is one of the most common malignant neoplasms in the world (73), there are relatively few patients with HCC who are candidates for curative surgical resection because of severe liver dysfunction caused by underlying liver cirrhosis (74).

Percutaneous ethanol injection (PEI) is now widely used in the treatment of HCC because of its ease of performance, safety, low cost, repeatability, therapeutic efficacy, and survival rates comparable to those of surgical resection. This was demonstrated in a recent study where the 5 year survival rates for small (<3 cm) HCCs were 59% in the PEI group as compared with 61.5% in the surgery group (75). The injection is best administered under sonographic guidance, because this real-time control allows for continuous monitoring of the procedure until the tumoral flow signal completely disappears. Residue of flow signals, which may be enhanced by micro-bubble ultrasound contrast, suggests incomplete ablation of the tumor and that ethanol injection must be continued. The inclusion criteria for PEI include a detectable lesion on sonography, no evidence of portal vein thrombosis, extrahepatic metastasis, or ascites.

In the differentiation between benign liver lesions such as focal fatty changes, adenomas, focal nodular hyperplasia, lipoma, hemangioma and malignant lesions consisting of hepatocellular carcinoma (HCC), cholangiocarcinoma and liver metastases, contrast-enhanced US may significantly improve diagnosis. This was illustrated in a recent study of tumor vascularity. By the integrated use of all three US methods, gray-scale, conventional power Doppler, and micro-bubble contrast enhanced power Doppler, a correct diagnosis was obtained in 86% of 85 liver lesions (76). In this study tumor vascularity was divided into different patterns: (1) radial arterial vascularity; (2) central artery; (3) irregular chaotic intratumoral vascularity; (4) circular vascularity pattern with or without branching vessels into the center of the lesion (76).

The so-called basket pattern of a fine peripheral network of vessels surrounding and penetrating a lesion on color Doppler may be seen in up to 75% of HCCs (19).

The different patterns found in the arterial phase are not specific. Radial centrifugal arterial vascularity with a central artery, regarded as typical of FNH, may be found in as many as 86% of the HCC patients (76). The circular vascularity pattern without branching vessels into the center of the lesion, regarded as typical of hemangiomas, may be seen in only 56% of the hemangiomas as compared with 33% in the patients with metastases (76). Irregular chaotic intramural vascularity with or without circular vascularity pattern, is considered characteristic for malignancy (e.g. hepatocellular carcinoma in cirrhotic liver or metastasis in noncirrhotic liver) (76). Most useful in the differentiation of HCC from regenerating nodules and focal nodular hyperplasia seems to be imaging with phase inversion sonography during the liver-specific late phase. Here HCCs, which contain abnormal liver cells, show enhancement defects.

### 1.3.2. *Biliary duct neoplasms*

Tumors arising within intrahepatic ducts are rare. They consist of the benign cystadenoma and the malignant cystadenocarcinoma and cholangiocarcinoma (19). The cystadenoma and cystadenocarcinoma, which can only be differentiated from each other by histology, usually appear as large intrahepatic multilocated septated cystic masses. It is important to look for intracystic papillae.

Cholangiocarcinoma is the commonest malignant tumor of the bile ducts. Only one-third are intra-hepatic (19). The tumor, which not infrequently is overlooked by US, tends to be ill-defined with low level echoes and may be detected by following the dilated ducts to where they terminate. The tumor infiltration may be limited to the duct lumen or just represent a thickening of the duct walls. In the latter type of patients, recent developments such as intraductal US may be helpful. Sonographic findings indicating inoperability of a primary liver or biliary tumor are invasion of the hepatic artery, portal vein and adjacent liver as well as hepatic or lymph node metastases.

### 1.3.3. *Metastatic tumors*

Liver metastases take most of their blood supply from the hepatic artery rather than the portal vein (77). However, these lesions are generally not particularly vascular lesions.

Echo-poor lesions, which may be produced by any type of primary tumor, are typical of most malignancies, such as carcinoma of the breast and bronchus. Echogenic metastases are generally easier to detect than those that are hypoechoic.

The appearance of metastases may differ widely within the same liver (Fig. 8). Echogenic lesions may be surrounded by a broad echo-poor band several millimeters thick and thus

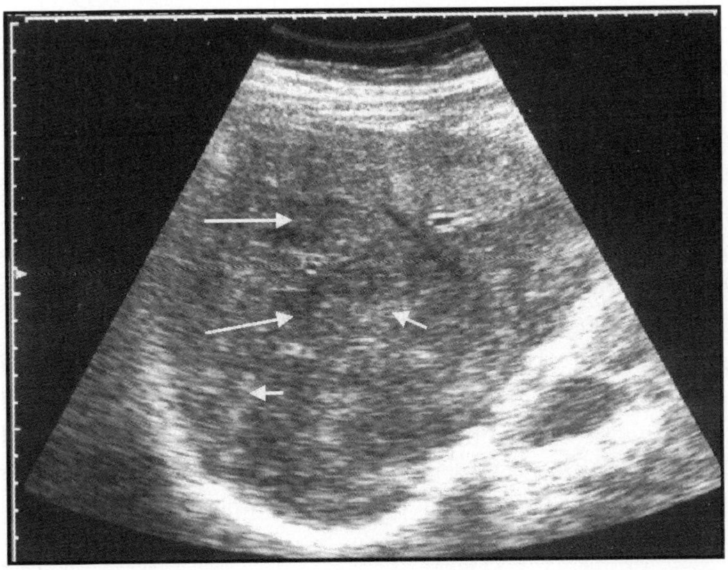

Fig. 8. Subcostal view of the right lobe of the liver containing innumerable metastases which represent a mixture of hypo-echogenic (long arrows) and hyper-echogenic metastases (short arrows).

present with the appearance of a target or "bull's-eye", or the tumor may be limited merely by a fine line (halo). Tumors originating in the gastrointestinal and urogenital tracts such as colorectal carcinomas and carcinoma of the ovary, pancreas and kidney tend to be associated with echogenic and target lesions, but may also produce echo-poor lesions or a mixture of both within the same liver.

In contrast to true cysts, the cystic area of central necrosis is surrounded by a shaggy wall and may be mistaken for an abscess. To reveal its progressive enlargement, repeated examinations over a period of months may be needed.

Calcified lesions have very intense echoes and may produce shadowing if the foci of calcium are sufficiently large. Calcification commonly occurs in metastases from colorectal and gastric carcinomas, as well as in neuroblastomas.

Diffuse involvement of the liver is a common feature of the lymphomas and leukemias, though in the former there may also be focal involvement (78). The leukemias and lymphomas tend to cause hypo-echogenic enlargement which involve both the liver and the spleen.

### 1.3.4. *Accuracy of ultrasound in liver malignancy*

HCCs have variable echogenicity and may be indistinguishable from dysplastic nodules and larger regenerative nodules because there is considerable overlap in their sonographic characteristics (68). The true sensitivity of sonography in a screening population is unknown because the frequency of false negatives cannot be assessed, but studies based on histological correlation of whole livers in transplanted patients show the sensitivity of sonography for HCCs to range from 30 to 50% (68). Improved triphasic helical CT techniques is slightly better than sonography, but still 60–70% of HCCs in explants remain undetected.

In small HCCs the detection rate may be even lower (40%) (68). Although MRI with dynamic super paramagnetic iron oxide (SPIO) enhancement detects more and smaller lesions, CT and MR are comparable in terms of classification for management (79).

In hepatic metastases sonographic detection is relatively poor (53–77%) (22). Most of the lesions not visualized on sonography are either small or isoechoic with the surrounding liver. The diagnostic sensitivity in lesions less than 1 cm is only 20% (22).

In a recent study, pathological analysis of explants showed that US did not detect HCC in more than 38% of the patients with this lesion and none of the patients with dysplastic nodules (80). Low diagnostic sensitivity of US (58%) with regard to HCC in cirrhotic livers has also been found by others (81).

The new liver-specific micro-bubble contrast agents such as Levovist used together with pulse inversion technique may significantly increase the detection rate of malignant liver lesions from 85% obtained by conventional B-scan to near 100% using liver-specific late phase contrast enhancement (82). All lesions showing enhancement in the late phase seem to be benign, while 90% of the lesions lacking enhancement seem to be malignant. All iso-echoic (invisible) lesions on conventional B-scans becoming visible in the late phase because lack of contrast enhancement seem to be malignant (82).

## References (liver section)

1. Couinaud, C.: Le foie: Etudes anatomiques et chirurgicales. Paris, Masson, 1957.
2. Bismuth, H., Surgical anatomy and anatomical surgery of the liver. World J Surg 1982; 6: 3–9.
3. Meyer, C. A., Colon, E., Provost, T. and Sherman, J. L., Delineation of surgical segmental liver anatomy: Value of PRISE, an MR fast scanning technique. AJR 1992; 158: 299–301.
4. Smith, D., Downey, D., Spouge, A. and Soney, S., Sonographic demonstration of Couinaud's liver segments. J Ultrasound Med 1998; 17: 375–381.
5. Tchelepi, H., Ralls, P. W., Radin, R. and Grant, E., Sonography of diffuse liver disease. J Ultrasound Med. 2002; 21: 1023–1032.
6. Niederau, C., Sonnenberg, A., Muller, J. E., Erchenbrecht, J. F., Scholten, T. and Frisch, W. P., Sonographic measurements of the normal liver, spleen, pancreas and portal vein. Radiology 1983; 149: 537–540.
7. Taylor, K. J. W., Riely, C. A., Flax, S., Weltin, G., Kuc, R. and Barwick, K. W., Quantitative US attenuation in normal liver and in patients with diffuse liver diseas: Importance of fat. Radiology 1986; 160: 65–71.
8. Shepherd, D. F. C. and Dewbury, K. C., Sequential imaging of the process of acute alcoholic hepatitis with ultrasound and isotopes. Br J Radiol 1980; 53: 163–165.
9. Taylor, K. J. W., Gorelick, F. S., Rosenfield, A. T. and Riely, C. A., Ultrasonography of alcoholic liver disease with histological correlation. Radiology 1981; 141: 157–161.
10. Dietrich, C. F. and Zeuzem, S., Sonographic detection of perihepatic lymph nodes: Technique and clinical value. Zeitschr Gastroenterol 1999; 37: 141–151.
11. Cassani, F., Valentini, P., Cataleta, M. *et al.*, Ultrasound detected abdominal lyphadenopathy in chronic hepatitis C: High frequency and relationship with viremia. J Hepatol 1997; 26: 479–483.
12. Scatarige, J. C., Scott, W. W., Donowan, P. J., Siegelman, S. S. and Sanders, R. C., Fatty infiltration of the liver: Ultrasonographic and computed tomographic correlation. J Ultrasound Med 1984; 3: 9–14.
13. Bashist, B., Hecht, H. L. and Harley, W. D., Computed tomographic demonstration of rapid changes in fatty infiltration of the liver. Radiology 1982; 142: 691–692.
14. Joseph, A. E. A., Saverymuttu, S., Al-Sam, S., Cook, M. G. and Maxwell, J. D., Comparison of liver histology with ultrasonography in assessing diffuse parenchymal liver disease. Clin Radiol 1991; 43: 26–31.
15. Goyal, A. K., Pokharna, D. S. and Sharma, S. K., Ultrasonic diagnosis of cirrhosis: Reference to quantitative measurements of hepatic dimensions. Gastrointest Radiol 1990; 15: 32–34.
16. Ward, B., Baker, A. C. and Humphrey, V. F., Nonlinear propagation applied to the improvement of resolution in diagnostic medical ultrasound. J Acoust Soc Am 1997; 101: 143–154.
17. Tanaka, S., Oshikawa, O., Sasaki, T., Ioka, T. and Tsukuma, H., Evaluation of tissue harmonic imaging for the diagnosis of focal liver lesions. Ultrasound Med Biol 2000; 26: 183–187.
18. Choudry, S., Gorman, B., Charboneau, J. W., Tradup, D. J., Beck, R. J., Kofler, J. M. and Groth, D. S., Comparison of tissue harmonic imaging with conventional US in abdominal disease. Radiographics 2000; 20: 1127–1135.
19. Harvey, C. J., Blomley, M. J. K., Eckersley, R. J. and Cosgrove D. O., Developments in ultrasound contrast media. Eur Radiol 2001; 11: 675–689.
20. Harvey, C. J., Blomley, M. J., Eckersley, R. J., Heckemann, R. A., Butler-Barnes, J. and Cosgrove, D. O., Pulse-inversion mode imaging of liver specific microbubbles: Improved detection of subcentimetre metastases. Lancet 2000; 355: 807–808.
21. Lencioni, R., Cioni, D. and Bartolozzi, C., Tissue harmonic and contrast-specific imaging: Back to gray scale in ultrasound. Eur Radiol 2002; 12: 151–156.

22. Albrecht, T., Hoffman, C. W., Scmitz, S. A., Schettler, S., Overberg, A., Christoph, T., and Wolf, H. K. J., Phase-inversion sonography during the liver-specific late phase of contrast enhancement: Improved detection of liver metastases. AJR Am J Roentgenol 2001; 176: 1191–1198.
23. Blomley, M. J. K., Albrecht, T., Cosgrove, D. O. *et al.*, Improved detection of liver metastases with stimulated acoustic emission in the late phase of enhancement with the sonography contrast agent SH U 508A: Early experience. Radiology 1999; 210: 409–416.
24. Kissin, C. M., Bellamy, E. A., Cosgrove, D. O., Slack, N. and Husband, J. E., Focal sparing in fatty infiltration of the liver. Br Radiol 1986; 59: 25–28.
25. Halvorsen, R. A., Korobkin, M., Ram, P. C. and Thompson, W. M., CT appearances of focal fatty infiltration of the liver. AJR Am J Roentgenol 1982; 139: 277–281.
26. Swobodnik, W., Wechsler, J. G., Manne, W. and Ditschuneit, H., Multiple regular circumscript fatty infiltrations of the liver. J Clin Ultrasound 1985; 13: 577–580.
27. Wilson, S. R., Rosen, I. E. and Chin Sang, H. B., *et al.*, Fatty infiltration of the liver: An imaging challenge. J Can Assoc Radiol 1982; 22: 7–32.
28. Filly, R. A., Shireesha, G., Reddy, S. G., Nalbandian, A. B., Lu, Y. and Callen, P. W., Sonographic evaluation of liver nodularity: Inspection of deep versus superficial surfaces of the liver. J Clin Ultrasound 2002; 30: 399–407.
29. Ward, J. and Robinson, P. J., How to detect hepatocellular carcinoma in cirrhosis. Eur Radiol 2002; 12: 2258–2272.
30. Sanford, N. L., Walsh, P., Matis, C., Baddeley, H. and Powell, L. W., Is ultrasonography useful in the assessment of diffuse parenchymal liver disease? Gastroenterology 1985; 89: 186–191.
31. Needleman, L., Kurtz, A. B., Rifkin, M. D., Cooper, H. S., Pasto, M. E. and Goldberg, B. B., Sonography of diffuse benign liver disease: Accuracy of pattern recognition and grading. AJR Am J Roentgenol 1986; 146: 1011–1015.
32. Gosink, B. B., Lemon, S. K., Scheible, W. and Leopold, G. R., Accuracy of ultrasonography in diagnosis of hepatocellular disease. AJR Am J Roentgenol 1979; 133: 19–23.
33. Garra, B. S., Insana, M. F., Shawker, T. H. and Russell, M. A., Quantitative estimation of liver attenuation and echogenicity: Normal state versus diffuse liver disease. Radiology 1987; 162: 61–67.
34. Ralls, P. W., Color Doppler sonography of the hepatic artery and portal venous system. AJR Am J Roentgenol 1990; 155: 517–525.
35. Roemer, C. E., Ferruchi, J. T., Jr., Mueller, P. R., Simeone, J. F., vanSonnenberg, E. and Wittenberg, J., Hepatic cysts: Diagnosis and therapy by sonographic needle aspiration. AJR Am J Roentgenol 1981; 136: 1065–1070.
36. Larssen, T. B., Viste, A., Jensen, D. K., Sondenaa, K., Rokke, O. and Horn, A., Single-session alcohol sclerotherapy in benign symptomatic hepatic cysts. Acta Radiol 1997; 38: 993–997.
37. Choliz, J. D., Olaverri, F. J. L., Casas, T. F. and Zubieta, S. O., Computed tomography in hepatic echinococcosis. AJR Am J Roentgenol 1982; 139: 699–702.
38. Itzchuk, Y., Rubinstein, Z. and Shilo, R., Ultrasound in tropical diseases. In Sanders R. C., Hiløl M. C., eds. Ultrasound annual. New York: Raven Press, 1983: 69.
39. Babcock, D. S., Kaufman, L. and Cosnow, I., Ultrasound diagnosis of hydatid disease (echinococcosis) in two cases. AJR Am J Roentgenol 1978; 131: 895–897.
40. Salama, H. M., Ahmed, N. H., Deeb, N. E. and Ahmed, R., Hepatic hydatid cysts: Sonographic follow-up after percutaneous sonographically guided aspiration. J Clin Ultrasound 1998; 26: 455–460.
41. Kaul, V. V., Friedenberg, F. and Rotstein, K. D., Hepatic cysts. Curr Treat Options Gastroenterol 2000; 3: 439–444.

42. Khuroo, M. S., Wani, N. A., Javid, G., Khan, B. A., Yattoo, G. N., Shah, A. H. and Jeelani, S. G., Percutaneous drainage compared with surgery for hepatic hydatid cysts. N Engl J Med 1997; 337: 881–887.
43. Mohsen, A. H., Green, S. T., Read, R. C. and McKendrick, M. W., Liver abscess in adults: Ten years experience in a UK centre. QJM 2002; 95: 797–802.
44. Wong, W. M., Wong, B. C., Hui, C. K., Ng, M., Lai, K. C., Tso, W. K., Lam, S. K. and Lai, C. L., Pyogenic liver abscess: Retrospective analysis of 80 cases over 10-year period. J Gastroenterol Hepatol 2002; 17: 1001–1007.
45. Terrier, F., Becker, C. D. and Triller, J. K., Morphologic aspects of hepatic abscesses at computed tomography and ultrasound. Acta Radiol 1983; 24: 129–137.
46. Powers, T. A., Jones, T. B. and Carl, J. H., Echogenic hepatic abscess without radiographic evidence of gas. AJR Am J Roentgenol 1981; 137: 159–160.
47. vanSonnenberg, E., Wittich, G. R., Goodacre, B. W., Casola, G. and D'Agostino, H. B., Percutaneous abscess drainage: Update. World J Surg 2001; 25: 362–369.
48. Ralls, P. W., Colletti, P. M., Quinn, M. F. and Halls, J., Sonographic findings in hepatic amoebic abscess. Radiology 1982; 145: 123–126.
49. Goessling, W. and Chung, R. T., Amebic liver abscess. Curr Treat Options Gastroenterol 2002; 5: 443–449.
50. Kurdziel, J. C., Itines, J., Parache, R. M. and Chaulieu, C., Adenolipoma of the liver: A unique case with ultrasound and CT pattern. Eur J Radiol 1984; 4: 45–46.
51. Ishak, K. G. and Rabin, L., Benign tumors of the liver. Med Clin North Am 1975; 995–1013.
52. Taboury, J., Porcel, A., Tubiana, J. M. and Monnier, J. P., Cavernous haemangiomas of the liver studied by US. Radiology 1983; 149: 781–785.
53. Caturelli, E., Pompili Maurizio, Bartolucci, F., Siena, D. A., Sperandeo, M., Andriulli, A. and Bisceglia, M., Hemangioma-like lesions in chronic liver disease: Diagnostic evaluation in patients. Radiology 2001; 220: 337–342.
54. Fornari, F., Filice, C. and Rapaccini, G. L. *et al.*, Small ($\leq$3 cm) hepatic lesions: Results of sonographically guided fine needle biopsy in 385 patients. Dig Dis Sci 1994; 39: 2267–2275.
55. Scatarige, J. C., Fishman, E. K. and Sanders, R. C., The sonographic "scar sign" in focal nodular hyperplasia of the liver. J ultrasound Med 1982; 1: 275–278.
56. Rogers, J. V., Mack, L. A., Freeny, P. C., Johnson, M. L. and Sones, P. J., Hepatic focal nodular hyperplasia: Angiography, CT, sonography, and scintigraphy. AJR Am J Roentgenol 1981; 137: 983–990.
57. Sandler, M. A., Petrocelli, R. D., Marks, D. S. and Lopez, R., Ultrasonic features and radionuclide correlation in liver cell adenoma and focal nodular hyperplasia. Radiology 1980; 135: 393–397.
58. Yoshida, T., Matsue, H., Okazaki, N. and Yoshino, M., Ultrasonographic differentiation of hepatocellular carcinoma from metastatic liver cancer. J Clin Ultrasound 1987; 15: 431–437.
59. diStasi, M., Caturelli, E., de. Sio, I., Salmi, A. and Buscarini. L., Natural history of focal nodular hyperplasia of the liver: An ultrasound study. J Clin Ultrasound 1996; 24: 345–350.
60. Kudo, M., Tomita, S., Tochio, H., Kashida, H., Hirasa, M. and Todo, A., Hepatic focal nodular hyperplasia: Specific findings at dynamic contrast-enhanced US with carbon dioxide microbubbles. AJR Am J Roentgenol 1991; 179: 377–382.
61. Strobel, D., Hoefer, A., Martus,, P., Hahn, E. G. and Becker, D., Dynamic contrast-enhanced power Doppler sonography improves the differential diagnosis of liver lesions. Int J Colorectal Dis 2001; 16: 247–256.

62. Dill-Macky, M. J., Burns, P. N., Khalili, K. and Wilson, S. R., Focal hepatic masses: Enhancement patterns with SH U 508A and pulse-inversion US. Radiology 2002; 222: 95–102.
63. Okuda, K., Kubo, Y. and Okazaki, N. *et al.*, Clinical aspects of intrahepatic bile duct carcinoma including hilar carcinoma. A study of 57 autopsy-proven cases. Cancer 1977; 39: 232–246.
64. Klatskin, G., Hepatic tumours: Possible relationship to use of oral contraceptives. Gastroenterology 1977; 73: 386–394.
65. Ishiguchi, T., Shimamoto, K., Fukatsu, H., Yamakawa, K. and Ishigaki, T., Radiologic diagnosis of hepatocellular carcinoma. Semin Surg Oncol 1996; 12: 164–169.
66. Wernecke, K., Vassallo, P., Bick, U., Diedrich, S. and Peters, P. E., The distinction between benign and malignant liver tumors on sonography: Value of a hypoechoic halo. AJR Am J Roentgenol 1992; 159: 1005–1009.
67. Ho, S., Lau, W. Y., Leung, W. T., Chan, M., Chan, K. W., Johnson, P. J. and Li, A. K., Arteriovenous shunts in patients with hepatic tumors. J Nucl Med 1997; 38: 1201–1205.
68. Ward, J. and Robinson, P. J., How to detect hepatocellular carcinoma. Eur Radiol 2002; 12: 2258–2272.
69. Sheu, J. C., Sung, J. L., Chen, D. S., Yu, J. Y., Wang, T. H., Su, C. T. and Tsang, Y. M., Ultrasonograhy of small hepatic tumors using high-resolution linear-array real-time instruments, Radiology 1984; 150: 797–802.
70. Oka, H., Kurioka, N. and Kim, K. *et al.*, Prospective study of early detection of hepatocellular carcinoma in patients with cirrhosis. Hepatology 1990; 12: 680–687.
71. Tanaka, S., Kitamura, T. and Nakanishi, K. *et al.*, Effectiveness of periodic checkup ultrasonography for the early diagnosis of hepatocellular carcinoma. Cancer 1990; 66: 2210–2214.
72. Shirato, K., Manabu, M. and Naohiko, T. *et al.*, Hepatocellular carcinoma. Therapeutic experience with percutaneous ethanol injection under real-time contrast-enhanced color Doppler sonography with the contrast agent Levovist. J Ultrasound Med 2002; 21: 1015–1022.
73. Simonetti, R. G., Camma, C., Fiorello, F., Politi, F., Dàmico, G. and Pagliaro, L., Hepatocellular carcinoma: A world-wide problem and the major risk factors. Dig Dis Sci 1991; 36: 962–972.
74. Okuda, K., Ohnishi, K. and Kimura, K. *et al.*, Incidence of portal vein thrombosis in liver cirrhosis. Gastroenterology 1985; 89: 279–286.
75. Yamamoto, J., Okada, S., Shimada, K., Okusaka, T., Yamasaki, S., Ueno, H. and Kosuge, T., Treatment strategy for small hepatocellular carcinoma: Comparison of long-term results after percutaneous ethanol injection therapy and surgical resection. Hepatology 2001; 34: 707–713.
76. Strobel, D., Hoefer, A., Martus, P., Hahn, E. G. and Becker, D., Dynamic contrast-enhanced power Doppler sonography improves the differential diagnosis of liver lesions. Int J Colorectal Dis 2001; 16: 247–256.
77. Ackerman, N. B., The blood supply of experimental liver metastases. Surgery 1974; 75; 589–596.
78. Scholmerich, J., Volk, B. A. and Gerok, W., Value and limitations of abdominal ultrasound in tumor staging — liver metastases and lymphoma. Eur J Radiol 1987; 7: 243–245.
79. Stoker, J., Romijn, M. G., de Man, R. A., Brouwer, J. T., Weverling, G. J., van Muiswinkel, J. M., Zondervan, P. E., Lameris, J. S. and Ijzermans, J. N., Gut 2002; 51: 105–107.
80. Kim, C. K., Lim, J. H. and Lee, W. J., Detection of hepatocellular carcinomas and dysplastic nodules in cirrhotic liver: Accuracy of ultrasonography in transplant patients. J Ultrasound Med 2001; 20: 99–104.
81. Gambarin-Gelwan, M., Wolf, D. C., Shapiro, R., Schwartz, M. E. and Min, A. D., Sensitivity of commonly available screening tests in detecting hepatocellular carcinoma in cirrhotic patients undergoing liver transplantation. Am J Gastroenterol 2000; 95: 1535–1538.

82. von Herbay, A., Vogt, C. and Haussinger, D., Late-phase pulse-inversion sonography using the contrast agent Levovist: Differentiation between benign and malignant focal lesions of the liver. AJR Am J Roentgenol 2002; 179: 1273–1279.

## 2. Gallbladder and Biliary System

### 2.1. *Jaundice*

Jaundice can be classified into three main groups: hemolytic (pre-hepatic); hepatocellular (or hepatic); and obstructive. It is caused by an increase in the serum bilirubin level above the normal range of 1–15 mg/l (1.7–25 mikro mol/l). The ultrasonographic features of parenchymal liver disease in jaundiced patients is mainly dependent on the underlying cause, most frequently hepatitis, cirrhosis, or primary or secondary malignant disease. Obstructive jaundice is due to the obstruction of the bile ducts between the liver cells and the duodenum.

### 2.2. *Biliary obstruction — cause and level*

Common causes of biliary obstruction include: choledocholithiasis; pancreatitis; sclerosing cholangitis; primary neoplasm; metastatic neoplasm. The level of obstruction may be divided into: porta hepatis (involving the confluence of the right and left hepatic ducts or the proximal 2 cm of the common hepatic duct); suprapancreatic (between the porta hepatis and the pancreas); pancreatic (within the pancreas) (1, 2).

#### 2.2.1. *Choledocholithiasis*

An estimated 15% of patients undergoing cholecystectomy for symptomatic or complicated gallstones have choledocholithasis (3). Despite absence of cholelithiasis, common duct stones may be present in as many as 4% of post-cholecystectomy cases (4), many of whom will present with abdominal symptoms without jaundice (5). The classic clinical presentations of choledocholithiasis include biliary colic, jaundice and fluctuating fever.

#### 2.2.2. *Sclerosing cholangitis*

Sclerosing cholangitis, both primary and secondary, may cause extrahepatic cholestasis as well as focal areas of dilatation within the liver. Due to the intrahepatic duct strictures, the irregularities of the duct lumen may give the ducts a beaded appearance (6). This appearance of the intrahepatic ducts may be mimicked by the rarely occurring diffuse form of cholangiocarcinoma (6).

#### 2.2.3. *Choledochal cyst*

Choledochal cyst, which is rarely diagnosed in adulthood, is also a potential cause of bile duct obstruction. In contrast to jaundice and abdominal mass found in children, the clinical symptoms in adults tend to be nonspecific (7). The diagnosis should not be delayed, as there is a 10 to 16% chance of malignancy in the cyst (7, 8).

### 2.2.4. *Caroli's disease*

Caroli's disease is a rare congenital hepatobiliary disease characterized by multifocal segmental dilatation of intrahepatic bile ducts affecting all or parts of the liver (9). In contrast to magnetic resonance cholangiography (MRCP) and endoscopic retrograde cholangiopancreatography (ERCP), sonographic diagnosis is difficult due to the need for demonstration of communication between the different cysts and the biliary tree, necessary for differentiation of Caroli's disease from other cystic diseases of the liver (9).

### 2.2.5. *Other non-neoplastic causes*

Bile duct obstruction may also occur at the level of the pancreas or the ampulla in cases of pancreatic inflammation or malignancy causing compression of the intrapancreatic part of the common duct. While the dilatation in acute pancreatitis tend to be transient and moderate, usually without involving the intrahepatic bile ducts, the fibrous strictures in chronic pancreatitis usually is more extensive and involve both extra- and intra-hepatic bile ducts. The sonographic appearance of the bile duct obstruction may be indistinguishable from malignant disease both on ultrasound and in surgery. Functional obstruction may also occur at the level of the papilla of Vater due to malfunction or strictures, sometimes being the cause of recurrent acute pancreatitis.

### 2.2.6. *Benign tumors*

Benign tumors of the bile ducts are rare. They include papillomas, adenomas, cystadenomas and granular cell myoblastomas. Papillomas and solid adenomas appear as solid, intraluminal masses that lack the shadow associated with stones. The cystadenomas are multiloculated cystic masses that originate from the bile duct epithelium. They usually do not communicate with the biliary tree and are most frequently found in young females. They need to be differentiated from other cystic lesions including among others echinococcal cysts, cystic metastases, and abscesses (10).

### 2.2.7. *Malignant Tumors*

Although rare, cholangiocarcinomas are much more common than benign tumors and account for about 20 percent of all "primary liver tumors". However, unlike the more common hepatocellular carcinomas, association with prior cirrhosis or hepatitis is not evident (11, 12). The anatomic distribution of cholangiocarcinoma is: the hepatic ducts, 15 percent; common hepatic duct, 35 percent; mid common bile duct, 32 percent; and periampullary, 15 percent (13).

Cholangiocarcinomas may develop at any level within the biliary tree, but demonstrate a tendency to occur at the junction of ducts within bile cysts, and in patients with ulcerative colitis, a disease known to be associated with sclerosing cholangitis (14). When cholangiocarcinomas involve the confluence of the right and left hepatic duct at the porta hepatis, they are referred to as "Klatskin tumors" (15).

Biliary obstruction due to lymphoma can be diagnosed on the basis of the extensive involvement of nodes in the area of the porta hepatis, associated with the involvement of other organs.

Most bile duct carcinomas are diagnosed at an advanced stage, after the appearance of jaundice in 80 to 100% of the cases. Early clinical mis-diagnosis of cholangiocarcinoma is a problem as approximately 60 percent of the more peripheral intrahepatic lesions present prior to the onset of jaundice (16, 17). At this stage there is a 83% resectability and 50% five-year survival rate versus a 58% resectability and 22% five-year survival rate in the jaundiced patients (16). Thus, for the early diagnosis of bile duct carcinomas detailed sonographic examination is necessary, and subtle changes should be subjected to direct cholangiography (16).

The nonspecific symptoms of cholangiocarcinoma such as pruritus, malaise, abdominal pain, and fever, may simulate the symptoms of cholecystitis, common duct stones, benign stricture, sclerosing cholangitis, and pancreatic tumors. In cases of necrosis of the tumor and relief of the obstruction, cholangiocarcinoma may also mimic gallstones.

Multifocal development may make cholangiocarcinoma indistinguishable from hepatic metastastatic disease on ultrasound, and from sclerosing cholangitis on cholangiography due to multiple bile duct strictures. In some cases, fibrosis may predominate, leaving hardly any neoplastic cells (17).

The ultrasound appearance of the cholangiocarcinoma may be that of an hypoechogenic, solid, mass with ill-defined margins or just as an area of infiltrated submucosa where the thickening of the duct wall constitutes a few millimeters. In these cases, the cholangiocarcinoma may be undetectable to both palpation by the surgeon and naked eye inspection by the pathologist (18–20).

In patients where the malignant lesion is limited to parts of the duct wall, new technology such as high frequency (20 MHz) intraductal and endoscopic ultrasound may be of great help due to its ability to visualize the different layers of the duct wall.

### 2.2.8. *Tumors derived from non-biliary duct tissue*

Obstruction from tumors derived from non-duct tissue include intrahepatic tumors, enlarged lymph nodes at the porta hepatis, carcinoma of the head of the pancreas, and ampullary tumors. The nodal nature of an obstructing mass at the porta hepatis may be suspected when the mass is divided into several discrete more or less oval masses. Biopsy is required for accurate distinction between lymphoma and metastases which most frequently come from the stomach, pancreas, colon, and breast.

Surgically, the periampullary tumors form a subgroup that is clinically, and even histologically, indistinguishable and comprise tumors derived from the common bile duct, pancreas, and duodenum. Those derived from the common bile duct constitute only 8 percent of the tumors. Cancers that grow from the ampulla nearly always can be removed, and survival rates are acceptable (33% at 5 years) (6). The ampullary cancers are difficult to identify on ultrasound. Their existence, however, may be suspected in the presence of a dilated common duct and a normal head of the pancreas, especially if pancreatic duct dilatation is also detected.

Ultrasound is also important in the assessment of tumor resectability, which includes information about portal vein involvement and the proximal extent of bile duct involvement by tumor, liver affection as determined by lobar liver atrophy indicated by a small lobe with dilated intrahepatic ducts, with or without compensatory hypertrophy of the contralateral lobe. Hilar tumors are judged to be potentially resectable if it is possible to excise the tumor completely and still leave at least one lobe of nonatrophic and tumor-free liver with an intact portal vein (2).

Nonhilar tumors, are judged to be unresectable if any of the following are present: hepatic metastases; remote or marked lymphadenopathy diagnosed as malignant by fine-needle aspiration cytology; tumor involvement of the superior mesenteric vessels, portal vein, or gastroduodenal artery (2). Vessel affection can often be assessed by color Doppler imaging. Important are severe narrowing or occlusion of the vessel and if the tumor has continuity with the echogenic vessel wall, especially if there is disruption of the wall echoes at the tumor/vessel interface. Portal venous involvement can be assessed by color Doppler imaging with high accuracy (91%) (21).

### 2.2.9. *Bile ducts — sonography*

The intrahepatic ducts all drain into the right and left main hepatic ducts. After having emerged from the liver substance these ducts join to form the common hepatic duct. With the exception of the right and left hepatic ducts, non-dilated intrahepatic bile ducts are usually not visualized separately from portal and hepatic artery radicals.

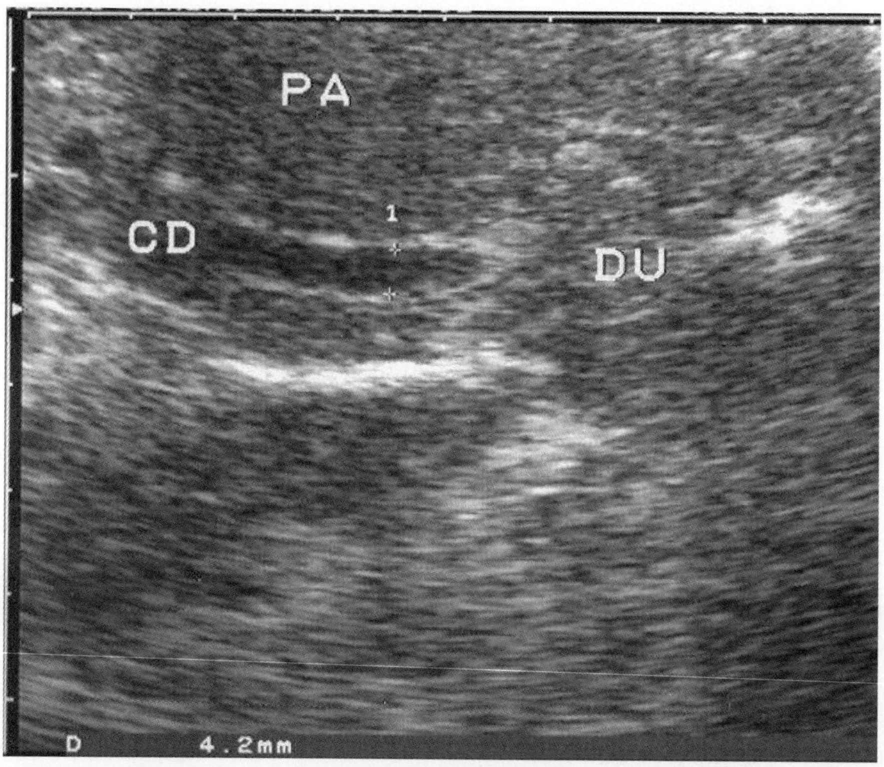


Fig. 1. Longitudinal view of the distal part of the common duct (CD) running through the dorsal part of the pancreatic head (PA) to enter the second part of the duodenum (DU). 1 — CD diameter = 4.2 mm.

Approximately 3 cm below the porta hepatis, the cystic duct joins the common hepatic duct to become the common bile duct. The exact point at which the cystic duct joins the common hepatic duct, however, may vary considerably and is difficult to establish. It may even unite with the right hepatic duct or join the common duct at the level of the pancreatic head. Therefore, the common hepatic and the common bile duct are often referred to as the common duct (CD).

The CD courses caudally, medially, and dorsally, for approximately 7 cm in the hepatoduodenal ligament. Here it lies ventrally and laterally to the portal vein and laterally to the hepatic artery. At the termination of the hepatoduodenal ligament, the duct dives dorsally and runs through the dorsal part of the pancreatic head (Fig. 1) until it turns right and empties into the second part of the duodenum at the ampulla/papilla of Vater. This last part of the CD is often insufficiently visualized by conventional transabdominal ultrasonography. This is an important reason why the diagnostic accuracy regarding the specific cause of obstruction is relatively low.

The cystic duct is a 3 to 4 cm long tubular structure, which may be visualized in approximately half of patients with a normal gallbladder and common bile duct. It is lined by mucosal folds which run in a spiral fashion termed the "spiral valve". These folds may sometimes cause an acoustic shadow, falsely suggesting the presence of a stone (22).

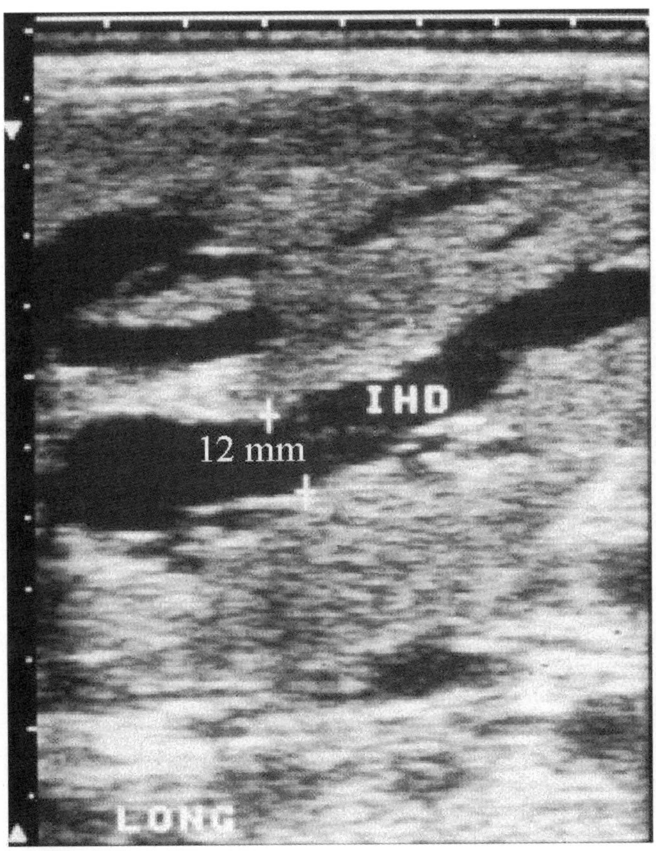


Fig. 2. Dilated intra-hepatic ducts (IHD). Note their irregular course.

### 2.2.10. *Dilated intrahepatic bile ducts*

Normal intrahepatic bile ducts are generally too small to be visualized on ultrasound. The larger main bile ducts, however, can be identified as tubular structures running anterior and parallel to the right and left branches of the portal vein. Dilatation of the intrahepatic bile ducts (Fig. 2) is indicated by the occurrence of multiple irregular anechoic channels without wall echoes, running parallel to portal vein radicals. Bile transmits ultrasound without attenuation and thus gives rise to increased through-transmission of sound. Dilated bile ducts are especially characteristic due to their extremely irregular course within the liver parenchyma, sometimes resembling the antler of a deer. Differentiation of bile ducts from hepatic veins, which both lack wall echoes on ultrasound images, is easy because the veins run in a straight or slightly curved fashion towards the superior part of the inferior vena cava while the bile ducts have a very irregular course and run towards the porta hepatis.

Diagnosis of bile duct dilatation relies on several sonographic signs including the "parallel channel sign" (23), which consists of longitudinal sections of the portal vein running parallel with a dilated CD of similar size and the "double-barrel shotgun sign", which is the same when visualized in cross section (24). The "too many tubes" sign relates to the added number of biliary ducts at the porta hepatis.

According to animal studies, bile duct dilatation spreads in a centrifugal fashion, starting with the common bile duct (Fig. 3) and ending with the most peripheral intrahepatic ducts near the liver surface (25). This sequence of bile duct dilatation, which is consistent with

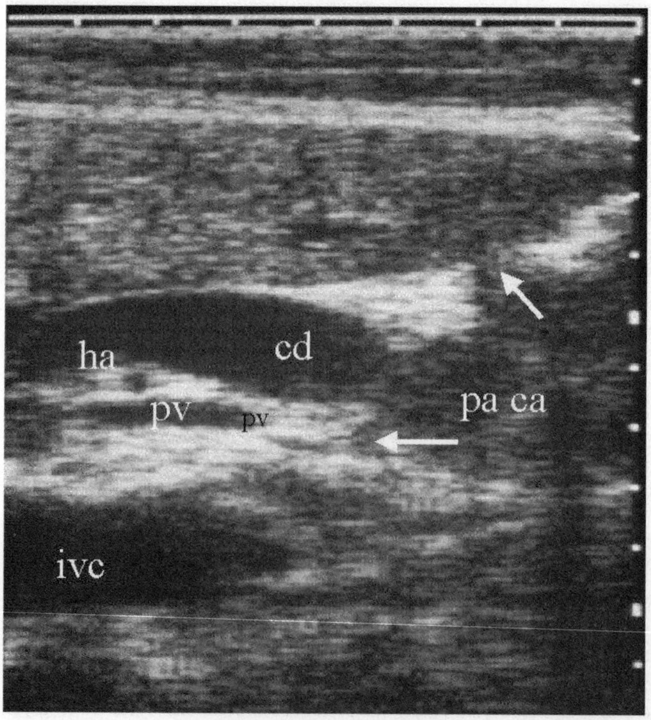


Fig. 3. Dilated common duct (cd) ending abruptly at a carcinoma of the pancreatic head (pa ca). Arrows show extensions of malignant tissue. ha — hepatic artery. pv — portal vein. ivc — inferior vena cava.

the law of Laplace, has also been observed in patients who had a mildly dilated CD in the presence of non-dilated intrahepatic bile ducts (26, 27).

### 2.2.11. *Dilated extrahepatic ducts*

Despite the obvious need for consensus, no upper limit for the normal CD diameter, measured at a standard position, has yet gained general acceptance (28). In standard textbooks, it says that the normal common duct should not exceed 6 mm and should be considered enlarged if 7 mm or more. Especially two papers are cited as the source for this upper limit. They represent two different ways of measuring the CD diameter (29, 30). In the first study by Sample *et al.*, the common bile duct was measured in the postero-lateral aspect of the head of the pancreas and/or the antero-lateral aspect of the hepato-duodenal ligament. Longitudinal scans of the common bile duct were inclined according to a line passing through the common bile duct and the main portal vein. The maximal inner diameter of the extrahepatic biliary system was determined anywhere along its course in either the transverse or longitudinal scan. The right and left hepatic ducts were considered part of the intrahepatic biliary system because they are located adjacent to their intrahepatic portions of the portal venous system (29). In the 17 patients with medical jaundice and measurable CD, the mean diameter was 3.6 mm, range 1 to 7 mm ($n = 1$). The size criterion, which would optimize the nosological probabilities important to screening, was 6 mm. The authors, however, pointed out that the 6–8 mm range must be regarded as equivocal where cases of surgical and medical jaundice would tend to overlap (29-Sample, 1978). The other frequently cited study is that of Cooperberg *et al.* also published in 1978 (30). In this study ($n = 100$), the common hepatic duct was measured in longitudinal sections at a point where the duct passes anterior to the right portal vein, visualized in cross-section. At this point, the right branch of the hepatic artery may be visualized in cross section as a circle appearing between the bile duct and the portal vein (30). The internal diameter of the common hepatic duct in this position measured from 1 to 4 mm, mean 3.2 mm.

When taking into consideration 95% confidence intervals for the number of subjects having CDs of 7 mm or more in these and other studies of normal patients, the upper limit most probably should be extended to include 7 mm (28, 31). This is especially obvious in patients over the age of 65 years (28).

The influence of increasing age on the caliber of the CD has been assessed in a large longitudinal study (4 years) in 1,018 patients aged 60 to 96 years. During the observation period the CD diameter increased with mean 0.4 mm, from mean 3,6 mm, SD 0.2 mm to mean 4.0 mm, SD 0.2 mm. This increase is equivalent to 1 mm increase per decade of increase in age (32). These figures are consistent with those found in cross-sectional studies of patients 65 years or older where the CD diameter ranged between 1 and 10 mm (31).

Another controversy is the influence of cholecystectomy on CD caliber. Recent longitudinal studies indicate that post-cholecystectomy enlargement, if there is any at all, is clinically insignificant (33–35). However, several authors have found wider non-obstructed CDs in cholecystectomy patients than in patients with an intact gallbladder. The upper limit of the CD in the cholecystectomy patients ranged from 10 to 13 mm (36, 37). The explanation for a larger caliber of the CDs in postcholecystectomy patients might be that they represent a different patient population, possibly with more severe disease.

### 2.2.12. *Factors that may influence the assessment of the common duct caliber*

Firstly, the CD diameter must be measured correctly. It is vital that longitudinal sections intersect the long axis of the CD. If not, the wall echoes no longer appear parallel and the lumen may appear smaller. Static B-scanners, used in the earliest studies of the CD size, were connected to a rigid scanning arm, which did not allow the same degree of freedom to adjust the scanning plane as when using real-time scanners. In transverse sections, the transecting plane must be perpendicular to the long axis of the CD. If not, the duct appears oval instead of circular, possibly leading to an overestimation of the CD caliber.

Although the gain settings of the scanner might be ideal for studying liver parenchymal disease, the settings can be much too high for optimal display of bile duct lumen, especially important when estimating CD caliber. Excessive gain tends to cause a "bloom" effect where the echogenic CD walls appear broader than their true anatomic thickness. This artifact of broadening which encroaches on the duct lumen may lead to an underestimation of the CD diameter (30)). This problem was especially related to the US scanners of the late seventies and early eighties. The artifact of broadening of the CD walls, therefore, must be taken into consideration when criteria for CD dilatation established at that time is applied to measurements by modern US scanners with tissue harmonic imaging (THI), where vessel walls in general appear thinner due to both better axial resolution and less side-lobe artifacts.

The walls of the extrahepatic biliary ducts are composed mainly of elastic fibers and connective tissue, little or no smooth muscle (38). Due to this elasticity of the duct walls, the CD caliber may change with the time of the day, respiration, meals, valsalva maneuver or patient positioning during the examination (32).

Passing of choledocholithiasis has shown that the CD may change in diameter by more than 50% within one week and sometimes within days or hours (38). Animal studies have demonstrated that the CD start to dilate as early as 4 hours after biliary obstruction and before significant elevation of serum bilirubin and even before dilatation of the intrahepatic ducts become evident (26). This elasticity of the CD walls limits comparison of CD diameters obtained by sonography with those gained by direct cholangiography where the contrast is injected under pressure (38).

### 2.2.13. *Sonography of the common duct — scanning techniques*

The ultrasound examination of the CD may first commence with transverse sections through the pancreatic head and uncinate process with the patient in a semierect position approximately 60 degrees to the vertical and in a right posterior oblique (RPO) position (45 degrees to the vertical) (39).

If overlying bowel gas obscures this region, the patient is given tap water or degassed fluid to drink, is then placed into a right lateral decubitus position for 2–3 minutes and is then rescanned in the semierect position. Transverse and longitudinal scans of the head and body of the pancreas are also obtained with the patient in this position (39). In difficult patients, intercostal views through the liver usually provides a good overview of the bile ducts and blood vessels at the porta hepatis. Color Doppler can be useful in differentiating blood vessels from bile ducts.

Sonographic detection of CD stones, especially in the distal part of the duct, is still regarded as difficult. This is especially due to gas in the first and second parts of the duodenum. The pancreatic part of the CD is usually well visualized, but the difficulty lies in being able to follow the distal part as it turns away from the pancreas to enter the duodenum at the ampulla (Fig. 4). The best views of the proximal CD are usually obtained with the patient in a supine left posterior oblique position or in the erect position.

Detection of choledocholithiasis can be substantially improved by scanning the intrapancreatic part of the bile duct alteratively in transverse and longitudinal fashion. In transverse sections, the CD is most easily identified at the posterior surface of the pancreatic head just in front of the inferior vena cava (Fig. 5), which is an especially important landmark when scanning the CD in longitudinal fashion. Longitudinal sections are obtained by turning the transducer slowly clockwise into a parasagital position. The ampulla/papilla is identified by following the parallel echoes of the CD wall towards the duodenum, which may be localized due to movements of its contents. A fluid load may further enhance definition of the duodenal wall.

In the assessment of level and cause of CD obstruction, it is important to find the transition point from dilated to narrowed/obliterated duct lumen. At this point careful attention should be paid to the appearance of the obstruction as this may provide information about the nature of the obstruction. Abrupt transition from dilated to obliterated would predict neoplasm, while gradual tapering of the common duct into and through the pancreatic head would suggest narrowing due to chronic pancreatitis (6).

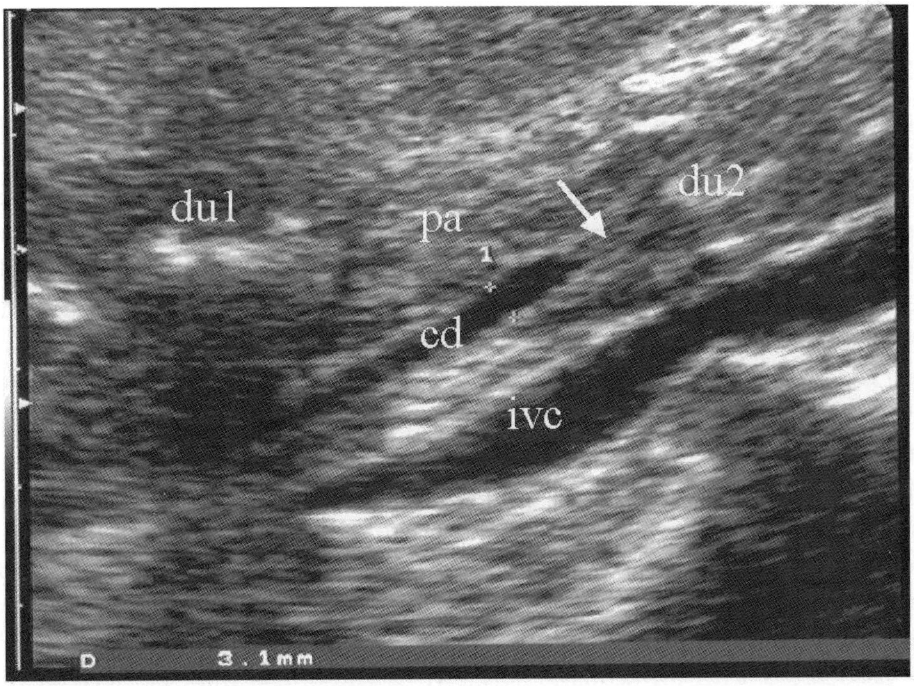


Fig. 4. Common duct (cd) as it passes behind the first part of the duodenum (du 1) to enter the second part of the duodenum (du 2) at the papilla of Vater (arrow). pa — pancreas. ivc — inferior vena cava.

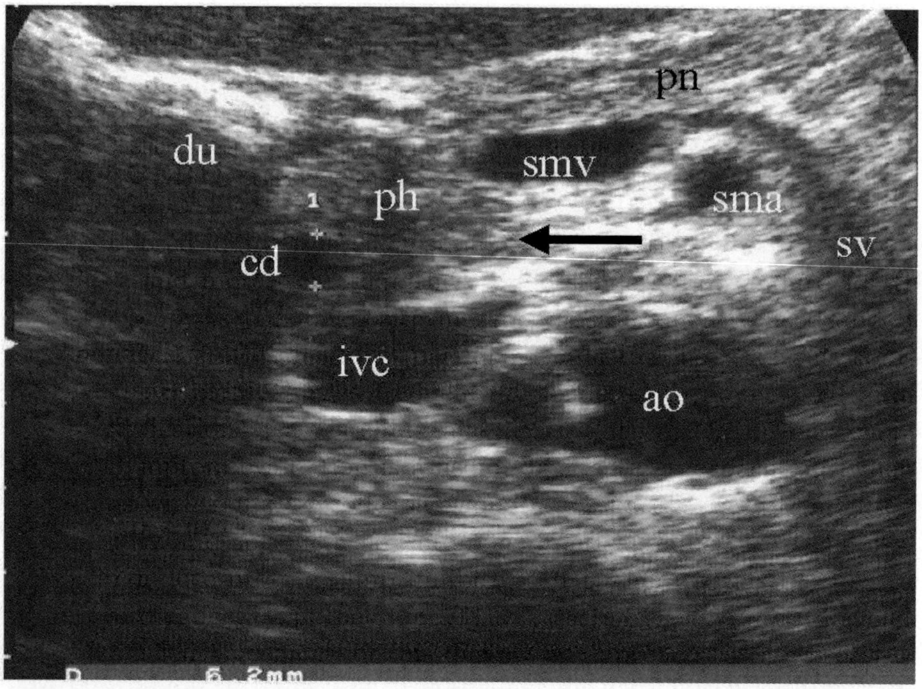


Fig. 5. Transverse section through the intra-pancreatic part of the common duct (cd). 1 — common duct = 6.2 mm. ph — pancreatic head. pn — pancreatic neck. Arrow — uncinate process. du — first part of the duodenum. smv – superior mesenteric vein. sv — splenic vein. sma — superior mesenteric artery. ivc — inferior vena cava. ao — aorta.

### 2.2.14. *The value of bile duct dilatation as sign of bile duct obstruction*

While the results of most studies show that the number of false positive sonographic diagnosis of bile duct obstruction is low, the opposite is well documented (6, 27, 40–42). False negative diagnosis of bile duct obstruction is mainly linked to choledocholithiasis causing intermittent obstruction. The stones, acting as a "ball valve", are often located at the very end of the CD and may not be detectable by sonography due to interfering gas-filled bowel (42). The number of patients with choledocholithiasis lacking bile duct dilatation range from 20 to 36% (27, 43–47). In one study, 9 of 10 patients with false negative obstructive jaundice had choledocholithiasis (27). On the other hand, choledocholithiasis may not infrequently (35%) have the opposite effect causing CD dilatation without jaundice (48).

Visualization of choledocholithiasis in normal sized CDs is very difficult, especially when the stones are small. These are also more apt to cast indistinct shadows or no shadows at all. Common duct stones that do not cast ultrasonic shadows, the hallmark of a biliary stone, represent a diagnostic problem. In such cases, the stone echoes may be impossible to differentiate from the relatively strong echoes of the surrounding tissues, including gas-filled bowel. The predictive value of non-shadowing stone-like echoes is considerably lower than echoes associated with an acoustic shadow, as these also may be derived from other intraduct pathology including blood clot, tumor or parasitic infestation. The frequency of non-shadowing CD stones may be as high as 21% to 33% (44, 49). Usually these stones are smaller than 3 or 4 mm but this phenomenon has also been observed in patients with larger stones. In such cases, the stone or stones may be mistaken for a tumor (50). Stones located higher up in the CD are more easily detected, but may not necessarily represent the true cause of the obstruction remaining undetected at the ampulla (44).

Therefore, the diagnosis of biliary obstruction seldom has to rely on detection of CD dilatation alone, which not infrequently leads to false negative diagnosis. At the time of US examination, the CD may appear normal or borderline dilated due to intermittent obstruction, the intrahepatic ducts appearing normal. Due to the lagtime in the rise and fall of serum bilirubin and liver enzymes, the patient may still be jaundiced despite complete relief of the obstruction having occurred days before. However, a fall in serum bilirubin levels prior to the US examination provides an indication of what has happened. In these patients with no or just borderline dilatation of the CD, the criteria set for enlargement become crucial (27).

Until recently, choledocholithiasis has largely been diagnosed by endoscopic retrograde cholangiopancreatography (ERCP). This modality has the advantage of accurate diagnosis, and treatment can be instituted at the same time. However, ERCP is invasive and associated with a morbidity of about 5%, and complications tend to occur more frequently in patients without stones (51). In several studies of suspected choledocholithiasis, ERCP was negative in approximately 60% of the patients (52). For these reasons, unnecessary ERCPs should be avoided and substituted for endoscopic ultrasound whenever possible.

Due to well-established benefits of laparoscopic cholecystectomy, this method has become the new gold standard for the treatment of symptomatic gallbladder disease. Although perioperative cholangiography is valuable and highly accurate in the detection of CD stones, its routine use is controversial because of its inherent disadvantages (53). Recent studies, however, indicate that ultrasound together with liver enzymes may predict which patients have a low risk of choledocholithiasis, thus avoiding perioperative cholangiography. This was demonstrated in a large study of 561 patients undergoing cholangiography before laparoscopic cholecystectomy where a CD >10 mm represented an independent risk factor regarding the presence of preoperative choledocholithiasis. Three levels of risk concerning the presence of choledocholithiasis were determined: (1) low risk group with CD less than 10 mm (73.8%), the prevalence of choledocholithiasis being 1.5%; (2) moderate risk group with dilated CD and normal liver function tests (18.4%), the prevalence of CD stones being 48.8%; and (3) the high risk group with dilated CD and abnormal liver function tests (18.4%), the prevalence of CD stones being 66.7% (53). In their following prospective study of 153 consecutive low-risk patients (CD <10 mm) who underwent laparoscopic cholecystectomy without perioperative cholangiography, there were only 2 cases of symptomatic choledocholithiasis. These were diagnosed postoperatively by ERCP and retrieved by endoscopic sphincterotomy (53).

In another prospective study, perioperative cholangiography was omitted in 57% of 1050 cholecystectomy patients. In these patients who met the criteria of low risk for common bile duct stones defined as common bile duct less than 5 mm, normal liver enzymes, and no history of acute cholecystitis, jaundice, or pancreatitis, there were no clinical signs of common bile duct stones on follow-up (54).

Another rare condition where cholestasis is associated with a normal calibered CD is when dilatation is impaired due to encasement of the common duct by tumor or fibrosis of the CD duct wall, as in sclerosing cholangitis (29, 55, 56). Similar impairment of bile duct dilatation has also been observed within the liver where the impairment of dilatation is caused by rigidity of the surrounding liver parenchyma in association with chronic hepatitis or cirrhosis (44).

## 2.3. *Sonography — Diagnostic accuracy*

### 2.3.1. *Medical versus surgical jaundice*

The reported sensitivity of sonography in diagnosing biliary obstruction varies considerably, ranging from 65% and 99% (23, 26, 27, 57, 58). Although, skill and equipment play an important role, most of the difference in results is most probably due to differences in patient material, especially with regard to the number of patients with obstructing choledocholithiasis. This may lower the diagnostic sensitivity to 80% in these patients as compared with 98.4% sensitivity in patients with obstruction due to other causes, mainly cancer (27).

Most studies report high diagnostic specificity (few patients with false positive US diagnosis of biliary obstruction) ranging from 87% to 100% (23, 26, 27, 57, 58). Also the diagnostic specificity can be influenced by the patient material, especially the number of patients with gallstone disease, as these tend to have a slightly wider CD than that found in normal subjects, irrespective of the presence of choledocholithiasis or not. False positive diagnosis of obstructive jaundice may also occur when an obstructing stone passes in the time between sonographic examination and confirmatory cholangiography.

### 2.3.2. *Level of obstruction*

The success rate regarding correct level of obstruction varies between 27% and 92% (1–3, 23, 59). The difference in results may partly be related to different definitions of terms such as "exact level" and "exact cause" of obstruction. Some of these definitions require complete visualization of the CD and detailed description of the obstructing lesion which may not be possible by conventional transabdominal US. Also, regarding the level of obstruction, the number of patients with choledocholithiasis plays a great role, as a substantial number of these patients tend to be without bilary dilatation.

### 2.3.3. *Cause of obstruction*

Concerning the cause of biliary obstruction, the results of sonography also vary considerably, ranging from 23% to 88% (1, 2, 23, 59). Common causes include benign stricture, gallstones, juxtapapillary duodenal diverticulum, bile duct mass, choledochal cyst with or without anomalous union of the pancreaticobiliary duct and ova of Ascaris. Obviously, conventional transabdominal US is bound to fail in patients with many of these lesions (60).

Thus, accuracy of US regarding differentiation between medical and obstructive jaundice, the level of obstruction and the cause of obstruction is closely linked to the patient material, especially the number of patients with obstruction due to choledocholithiasis (27). Sonographic detection of choledocholithiasis still constitutes a diagnostic problem.

Improvements of equipment and application of meticulous scanning techniques, however, has led to increased detection rate which may exceed 80% (1, 61).

## 2.4. *Gallbladder*

### 2.4.1. *Anatomy*

The gallbladder (GB) is located in a fossa under the right lobe of the liver. It has a thin, maximum 2 mm, smooth wall composed of an outer serosal layer, a middle fibromuscular layer and an inner mucosa. The bulbus usually represents the most caudal and anterior part of the gallbladder, which tapers into the body and finally the neck before joining the cystic duct.

The shape, size and position of the gallbladder are highly variable. The gallbladder may be totally absent, single, duplicate or triplicate, with a single cystic duct or with multiple separate cystic ducts. Sometimes the gallbladder is attached to the liver by a long mesentery and may be found as far down as the right iliac fossa. The neck, however, may still be found at the porta hepatis.

### 2.4.2. *Sonography — scanning techniques*

The sonographic examination of the GB should ideally be performed after a night's fast because in the non-fasted state the normal gallbladder is contracted and thick-walled, similar to a pathologically contracted GB. The thickness of the gallbladder wall is usually measured in the transverse section with the beam perpendicular to the long axis of the GB because oblique sections may give a false impression of wall thickening.

The gallbladder must be examined in both longitudinal and transverse sections. When viewing from the fundus with the transducer aligned along the long axis of the gallbladder, the whole lumen may be visualized by angulation of the scanning plane from side to side.

Intercostal or subcostal views (deep inspiration), using the liver as an ultrasonic window, allow the GB to be seen with minimum disturbance from adjacent gas-filled bowel.

The posterior wall of the GB is often located adjacent to the duodenum, which may cause acoustic shadowing that can be difficult to differentiate from that of GB pathology. In these cases a drink of water, which outlines the duodenum, may help rule out shadowing caused by multiple small stones.

Folding over of the fundus may mimic septation in some patients. However, rotating the patient into the left lateral decubitus position or prolonging the fast, may unfold the gallbladder. True septa are uncommon.

The GB volume is usually assessed after an overnight fast at increments of time (10 min intervals) after a standard fatty meal has been given. Fasting gall bladder volume, residual volume and ejection fraction may then be calculated using the ellipsoid model for volume calculation.

Detection of possible gallbladder stones usually involves scanning the patient in the supine, right anterior oblique and erect positions. However, there is a minority (4%) who benefits from examination in the prone position also. The patients are placed in the prone position for 1 min before the right side is elevated just enough to allow scanning from the midclavicular line, intercostally or subcostally (62). The use of different positions is especially important in differentiating small mobile stones from non-mobile polyps.

The GB may be successfully examined by many different transducers, most commonly by a curved linear array transducer with a transmitting center frequency of 5 MHz. In patients who are difficult to examine with US, however, there may be a need for linear array and sector transducers. These may have advantages regarding higher resolution and smaller "foot print". In patients with deeply located gallbladders, there is often a need for lower transducer frequencies.

### 2.4.3. *Gallbladder stones*

The prevalence of gallstones in the western world is approximately 10%. Of these, two-thirds are asymptomatic (63). The probability of silent stones becoming symptomatic is not more than 18% in 24 years (64).

Sonography is the preferred initial examination in patients with right upper abdominal pain or signs of gallbladder disease. The method provides valuable information on gallbladder and duct morphology, as well as contents. A suspected hydrops of the GB is an important indication for ultrasound examination. Because of variations in size and shape of the GB, it is difficult to diagnose a hydrops on shape and size alone. However, an obstructed GB typically appears more spherical than one merely physiologically distended. When the longitudinal axis of the GB exceeds 12 cm, physiological dilatation is unlikely.

The ultrasound images of GB stones vary according to composition, size, shape and number. The most common appearance is that of a highly reflective intraluminal structure which is gravity dependent and casts an acoustic shadow (Fig. 6). The predictive value of all these findings together is nearly 100% (17).

The appearance of an acoustic shadow behind a tissue structure depends upon how this structure absorbs and reflects ultrasound. However, whether a gall stone is going to cast a shadow or not is usually not dependent on its chemical composition. It is rather dependent on whether or not the stone occupies the full width of the ultrasound beam. Therefore, in order to increase the chances of a common duct stone casting a shadow, it is important to pay attention to the beam focus. While stone shadows tend to be sharply limited and nearly anechoic, the shadow due to reverberations appearing behind gas filled loops of bowel (Fig. 7) is usually weakly echogenic and more diffuse in its limitation.

The size of an echo-producing structure within the GB lumen is not a limitation, as it has been shown that particles as small as 5–10 mikro meter ($\mu$) will produce echoes within the bile (65). These particles do not produce acoustic shadows and thus do not fulfill the diagnostic criteria given above. Recently, tissue harmonic imaging has demonstrated advantages over conventional fundamental (frequency) imaging regarding lateral resolution, side lobe artifacts, and signal-to-noise ratio which tend to enhance shadow formation behind small gallstones (66). Repositioning of the patient may help small stones to be collected into a group, thus fascilitating acoustic shadowing. Small stones lying on the posterior wall of the GB, adjacent to bowel gas, may be easier to distinguish if the gain is turned down.

The gravity dependence of stones can be demonstrated by letting the patient take different positions including sitting and standing. Stones hidden in the the neck of the GB may thus come into view. Demonstration of stone motility is not always easy. This was

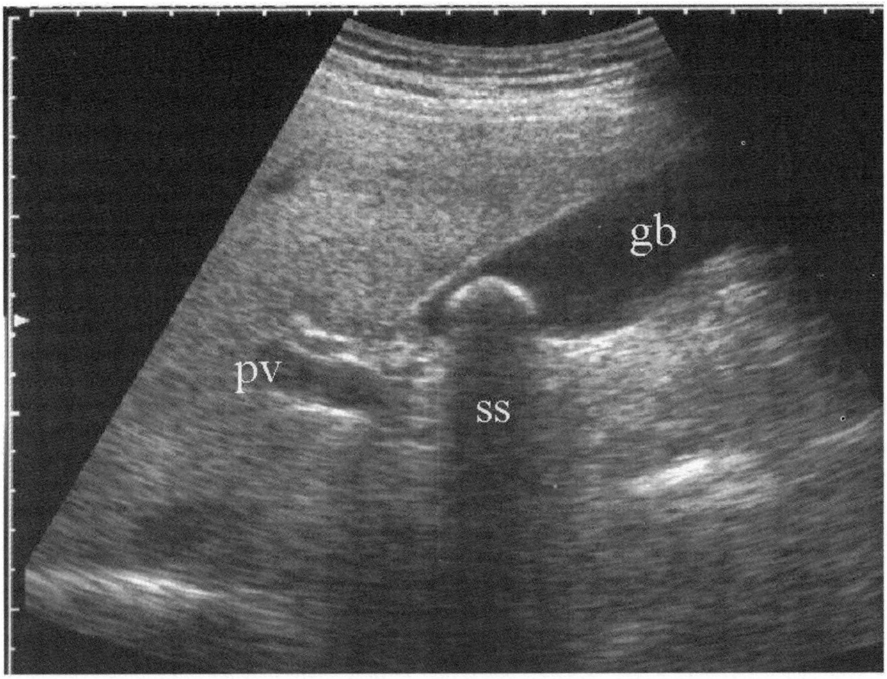


Fig. 6. Highly reflective gallstone located near the neck of the gallbladder (gb). ss — stone shadow. pv — portal vein.

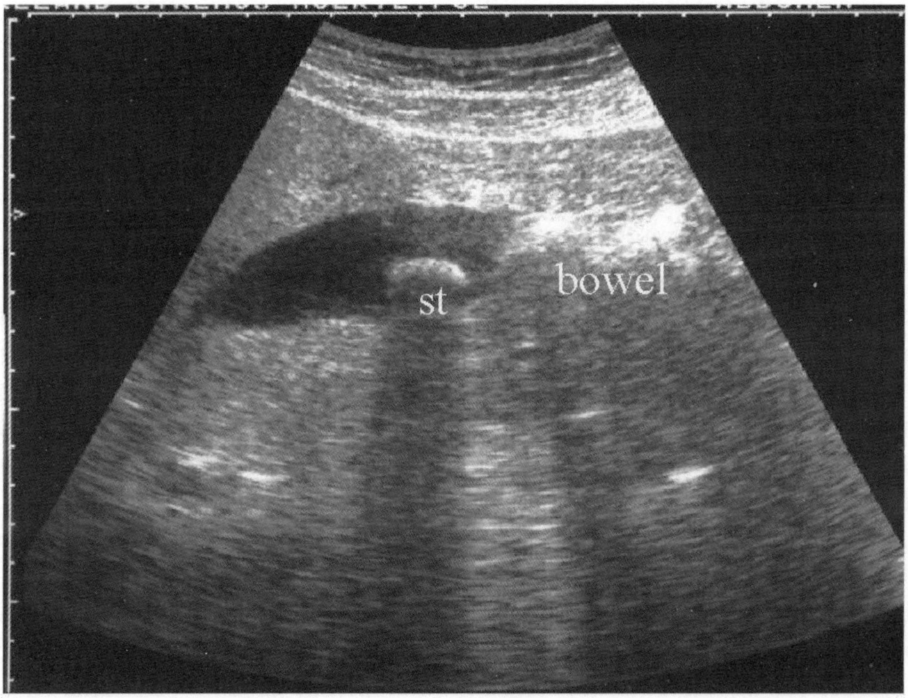


Fig. 7. Comparison of acoustic shadows derived from a gallstone (st) versus the less well defined shadow caused by gas-filled loops of bowel (bowel).

demonstrated in a histopathologic study of polypoid lesions, where 37% represented cholelithiasis, 41% cholesterolosis and only 5% true polyps. Therefore, many of the small polyps seen on sonography most likely represent a stone embedded in the gallbladder wall or other abnormality (67).

### 2.4.4. *Contracted gallbladder*

Congenital absence of the gallbladder is rare, being present in less than one percent. Thus, non-visualization of the gallbladder lumen on sonography indicates pathology. This may include a gallbladder totally filled with stones, or the GB wall has become fibrotic as a result of chronic inflammation, or bile is lacking due to obstruction of the cystic duct. Its presence may still be indicated by a distal acoustic shadowing emanating from the gallbladder fossa, representing a stone-filled lumen or a "porcelain" GB where the wall is completely calcified. This condition, however, is associated with an increased prevalence of cancer.

### 2.4.5. *Echogenic bile*

Non-shadowing, gravity dependent, echoes within the GB is commonly referred to as "biliary sludge" or "echogenic bile", which may arise from pus or blood in the bile or it may be seen in association with obvious stones in the gallbladder (68). However, echogenic bile may also be seen in the absence of stone disease, when there is bile stasis or in patients who are on parenteral nutrition (69, 70) or after surgery on the gastrointestinal tract (71). *In vitro* studies have shown that the echoes in "biliary sludge" are caused by particles 5–10 micro-meter in size, and chemical analysis reveals calcium crystals (65).

Occasionally non-shadowing echoes within the GB may clump together. These so-called "sludge balls" may mimic a soft tissue mass projecting into the GB lumen. Movement may be very slow due to thick and viscid bile. All solid appearing lesions should be tested with regard to Doppler signals as detection of blood vessels within the lesion would indicate a solid lesion.

### 2.4.6. *Wall thickening*

In the fasting state, the normally distended gallbladder usually has a wall thickness of 2 mm or less. Thickening of the GB wall may be defined as a focal or diffuse thickness of more than 3 mm (72). When contracted the normal GB wall becomes thicker, and might display three distinct zones (Fig. 8), strongly reflecting outer and inner layers and an echo-poor intermediate layer (73). Measurements of GB wall thickness is preferably performed on the anterior wall, which normally appears as a single, smooth, well defined reflecting structure. In contrast, the posterior wall may be more difficult to measure due to frequent contact with gas-filled bowel.

The GB wall may be thickened in several conditions, including ascites, hypo-albuminaemia in chronic alcoholics, liver cirrhosis, portal hypertension, cholecystitis (acute and chronic), sclerosing cholangitis, AIDS, adenomyomatosis, carcinoma of the GB, leukaemia, multiple myeloma, renal disease and others. Also nearby inflammatory disease such as hepatitis (viral and alcoholic), acute pancreatitis, and pericholecystic abscesses may cause thickening of the GB wall.

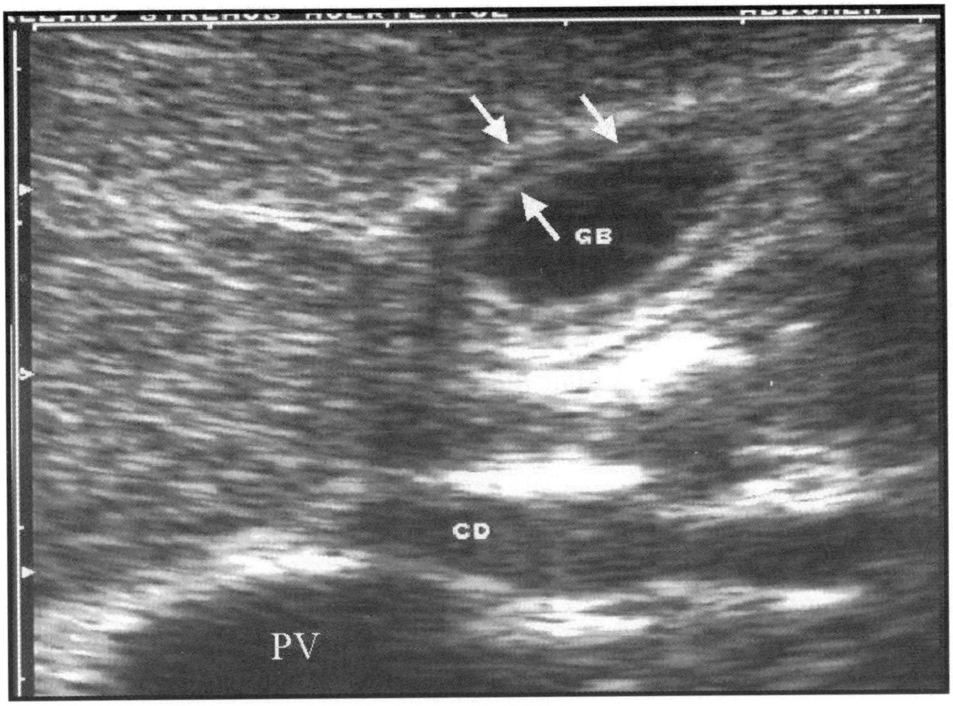


Fig. 8. Postprandial contraction of the gallbladder (GB) demonstrating three distinct zones within its wall (arrows), a strongly reflecting outer and inner layer and an echo-poor intermediate layer. CD — common duct. PV — portal vein.

### 2.4.7. *Acute cholecystitis*

There is no single sonographic sign specific for the diagnosis of acute cholecystitis. However, together the following (major) signs may be both sensitive and specific. These are: the presence of (1) stones in the GB. It is important to remember that acute cholecystitis may be acalculous in 5–10% of cases (74). Gallbladder inflammation without gallstones typically occurs in critically ill patients and is consequently associated with a high mortality rate (75). The histologic changes in the GB wall, however, are similar to those found in calculous cholecystitis; (2) edema of the GB wall (39%) visualized as an anechoic (sonolucent) layer in the gallbladder wall (76); (3) gas in the GB wall (emphysematous cholecystitis) recognized as areas of high echogenicity within a thickened gallbladder wall. These pockets of gas may cause shadowing and reverberations distally (77, 78). Gas within the gallbladder lumen may also occur making the gallbladder look like a loop of bowel. However, while gas in the GB tend to shift with gravity bowel gas does not. (79); (4) gallbladder tenderness or "sonographic Murphy's sign", which must be elicited during image-verified deformation of the gallbladder (80–82). In contrast to the high frequency of positive Murphy's sign (95%) in acute non-gangrenous cholecystitis, this sign may be present in only 33% of patients with gangrenous gallbladders (80, 83).

The following signs of acute cholecystitis may be characterized as somewhat less reliable or minor: (1) wall thickening present in 46% to 80% and increased volume in 64%

(76, 82, 84); (2) pericholecystic fluid collections. This fluid may be associated with localized peritonitis, or be due to acute cholecystitis having progressed to gangrenous cholecystitis and ultimately to perforation with the development of pericholecystic abscess. These fluid collections may vary from a small bile collection as a result of a microperforation to a true pericholecystic abscess. The echogenicity of the fluid may range from predominantly echo-free to predominantly echogenic, although increased through transmission of sound remains apparent (85); (3) enlargement of the GB reported in 60% of the patients (76); (4) hyperemia in the gallbladder wall assessed by color or power Doppler. Power Doppler has several advantages over color Doppler, including high sensitivity to slow flow, no angle dependency and no aliasing (86, 87).

Empyema of the gallbladder is difficult to differentiate from several other conditions which may also be associated with sludge (non-shadowing gravity-dependent echoes). Gangrene of the gallbladder, however, may be indicated by intraluminal membranes, caused by fibrinogenous strands, and sloughing of the gallbladder mucosa. As mentioned above, only a minority (30%) has a positive sonographic Murphy's sign, possibly due to the destruction of nerve endings (82).

Recently, sonography has proved to be useful as an adjuvant to fluoroscopy in performing guided palliative percutaneous transhepatic drainage of gallbladder empyema before laparoscopic cholecystectomy, which appears to be a safe and effective procedure for the initial management of GB empyema (88).

### 2.4.8. *Chronic cholecystitis*

In chronic cholecystitis all layers of the GB wall tend to be infiltrated by inflammatory cells which eventually may lead to thickening of the gallbladder wall and ultimately to fibrosis and shrinkage of the GB. In a study of 412 patients with chronic cholecystitis wall thickening was found in 18%, wall sonolucency 4%, GB dilatation 12%, sludge 13%, stones 93% of the patients (76).

### 2.4.9. *Cholecystectomy*

Laparoscopic cholecystectomy is considered the treatment of choice for symptomatic gallbladder stones. The method has advantages over the traditional open cholecystectomy in terms of minimal postoperative pain, shorter hospitalization, earlier recovery and resumption of activity (89).

Conversion to open cholecystectomy is sometimes necessary. Studies indicate that ultrasound may play an important role in predicting which patients might need conversion (89, 90). In a series of 738 patients, the overall conversion rate was 3.5%. The factors found to increase significantly the risk of conversion to open surgery were patient age (>70 years), a stone at least 20 mm in diameter, a gallbladder wall thicker than 4 mm, a common bile duct wider than 6 mm and contracted gallbladder on ultrasound. In these high risk patients, the conversion rate was 15.3% while in the low risk group without these signs, the conversion rate was only 1.3%. According to multivariate analysis, gallbladder wall thickening seems to be important. Pericholecystic fluid, however, seems to be a very specific predictor of conversion to open cholecystectomy (91–93).

### 2.4.10. *Hyperplastic cholecystoses — cholesterolosis and adenomyomatosis*

Cholesterolosis and adenomyomatosis represent two diseases of the GB that are unrelated to cholelithiasis or cholecystitis. Cholesterolosis is the result of the accumulation of triglycerides and esterified sterols in macrophages in the lamina propria. The abnormality is unassociated with cholesterol gallstones, supersaturation of bile with cholesterol, hyperlipidemia, obesity, or atherosclerosis. Adenomyomatosis involves hyperplasia of the tissues of the gallbladder wall with outpouches of the mucosa similar to diverticula of the colon (94).

Cholesterolosis ("strawberry gallbladder") is difficult to detect by ultrasound preoperatively as the resulting surface nodules are usually less than 1 mm in diameter. However, larger polypoid excrescences or cholesterol polyps sometimes develop. These may be revealed by ultrasonography as single or multiple polypoid densities (reflective foci) attached to the wall of the gallbladder. They are usually without shadows and do not move within the GB when the patient changes position (95). Cholecystography reveals cholesterolosis as contrast medium defects attached to the gallbladder wall (96). Adenomyomatosis of the GB, which is characterized by diffuse or segmental thickening of the gallbladder wall, with intramural diverticula, may also be visualized by ultrasound. Diverticula containing bile appear anechoic. Diverticula containing sludge or stones, however, appear echogenic, with or without acoustic shadows or reverberation artifacts (97). The clinical significance of this lesion of the gallbladder is controversial as it also may be found in asymptomatic individuals.

### 2.4.11. *Polyps of the gallbladder*

Benign polyps of the gallbladder consist of true polyps and pseudopolyps. The most frequently occurring type of true polyp in the gallbladder is the adenoma. Pseudo-polyps consist of cholesterol polyps, inflammatory polyps, and the localized form of adenomyomatosis. The cholesterol polyp is the commonest form of polyp in the gallbladder, responsible for over 60% of resected lesions (98).

On sonography, the true polyp typically appears as a tissue mass projecting into the gallbladder lumen (Fig. 9). It is usually solitary and can be either sessile or papillary (99). It neither moves with repositioning of the patient nor casts an acoustic shadow. It is very difficult to distinguish between benign and malignant or potentially malignant polyps on ultrasonography. Sonographic factors that indicate possible malignancy include age greater than 50 years, the presence of a single polyp, a polyp greater than 1.0 cm, the presence of gallstones, a sessile lesion even less than 1.0 cm in size, and rapid change in size of a polyp on follow-up ultrasonography (98). Several reports indicate that sessile lesions less than 1.0 cm have an increased incidence of malignancy compared with those with a stalk (98).

Because of the increased risk of malignancy in true polyps, several authors have recommended that any polyp of the gallbladder greater than 1 cm should be removed (97–100).

Other benign neoplasms of the gallbladder include fibroma, lipoma, myoma, carcinoid and haemangioma — all extremely rare (101).

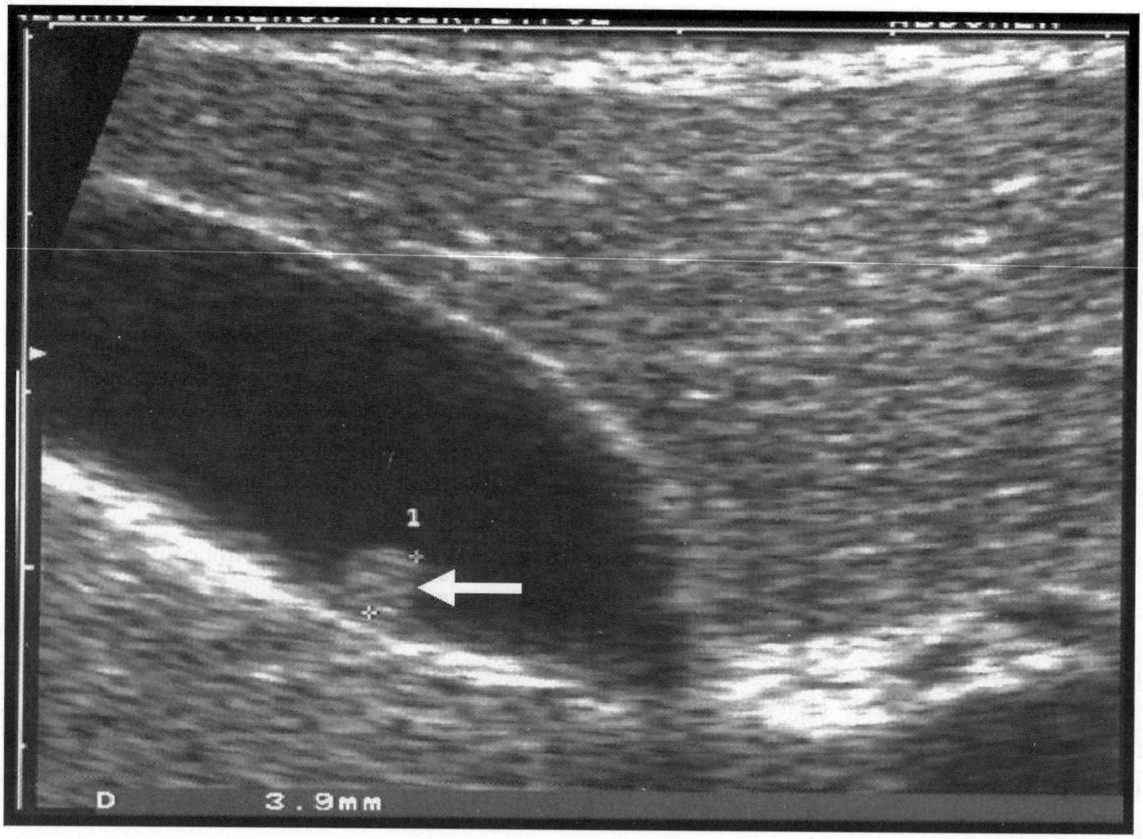


Fig. 9. Tissue mass projecting into the gallbladder lumen (arrow). Consistent with a true polyp the mass does not cast an acoustic shadow. 1 — mass = 3.9 mm.

### 2.4.12. *Carcinoma of the gallbladder*

Over 90% of gallbladder carcinomas are adenocarcinomas and advanced local and regional disease is usually present at the time of diagnosis (102). It affects females four times as commonly as males; its prevalence increases with age. Chronic cholecystitis, choledochal cysts and significantly high body mass index are associated risk factors (102). Overall, the curative resection rates for gallbladder carcinoma range from 10% to 30%. (102). The most common sonographic finding is that of a large solid mass filling the gallbladder bed (103). The tumor may also appear as an irregular polypoid mass within the gallbladder lumen, or as irregular thickening of the gallbladder wall which may be focal or diffuse. CT is still the method of choice for staging malignancy, particularly the detection of lymphatic and peritoneal spread. Approximately 25% of patients with a porcelain gallbladder (calcification of the gallbladder wall) will have associated carcinoma, which may be obscured by the acoustic shadow arising from the calcified anterior wall.

Differentiating a porcelain gallbladder from a gallbladder full of stones is important because of this high risk of malignancy. The development of a carcinoma within a porcelain gallbladder can be detected if there is a thickening of the gallbladder wall external to the calcified portion or an eccentric mass arising from the gallbladder wall. It is also important to look for other manifestations of malignancy such as biliary obstruction, porta hepatis or peripancreatic lymphadenopathy, or liver metastases.

The gallbladder may also be subject to metastases causing asymmetric wall thickening or polypoid intraluminal masses which can be indistinguishable from primary gallbladder cancer (104). Malignant melanoma is the most common source of gallbladder metastases (105).

Although, a variety of techniques for visualizing the biliary tree are now available, sonography is still the preferred initial imaging procedure on the grounds of safety, simplicity, cost and accuracy.

## References (gall bladder and biliary tract section)


1. Laing, F. C., Jeffrey, R. B., Wing, V. W. and Nyberg, D. A., Biliary dilatation: Defining the level and cause by real time ultrasound. Radiology 1986; 160: 39–42.
2. Gibson, R. N., Yeung, E., Thompson, J. N., Carr, D. H., Hemingway, A. P., Bradpiece, H. A. *et al.*, Bile duct obstruction: Radiologic evaluation of level, cause, and tumor resectability. Radiology 1986; 160: 43–47.
3. Baron, R. L., Stanley, R. J., Lee, J. K., Koehler, R. E., Melson, G. L., Balfe, D. M. and Weyman, P. J., A prospective comparison of the evaluation of biliary obstruction using computed tomography and ultrasonography. Radiology 1982; 145: 91–98.
4. Glenn, F., Postcholecystectomy choledocholithiasis. Surg Gynecol Obstet 1972; 134: 249–252.
5. Ruddell, W. S., Lintott, D. J., Ashton, M. G. and Axon, A. T., Endoscopic retrograde cholangiography and pancreatography in investigation of post-cholecystectomy patients. Lancet 1980; 1: 444–447.
6. Ferruchi, J. T., Jr., Adson, M. A., Mueller, P. R., Stanley, R. J. and Stewart, E. T., Advances in the radiology of jaundice: A symposium and Review. AJR Am J Roentgenol 1983; 141: 1–20.
7. Jan, Y. Y., Chen, H. M. and Chen, M. F., Malignancy in choledochal cysts. Hepatogastroenterology 2002; 49: 100–103.
8. Shi, L. B., Peng, S. Y., Meng, X. X. *et al.*, Diagnosis and treatment of conmgenital choledochal cyst: 20 years experience in China. World J Gastroenterol 2001; 7: 732–734.
9. Hussain, S. Z., Bloom, D. A. and Tolia, V., Caroli's disease diagnosed in a child by MRCP. Clin Imaging 2000; 24: 289–291.
10. Carroll, B. A., Biliary cystadenoma and cystadenocarcinoma: Gray scale ultrasound appearance. J clin Ultrasound 1978; 6: 337–340.
11. Patton, R. B. and Horn, R. C. Jr., Primary liver carcinoma. Autopsy study of 60 cases. Cancer 1961; 17: 757–768.
12. Okuda, K., Kubo, Y., Okazaki, N. *et al.*, Clinical aspects of intrahepatic bile duct carcinoma including hilar carcinoma. A study of 57 autopsy proven cases. Cancer 1977; 39: 232–246.
13. McDermott, W. V. and Peinert, R. A., Carcinoma in the supra-ampullary portion of the bile ducts. Surg Gynecol Obstet 1979; 149: 681–686.
14. Broomè, U., Løfberg, R., Veress, B. and Eriksson, L. S., Primary sclerosing cholangitis and ulcerative colitis: Evidence for increased neoplastic potential. Hepatology 1995; 22: 1404–1408.
15. Klatskin, G., Adenocarcinoma of the hepatic duct at its bifurcation within the porta hepatis. Am J Med 1965; 38: 241–256.
16. Sugiyama, M., Atomi, Y., Kuroda, A. and Muto, T., Bile duct carcinoma without jaundice: Clues to early diagnosis. Hepatogastroenterology 1977; 44: 1477–1483.

17. Crade, M., Taylor, K. J. W., Rosenfield, A. T., de. Graf, C. S. and Minihan, P., Surgical and pathologic correlation of cholecystosonography and cholecystography. AJR Am J Roentgenol 1978; 131: 227–229.
18. Dillon, E., Peel, A. L. G. and Parkin, J. G. S., The diagnosis of primary bile duct carcinoma (cholangiocarcinoma) in the jaundiced patient. Clin Radiol 1981; 32: 311–317.
19. Subramanyam, B. R., Raghavendra, B. N., Balthazar, E. J. *et al.*, Ultrasonic features of cholangiocarcinoma. J Ultrasound Med 1984; 3: 405–408.
20. Yeung, E. Y., McCarthy, P., Gompertz, R. H., Benjamin, I. S., Gibson, R. N. and Dawson, P., The ultrasonographic appearance of hilar cholangiocarcinoma (Klatskin tumours). Br J Radiol 1988; 61: 991–995.
21. Smits, N. J. and Reeders, J. W., Imaging and staging of biliopancreatic malignancy: Role of ultrasound. Ann Oncol 1999; 10 Suppl 4: 20–24.
22. Parulekar, S. G., Sonography of the distal cystic duct. J Ultrasound Med 1989; 8: 367–373.
23. Weill, F., Eisencher, A. and Zeltner, F., Ultrasound study of the normal and dilated biliary treee. Radiology 1978; 127: 221–224.
24. Conrad, M. R., Landay, M. J. and James, J. O., Sonographic "parallel channel" sign of biliary tree enlargement in mild to moderate obstructive jaundice. AJR Am J Roentgenol 1978; 130: 279–286.
25. Shawker, T. H., Jones, B. L. and Girton, M. E., Distal common bile duct obstruction: An experimental study in monkeys. J Clin J Ultrasound 1981; 9: 77–82.
26. Zeman, R. K., Dorfman, G. S., Burrell, M. I., Stein, S., Berg, G. R. and Gold, J. A., Disparate dilatation of the intrahepatic and extrahepatic bile ducts in surgical jaundice. Radiology 1981; 138: 129–136.
27. Pedersen, O. M., Nordgård, K. and Kvinnsland, S., Value of sonography in obstructive jaundice. Limitations of bile duct caliber as an index of obstruction. Scand J Gastroenterol 1987; 22: 975–981.
28. Bowie, J. D., What is the upper limit of normal for the common bile duct on ultrasound: How much do you want it to be? Am J Gastroenterol 2000; 95: 897–900.
29. Sample, W. F., Sarti, D. A., Goldstein, L. I., Weiner, M. and Kadell, B. M., Gray-scale ultrasonography of the jaundiced patient. Radiology 1978; 128: 719–725.
30. Cooperberg, P. L., High-resolution real-time ultrasound in the evaluation of the normal and obstructed biliary tract. Radiology 1978; 129: 477–480.
31. Wu, C. C., Ho, Y. H. and Chen, C. Y., Effect of aging on common bile duct diameter: A real-time ultrasonographic study. J Clin Ultrasound 1984; 12: 473–478.
32. Perret, R. S., Sloop, G. D. and Borne, J. A., Common bile duct measurements in an elderly population. J Ultrasound Med 2000; 19: 727–730.
33. Feng, B., Song Qiumei. Does the common bile duct dilate after cholecystectomy? Sonographic evaluation in 234 patients. AJR Am J Roentgenol 1995; 165: 859–861.
34. Majeed, A. W., Ross, B. and Johnson, A. G., The preoperatively bile duct does not dilate after cholecystectomy: Results of a five year study. Gut 1999; 45: 741–743.
35. Bucceri, A. M., Brogna, A. and Ferra, R., Common bile duct caliber following cholecystectomy: A two-year sonographic survey. Abdom Imaging 1994; 19: 251–252.
36. Niederau, C., Muller, J., Sonnenberg, A., Scholten, T., Erckenbrecht, J., Fritsch, W. P., Bruster, T. and Strohmeyer, G., Extrahepatic bile ducts in healthy subjects, in patients with cholelithiasis, and in postcholecystectomy patients: A prospective ultrasonic study. J Clin Ultrasound 1983; 11: 23–27.

37. Kaim, A., Steinke, K., Frank, M., Enriquez, R., Kirsch, E., Bongartz, G. and Steinbrich, W., Diameter of the common bile duct in the elderly patient: Measurement by ultrasound. Eur Radiol 1998; 8: 1413–1415.
38. Mueller, P. R., Ferruchi, J. T., Simeone, J. F., vanSonnenberg, E., Hall, D. A. and Wittenberg, J., Observations on distensibility of the common bile duct. Radiology 1982; 142: 467–472.
39. Faye, C. L., Jeffrey, R. B., Wing, V. W. and Nyberg, D. A., Biliary dilatation: Defining the level and cause by real-time US. Radiology 1986; 160: 39–42.
40. Muhletaler, C. A., Gerlock, A. J. Jr., Fleischer, A. C. and James, A. E. Jr., Diagnosis of obstructive jaundice with nondilated bile ducts. AJR Am J Roentgenol 1980; 134: 1149–1152.
41. Thomas, J. L. and Zornoza, J., Obstructive jaundice in the absence of sonographic biliary dilatation. Gastrointest Radiol 1980; 5: 357–360.
42. Greenwald, R. A., Pereiras, R., Morris, S. J. and Schiff, E. R., Jaundice, choledocholithiasis, and a non-dilated common duct. JAMA 1978; 240: 1983–1984.
43. O'Connor, K. W., Snograss, P. J., Swonder, J. E., Mahoney, S., Burt, R., Cockerill, E. M. and Lumeng, L., Gastroenterology 1983; 84: 1498–1504.
44. Einstein, D. M., Lapin, S. A., Ralls, P. W. and Halls, J. M., The insensitivity of sonography in the detection of choledocholithiasis. AJR Am J Roentgenol 1984; 142: 725–728.
45. Laing, F. C. and Jeffrey, R. B., Choledocholithiasis and cystic duct obstruction: Difficult ultrasonographic diagnosis. Radiology 1983; 146: 475–479.
46. Cronan, J. J., Mueller, P. R., Simeone, J. F. *et al.*, Prospective diagnosis of choledocholithiasis. Radiology 1983; 146: 467–469.
47. Cronan, J. J., US diagnosis of choledocholithiasis: Reappraisal. Radiology 1986; 161: 133–134.
48. Weinstein, B. J. and Weinstein, D. P., Biliary tract dilatation in the nonjaundiced patient AJR Am J Roentgenol 1980; 134: 899–906.
49. Parulekar, S. G. and McNamara, M. P. Jr., Ultrasonography of choledocholithiasis. J Ultrasound Med 1983; 2: 395–400.
50. Dewbury, K. C. and Smith, C. L., The misdiagnosis of common bile duct stones with ultrasound. Br J Radiol 1983; 56: 625–630.
51. Pickuth, D., Radiologic diagnosis of common bile duct stones. Abdom Imaging 2000; 25: 618–621.
52. Neitlich, J. D., Topazian, M., Smith, R. C., Gupta, A., Burrell, M. I. and Rosenfield, A. T., Detection of choledocho-lithiasis: Comparison of unenhanced helical CT and endoscopic retrograde cholangiopancreatography. Radiology 1997; 203: 753–757.
53. Kim, K. H., Kim, W., Lee, H. I. and Sung, C. K., Prediction of common bile duct stones: Its validation in laparoscopic cholecystectomy. Hepatogastroenterology 1997; 44: 1574–1579.
54. Voyles, C. R., Sanders, D. L. and Hogan, R., Common bile duct evaluation in the era of laparoscopic cholecystectomy 1050 cases later. Ann Surg 1994; 219: 744–750.
55. Beinart, C., Efremidis, S., Cohen, B. and Mitty, H. A., Obstruction without dilatation, JAMA 1981; 245: 353–356.
56. Carroll, B. A. and Oppenheimer, D. A., Sclerosing cholangitis: Sonographic demonstration of bile duct wall thickening. Am J Roentgenol 1982; 139: 1016–1018.
57. Cooperberg, P. L., Li, D., Wong, P., Cohen, M. M. and Burhenne, H. J., The accuracy of common hepatic duct size in the evaluation of extrahepatic biliary obstruction. Radiology 1980; 135: 141–144.
58. Borsch, G., Wegner, M., Wedmann, B., Kissler, M. and Glocke, M., Clinical evaluation, ultrasound, cholescintigraphy, and endoscopic retrograde cholangiography in cholestasis. A prospective comparative clinical study. J Clin Gastroenterol 1988; 10: 185–90.

59. Honickman, S. P., Mueller, P. R., Wittenberg, J., Simeone, J. F., Ferruchi, J. T. Jr., Cronan, J. J. and vanSonnenberg, E., Ultrasound in obstructive jaundice: Prospective evaluation of site and cause. Radiology 1983; 147: 511–515.
60. Kim, J. E., Lee, J. K., Lee, J. K. *et al.*, The clinical significance of common bile-duct dilatation in patients without biliary symptoms or causative lesions on ultrasonography. Endoscopy 2001; 33: 495–500.
61. Lindsell, D. R., Ultrasound imaging of pancreas and biliary tract. Lancet 1990; 335: 390–393.
62. Hough, D. M., Glazebrook, K. N., Paulson, E. K., Bowie, J. D. and Foster, W. L., Value of prone positioning in the ultrasonographic diagnosis of gallstones: Prospective study. J Ultrasound Med. 2000; 19: 633–638.
63. GREPCO. Prevalence of gallstone disease in an italian adult female population. Am J Epidemiol 1984; 119: 796–805.
64. Gracie, W. A. and Ransohoff, D. F., The natural history of silent gallstones: The innocent gallstone is not a myth. N Engl J Med 1987; 307: 798–800.
65. Filly, R. A., Allen, B., Minton, M. J., Bernhoft, R. and Way, L. W., *In vitro* investigation of the origin of echoes within biliary sludge. J Clin Ultrasound 1980; 8: 193–200.
66. Ward, B., Baker, A. C. and Humphrey, V. F., Nonlinear propagation applied to the improvement of resolution in diagnostic medical ultrasound. J Acoust Soc Am 1997; 101: 143–154.
67. Damore, L. J. 2nd, Cook, C. H., Fernandez, K. L., Cunningham, J., Ellison, E. C. and Melvin, W. S., Ultrasonography incorrectly diagnoses gallbladder polyps. Surg Laparosc Endosc Percutan Tech 2001; 11: 88–91.
68. Conrad, M. R., Janes, J. O. and Dietchy, J., Significance of low level echoes within the gallbladder. AJR Am J Roentgenol 1979; 132: 967–972.
69. Simeone, J. F., Mueller, P. R., Ferruchi, J. T., Harbin, W. P. and Wittenberg, J., Significance of non-shadowing focal opacities at cholecystography. Radiology 1980; 137: 181–185.
70. Messing, B., Bories, C., Kunstlinger, F. and Bernier, J. J., Does total parenteral nutrition induce gallbladder sludge formation and lithiasis? Gastroenterology 1983; 84: 1012–1019.
71. Bolondi, L. *et al.*, Early detection of biliary sludge and gallstones after surgery of the GI tract. In: Barbara, L., Dowling, R. H., Hofman, A. F., Roda, E., eds. Recent advances in bile acid research. New York Raven Press. 1985; 281–285.
72. Engel, J. M., Deitch, E. A. and Sikkema, W., Gallbladder wall thickness: Sonographic accuracy and relation to disease. AJR Am J Roentgenol 1979; 134: 907–909.
73. Marchal, G., Van, de. Voorde, P., Van, Dooren, W., Ponette, E. and Baert, A., Ultrasonic appearance of the filled and contracted normal gallbladder. J Clin Ultrasound 1980; 8: 143–146.
74. Deitch, E. A. and Engel, J. M., Acute acalculous cholecystitis: An ultrasonic diagnosis. AJR Am J Roentgenol 1981; 142: 290–292.
75. Trowbridge, R. L., Rutkowski, N. K. and Shojania, K. G., Does this patient have acute cholecystitis? JAMA 2003; 289: 80–86.
76. Paivansalo, M. and Myllyla, V., Sonographic and cholecystographic diagnosis of cholesterolosis of the gallbladder. Rontgenblatter 1984; 37: 357–358.
77. Blaquierer, R. M. and Dewbury, K. C., The ultrasound diagnosis of emphysematous cholecystitis. Br J Radiol 1982; 55: 114–116.
78. Parulekar, S. G., Sonographic findings in acute emphysematous cholecystitis. Radiology 1982; 145: 117–119.
79. Bloom, R. A., Fisher, A., Pode, D. and Asaf, Y., Shifting intramural gas: A new ultrasound sign of emhysematous cholecystitis. J Clin Ultrasound 1984; 12: 40–42.

80. Ralls, P. W., Halls, J., Lapin, S. A., Quinn, M. F., Morris, U. L. and Boswell, W., Prospective evaluation of the sonographic Murphy sign in suspected acute cholecystitis. J Clin Ultrasound 1982; 10: 113–115.
81. Finberg, H. J. and Birnhotz, J., Ultrasound evaluation of the gallbladder wall. Radiology 1979; 133: 693–698.
82. Soiva, M., Suramo, I. and Taavitsainen, M., Ultrasonography of the gallbladder in patients with a clinical suspicion of acute cholecystitis. Diagn Imaging Clin Med 1986; 55: 337–342.
83. Simeone, J. F., Brink, J. A., Mueller, P. R. *et al.*, The sonographic diagnosis of acute gangrenous cholecystitis: Importance of the Murphy sign AJR Am J Roentgenol 1989; 152: 289–290.
84. Sariego, J., Matsumoto, T. and Kerstein, M., Significance of wall thickness in symptomatic gallbladder disease. Arch Surg 1992; 127: 1216–1218.
85. Madrazo, B. L., Francis, L., Hricak, H., Sandler, M. A., Hudak, S. and Gitschlag, K., Sonographic findings in perforation of the gallbladder. AJR Am J Roentgenol 1982; 139: 491–496.
86. Kim, A. Y., Choi, B. I., Kim, T. K., Han, J. K., Yun, E. J., Lee, K. Y. and Han, M. C., Hepatocellular carcinoma: Power Doppler US with a contrast agent — preliminary results. Radiology 1998; 209: 135–140.
87. Draghi, F., Ferrozzi, G., Callida, F., Solcia, M., Madonia, L. and Campani, R., Power Doppler ultrasound of gallbladder wall vascularization in inflammation: Clinical implication. Eur Radiol 2000; 10: 1587–1590.
88. Tseng, L. J., Tsai, C. C., Mo, L. R. *et al.*, Palliative percutaneous transhepatic gallbladder drainage of gallbladder empyema before laparoscopic cholecystectomy. Hepatogastroenterology 2000; 47: 932–936.
89. Corr, P., Tate, J. J. T., Lau, W. Y., Dawson, J. W. and Li, A. K. C., Preoperative ultrasound to predict technical difficulties and complications of laparoscopic cholecystectomy. Am J Surg 1994; 168: 54–56.
90. Jansen, S., Jorgensen, J., Caplehorn, J. and Hunt, D., Preoperative ultrasound to predict conversion in laparoscopic cholecystectomy. Surg Laparosc Endosc 1997; 7: 121–123.
91. Daradkeh, S. S., Suwan, Z. and Abu-Khalaf, M., Preoperative ultrasonography and prediction of technical difficulties during laparoscopic cholecystectomy. World J Surg 1998; 22: 75–77.
92. Alponat, A., Kum, C. K., Koh, B. C. and Rajnakova, A., Predictive factors for conversion of laparoscopic cholecystectomy. World J Surg 1997; 21: 629–633.
93. Dinkel, H. P., Kraus, S., Heimbucher, J., Moll, R., Knupffer, J., Gassel, H. J., Freys, S. M., Fuchs, K. H. and Schindler, G., Sonography for selecting candidates for laparoscopic cholecystectomy: A prospective study. Am J Roentgenol 2000; 174: 1433–1439.
94. Berk, R. N., van der Vegt, J. H. and Lichtenstein, J. E., The hyperplastic cholecystoses: Cholesterolosis and adenomyomatosis. Radiology 1983; 146: 593–601.
95. Price, R. J., Stewart, E. T., Foley, W. D. and Dodds, W. J., Sonography of polypoid cholesterolosis. AJR Am J Roentgenol 1982; 139: 1197–1198.
96. Paivansalo, M., Siniluoto, T., Myllyla, V., Kairaluoma, M. I. and Kallioinen, M., Ultrasound in acute and chronic cholecystitis. Am J. Roentgenol 1987; 147: 84–87.
97. Raghavendra, B. N., Subramanyam, B. R., Balthazar, E. J., Horii, S. C., Megibow, A. J. and Hilton, S., Sonography of adenomyomatosis of the gallbladder: Radiologic-pathologic correlation. Radiology 1983; 146: 747–752.
98. Mainprize, K. S., Gould, S. W. T. and Gilbert, J. M., Surgical management of polypoid lesions of the gallbladder. Br J Surg 2000; 87: 414–417.

99. Carter, S. J., Rutledge, J. and Hirsch, J. H., Papillary adenoma of the gallbladder: Ultrasonic demonstration. J Clin Ultrasound 1978; 6: 433–435.
100. Donohue, J. H., Present status of the diagnosis and treatment of gallbladder carcinoma. Hepatobiliary Pancreat Surg 2001; 8: 530–534.
101. Majeski, J. A., Polyps of the gallbladder. J Surg Oncol 1986; 32: 16–18.
102. Levin, B., Gallbladder carcinoma. Ann Oncol 1999; 10 suppl 4: 129–130.
103. Yum, H. Y. and Fink, A. H., Sonographic findings in primary carcinoma of the gallbladder. Radiology 1980; 134: 693–696.
104. Phillips, G., Pochaczevsky, R., Goodman, J. *et al.*, Ultrasound patterns of metastatic melanoma presenting as acute cholecystitis. J Clin Ultrasound 1982; 10: 285.
105. Bundy, A. L. and Richie, W. G. M., Ultrasonic diagnosis of metastatic melanoma presenting as acute cholecystitis. J Clin Ultrasound 1982; 10: 379.

## 3. The Pancreas

### 3.1. *Anatomy*

The pancreas is situated retroperitoneally, extending transversely across the abdomen from the concavity of the duodenum to the splenic hilum. Its size and configuration varies considerably from person to person. In normal adults, the pancreas is 12 to 15 cm long, 3 to 5 cm wide and approximately 2 cm thick (1). Anatomically, it is divided into head, neck, body and tail. The head of the pancreas lies in the duodenal loop extending a few cm to the right of the vertebral column. The first part of the duodenum and the pyloric part of the stomach is often found anterior to the superior portion of the head.

On ultrasound images the pancreas is most easily found by first trying to establish the location of its surrounding arteries and veins (Figs. 1 and 2). The pancreatic head, usually the broadest part of the gland, is located anterior to the inferior vena cava and caudal to the portal vein. The uncinate process, an extension of the posterior part of the pancreatic head, extends medially behind the superior mesenteric vein. Moving medially, the head tapers to form the neck, which is found immediately anterior to the superior mesenteric artery and vein and posterior to the antrum of the stomach.

The body of the pancreas passes to the left, slightly cranial and after crossing in front of the aorta it extends slightly posteriorly. Another very useful landmark is the splenic vein, which runs medially along the dorso-cranial part of the pancreatic body where it meets the superior mesenteric vein to form the portal vein. This landmark is located just behind the neck of the pancreas. The upper border of the pancreatic body is limited by the often very tortuous splenic artery, which runs along its superior margin. The left renal vein passes between the superior mesenteric vessels and the aorta and thus may be used as a posterior landmark for body and tail. The tail of the pancreas extends to the left across the upper pole of the left kidney towards the hilum of the spleen.

The pancreatic duct runs along the length of the gland, tapering towards the pancreatic tail. The common bile duct runs anterior to and almost parallel to the portal vein and posterior to the head of the pancreas The distal part is embedded in the pancreatic tissue before entering the second part of the duodenum.

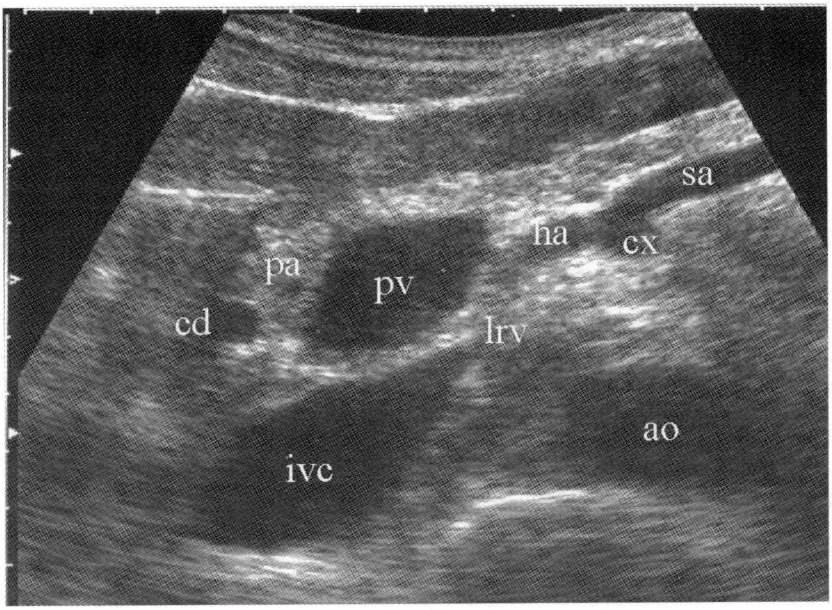


Fig. 1. Transverse section through pancreas, common duct (cd) and surrounding blood vessels, coeliac axis (cx), hepatic artery (ha), splenic artery (sa), portal vein (pv), inferior vena cava (ivc) receiving the left renal vein (lrv), and aorta (ao).

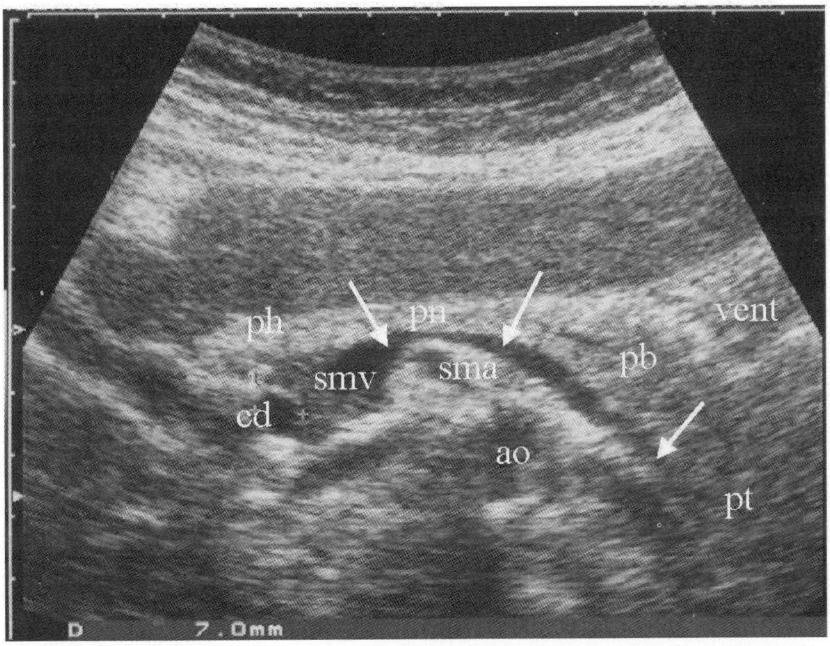


Fig. 2. Transverse section through pancreas, head (ph), neck (pn), body (pb) and tail (pt). The gas-filled ventricle (vent) constitutes the anterior border of the pancreatic body. The gland is posteriorly limited by the splenic vein (arrows) which medially, behind the neck of the pancreas, melts with the superior mesenteric vein (smv) to form the portal vein not visualized in the present section. cd — common duct (7.0 mm). sma — superior mesenteric artery. ao — aorta.

### 3.1.1. *Congenital anomalies*

The pancreas is formed from embryonic anlagen derived from the posterior wall of the duodenum and common bile duct. The uncinate process and part of the head develop from the ventral bud while the rest develops from the dorsal anlage. The ducts of the dorsal and ventral anlage fuse to form the main pancreatic duct (duct of Wirsung), which opens into the ampulla of Vater at the duodenum. The proximal portion of the dorsal duct usually disappears, but may remain as the accessory pancreatic duct (duct of Sartorini), opening into the duodenum a few centimeters proximal to the ampulla.

In cases of ectopic pancreas, pancreatic tissue can be found anywhere in the gut, the stomach wall, the small intestine, but rarely distal to Meckel's diverticulum. The commonest form of pancreatic ectopia is the annular pancreas, where a ring of pancreatic tissue encircles the second part of the duodenum where it can lead to varying degrees of obstruction (2). Congenital cysts may be solitary or multiple or may be found as isolated lesions of the pancreas or as part of polycystic kidney disease.

### 3.1.2. *Ultrasound examination*

Several different scanning methods may be used to visualize the pancreas, including transcutaneous or transabdominal (*B*-mode and Doppler), endoscopic, laparoscopic and intraoperative ultrasound. They may be equipped with color and power Doppler and recently also include tissue harmonic imaging, which facilitates the use of ultrasound contrast.

Transabdominal ultrasound is preferably conducted after an overnight fast to ensure that the stomach is empty and to reduce intestinal gas. The pancreas is examined both transversely and longitudinally using the above landmarks for identification. Sound transmission may be significantly reduced by intestinal gas which can be removed by gentle pressure of the transducer against the epigastrium. Sound transmission may also be improved by using liver, gallbladder, kidney or spleen as an ultrasonic window. It is very important to bring the left lobe of the liver down so that it covers the pancreas, either by deep inspiration or by examining the patient in the left lateral decubitus or erect position. The left kidney represents an important ultrasonic window to the pancreatic tail. This view usually requires the patient to be placed in a right lateral or prone position. Visualization of the pancreas is often further enhanced if the examination is performed after the patient has been given something to drink, preferably degassed, but tap water will often be sufficient. In order to fill the gastric fundus with fluid, the patient is usually turned into a slight left lateral position. The fluid-filled ventricle is especially helpful in visualization of the body and tail of the pancreas. Turning the patient on to the right side allows the fluid to pass into the antrum and duodenum. This facilitates a better view of the head and uncinate process.

### 3.1.3. *Ultrasound appearance*

The pancreas is usually located at the level of the 1st to 2nd lumbar vertebrae (3). Pancreatic measurements are usually not very important in clinical practice because of the wide normal variations, especially with regard to the distribution of volume between the pancreatic head, body and tail. It is far more important to study the contour and texture of the gland.

The pancreas tends to atrophy with age. A pancreas of normal size for a young patient may represent a diffusely enlarged gland in an elderly patient. The suggested maximum anterior-posterior diameters of the head, body and tail are 25, 15, and 35 mm, respectively (4, 5).

The assessment of size and appearance of the pancreatic duct (duct of Wirsung), however, is diagnostically much more important. With modern ultrasound equipment, parts of the pancreatic duct can be visualized in most patients as a tubular structure with reflective walls or just a thin line. The duct is most consistently visualized in the body of the pancreas (Fig. 3), where it has a relatively straight course, perpendicular to the ultrasound beams. The pancreatic duct, which dilates somewhat with increasing age, should not have a lumen that exceeds 3 mm in young adults and 5 mm in the elderly (3).

## 3.2. *Inflammatory disorders*

### 3.2.1. *Acute pancreatitis*

According to the Atlanta classification of 1992, acute pancreatitis is defined as an acute inflammatory process of the pancreas with variable involvement of peripancreatic tissues or remote organ systems (6).

In industrialized countries, the incidence of acute pancreatitis ranges from 5 to 70 cases per 100,000 inhabitants, with the severe form occurring in approximately 20% of all patients

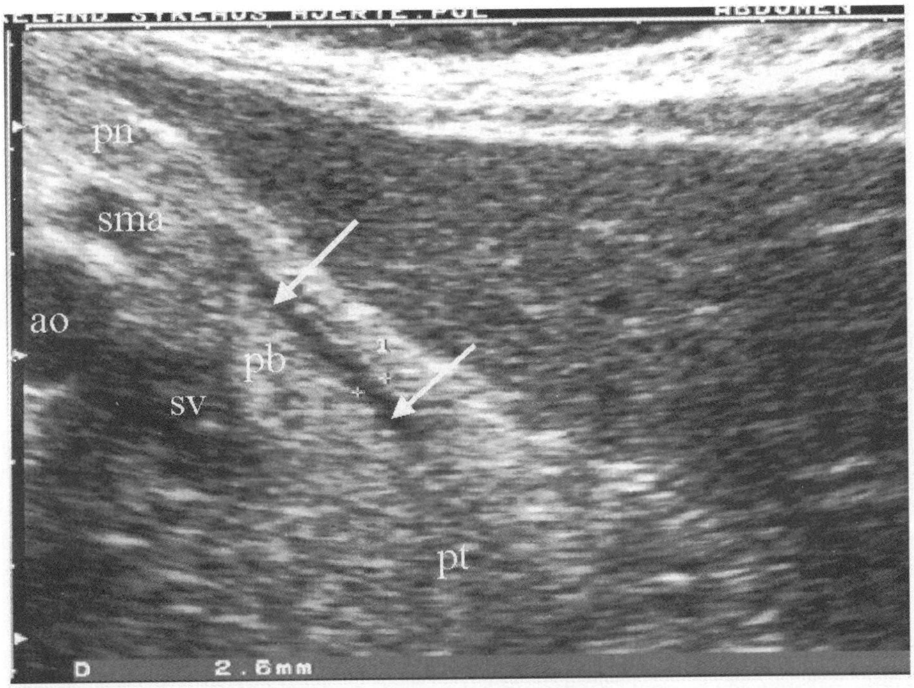


Fig. 3. The transducer is placed medially and angled to the left in order to avoid directing the ultrasound beams at the gas-filled ventricle. A normal appearing pancreatic duct (arrows) is demonstrated in the body of the pancreas (pb). 1 — diameter = 2.6 mm. pn — pancreatic neck. pt — pancreatic tail. sma — superior mesenteric artery. ao — aorta. sv — splenic vein.

(7). Alcohol abuse and gallstone disease are the most common causes of acute pancreatitis, accounting for more than 70% of all cases (7).

The causes of acute pancreatitis can be categorized into toxic-metabolic, mechanical, vascular, infectious, and drug-related. Toxic-metabolic causes include alcohol, hyperlipidemia, hypercalcemia and others. Mechanical causes include choledocholithiasis/microlithiasis, periampullary/ampullary obstruction, congenital malformations, and trauma, e.g. Vascular causes may include polyarteritis nodosa, atheroembolism and others. Infectious causes include viral infections such as mumps, Hepatitis B and others, bacterial infections such as Mycoplasma, Legionella, Leptospira, and Salmonella, as well as fungal and parasitic infections (7).

Drugs or chemical substances that may be associated with acute pancreatitis include L-asparaginase, azathioprine, calcium, estrogene, furosemide, salicylate, sulfonamide, tetracycline, thiazides e.g. (7).

The two most common patho-physiologic mechanisms of acute pancreatitis postulate either primary damage to the acinar cells or a ductal obstruction combined with reflux of bile. Both mechanisms lead to lipase-induced fat necrosis and its sequelae, which include necrosis of the adjacent vessels, acinar cells, and ducts.

The clinical findings in acute pancreatitis are associated with abdominal pain, tenderness on palpation, nausea, vomiting, fever, and tachycardia. The laboratory findings include elevated pancreatic enzymes (amylase and lipase), leucocytosis, and acute phase reactants.

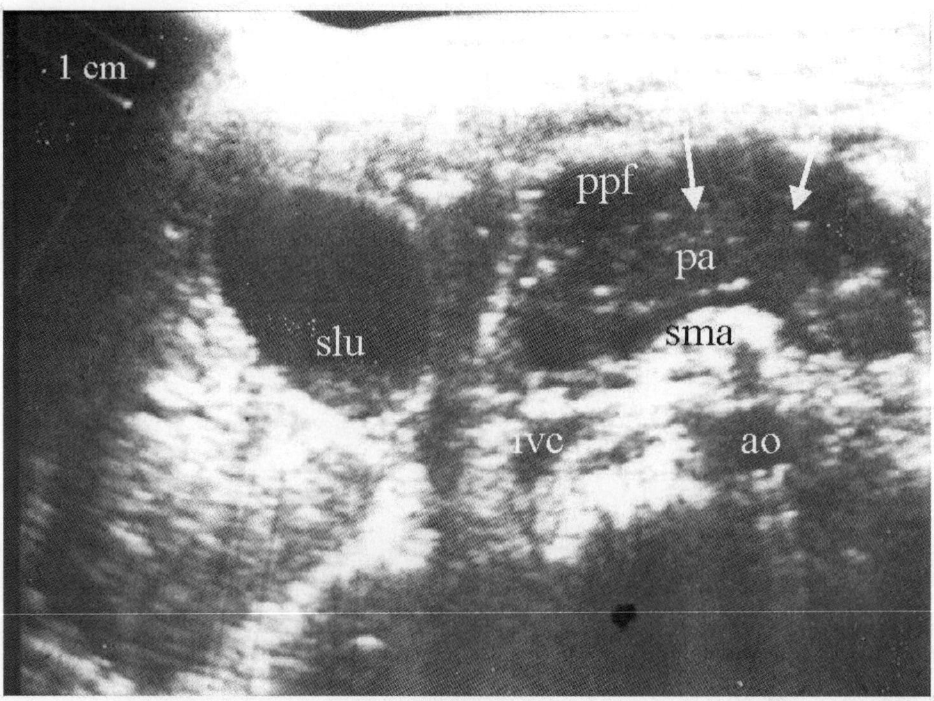


Fig. 4. Transverse view of an acutely inflamed echo-weak pancreas (pa) with peripancreatic anechoic fluid (ppf) anteriorly. Anterior border of pancreas marked by arrows. The gallbladder contains echogenic nonshadowing contents consistent with sludge (slu). sma — superior mesenteric artery. ivc — inferior vena cava. ao — aorta.

Morphologic findings range from interstitial edema and minimal necrosis in the mild form, to large confluent areas of necrosis and hemorrhage in the severe form. The latter form may also be associated with organ failure and the development of local complications such as pseudocyst and abscess formation. The most outstanding ultrasound features found in patients with acute pancreatitis is an enlarged (swollen) often strongly hypoechogenic gland with diffusely limited margins (Fig. 4).

### 3.2.2. *Complications in acute pancreatitis*

Acute fluid collections occur early in the course of acute pancreatitis in 30–50% of patients. They are located in or near the pancreas and, unlike pseudocysts or abscesses, they lack a wall of fibrous tissue. Spontaneous regression may be expected in more than half of the cases (7, 8). If peripancreatic fluid collections remain without resolvement, they may evolve into pancreatic pseudocyst (Fig. 5). These are round, encapsulated (non-epithelialized fibrous wall) collections of pancreatic fluid which may be detected 2–4 weeks from the onset of an episode of acute pancreatitis, or in the course of acute episodes associated with chronic pancreatitis. The wall thickens as the cyst mature.

Pseudocysts develop in up to 50% of patients after a severe attack of acute pancreatitis. They are usually easy to delineate as solitary or sometimes multiloculated fluid spaces with no or only low-level internal echoes. They may dissect along tissue planes and thus be found in quite unusual positions. The vast majority of pseudocysts lie close to the pancreas, most in the lesser sac. Rarely, a pseudocyst may rupture into the peritoneal space where its digestive enzymes produce severe acute peritonitis.

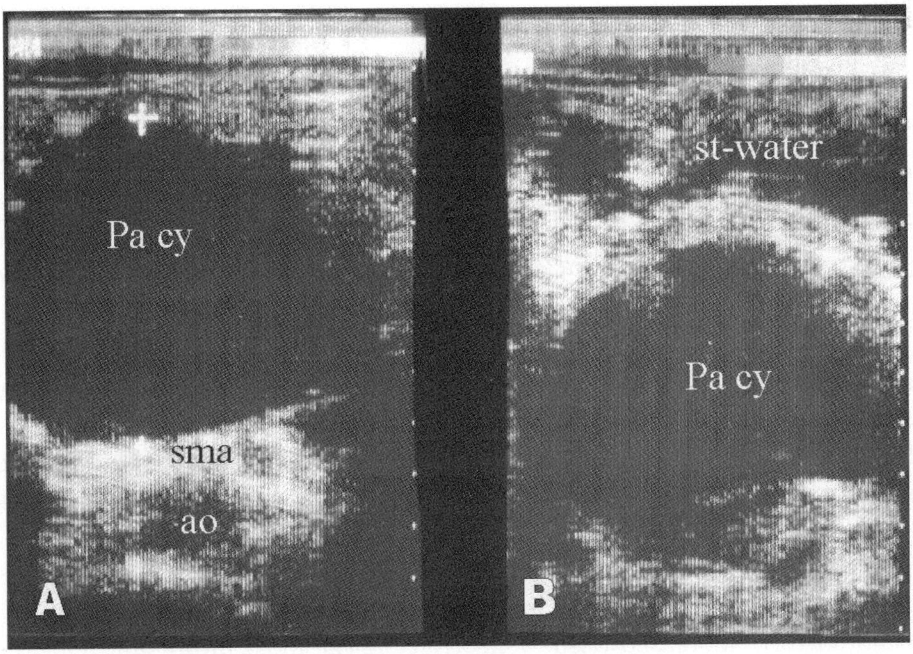


Fig. 5. Transverse section through a pancreatic pseudocyst (pa–cy), A without and B with fluid in the stomach (st-water). sma — superior mesenteric artery. ao — aorta.

In the early stages non-communicating pseudocysts may regress and disappear, but if there is no improvement by 6 weeks (9), percutaneous drainage is required and can be curative. Pseudocysts arising in the tail of the pancreas lie close to the spleen and its pedicle so that splenic vein thrombosis and splenic infarction are common complications. Both may be demonstrated with color Doppler. The thrombosis may extend to include the superior mesenteric and portal veins. Damage to the splenic artery may lead to pseudoaneurysm formation.

Pseudocysts may contain bacteria but usually as contamination only, without signs of clinical infection (7). When pus is present, the pseudocyst is termed pancreatic abscess.

Severe acute pancreatitis is a condition which is often associated with pancreatic necrosis involving both the pancreatic parenchyma as well as the peripancreatic fat. Contrast-enhanced CT imaging will usually establish the diagnosis. It is crucial to distinguish between sterile and infected necrosis because infected necrosis may triple the mortality risk and requires surgical debridement. The diagnosis of infection may be established by performing an image guided needle aspiration bacteriology.

Pancreatic abscesses represent circumscribed intra-abdominal collections of pus mostly located in the peripancreatic space. They may arise as a consequence of acute pancreatitis or pancreatic trauma and usually takes several weeks to develop. They contain little or no pancreatic necrosis (7). The distinction between infected necrosis and an abscess is important because the mortality risk of infected necrosis is twice that for pancreatic abscess.

Acute pancreatitis promotes translocation of gut-derived organisms to the inflamed pancreas and peripancreatic region, which in cases of severe acute pancreatitis may lead to development of severe sepsis in 40% to 70% of the patients, the frequency increasing with time after onset of symptoms (8).

### 3.2.3. *Chronic pancreatitis*

The features of advanced chronic pancreatitis are irregular scarring of the pancreatic parenchyma, strictures of the main pancreatic duct and stenosis of the side branches (usually at their junctions with the main duct). This mixture of narrow and dilated areas of the pancreatic duct may give the duct a beaded appearance on ultrasonography (Fig. 6). Intraductal protein plugs are a common finding, and these frequently calcify in severe disease. Many cases show focal necrosis with intrapancreatic pesudocyst formation. Chronic pancreatitis has various causes, the most common cause is chronic alcoholism for 6–12 years (8).

Patients usually present with recurrent abdominal pain and exocrine or endocrine dysfunction after the subclinical phase. Most common complications are obstructive jaundice, ileus, pseudocyst formation, pancreatic abscess, thrombosis of the portal venous system, and gastrointestinal bleeding. Pancreatic cancer develops in approximately 4% of patients within 20 years (8).

Chronic quiescent pancreatitis without pseudocysts is characterized by changes in the contours, the tissue echopattern, and to a lesser degree, the size of the gland. Of the changes in echo pattern, increased tissue reflectivity is the most important feature, particularly obvious in calcific pancreatitis. Increased pancreatic echogenicity, most probably due to fibrosis, may also be encountered in noncalcific pancreatitis. Ultimately, these changes

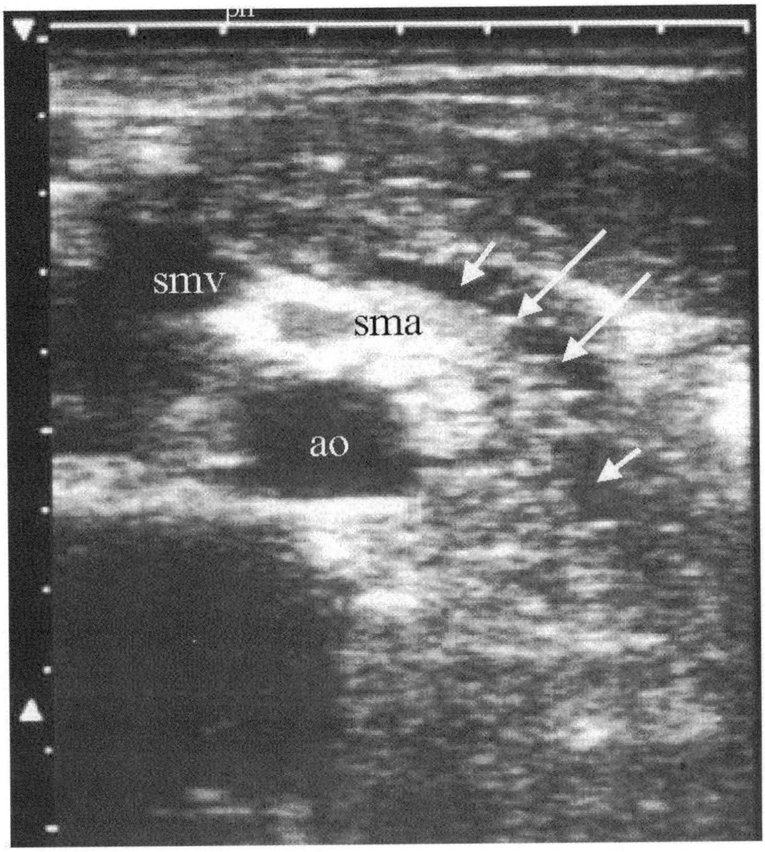


Fig. 6. Pancreatic duct in chronic pancreatitis demonstrating how dilated parts (long arrow) may be mixed with strictures (short arrow) which gives the duct a beady appearance. smv — superior mesenteric vein. sma — superior mesenteric artery. ao — aorta.

give rise to a gland that is ultrasonically heterogeneous, with areas of intense reflectivity, irregular shape, and variable size scattered in the pancreatic tissue. On sagittal scans the superior mesenteric vein may be depressed or displaced. In quiescent chronic pancreatitis it is unusual to find a sonolucent echopattern except when a superimposed acute or subacute process is involved (Fig. 7). Another important sign of superimposed acute changes is changes in contour of the gland. In chronic pancreatitis, these are characteristically irregular, if not spiky, which makes them different from the more regular, rounded and bulgy changes associated with carcinoma. However, in patients where there is an acute inflammatory process superimposed on the typical changes of chronic pancreatitis, the parenchyma becomes sonolucent and the contour of the pancreas becomes more regular and thus make the inflammatory changes difficult to differentiate from a carcinoma.

In quiescent chronic pancreatitis, the size of the gland tends to be subnormal with reflective heterogeneous echopattern with micronodules and an irregular, spiky contour. Atrophy, which is a late feature of chronic disease, may not be readily apparent

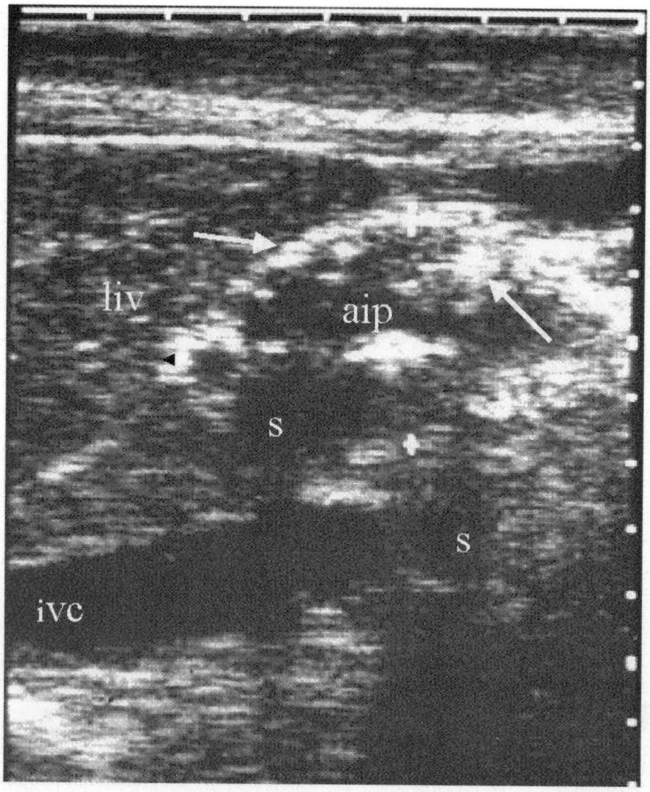


Fig. 7. Longitudinal section of the pancreas where an echo-weak acute inflammatory process (aip) is superimposed on echo-rich chronic calcific pancreatitis. Shadow-producing calcifications are marked by arrows. s — shadow from calcifications. liv — liver. ivc — inferior vena cava.

because peripancreatic fat and fibrotic gland tissue both are visualized as an hyperechogenic area with only minor structural changes (8). In the early stages of chronic pancreatitis, endoscopic retrograde cholangio-pancreography (ERCP) has demonstrated that although the main pancreatic duct appears normal (diameter <3 mm), there may be side branch dilatation with or without stenosis, irregular lining, intraluminal filling defects, and small calcified stones. In the later stages, the main pancreatic duct also becomes abnormal showing diffuse, focal or multisegmental changes detectable by sonography (8). Regularly lined cavities, which fill with contrast usually represent pseudocysts. Pseudocysts may measure from 1 to 20 cm, or even larger. They may be located in or around the pancreas. Such cavities are only filled with contrast when they communicate with the main pancreatic duct or a side branch (8). CT findings of chronic pancreatitis are primarily dilatation of the main pancreatic duct, parenchymal atrophy, pancreatic calcifications and pseudocysts.

Color Doppler ultrasound plays an important part in the diagnosis of vascular complications such as formation of pseudoaneurysm of the peripancreatic arteries, thromboses of portal system, and the presence of collateral pathways (8).

Carcinomas are relatively uncommon in patients with known chronic pancreatitis but are hard to diagnose when they coexist. Moreover, tumors are difficult to differentiate from focal areas of chronic pancreatitis. The presence of ductal calcification or stone is suggestive of a benign lesion.

### 3.3. *Pancreatic trauma*

Severe pancreatic traumas produce ultrasonic features typical of acute pancreatitis including an enlarged, dark gland, sometimes containing traumatic necrosis (10). Because the duct is usually disrupted, large pseudocysts often form. With penetrating injuries the interruption can occur at any point (11). In blunt injuries, however, the neck of the pancreas is most vulnerable and tends to tear where it is compressed against the aorta and the spine. Abdominal trauma is the commonest cause of pancreatitis in the pediatric age group (12). Even complete transection of the pancreas can be clinically silent until pancreatic ascites or a large pseudocyst develop. Distal pancreatectomy is required if there has been complete disruption of the main pancreatic duct.

Finally Color-Doppler may be used to look for vascular complications, such as portal venous thrombosis and resulting venous collateral pathways or the formation of pseudoaneurysms of the peripancreatic arteries, gastro-duodenal and splenic artery (7). CT is less sensitive in showing the intrapancreatic changes in mild acute interstitial pancreatitis (AIP) but demonstrates the effects on the surrounding tissues better (13).

Other complications are biliary obstruction, obstruction to the gastrointestinal tract, renal obstruction, or aneurysm formation. Of these, aneurysms are the most important as they may cause fatal hemorrhage. They take 2–3 weeks to develop and should be searched for by color Doppler in any case of severe pancreatitis (14, 15).

Mild acute interstitial pancreatitis causes swelling of the pancreatic parenchyma, which may be focal or lobular in distribution. The pancreatic duct system becomes compressed. Together with edema accumulating in the peripancreatic fat spaces and in the lesser sac, there is a general reduction in the echogenicity of the pancreas and its surroundings. In the initial phase of severe acute pancreatitis, the pancreas is often difficult to visualize as the view may be obscured by overlying gas due to an adynamic ileus.

In early acute pancreatitis, the gland may appear normal with regard to size, echogenicity and echotexture, but as interstitial edema increases the pancreatic parenchyma becomes diffusely enlarged and echo-weak. These changes lead to a relative increase in the reflectivity of the walls of a normal or narrowed pancreatic duct system.

Color Doppler frequently shows hyperemia in and around the poorly reflective regions of acute pancreatitis. Acute interstitial pancreatitis may also be focal, demonstrating areas of circumscribed acute pancreatitis, possibly accompanied by acute fluid collections, necrosis and hemorrhage (7). Sometimes the echo-poor mass may be difficult to distinguish from a tumor.

Ultrasound visualizes peripancreatic fluid collections as anechoic areas. Free intraperitoneal fluid should be searched for in the pouches of Morrison and Douglas. At a later stage, ultrasound may detect formation of pseudocysts and abscesses.

Gas is a valuable telltale sign of infected pancreatic necrosis, which usually is an indication for surgery as percutaneous catheter drainage is rarely effective because of the viscid nature of the fluid.

## 3.4. *Pancreatic masses*

### 3.4.1. *Carcinomas*

Pancreatic carcinoma is the third most common malignancy of the gastrointestinal tract. Unfortunately, this lesion is associated with an extremely poor prognosis. The highest cure rate occurs in the less than 20% of the patients who have a pancreatic cancer of less than 2.0 cm (greatest dimension) and which is truly localized to the pancreas (16). In those with completely resected tumors, there is approximately a 20% 5-year survival rate as compared with only a 4 to 5% for all patients with pancreatic cancer. Of these, fewer than 20% survive the first year after diagnosis (17).

In patients with minute pancreatic cancer of less than 1.0 cm, however, the 5-year survival rate has been reported significantly higher. The 5-year survival rate was 34% in 13 patients with jaundice and/or tumor mass at presentation as compared with 69% in 22 patients where the first signs of pancreatic pathology was elevated serum pancreatic enzyme levels, glucose intolerance, and or duct dilatation (18).

However, since initial symptoms are usually nonspecific (abdominal pain and weight loss) and are frequently disregarded, some 80% to 90% of the patients have regional and distant metastases (stage IV B), which render them inoperable by the time the pancreatic cancer is diagnosed (19). Of pancreatic adenocarcinomas, which account for more than 90% of all pancreatic neoplasms (19), only about 4–16% are resectable at diagnosis (20–24). Criteria for unresectability include presence of distant metastases, multiple liver metastases, peritoneal involvement with massive ascites, or invasion of peripancreatic vessels (25).

The most common symptoms associated with pancreatic carcinoma at the time of presentation are weight loss, abdominal pain and jaundice. Often these symptoms have been present for several months (26). Pain is most often epigastric and radiates to the back in 60% of patients. Jaundice occurs at some time in the condition in 90% of cases and is progressive, although initially it may fluctuate in severity.

Pancreatic tumors are chiefly ductal carcinomas, but there is no ultrasonic method of differentiating a true pancreatic carcinoma from an ampullary tumor or from a cholangiocarcinoma arising from the intra-pancreatic segment of the common bile duct. More rarely, cystadenomas or islet cell tumors are encountered.

The distribution of pancreatic cancer is 61% in the head, 13% in the body and 5% in the tail and a combination of these in 21%. Those arising in the head of the pancreas are more likely to be detected at an earlier stage due to their potential of obstructing the common bile duct or the main pancreatic duct. Therefore, tumors as small as 1 cm can be identified in the head of the pancreas and the presence of even smaller lesions inferred, when both duct systems are dilated, the "double duct sign" (27).

Both the normal and the enlarged pancreatic head are often better demonstrated in longitudinal scans as compared with transverse and oblique scans which tend to underestimate the size of the head. Since most adenocarcinomas involve the head, there is a high incidence of obstructive jaundice. Nodal metastases located at the porta hepatis, however, may also cause obstruction of the biliary tree, which may lead to dilatation of the intrahepatic bile ducts while the common bile duct remains normal.

Adenocarcinomas of the body and the tail, however, are usually not associated with early warning signs, frequently resulting in delay of diagnosis. Tumors in the tail of the pancreas are especially difficult to visualize due to gas collections in the colon. The threshold visibility of a mass in the pancreatic tail, therefore, may be considerably higher than that of the head. Using the left kidney and spleen as ultrasonic windows, however, may facilitate an earlier diagnosis.

Ultrasonographic detection of pancreatic malignancy is mainly dependent on differences in echogenicity, especially hypo-echogenicity. Even when the total volume of the pancreas is within normal range, sonography may predict malignancy due to irregularities of the normal pancreatic contour (Fig. 8) caused by partial enlargement of the head, body, or tail.

Reduced echogenicity of the pancreatic parenchyma is a typical sign of inflammation or infiltration of malignant tissue. Areas of reduced echogenicity may allow differentiation of even minute tumors less than 1.0 cm despite lack of changes in the shape of the gland.

Unfortunately, the hypoechogenicity, typical of pancreatic adenocarcinoma, is not specific, but may also be seen in association with other tumors and chronic pancreatitis. The majority of pancreatic cancers are poorly reflective mass lesions with a homogenous echo texture. The larger tumors, however, may be more heterogeneous in appearance. Strongly echogenic adenocarcinomas, however, are rare.

Due to the invasiveness of the adenocarcinomas, the margins of the tumor can be quite irregular and take the form of fingers or pseudopods, which look different from the more

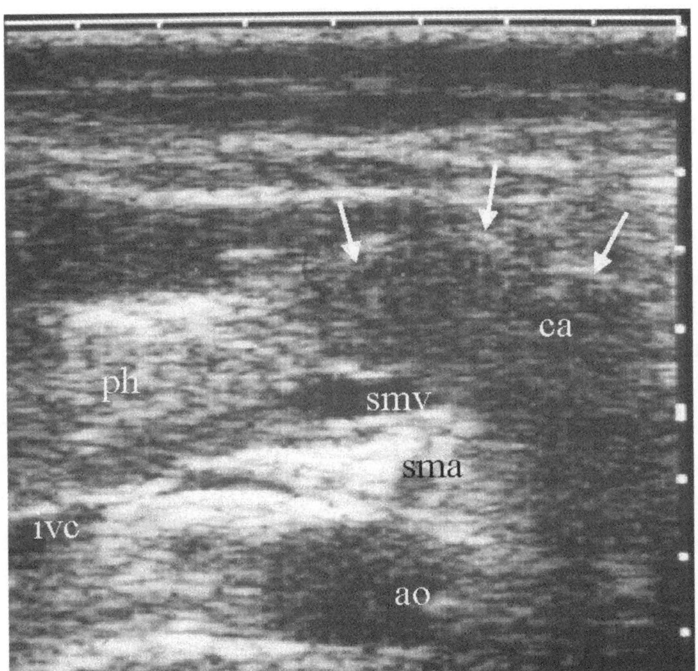


Fig. 8. Transverse section of the head and body of pancreas where a carcinoma (ca) of the body can easily be detected due to both its hypo-echogenicity and the changes in pancreatic contour (arrows) it causes. smv — superior mesenteric vein. sma — superior mesenteric artery. ivc — inferior vena cava. ao — aorta.

*spiky* irregularities of the pancreatic contour seen in patients with chronic pancreatitis. Most adenocarcinomas are similar to other solid structures in their attenuation of sound energy (28). The absence of ultrasound enhancement behind a tumor that appears to be devoid of internal echoes, is a valuable sign in differentiating cancer from a cystic lesion. A peculiar phenomenon is the echo texture of the adenocarcinoma which quite often bears a resemblance to the echo texture found behind adjacent gas collections. In these cases, it is important to demonstrate "through transmission" by visualizing tissue structures behind the tumor.

Ultrasound may also provide valuable information concerning resectability of a cancer in the pancreas. The TNM definition regarding staging (I-IVB) of malignancy takes into consideration the size of the tumor ($\leq$2 cm or >2 cm), extension of tumor outside the pancreas and whether there are local ($N$) or distant metastases ($M$). With the different tumor stages in mind, it is easier to perform a systematic assessment of the tumor. Patients with stage I cancer have no involvement of lymph nodes. When the tumor is limited to the pancreas and is equal to or less than 2 cm in diameter it is classified as $T1$, $N0$, $M0$ and $T2$, $N0$, $M0$ when the tumor is still limited to the pancreas but measures more than 2 cm. In stage II ($T3, N0, M0$) cancers extends directly into any of the following: duodenum, bile duct, or peripancreatic tissue but lack metastases ($N0, M0$). Regardless of tumor extension ($T1$–3), the cancer moves to stage III ($T1$–3, $N1$, $M0$) when local lymph node metastases has been detected. At stage IVA ($T4$, Any $N$, $M0$) there are local lymph node metastastases as well as direct extension into the stomach, spleen, colon or adjacent large vessels. The last and most severe stage IV B (Any $T$, Any $N$, $M1$) includes cancers with distant metastases ($M1$), nodes of the liver hilum or liver parencyma.

Vascular invasion may be detected on grey-scale ultrasound but is better assessed with color or power Doppler. In patients with cancer of the pancreatic head and neck, it is particularly important to examine the portal vein, superior mesenteric vein and artery, celiac trunk, and hepatic artery. In cancer of the body or tail, the examination should be extended to splenic vessels as well.

Involvement of the portal vein by tumor is common, occurring in 65% of pancreatic and 40% of bile duct cancers. Compression of the vein produces high velocity jet through the narrowed area, which may be quite obvious on color Doppler (29). Portal vein occlusion obliterates the Doppler signal, but the diagnosis may be indicated by demonstration of collateral vessels (30).

Absence of direct vascular involvement is indicated by the presence of unaffected pancreatic tissue located between the echo-poor tumor and the vessel wall. Vessel involvement is indicated when the vessel lumen is reduced or when the vessel is encased by tumor, partially or completely. The degree of involvement may be given as percentage of the vessel periphery being in direct contact with the tumor (31).

### 3.4.2. *Non-pancreatic periampullary tumors*

Tumors arising from the duodenum, extrahepatic bile duct, or ampulla of Vater have a clinical presentation similar to that of the adenocarcinoma of the pancreatic head. Due to their significantly better prognosis, non-pancreatic periampullary cancers need to be differentiated from pancreatic adenocarcinoma, which is impossible by transabdominal ultrasound.

### 3.4.3. *Cystic masses*

Cystic mass lesions of the pancreas include congenital cysts, retention cysts, neoplastic cysts and the most common cyst — the pseudocyst. Although uncommon, cystic neoplasms of the pancreas represent 10–15% of all pancreatic neoplasm (3). A cystic neoplasm is classified as benign (serous microcystic adenoma), malignant, or potentially malignant (mucinous cystic neoplasm) (32). Serious microcystic adenoma is a benign, glycogen rich, lesion found more commonly in the head of the pancreas (70%) in females above the age of 60 (3). These microcystic adenomas are defined by having more than six small cysts ($<$2 cm) and often have central, stellate scars that may be calcified. Due to the sum of small cysts, scar, and calcification, ultrasound usually visualize these tumors as hyperechoic complex masses. Cystadenocarcinoma should be considered when the cysts are large and few, less than 6, diameters more than 2 cm. They are predominantly located in the pancreatic tail and body of younger patients, especially females. In contrast to adenocarcinomas, the cystadenocarcinoma is predominantly cystic with decreased attenuation. As in the case of an islet cell carcinoma, cystadenocarcinoma has a much better prognosis than adenocarcinoma.

### 3.4.4. *Endocrine tumors*

The islet cell neoplasm which arises from multi-potential stem cells may be solitary or multi-centric, which is common in patients with multiple endocrine neoplasm. The most important functional tumors are insulinoma with a mean size of $<$2 cm and gastrinoma with a mean size near 3.5 cm. The islet cell tumors are classified as functional in 85% of the patients and non-secreting in 15%. The non-functional islet cell tumors are clinically silent until their volume is large enough to give rise to functional disturbances by compression. They have a higher malignant potential and are more often located in the head of the pancreas (3). Localization of islet cell tumors can be extremely difficult because of their small size (33).

Ultrasound detects islet cell neoplasm chiefly because it appears hypoechogenic in relation to the surrounding pancreatic tissue. However, in young patients (under 30) the normal pancreas is relatively echo poor, making it difficult to distinguish the tumor from normal parenchyma. In addition, the neoplasms are often small and may be multiple. The pancreatic tail remains an area of particularly difficulty. Detection rates for small insulinomas with modern transabdominal ultrasound equipment and techniques compare favorably with both CT and angiography (all approximately 60%). Endoscopic and intra-operative ultrasound, which can detect tumors down to a few millimeters, are significantly better at detecting these small islet cell neoplasm (34, 35).

### 3.4.5. *Other tumors*

Primary pancreatic tumors can be classified by their cell type into ductal, acinar and connective tissue types. Metastases constitute up to 7% of pancreatic tumors in some studies. Lymphoma which is the most common metastasis tend to form large, lumpy, hypoechoic masses.

### 3.4.6. *Biopsy*

Histological diagnosis is important for determining the management of a tumor suspect lesion due to the much better prognosis of malignancy of other histological types than adenocarcinoma. Real-time ultrasound has been used extensively to guide fine-needle aspiration for cytology. Although false positives are rare, the sensitivity of the method with regard to acquiring diagnostic material is disappointing at around 75% (36). This low detection rate is partly explained by the extensive desmoplastic reaction that adenocarcinomas of the pancreas cause. However, tissue specimens obtained by both tru-cut biopsy and biopsies using the Biopty® Gun, and biopsies directed by endoscopic ultrasound provide better specimens (37).

## References (pancreas section)

1. Holm, H. H., Kristensen, K. J., Rasmussen, S. N., Pedersen, J. F., Hancke, S., Jensen, F., Gammelgaard, J. and Smith, E. H., Abdominal ultrasound. Static & dynamic scanning. 2nd. ed. Munksgaard. 1980; 113–125.
2. Hyden, W. H., The true nature of annular pancreas. Ann Surg 1963; 157: 71–77.
3. Martinez-Noguera, A., Montserrat, E., Torrubia, S., Monill, J. M. and Estrada, P., Ultrasound of the pancreas: Update and controversies, Eur Radiol 2001; 11: 1594–1606.
4. DeGraff, C., Taylor, K. J. W., Simmonds, B. and Rosenfield, A., Gray scale echography of the pancreas and portal vein. Radiology 1978; 129: 157–161.
5. Niederau, C., Sonnenberg, A., Muller, J., Erkenbrecht, J., Scholten, T. and Frisch, W., Sonographic measurements of the normal liver, spleen, pancreas and portal vein. Radiology 1983; 149: 537–540.
6. Bradley, E. L., A clinically based classification system for acute pancreatitis. Summary of the international symposium on acute pancreatitis, Atlanta, GA, September 11 through 13, 1992. Arch Surg 128; 586–590.
7. Merkle, E. M. and Gørich, J., Imaging of acute pancreatitis. Eur Radiol 2002; 12: 1979–1992.
8. Elmas, N., The role of diagnostic radiology in pancreatitis. Eur J Radiol 2001; 38: 120–132.
9. Bradley, E. L. 3rd and Clements, L. J., Spontaneous resolution of pseudocysts. Am J Surg 1975; 129: 23–28.
10. Yoshi, H., Sato, M., Yamamoto, S. *et al.*, Usefulness and limitations of ultrasonography in the initial evaluation of blunt abdominal trauma. J Trauma 1998; 45: 45–50.
11. Warren, P., Garret, W. and Kossoff, G., The liquid filled stomach: An ultrasonic window to the upper abdomen. J Clin Ultrasound 1978; 6: 315–320.
12. Cabrera, R., Otero, H., Blesa, E., Jiminez, C. and Nunez, R., Pancreatic pseudocyst. Review of 22 cases. Chir Ped 1997; 10: 49–53.
13. Choi, Y. H., Rubenstein, W. A., Ramirez De Arellano, E., Intriere, L. and Kazam, E., CT and US of the pancreas. Clin Imag 1997; 21: 414–440.
14. Waslen, T., Wallace, K., Burbridge, B. and Kwauk, S., Pseudoaneurysm secondary to pancreatitis presenting as GI bleeding. Abdom Imag 1998; 23: 318–321.
15. Dirks, K., Schuler, A. and Lutz, H., An unusual cause of gastrointestinal hemorrhage: Pseudoaneurysm of the gastroduodenal artery in chronic pancreatitis. Zeitschr Gastroenterol 1999; 37: 489–493.
16. Parker, S. L., Tong, T., Bolden, S. and Wingo, P. A., Cancer Statistics, 1997. Cancer J Clin 1997; 47: 5–27.

17. Taylor, W. F. and Everhart, J. E., Pancreatic cancer. Bethesda, MD: US Department of Health and Human Services 1994; 249. National Institutes of Health publication 94–1447.
18. Ishikawa, O., Ohigashi, H., Imaoka, S. *et al.*, Minute carcinoma of the pancreas measuring 1 cm or less in diameter- collective review of Japanese case reports. Hepatogastroenterology 1999; 46: 8–15.
19. Arnar, D. O., Theodors, A., Isaksson, H. J. *et al.*, Cancer of the pancreas in Iceland. An epidemiologic and clinical study, 1974–85. Scand J Gastroenterol 1991; 26: 724–730.
20. Gudjonsson, B., Cancer of the pancreas — 50 years of surgery. Cancer 1987; 60: 2284–2303.
21. Michelassi, F., Erroi, F., Dawson, P. J. *et al.*, Experience with 647 consecutive tumors of the duodenum, ampulla, head of the pancreas, and distal common bile duct. Ann Surg 1989; 210: 544–556.
22. Bottger, T., Zech, J., Weber, W. *et al.*, Relevant factors in the prognosis of ductal pancreatic carcinoma. Acta Chir Scand 1990; 156: 781–788.
23. Russel, R. C. G., Surgical resection for cancer of the pancreas. Baillieres Clin Gastroenterol 1990; 4: 889–916.
24. Nix, G. A. J. J., Dubbelman, C., Wilson, J. H. P. *et al.*, Prognostic implications of tumor diameter in carcinoma of the head of the pancreas. Cancer 1991; 67: 529–535.
25. Ozava, Y., Numata, K., Tanaka, K. *et al.*, Contrast-enhanced sonography of small pancreatic mass lesions. J Ultrasound Med 2002; 21: 983–991.
26. Puchalski, Z., Ladny, J. R., Polakow, J., Razak, H. and Deeb, A., Diagnosis and surgical treatment of pancreatic carcinoma. Roczniki Akademii Medycznej W Bialymstoku 1996; 41: 210–217.
27. Lees, W. R., Pancreatic ultrasonography. Clin Gastroenterol 1984; 13: 763–789.
28. Weinstein, D. P., Wolfman, N. T. and Weinstein, B. J., Ultrasonic characteristics of pancreatic tumors. Gastrointest Radiol 1979; 4: 245–251.
29. Casadei, R., Ghigi, G., Gullo, L. *et al.*, Role of color Doppler ultrasonography in the preoperative staging of pancreatic cancer. Pancreas 1998; 16: 26–30.
30. Kane, R. A. and Katz, S. G., The spectrum of sonographic findings in portal hypertension: A subject review and new observations. Radiology 1982; 142: 453–458.
31. Angeli, E., Venturini, M., Angelo, V. *et al.*, Color Doppler imaging in the assessment of vascular involvement by pancreatic carcinoma. AJR Am J Roentgenol 1997; 168: 193–197.
32. Compagno, J. and Oertel, J. E., Mucinous cystic neoplasms of the pancreas with overt and latent malignancy. (cystadenocarcinoma and cystadenoma.) A clinicopathologic study of 41 cases. Am J Clin Pathol 1978; 69: 573–580.
33. Ardengh, J. C., Rosenbaum, P., Gane, A. J., Goldenberg, A., Lobo, E. J., Malheiros, C. A., Rahal, F. and Ferrari, A. P., Gastrointest Endosc 2000; 51: 552–555.
34. Kuzin, N. M., Egorov, A. V., Kondrashin, S. A., Lotov, A. N., Kuznetzov, N. S. and Majorova, J. B., Preoperative and intraoperative topographic diagnosis of insulinomas. World J Surg 1998; 22: 593–597; discussion 597–598.
35. Nesje, L. B., Varhaug, J. E., Husebye, E. S. and Odegaard, S., Endoscopic ultrasonography for preoperative diagnosis and localization of insulinomas. Scand J Gastroenterol 2002; 37: 732–737.
36. Di, Stasi, M., Lencioni, R., Solmi, L. *et al.*, Ultrasound-guided fine needle biopsy of pancreatic masses: Results of a multicenter study. Am J Gastroenterol 1998; 93: 1329–1333.
37. Suits, J., Franzee, R. and Erickson, R. A., Endoscopic ultrasound and fine needle aspiration for the evaluation of pancreatic masses. Arch Surg 1999; 134: 639–642; discussion 642–643. Ann Intern Med 1988; 109: 722–727.

CHAPTER 4

# ULTRASONOGRAPHIC ASSESSMENT OF ESOPHAGEAL MORPHOLOGY AND FUNCTION

SVEIN ØDEGAARD AND HANS GREGERSEN

Esophagus is a tube that is approximately 20 cm long with an upper and a lower sphincter. The esophageal wall consists of mucosa, submucosa, muscularis propria and adventitia. Muscularis propria has an inner circular and an outer longitudinal layer that is separated by the myenteric plexus. Adventitia is an external layer that contains relatively numerous fibers. Peristaltic contractions of the esophageal wall muscles regulate the transport of food through esophagus into the stomach.

Techniques currently used to study esophageal disorders include barium contrast radiography, endoscopy (Fig. 1), radionuclide studies, electromyography, and manometry. However, these techniques do not allow for the specific analysis of structural changes occurring within the esophageal wall. Technical improvement of ultrasound machines has made it possible to obtain detailed transabdominal images of the gastrointestinal tract and to examine gastrointestinal motility using different ultrasound modalities. Esophagus is not accessible for external ultrasound imaging. However, intraluminal ultrasound (endosonography — ES) probes have become an important tool for ultrasound imaging of this organ (1–5).

Endosonography of the esophagus is a method by which an ultrasound (US) probe is inserted into the esophagus. Since the US transducer is placed close to the esophageal wall, high ultrasound frequencies can be applied which improves the image resolution. ES can either be performed by placing the US transducer close to or directly on the mucosa

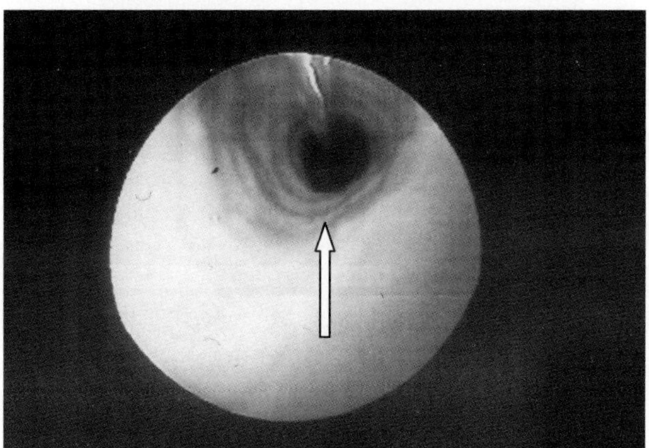

Fig. 1. Endoscopic image of small peristaltic esophageal contractions (arrow).

or using a waterfilled balloon around the US transducer. Esophagus and mediastinum constitute major targets for ES, which is regarded to be an important imaging modality in the evaluation of several esophageal diseases.

## 1. Endosonography Systems

Echoendoscopes combine endoscopy with integrated ultrasound transducers. These instruments can be classified both according to the type of endoscope and US system. Echoendoscopes have either radial or curvilinear array US transducers with frequencies between 7.5 and 30 MHz (Figs. 2(A) and 2(B)). These systems are being continuously improved, and the possibility to combine echoendoscopes with conventional ultrasound machines has made it possible to apply different ultrasound modalities like *B*-mode, *M*-mode and Doppler technology.

US miniprobes have a diameter which allows the probe to be inserted through the biopsy channel of a conventional endoscope or through a suitable catheter (Fig. 2(C)). Currently

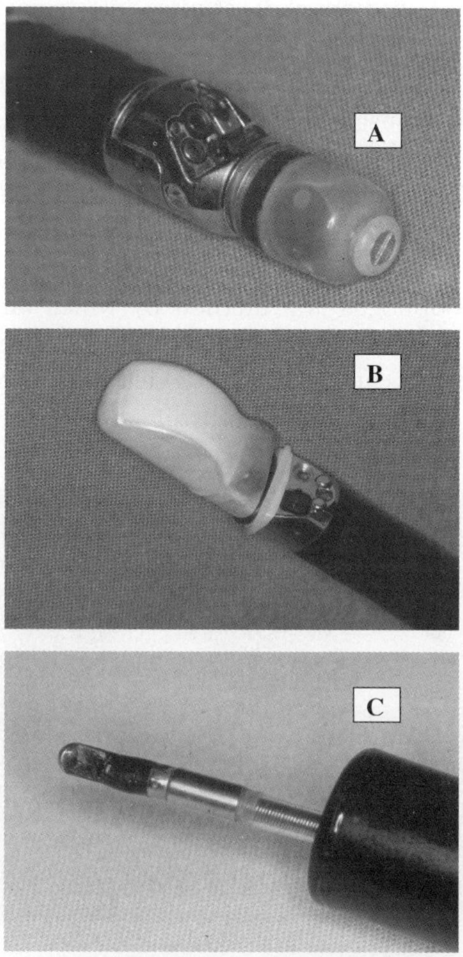


Fig. 2. Echoendoscopes with rotating (A) and linear transducers (B). Transendoscopic miniprobe (C).

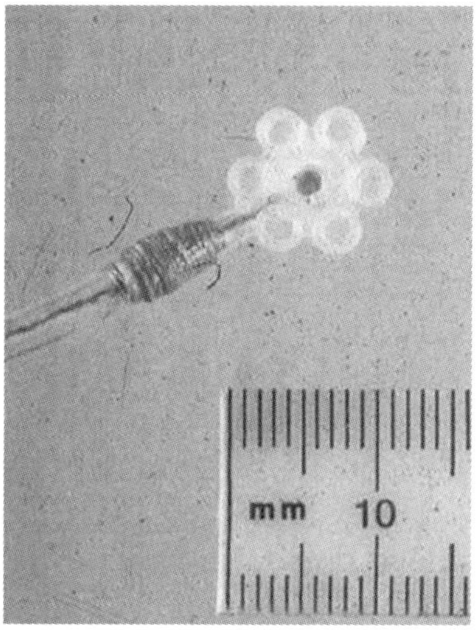


Fig. 3. Ultrasound $M$-mode device for motility examination of the gastrointestinal wall. Six suction cups are surrounding the ultrasound transducer in the centre (Courtesy RW Martin).

available US miniprobes are mechanical sector, electronic phased arrays, or single crystal linear compound systems operating with frequencies between 12 and 30 MHz. Systems that combine linear compound scanning with mechanical sector scanning or $M$-mode registration are also available making it possible to switch between these modalities. A device combining ultrasound and intraluminal pressure registration has been developed for esophageal motility studies. Suction cups attached to the mucosal surface of the gastrointestinal tract make the device stay in position during contractions (Fig. 3) (6).

The small size and high frequencies of miniature probes reduce the size of the US image and the penetration depth of the US beam into the tissue as compared to images produced by echoendoscopes. In most cases, useful information will be obtained from tissue within 2–3 cm from the transducer. The small diameter probes can also be passed into stenotic areas not traversable with conventional echoendoscopes.

Doppler sonography may provide important information about vascular flow and in separating vessels from other echo-poor structures. Some echoendoscopes have integrated Doppler technology and Doppler miniprobes for transendoscopic use have also been developed. External ultrasonography has also been used for motility studies of the gastrointestinal tract. Hausken *et al.* (7) examined gastroduodenal transpyloric flow of a meat soup using Duplex sonography including both spectral and color Doppler examination. Thus, both external and intraluminal ultrasound have potential in the evaluation of gastrointestinal physiology mechanisms.

## 2. Ultrasound Imaging of the Normal Esophageal Wall

High frequency ultrasound gives a detailed image of the layers (mucosa, submucosa, and muscularis propria) of the gastrointestinal wall. However, the layers do not correspond exactly to the histological layers due to the different imaging principles involved. The ultrasound layers result from a combination of interface echoes and echoes from the tissue. Kimmey *et al.* (8) have defined the interpretation of US images of the gastrointestinal tract and that of interface echoes between the wall layers. Interface echoes have an important impact on images of the gastrointestinal wall because the thickness of these echoes represents a relatively major part of the US image compared to the thickness of the anatomical layers.

The layers of the esophageal wall are usually interpreted as follows: the innermost layer is echogenic and represents the interface echo covering the top of the mucosa, and the second, hypoechoic layer is the rest of the mucosa. The third layer is also echogenic and corresponds mainly to the submucosa, and the fourth echopoor layer, mainly to the muscularis propria (Fig. 4). The fifth layer is echogenic and represents adventitia. Seven layers may be seen when an echogenic layer separates the inner and outer parts of the muscularis propria. Even nine and eleven layers have been described using high (over 20 MHz) US frequencies (9). The identification of the muscularis mucosae on US images has been a matter of debate. The interface echo between the lamina propria and the muscularis mucosae obscures this layer unless muscularis mucosa is thicker than the wavelength of the US beam (10).

The clarity of the layers and other details in the ultrasound images are related to a number of factors especially the resolution of the ultrasound system. ES systems with US frequencies between 7.5 and 30 MHz make it possible to resolve two points as close as 0.2 mm from each other in the axial dimension. The axial resolution is related to the duration of the ultrasound pulse and the frequency of the transducer and the lateral resolution to the size and focusing characteristics of the transducer. Thin miniprobes may be inserted into areas which cannot be passed by the endoscope, thus giving more precise images regarding some disorders (Fig. 5). It is crucial to achieve perpendicular scanning planes to the tissue surface to avoid artifacts.

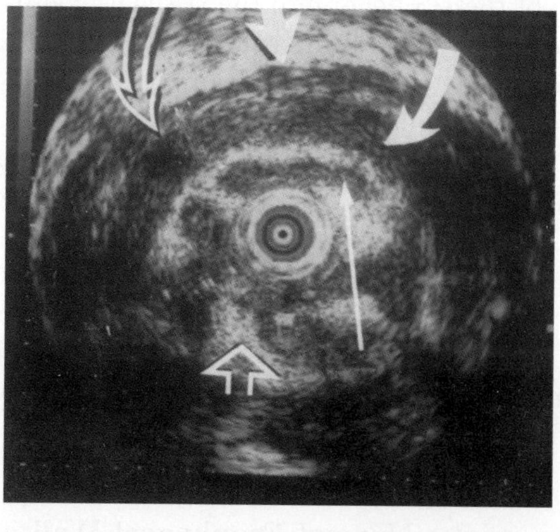

Fig. 4. Ultrasound image of a normal lower esophagel sphincter. Mucosa (thin arrow), submucosa (short open arrow), circular muscle (curved arrow), longitudinal muscle (short arrow), myenteric plexus interface (open curved arrow).

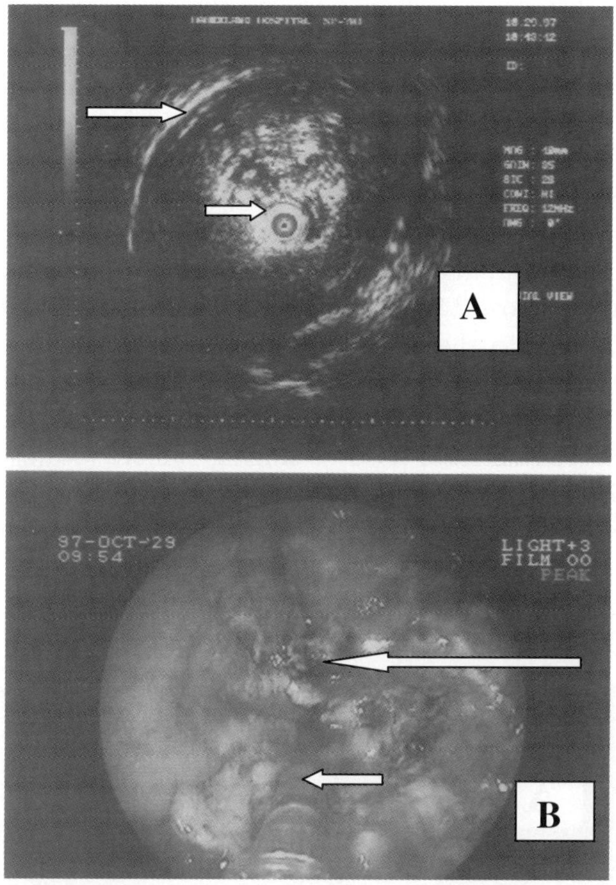


Fig. 5. (A) A circular ultrasound image obtained with an ultrasound probe (short arrow) within an esophageal stenosis showing a thickened esophageal wall (arrow). (B) Corresponding endocopic image with stenosis (arrow) and ultrasound miniprobe (short arrow).

## 3. Endosonography in Diseases of the Esophagus

The development of endoscopic ultrasound which combines ultrasonography and endosopy (EUS), has given the gastroenterologist a valuable tool to examine the surface of the gastrointestinal tract and look beneath the surface of the gastrointestinal mucosa. The method is today regarded as the best imaging modality in the evaluation of several esophageal diseases. The diagnosis and follow-up of precancerous conditions in the esophagus like Barrett's epithelium and esophagitis with dysplasia using EUS is difficult, especially because inflammatory changes cannot be reliably distinguished from tumor ingrowth. Nevertheless, EUS may be helpful in patients with precancerous conditions in the esophagus who have endoscopically visible nodules or ulcers and may also help find the optimal location for biopsies (1, 2, 5).

The diagnosis of esophageal carcinoma is usually not difficult using barium radiography or routine endoscopy and biopsy. Staging of the tumor in order to plan appropriate therapy is, however, a problem. EUS is currently regarded as the most accurate imaging modality for staging esophageal cancer. The prognosis of this disease depends on the tumor stage. EUS is especially valuable in staging early and locally advanced esophageal cancer. EUS using echoendoscopes has been used to evaluate depth of invasion into the esophageal wall, detect spread to mediastinal and coeliac lymph nodes, and to detect invasion of other mediastinal and thoracic structures.

All currently available miniprobes can visualize the esophageal wall and its nearest surroundings in detail. However, imaging of the mediastinum and adjacent organs is limited, especially with frequencies above 15 MHz. When a tumor is seen at endoscopy, the use of a miniprobe as an accessory to the endoscopic procedure can often stage a tumor up to at least T3N1 (Fig. 6). Hasegawa *et al.* (11) compared a US miniprobe (15 MHz) with a radial echo-endoscope in the staging of superficial esophageal carcinoma. The US miniprobe was more accurate than conventional EUS in staging tumors localized to the mucosa and submucosa (92% vs 76%).

A diagnostic challenge occurs during endoscopy when a bulge covered with normal mucosa is seen, suggesting the presence of a mass within or outside the gastrointestinal wall. The underlying nature of such changes can usually not be elucidated by endoscopy alone.

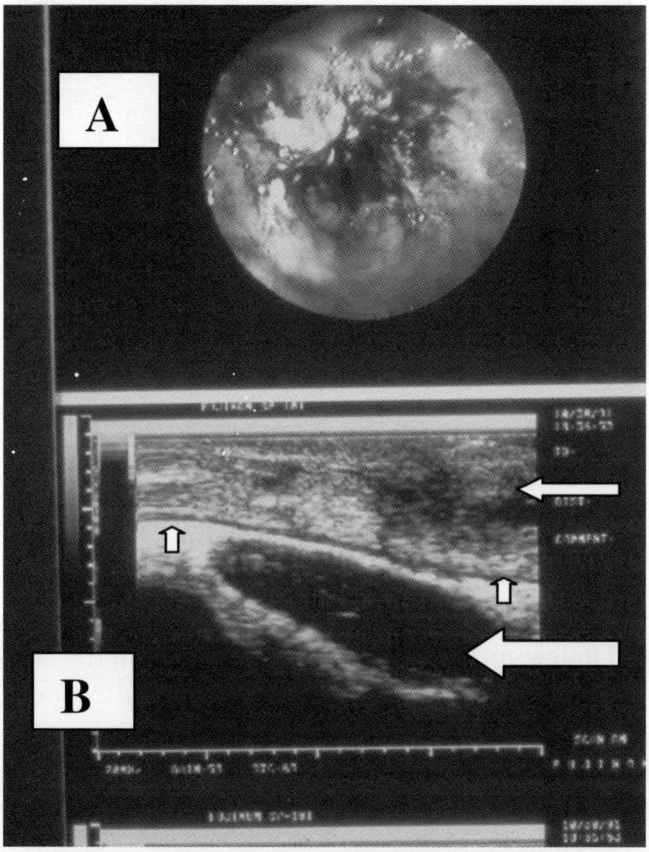


Fig. 6. (A) Endoscopic image of esophageal cancer. (B) Linear ultrasound image (20 MHz) of a T2N1 tumor (arrow), Lymph node (thick arrow), muscularis propria (small arrows).

It may be clinically important to determine whether a subepithelial mass is intramural or extramural and to describe the structural nature of a pathologic lesion.

The major and most difficult diagnostic issue concerning subepithelial lesions is to assess the malignant potential of stromal cell tumors, which may develop from myogenic or neurogenic tissue in the gastrointestinal wall. Large tumor size, ulceration, heterogeneous echo pattern, cystic spaces and irregular tumor border have been associated with risk of malignancy.

Gastrointestinal stromal cell tumors are usually recognized as an echo-poor expansion of the ultrasound layer corresponding to the muscularis propria. Some of these tumors may also arise from the muscularis mucosae, which is normally difficult to define on EUS since it is covered by the acoustical interface echo arising between the mucosal and submucosal wall layers. These tumors can be seen located in the mucosa or the submucosa and can be difficult to distinguish from other intramural tumors like carcinoids.

Lipomas are benign lesions, and can usually be seen as echo-rich well-defined structures located in the submucosa. In most cases, they are easy to diagnose with EUS, and they can usually be left *in situ*. Other tumors, like carcinoids, may however show a similar echogenicity (12).

## 4. Ultrasound and Motility

Abnormal motility in the esophagus may be caused by different diseases that may be localized in the organ itself or related to the nearest surrounding or to systemic diseases. Luminal manometry has so far been the most widely used method to study physiology and pathophysiology of several areas of the gastrointestinal tract. Despite the development of high-resolution manometry systems, there are still problems in the investigation of esophageal motor function. Esophageal pressure recordings depend on the size of the probe and esophageal tone is not detected. Respiration and cardiac contractions affect the recordings to a varying degree. In esophagus the strength of a contraction may vary considerably, thus giving more or less reliable manometric registrations. The combination of manometry and imaging techniques may be a promising approach in order to obtain new knowledge of the mechanics of motility in humans.

Transabdominal real time *B*-mode (brightness) ultrasonography has been accepted as a valuable tool in motility examination of the gastrointestinal tract (7, 13–15). *M*-mode US (time-based ultrasound) is a modality which has been mostly used to study structural changes in the cardiac muscle during contractions through both a transcutaneous and transesophageal approach. Endosonography has the potential to contribute to the study of esophageal motility. The ability of ES to visualize the layers of the wall in real time and study contractile activity has been demonstrated in several settings. Different ultrasound modalities used at high frequency with high resolution provide a unique method to study structural changes in the layers of the gastrointestinal wall during peristalsis or other intestinal motor activities. However, the ultrasound device should ideally maintain a stationary position in relation to the intestinal wall to permit accurate analysis of any structural changes occurring over time (16–20).

Taniguchi *et al.* (16) showed changes occurring in the layers of the sheep esophageal wall during swallowing using a 20 MHz $M$-mode probe, which could detect structural changes occurring separately in the esophageal wall layers during peristalsis. They reported on the use of an $M$-mode ultrasound device attached directly to the mucosa by suction in the esophagus of an unanesthetized sheep. The device was introduced and attached to the esophagus of the sheep through the nasal passage. The ultrasound layers of the sheep esophagus identified by the suction device were similar to those obtained with intraluminal ultrasound devices at 20 MHz in the human esophagus. Luminal contraction or dilation may cause tilting of the transducer but this was avoided by locating the transducer at the center of circumferentially arranged suction cups (Fig. 7).

It was demonstrated that frequencies of 15 to 20 MHz used in the sheep esophagus revealed a thickening of the inner circular muscle during contractions. Also, the ultrasound device demonstrated isolated thickening of the outer longitudinal muscle layer, which is unlikely to be detected by other diagnostic modalities. These types of observations may be important in studying gastrointestinal muscle activity in the normal and diseased state.

The presence of an endoscope in the lumen of the esophagus has an influence on motility. Ideally, the esophagus should probably be examined without having a device in the lumen. However, this is at the present time difficult, but ultrasound imaging of mediastinum and esophagus from trachea is possible (Fig. 8). Ultrasound has been used in combination with other methods as manometry catheters and electromyography electrodes. These types of studies allow correlation of pressure and electric potential changes with structural changes in the gastrointestinal wall.

Miller and coworkers (20) combined manometry with a 20 MHz ultrasound transducer and were able to correlate wall thickness, luminal diameter and contractive activity in healthy volunteers. They also identified four sonographic phases of an esophageal peristaltic sequence and indicated that the increase in muscle width by ultrasonography correlated with the increase in luminal pressure by manometry.

Taniguchi *et al.* (6) also performed a study of the sheep esophagus recording $M$-mode echoesophagram and manometry. The goal was to measure simultaneous changes in the thickness of the individual esophageal wall layers and the corresponding changes in intraluminal pressure (Fig. 9). The maximum manometric pressure, the esophageal wall layer thickness, and the duration of contraction were measured. Swallowing events up to one hour

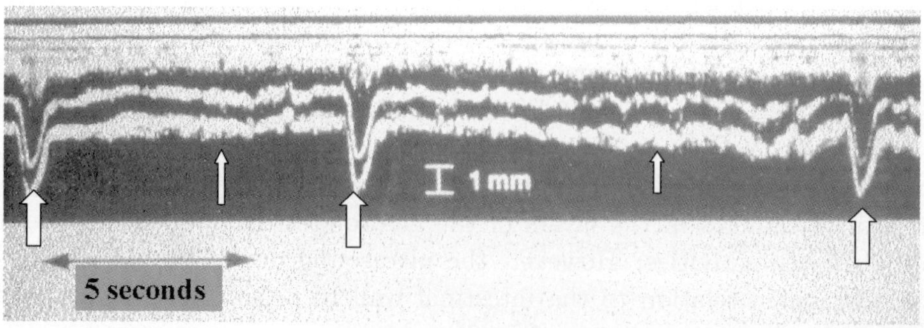


Fig. 7. $M$-mode ultrasound showing esophageal wall layers (arrows) and contractions (thick arrows).

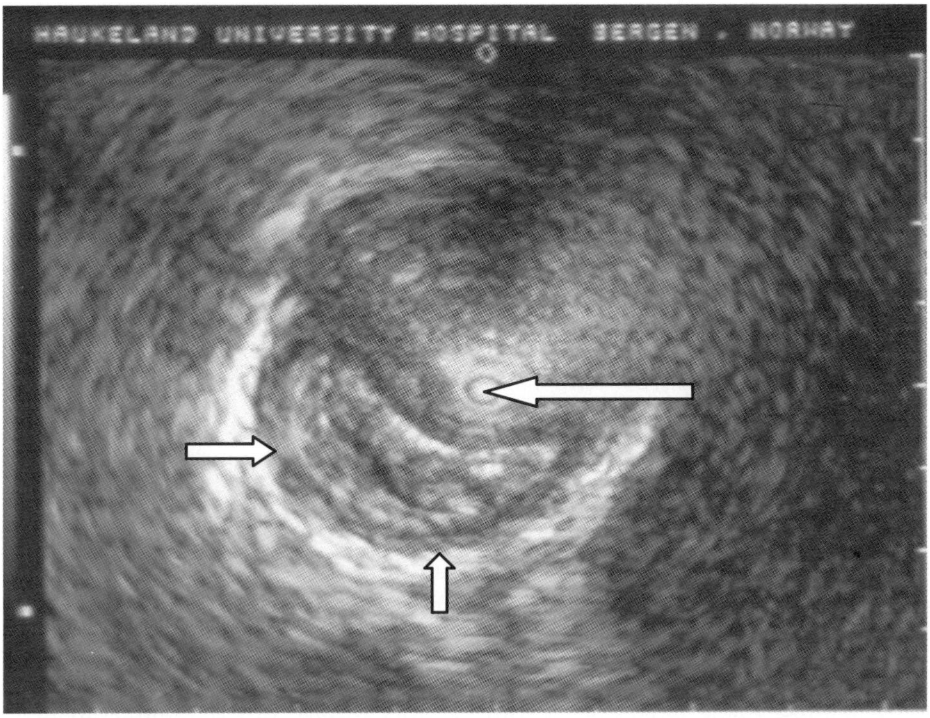


Fig. 8. Normal esophagus (arrows) imaged with an ultrasound transducer in the trachea (long arrow).

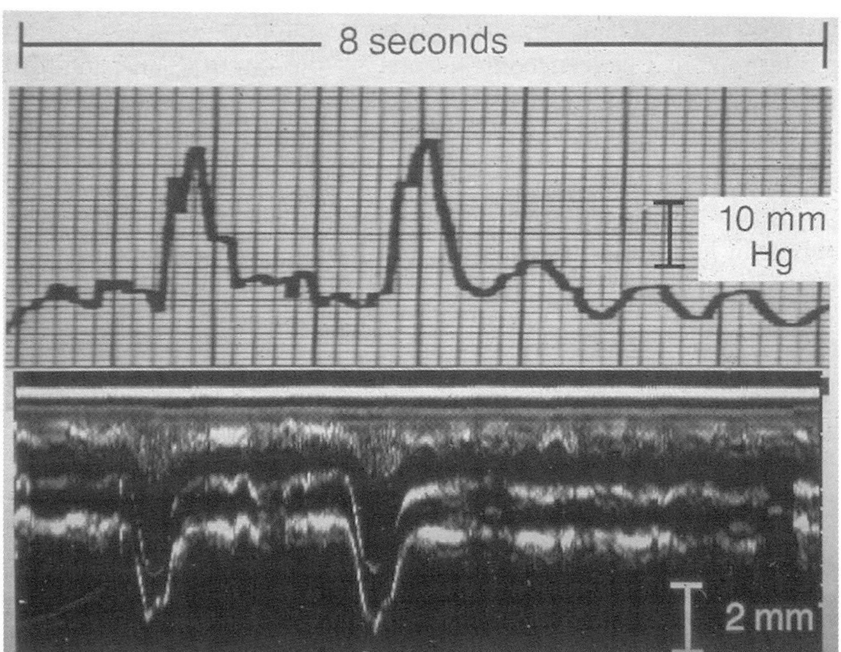


Fig. 9. Intraesophageal pressure (top) and corresponding $M$-mode ultrasound registration of the esophageal wall layers (bottom). (Courtesy RW Martin).

were recorded and in one trial both dry and wet swallows were compared. All swallowing events produced simultaneous increase in intraluminal pressure and esophageal wall thickness. The pressures recorded in dry swallows were lower than wet swallows. The thickness of the inner (circular) muscle layer increased for dry as well as wet swallows but most during wet swallows.

McCray *et al.* (18) studied the high pressure zone between the esophagus and stomach (lower esophageal sphincter and extrinsic crural diaphragm) in normal subjects with a dual high resolution endosonography–manometry catheter. This catheter recorded simultaneous manometric pressures and corresponding ultrasound images while being pulled through the distal esophagus. They found that simultaneous high-resolution endoluminal sonography and pressure manometry separate the two components of the high-pressure zone in the distal esophagus.

Technical pitfalls may bias results when using ES. This depends on the ES system and may be caused by the diameter of the ES equipment, overdistention of the balloon, and other reasons leading to compression of the esophageal wall (21). Thus, ultrasound miniprobes are regarded as superior to echoendoscopes in detailed imaging of the esophageal wall.

In recent years, ultrasound has been used in studies of the biomechanical function of the esophagus. In this sense biomechanics should be understood in a much broader sense than the term motility. Motility considers active properties such as peristaltic contractions whereas biomechanics deals with active and passive forces and deformation of the tissue. Balahan *et al.* (22) used endoscopic ultrasound to display the wall layers and suggested that there exist an association between sustained longitudinal layer contraction in the esophageal body and chest pain of unknown origin. Nicosia *et al.* (23) combined manometry and ultrasound and used conservation of mass principles to quantify local axial shortening of the esophagus. A relationship between contractions in the circular and longitudinal muscle layers during swallowing was established. Furthermore, they made 3D (space-time) reconstructions of the inner wall of the circular muscle layer for representative swallows. Takeda *et al.* (24) used combined ultrasound and manometry to determine circumferential stress-strain properties in the esophagus. Such studies will likely to advance our knowledge of esophageal function in health and disease.

## 5. Achalasia

Achalasia is a disorder of esophageal motility, with an incidence in the order of 6/100.000 adults per year. Dysphagia usually has a gradual onset and endoscopic findings are often normal in these patients. Achalasia is defined by its typical appearance at manometry and the diagnosis can be supported by findings at barium radiography that may show delayed passage through the lower esophageal sphincter and dilatation of the body of the esophagus. At manometry, achalasia is characterized primarily by aperistalsis of the esophageal body and incomplete relaxation of the lower esophageal sphincter. The diagnosis and therapy may, however, be delayed by several years. When achalasia is suspected, it is important to exclude other pathological processes. There are cases where typical achalasia is present manometrically, but the motility disturbance is secondary to other diseases like tumors ("pseudoachalasia") (Fig. 10).

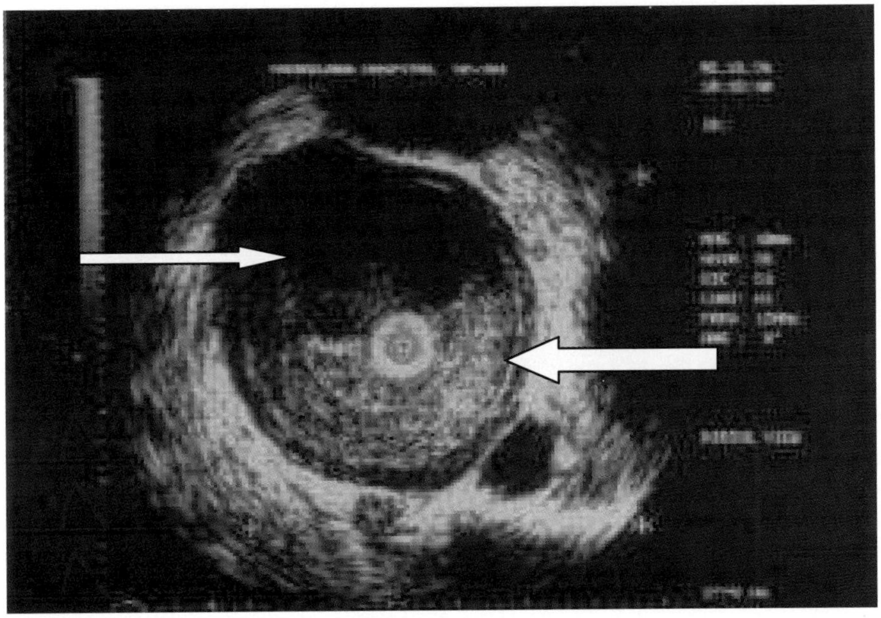

Fig. 10. Ultrasound image of a subepithelial lesion in the distal esophagus due to a leiomyoma (arrow) in a patient with suspected achalasia. Normal wall layers showing muscularis propria with the inner and outer muscular layers separated by the interface corresponding to the myenteric plexus (large arrow).

In autopsy studies of patients with achalasia the lower esophageal sphincter is increased in thickness. Using high frequency US probes, it has been shown that the thickened muscularis propria is in the inner circular portion of this layer (Fig. 11). Thickening of the circular layer of the muscularis propria at the cardia may support the diagnosis of evolving achalasia (25–32).

Deviere *et al.* (27) reported that by EUS the muscular layer was selectively thickened in 5/6 of their achalasia patients using a 7.5 MHz echoendoscope but later studies using similar echoendoscopes were unable to reproduce this high prevalence of a thickened esophageal wall.

Barthet *et al.* (25) reported a prospective study assessing systematic measurements of the esophageal wall in patients with newly diagnosed achalasia using a sector scanning echoendoscope with 12 MHz as working frequency. The endosonographic findings were correlated with manometric features and clinical symptoms. They demonstrated a significant increase in total wall thickness and thickness of the muscularis propria at the level of the lower esophageal sphincter and 5 cm more proximal in the group of achalasia patients. However, the variation made it difficult to diagnose pathology on EUS findings alone. At an early stage achalasia may be caused by dysfunction more than anatomical changes which can explain that EUS findings did not correlate well with clinical and some manometric findings.

Some studies have investigated the use of high-frequency ultrasound probes in achalasia patients. The high resolution of these probes allows us to measure the inner circular and outer longitudinal layers of the muscularis propria separately, which is of great interest.

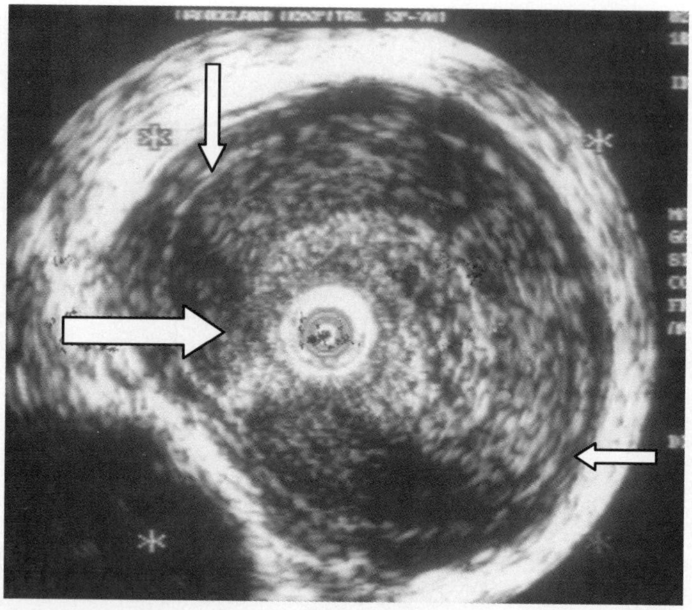

Fig. 11. The upper part of the lower esophageal sphincter in a patient with moderately increased pressure at manometry and symptoms indicating achalasia. An ultrasound miniprobe demonstrates a slightly thickened inner circular muscle (thick arrow) and a normal outer longitudinal muscle (small arrow) separated by an hyperechoic layer (interface) corresponding to the myenteric plexus (arrow).

Their small diameter and lack of a water-filled balloon makes it possible to avoid artifacts related to the compression of the tissue that would affect measurements.

High-frequency catheter-based ultrasound transducers can be inserted into the esophagus transnasally to evaluate esophageal wall structures. Lieu *et al.* (17) used this technique to examine eight patients with achalasia. Real-time US of the normal esophageal wall was performed during resting and swallowing. Thickening of the muscular layers at the lower esophageal sphincter was demonstrated.

Miller and coworkers (30) used a 20 MHz radial ultrasound transducer to examine the width of the total muscularis propria, and of the circular and longitudinal smooth muscles at the lower esophageal sphincter in 29 patients with achalasia and compared the measurements with corresponding findings in 19 normal subjects. They found that the mean width of these muscles was increased in patients with achalasia. However, because of overlap in muscle width thicknesses between these groups it was concluded that a thickened muscularis propria cannot be used to differentiate clinically between patients with achalasia and normal controls. Nevertheless, they found that both the mean longitudinal and mean circular smooth muscle layers at the lower esophageal sphincter are wider in patients with achalasia than in normal subjects.

Trowers and coworkers (31) used a single crystal transendoscopic probe giving linear images. Six achalasia patients were examined, finding the thickness of the muscularis propria to be increased.

EUS findings may predict the effect of pneumatic dilatation performed in patients with achalasia and visualization of the sphincter muscle by EUS can help guide therapeutic procedures like the injection of botulinum toxin (26, 33, 34).

## 6. Scleroderma (Systemic Sclerosis)

Patients suffering from systemic sclerosis have frequently clinical gastrointestinal manifestations, especially excessive deposition of collagen in the esophagus which may cause swallowing problems.

Lieu *et al.* (17) examined four patients with scleroderma of the esophagus. The US images obtained in these cases correlated with established pathologic descriptions like smooth muscle atrophy, variable fibrosis, and collagen deposition. Increased echogenicity and thinning of the muscularis propria, consistent with fibrosis and atrophy of the smooth muscle were observed. Endoluminal US is thus capable of defining morphologic as well as physiologic abnormalities of the esophagus in these patients. Further studies are necessary to evaluate the potential of EUS in examining swallowing events in these patients.

Miller *et al.* (35) used a 20 MHz ultrasound transducer in examining 13 patients suffering from systemic sclerosis and 13 healthy subjects. Also postmortem autopsy study was performed to compare histopathological abnormalities with sonographic findings in the esophagus. In the postmortem ultrasound study of two cases hyperechoic echoes were seen in the normally hypoechoic muscularis propria. These findings corresponded to fibrosis found in histological examinations. Hyperechoic abnormalities were ultrasonographically seen in the muscularis propria also in patients but not in normal controls. A strong positive correlation between esophageal hyperechoic and manometric abnormalities was also found.

## 7. Nutcracker Esophagus

Patients with nutcracker esophagus (NE) suffer from dysphagia and/or chest pain due to strong peristaltic contractions. High-pressure amplitudes are found using manometry. Melzer *et al.* (36, 37) used an echoendoscope to examine the thickness of the muscularis propria at the gastroesophageal junction and in the lower, middle, and upper esophagus in patients with nutcracker esophagus. The muscularis propria was thickened in one-third of the patients. This thickening, however, did not correspond to the location and the magnitude of the manometric abnormality and did not correlate with the clinical presentation. They also reported a patient with NE and esophageal pressures exceeding 800 mmHg in whom endoscopic ultrasonography demonstrated a markedly thickened esophageal muscularis propria. The hypertrophy of the muscularis propria extended from the gastroesophageal junction upwards to the middle esophagus. Thus, endosonography may be helpful in making therapeutic decisions in these patients. Pehlivanov *et al.* (38) confirmed that the muscle thickness often is increased in patients with esophageal spasms. Furthermore, they found a close association between the muscle thickness and the pressure.

## 8. Esophagitis

Esophageal dysfunction is a problem in reflux esophagitis. Important pathophysiological factors are impaired esophageal acid clearance and a hypotonic lower esophageal sphincter. The intraluminal esophageal pressure is related to the contraction of the inner circular smooth muscle. Defects of the lower esophageal sphincter area may cause esophageal reflux disease. Contraction of the longitudinal smooth muscle during swallowing may cause axial shortening of the esophagus. This muscle may stiffen the esophagus and thus generate intraluminal pressure during peristalsis. In patients with reflux esophagitis inflammatory changes are present, which may affect all or individual wall layers in the distal part of the esophagus. Periesophageal inflammation may also be present and depending on the degree of total inflammation may affect the esophageal motility and thus also acid clearance. These changes can be imaged by ultrasound miniprobes, which thus may offer new insights into the pathophysiology of reflux esophagitis.

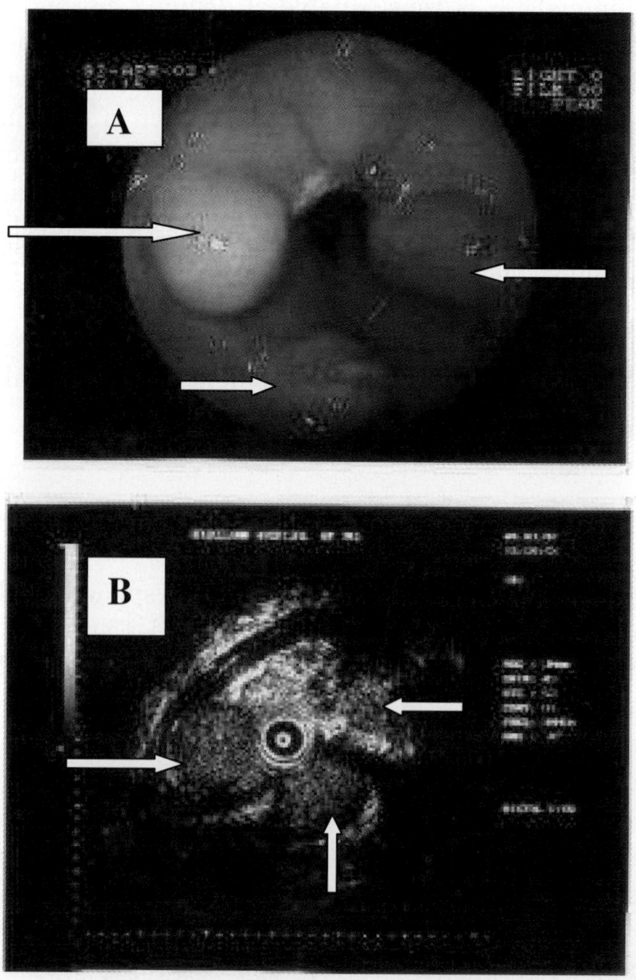


Fig. 12. Endoscopic therapy of gastro-esophageal reflux disease with implantation of Hypan prostheses (arrows) in the submucosa (A). Endosonograhic follows-up (B) to verify the position of implants (arrows).

Medical therapy for gastroesophageal reflux disease is effective, but is expensive, poses problems with compliance and causes worries about long-term side effects. Surgery is effective therapy for reflux symptoms but may create undesired symptoms in a significant proportion of patients.

Recently new endoscopic techniques have been introduced in the treatment of reflux disease. Implantation and follow-up of expandable prostheses in the distal esophagus under endoscopic and endosonographic guidance seems to be a promising method in the treatment of reflux disease (39) (Fig. 12).

## 9. Endosonography in Gastrointestinal Allergy

Adverse reactions to food and other substances may cause various intestinal (including esophagus) and extraintestinal symptoms. Based on the pathogenetic mechanisms involved, the reactions are classified as toxic or non-toxic. The latter is subdivided into immune-mediated and non-immune-mediated. Food allergy is by definition an immunologically mediated hypersensitivity reaction, whereas the term food intolerance includes pharmacological, enzymatic and other reactions due to irritants and stress.

Local allergen challenge of intestinal mucosa is associated with increased mucosal exudation of plasma, which is an immediate and non-injurious response to provocation. In allergy, luminal provocation may release various inflammatory mediators from the mucosa.

High frequency intraluminal ultrasonography has the potential to monitor wall thickening and other changes such as contractions of the gut in real time in response to provocation with food allergens. Arslan *et al.* (40) investigated duodenum with high frequency ultrasound to study wall layers and motility during allergen provocation. A 20 MHz miniature ultrasound probe was inserted through a nasoduodenal tube and ultrasound examination was performed before and after provocation. Clinical symptoms were recorded and the thickness of mucosa, submucosa and muscularis propria was measured directly on ultrasonographic images before and after allergen provocation. Endosonographic changes (i.e. any resolvable wall thickening, contraction or new echogenic layer) were observed in 15 of the 20 patients. Mucosal thickening, changes in the number of wall layers and sustained contractions of duodenum were observed in some patients after provocation. The mucosal thickening might represent mucosal edema in response to provocation. A new echorich layer was observed in two patients, which can be explained by an additional interface at the border of a thicker muscularis mucosa due to the allergic reaction. In a similar way as in duodenum, intraluminal sonography of the esophagus may show spasm and wall layer changes which may occur as a reaction to food, fluid or drug. Thus, ultrasound of the esophagus may, as in duodenum, help understand the pathophysiology behind symptoms like unexplained chest pain.

## 10. New Ultrasound Methods

Three-dimensional (3-D) endosonography is a new method which may improve the diagnostic potential of ES in imaging esophageal lesions (Fig. 13) and probably also in the evaluation of motility disorders (41–43). Thus, it is possible to estimate the volume of the

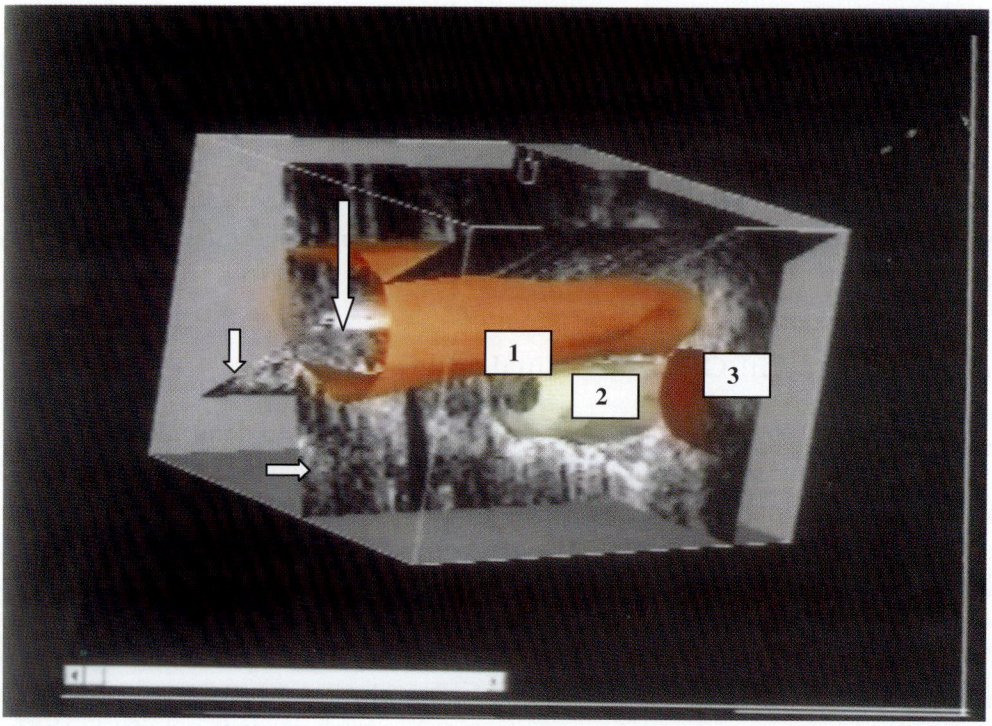


Fig. 13. Three-dimensional reconstruction of esophagus (1), lymph node (2) and aorta (3). Data obtained using a miniprobe in esophagus (long arrow). Two ultrasound planes (anyplane slicing) shown (small arrows).

inner and outer layer of muscularis propria over a defined length. The calculation of muscle volume in the distal 5 cm of the esophagus may help distinguish patients with achalasia from normal volunteers. 3-D ES probes and software programs are still research tools which are not widely available, but may be better suited to visualize the anatomy of the esophageal wall in motility disorders.

Strain rate imaging (SRI) is a novel technique to measure deformations in biological tissue. The technique is based on tissue velocity imaging, which is an ultrasound technique that provides quantitative information on the velocity of the tissue. By color-coded tissue velocity imaging, velocity samples from the whole field of view are available simultaneously. This allows for extraction of parameters such as strain and strain rate through spatial and temporal processing of the velocity data. The methods have primarily been used in echocardiography but measurements of gastric motor function have also been done recently (44).

Cardiac movement may influence accurate demonstration of the layers of the esophageal wall. In three-dimensional endosonography using high frequency probes, a "fuzzy" image may occur because of tissue movements during the cardiac cycle. A computer-controlled stepping motor device has been used in combination with echoendoscopes as well as miniprobes for serial acquisition of 2D images and 3D processing (45). Different methods for acquisition have been evaluated together with various settings based on ECG triggering. ECG — triggered 3D — ES acquisition seems to increase image resolution by reducing tissue dislocation due to cardiac movements. This results in greater accuracy in the evaluation of the esophageal wall.

## References

1. Ødegaard, S., Nesje, L. B., Ohm, M. and Kimmey, M. B., Endosonography in gastrointestinal diseases. Acta Radiologica 1999; 40: 119–34.
2. Nesje, L. B., Ødegaard, S. and Kimmey, M. B., Transendoscopic ultrasonography during conventional upper gastrointestinal endoscopy. Scand J Gastroenterol 1997; 32: 500–8.
3. Kimmey, M. B. and Ødegaard, S., High-resolution endoluminal sonography of the upper gastrointestinal tract: The linear scanning ultrasound probe. In: Van Dam J., Sivak, M. V., eds. Gastrointestinal endosonography. W.B. Saunders Company, Philadelphia. 1999. pp. 67–79.
4. Menzel, J. and Domschke, W., Gastrointestinal miniprobe sonography: The current status. Am J Gastroenterol 2000; 95: 605–16.
5. Nickl, N. J., Bhutani, M. S., Catalano, M., Hoffmann, B., Hawes, R., Chak, A. *et al.*, Clinical implications of endoscopic ultrasound: The American Endosonography Club study. Gastrointest Endosc 1996; 44: 371–7.
6. Taniguchi, D. K., Martin, R. W., Trowers, E. A. and Silverstein, F. E., Simultaneous $M$-mode echoesophagram and manometry in the sheep esophageus. Gastrointest Endosc 1995; 41: 582–586.
7. Hausken, T., Ødegaard, S., Matre, K. and Berstad, A., Antroduodenal motility and movements of luminal contents studied by Duplex sonography. Gastroenterology 1992; 102: 1583–1590.
8. Kimmey, M. B., Martin, R. W., Hagitt, R. C., Wang, K. Y., Franklin, D. W. and Silverstein, F. E., Histological correlates of gastrointestinal ultrasound images. Gastroenterology 1989; 96: 433–441.
9. Wiersema, M. and Wiersema, L., High-Resolution 25-Megahertz ultrasonography of the gastrointestinal wall: Histologic correlates. Gastrointest Endosc 1993; 39: 499–504.
10. Ødegaard, S. and Kimmey, M. B., Location of the muscularis mucosae on high frequency gastrointestinal ultrasound images. Eur J Ultrasound 1994; 1: 39–50.
11. Hasegawa, N., Niwa, Y., Arisawa, T., Hase, S., Goto, H. and Hayakawa T., Preoperative staging of superficial esophageal carcinoma. Comparison of an ultrasound probe and standard endocopic ultrasonography. Gastrointest Endosc 1996; 44: 388–393.
12. Yoshikane, H., Tsukamoto, Y., Niwa, Y., Goto, H., Hase, S., Mizutani, K. and Nakamura, T., Carcinoid tumors of the gastrointestinal tract: Evaluation with endoscopic ultrasonography. Gastrointest Endosc 1993; 39: 375–83.
13. Hausken, T., Gilja, O. H., Undeland, K. A. and Berstad, A., Timing of postprandial dyspeptic symptoms and transpyloric passage of gastric contents. Scand J Gastroenterol 1998; 33: 822–827.
14. Gilja, O. H., Hausken, T., Ødegaard, S. and Berstad, A., Monitoring postprandial size of the proximal stomach by ultrasonography. J Ultrasound Med 1995; 14: 81–89.
15. Berstad, A., Hausken, T., Gilja, O. H., Nesland, A. and Ødegaard, S., Imaging studies in dyspepsia. Eur J Surg (Suppl.) 1998. pp. 42–49.
16. Taniguchi, D. K., Martin, R. W., Trowers, E. A., Dennis, M. B., Ødegaard, S. and Silverstein, F. E., Changes in esophageal wall layers during motility: Measurements with a new miniature ultrasound suction device. Gastrointest Endosc 1993; 39: 146–152.

17. Liu, J. B., Miller, L. S., Goldberg, B. B., Feld, R. I., Alexander, A. A., Needleman, L., Castell, D. O., Klenn, P. J. and Millward, C. L., Transnasal US of the Esophagus: Preliminary Morphologic and Function Studies. Radiology 1992; 184: 721–727.
18. McGray, W. H., Chung, C., Parkman, H. P. and Miller, L. S., Use of simultaneous high-resolution endoluminal sonography (HRES) and manometry to characterize high pressure zone of distal esophagus. Dig Dis Sci 2000; 45: 1660–1666.
19. Manabe, N., Haruma, K., Hata, J., Kusunoki, H., Yoshida, S., Futagami, K., Tanaka, S. and Chayama, K., Evaluation of esophageal motility by endosonography using a miniature ultrasonographic probe in patients with reflux esophagitis. Scand J Gastroenterol 2002; 6: 674–678.
20. Miller, L. S., Liu, J.-B., Colizzo, F. P., Ter, H., Marzano, J., Barbarevech, C. *et al.*, Correlation of high-frequency endoscopic ultrasonography and manometry in the study of esophageal motility. Gastroenterology 1995; 109: 832–7.
21. Ødegaard, S., Kimmey, M. B., Martin, R. W., Yee, H. C., Cheung, A. H. S. and Silverstein, F. E., The effects of applied pressure on the thickness, layers, and echogenicity of gastrointestinal wall ultrasound images. Gastrointest Endosc 1992; 38: 351–6.
22. Balaban, D. H., Yamamoto, Y., Liu, J., Pehlivanov, N., Wisniewski, R., DeSilvey, D. and Mittal, R. K., Sustained esophageal contraction: A marker of esophageal chest pain identified by intraluminal ultrasonography. Gastroenterology. 1999; 116: 29–37.
23. Nicosia, M. A., Brasseur, J. G., Liu, J. B. and Miller, L. S., Local longitudinal muscle shortening of the human esophagus from high-frequency ultrasonography. Am J Physiol 2001; 281: G1022–G1033.
24. Takeda, T., Kassab, G., Liu, J., Puckett, J. L., Mittal, R. R. and Mittal, R. K., A novel ultrasound technique to study the biomechanics of the human esophagus *in vivo*. Am J Physiol 2002; 282: G785–G793.
25. Barthet, M., Mambrini, P., Audibert, P., Boustière, C., Helbert, T., Bertolino, J.-G. *et al.*, Relationships between endosonographic appearance and clinical or manometric features in patients with achalasia. Eur J Gastroenterol Hepatol 1998; 10: 559–564.
26. Birk, J. W., Brand, D. L., Georgesson, M., Hubbard, P., Quashie, A., Brugge, W. *et al.*, The use of endoscopic ultrasound, manometrics and esophogram to evaluate pneumatic dilatation in the treatment of achalasia. Gastroenterology 1995; 108: A59.
27. Deviere, J., Dunham, F., Rickhaert, F., Bourgeois, N. and Cremer, M., Endoscopic ultrasound in achalasia. Gastroenterology 1989; 96: 1210–1213.
28. Bertolino, J. G., Mambrini, P., Audibert, P., Zighed, D., Larroque, O., Boustière, C. *et al.*, Endoscopic ultrasonography of the distal esophagus in achalasia. Gastroenterology 1995; 108: A59.
29. Posat, P., Chaussade, S., Palazzo, L., Amouyal, P., Gaudric, M., Couturier, D. *et al.*, Endoscopic ultrasonography in achalasia. Gastroenterology 1990; 98: 253A.
30. Miller, L. S., Liu, J.-B., Barbarevech, C. A., Baranowski, R. J., Dhuria, M., Schiano, T. D., Goldberg, B. B. and Fischer, R. S., High-resolution endoluminal sonography in achalasia. Gastrointest Endosc 1995; 42: 545–9.
31. Trowers, E. A., Kimmey, M. B., Yee, H. C., Martin, R. W. and Taniguchi, D., Assessment of esophageal muscle thickness in achalasia using a high frequency linear endoscopic ultrasound probe. Gastrointest Endosc 1992; 38: 244A.
32. Hatlebakk, J. G. and Ødegaard, S., Endoscopic ultrasound — A new look at achalasia? Eur J Gastroenterol Hepatol 1998; 10: 543–545.
33. Hoffman, B. J., Bhutani, M. S., Verne, G. N. and Hawes, R. H., Treatment of achalasia by injection of botulinum toxin under endoscopic ultrasound guidance. Gastrointest Endosc 1997; 45: 77–79.

34. Hoffman, B. J., Knapple, W., Bhutani, M. S., Aabakken, L., Verne, G. N. and Hawes, R. H., EUS-guided injection of botulinum toxin (Botox) for achalasia: Final report of an open study. Am J Gastroenterol 1997; 92: 1593A.
35. Miller, L. S., Liu, J.-B., Klemm, P. J., Holahan, M. P., Varga, J., Feld, R. I. *et al.*, Endoluminal ultrasonography of the distal esophagus in systemic sclerosis. Gastroenterology 1993; 105: 31–39.
36. Melzer, E., Ron, Y., Tiomni, E., Avni, Y. and Bar-Meir, S., Assessment of the esophageal wall by endoscopic ultrasonography in patients with nutcracker esophagus. Gastrointest Endosc 1997; 46: 223–225.
37. Melzer, E., Tiomny, A., Coret, A. and Bar-Meir, S., Nutcracker esophagus: Severe muscular hypertrophy on endoscopic sonography. Gastrointest Endosc 1995; 42: 366–7.
38. Pehlivanov, N., Liu, J., Kassab, G. S., Beaumont, C. and Mittal, R. K., Relationship between esophageal muscle thickness and intraluminal pressure in patients with esophageal spasm. Am J Physiol 2002; 282: G1016–1023.
39. Fockens, P., Bruno, M. J., Gabbrielli, A., Ødegaard, S., Hatlebakk, J. *et al.*, Endoscopic augmentation of the lower esophageal sphincter for the treatment of gastroesphageal reflux disease: Multicenter study of the Gatekeeper reflux repair system. Endoscopy 2004; 36(8): 682–689. This paper is recently published.
40. Arslan, G., Ødegaard, S., Elsayed, S., Florvaag, E. and Berstad, A., Food allergy and intolerance: Response to intestinal provocation monitored by endosonography. Eur J Ultrasound 2002; 15: 29–36.
41. Molin, S. O., Nesje, L. B., Gilja, O. H., Hausken, T. and Ødegaard, S., Modalities for three-dimensional endoscopic and laparoscopic ultrasonography: *In vitro* and *in vivo* evaluation. Endoscopy 1996; 28: S38–39.
42. Liu, J. B., Miller, L. S., Chung, C. Y., Overton, D. A., Sheera, M., Forsberg, F. and Goldberg, B. B., Validation of volume measurement in esophageal pseudotumors using 3D endoluminal ultrasound. Ultrasound Med. Biol 2000; 26: 735–741.
43. Molin, S., Nesje, L. B., Gilja, O. H., Hausken, T., Martens, D. and Ødegaard, S., 3D-endosonography in gastroenterology: Methodology and clinical applications. Eur J Ultrasound 1999; 10: 171–177.
44. Gilja, O. H., Heimdal, A., Hausken, T., Gregersen, H., Matre, K., Berstad, A. and Ødegaard, S., Strain during gastric contractions can be measured using Doppler ultrasonography. Ultrasound Med Biol 2002; 28: 1457–1465.
45. Ødegaard, S., Nesje, L. B., Molin, S. O., Gilja, O. H. and Hausken, T., Three-dimensional intraluminal ultrasonography in the evaluation of gastrointestinal diseases. Abdom Imaging 1999; 24: 449–451.

Published with permission

0016-5107/93/3902-0146$1.00 + .10
GASTROINTESTINAL ENDOSCOPY


# Changes in esophageal wall layers during motility: measurements with a new miniature ultrasound suction device

Darik K. Taniguchi, MD, Roy W. Martin, PhD
Eugene A. Trowers, MD, Melvin B. Dennis, Jr., DVM
Svein Ødegaard, MD, Fred E. Silverstein, MD
*Seattle, Washington, and Bergen, Norway*

**We have developed a miniaturized ultrasound device that attaches to the gastrointestinal mucosa by suction and produces high-resolution (±0.1 mm) images of the layers of the intestinal wall. The esophageal wall layers in a single sheep were measured during 20 occlusive contractions observed with simultaneous endoscopy, which revealed thickening of the inner circular muscle layer from 1.2 ± 0.2 mm to 2.2 ± 0.4 mm ($p < 0.01$), and during 20 dilations demonstrating thinning of the full thickness of the esophageal wall from 3.6 ± 0.3 mm to 2.9 ± 0.3 mm ($p < 0.01$). Safety experiments performed in two canine stomachs demonstrated no erosions or ulceration at any level of suction. Our investigations indicate that the M-mode suction ultrasound device can safely assess changes occurring in the layers of the esophageal wall during contractions and dilations and should be evaluated for the study of human intestinal motility. (Gastrointest Endosc1993;39:146-52.)**

Abnormal motility of the gastrointestinal tract is a likely cause of symptoms in a large number of patients.[1-5] Techniques currently used to study gastrointestinal tract motility include barium contrast radiography, endoscopy, radionuclide studies, electromyography, and manometry.[6] However, these techniques do not allow for the specific analysis of structural changes occurring in the gastrointestinal wall.

For many years, the time-based ultrasound modality of M-mode has been used to study structural changes in the cardiac muscle during contractions through both a transcutaneous and a transesophageal approach.[7] This same ultrasound modality used at high frequency with high resolution provides a unique method to study structural changes in the layers of the gastrointestinal wall during peristalsis or other intestinal motor activities. However, the ultrasound device should maintain a stationary position in relation to the intestinal wall to permit accurate analysis of any structural changes occurring over time.

This study reports our investigation on the use of an M-mode ultrasound device developed by our research group. This miniaturized device attaches directly to the mucosa by suction and was studied in the esophagus of an unanesthetized sheep. M-mode images obtained in vivo with this device are compared to in vitro ultrasound images and to histologic images for correlation with known anatomic layers. We also present our findings regarding the safety of using suction to attach the device to the gastric mucosa for an extended period of time.

*Received September 21, 1992. Accepted November 16, 1992.*

*From the Department of Medicine, Division of Gastroenterology, the Department of Anesthesiology and Center for Bioengineering, and the Department of Comparative Medicine, University of Washington, Seattle, Washington, and the Section of Gastroenterology, Medical Department A, University of Bergan, Haukeland Hospital, Bergen, Norway.*

*Supported by National Institutes of Health grants R01 DK-34814-04A1, P40 RR01203-12, and T32 DK07247-14S1. Darik K. Taniguchi, MD, supported in part by a research grant from Glaxo Pharmaceuticals, Inc.*

*Reprint requests: Darik K. Taniguchi, MD, Department of Medicine, Division of Gastroenterology RG-24, University of Washington, Seattle, WA 98195.*

37/1/44235

## MATERIALS AND METHODS

### Suction device with ultrasound transducer

The device consists of four components: the suction apparatus, the ultrasound transducer and chamber, a coaxial ca-

Published with permission

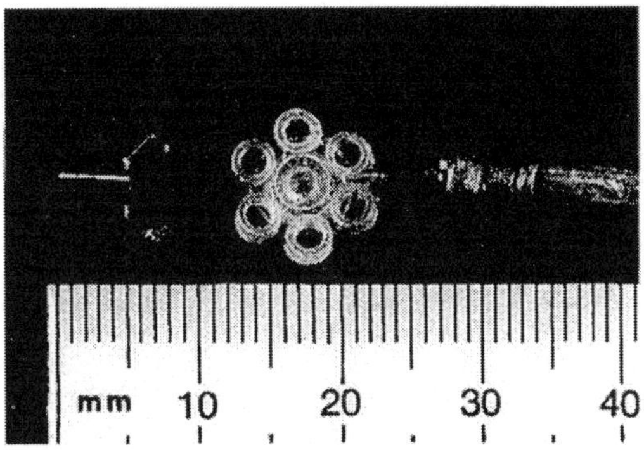


**Figure 1.** Photograph of suction ultrasound device from bottom view showing suction cup array surrounding separate transducer chamber. Open rat tooth forceps is shown for scale. Distance between tips of forceps is 5 mm.

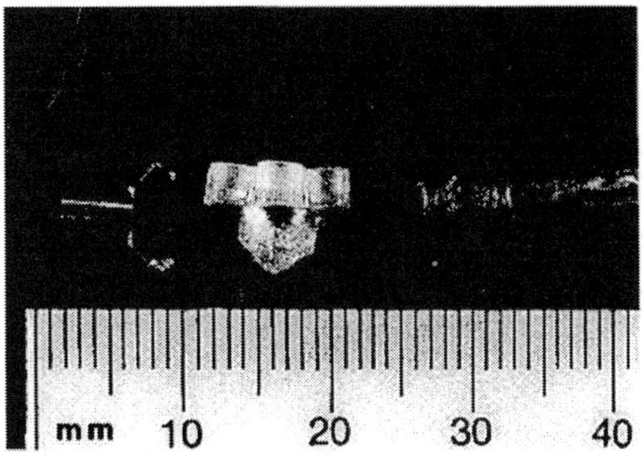


**Figure 2.** Photograph of suction ultrasound device from side view showing height of device. Open rat tooth forceps is shown for scale. Distance between tips of forceps is 5 mm.

ble for electrical connection, and the connection tubing for suction pressure and containment of the coaxial cable. The suction portion of the device is composed of silicone rubber (Silastic MDX4-4516, Dow Corning Medical Products Division, Midland, Mich.) molded to form an array of six suction cups. Each suction cup has an inner diameter of 2.1 mm and depth of 2.0 mm. The suction cups are connected to the suction tube through a common channel. The cups surround a separate central chamber for the ultrasound transducer. The chamber contains the piezoelectric transducer and distilled water to allow coupling of the ultrasound pulse from the transducer to the mucosal surface. The water is held in the chamber by a thin silicone membrane. The transducer was previously developed for a linear ultrasound imaging probe and is 1.8 mm in diameter and has a band width of 12 to 25 MHz. The axial resolution is 0.21 mm and lateral resolution is 0.45 mm at the focal region of 9 mm.[8] A coaxial cable, intertwined with an additional wire to act as a strain relief, attaches to the transducer to allow transmission of the signal. Silicone rubber tubing with an inner diameter of 1.1 mm attaches to the device to provide a channel for suction to be applied through the array of suction cups (Figs. 1 and 2).

### Image production and analysis

The M-mode ultrasound imaging unit permitted the generation of video images that were recorded on a standard videocassette recorder. The imaging unit consists of a high-frequency ultrasound transceiver and timing interface coupled with a frame grabber board (Oculus 200, Coreco Inc., Longueuil, Quebec, Canada) and a personal computer (International Business Machines Corporation, IBM-AT, Armonk, N.Y.), which uses an image-processing program to produce an image on a standard video monitor.[8] The M-mode ultrasound scans were made at a frequency of 20 MHz.

All ultrasound scans of tissue, including B-mode ultrasound images, were recorded on standard videotape. Ultrasound images were digitized for analysis by a personal computer (IBM-AT) with a frame grabber board (Oculus 200).

Histologic images of the sheep esophagus were digitized using a video microscope at an objective power of 2.5X coupled to an 8-bit (512 × 480 pixels) imaging system (Biosonics, Optical Pattern Recognition 513B, Seattle, Wash.). Visual correlation of the digitized ultrasound and histologic images was performed by placing a 2-mm scale bar on each image and adjusting the magnification to match the scale on the ultrasound image with the scale on the histologic image.

Measurement of the thickness of the layers on the digitized ultrasound images was performed with another personal computer (Apple Computer, Inc., Macintosh IIci, Cupertina, Calif.) with the National Institutes of Health Image program (version 1.44; Bethesda, Md.).

### Animals

Two sheep weighing 75 kg and 50 kg and two mongrel dogs weighing between 22 and 23 kg were obtained for the experiments. The sheep were fed alfalfa pellets, and the dogs were fed a commercial dog chow. Animals were housed individually in facilities accredited by the American Association for Accreditation of Laboratory Animal Care, and care was in accordance with the "Guide for the Care and Use of Laboratory Animals." All of the procedures were approved by the Institutional Animal Care and Use Committee of the University of Washington.

### M-mode and B-mode ultrasound image correlation with histologic images

The following experiment was performed to correlate the ultrasonic layers of the esophagus with the histologic layers. The suction M-mode ultrasound device was placed via a trans-nasal route in the mid-esophagus of the 50-kg sheep anesthetized with halothane, to a distance 45 cm from the nostril opening. Ultrasound images were generated with the M-mode ultrasound imaging unit at a frequency of 20 MHz. During continuous ultrasound monitoring, a surgical exploration of the neck was performed to identify the specific location of the device inside the esophagus. The area was identified by palpation of the device through the wall of the esophagus and was marked with a suture on the serosa. Subsequently, the animal was sacrificed and an esophagectomy

Published with permission

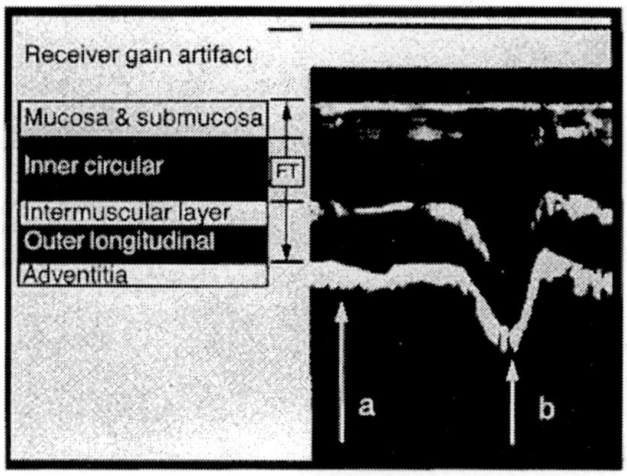


**Figure 3.** M-mode ultrasound image of sheep esophageal wall with corresponding schematic labeling of individual layers. Layers of sheep esophageal wall that were measured included full thickness *(FT)*, mucosa and submucosa, inner circular muscle, and outer longitudinal muscle. Measurements were made at baseline *(a)* and during peak of contraction *(b)*.

was performed. The area marked by the suture was excised and pinned flat to obtain in vitro ultrasound images, and histologic sections of the same portion of the esophagus from which the in vivo M-mode ultrasound images were obtained.

We performed the in vitro studies of this resected tissue with a modification of a technique previously described for obtaining correlation of the ultrasound image with the histologic samples of in vitro tissue.[9] A 20-MHz ultrasound transducer was used to obtain in vitro ultrasonic B-mode scans to compare to the in vivo M-mode ultrasound images generated with the suction device at a frequency of 20 MHz. After the ultrasound scans were completed, sections of the tissue were cut that corresponded closely to the same area and same plane of the in vitro B-mode ultrasound images. These sections were stained with Masson's trichrome stain to obtain maximal contrast between the esophageal layers. Subsequently, digitized images of the in vivo and in vitro ultrasound scans were compared with the digitized images of histologic samples of the sheep esophagus to assess the correlation of the ultrasonic and histologic layers.

### Measurements of the esophageal wall layers in the unanesthetized sheep

A single 74-kg adult sheep was used for three separate experiments to measure changes of thickness in the esophageal wall. The interval between each experiment was at least 3 weeks. No systemic or topical anesthesia was administered during the experiments. The sheep was trained to permit nasal passage of a small-diameter tube into the esophagus. After lubrication, the suction M-mode ultrasound device was placed into the nasal opening and advanced into the oropharynx and esophagus with the use of a snare or forceps to assist passage. The device was placed in the mid-esophagus at a distance of 45 to 50 cm from the nares in all experiments. The suction pump was activated at a suction level of 710 mm Hg, and the ultrasound imaging unit provided a continuous recording of the images. The rate of sweep of the M-mode imaging was 8 seconds for each video frame. After the training period, the sheep tolerated the procedure and was able to swallow liquids and solids during all experiments. Each of the three experiments had an approximate duration of 45 minutes.

The location and situation of the device was confirmed with a small-diameter (6 mm) endoscope (Fuji Photo Optical Co., Ltd., UGI-RU, Omiya City, Saitama, Japan) placed via the trans-nasal route. Complete endoscopy of the sheep esophagus revealed the junction between the esophagus and rumen (first compartment of the sheep stomach) was at 90 cm and the cricopharyngeus at 20 cm from the nares. The endoscope was placed approximately 5 cm proximal to the location of the suction ultrasound device. A single endoscopist monitored the changes occurring in the lumen of the esophagus. The esophagus was minimally distended to allow observation of the device during motility. The endoscopist was blinded to the ultrasound images during the observations. Three types of observed changes in the luminal diameter of the esophagus were seen during endoscopy and verbally noted by the endoscopist on the audio recording of the videotape. Complete obliteration of the lumen during endoscopy was designated as an occlusive contraction. A partial reduction in the luminal diameter was designated as a non-occlusive contraction, and an enlargement in the luminal diameter was designated as a dilation. Occlusive contractions could be seen after swallowing was induced by either digital stimulation of the oral cavity or introduction of water into the mouth. Correlation between the endoscopic events and the ultrasound images was obtained by synchronously recording the endoscopist's audio description of the luminal diameter and the video recording of the ultrasound M-mode images. At the conclusion of the experiment, the device was removed and the esophageal mucosa was inspected with the endoscope for any evidence of trauma or bleeding.

A total of 75 images from the three experiments corresponding to the identified endoscopic events were analyzed. Image analysis was performed by using the audio endoscopic recording to select the corresponding images from the video recording and digitizing the appropriate frames for measurement. Measurements of the ultrasonic layers were made at the resting baseline and during the endoscopic event for each image (Fig. 3).

### Statistical analysis

All data are expressed as the mean plus or minus standard deviation; $n$ represents the number of observations made. The paired $t$ test was used to determine significant differences between baseline measurements and the thickness during the observed contractions or dilations. A $p$ value of less than 0.01 was used to define a statistically significant difference.

### Safety of suction device

Two mongrel dogs were used to assess the potential for suction-induced injury with the prototype suction ultrasound device. The canine model was chosen because of the previous published experience in the assessment of injury to

Published with permission

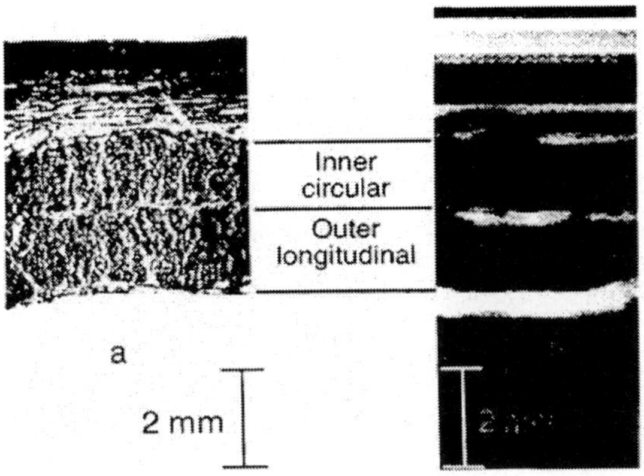


**Figure 4.** Comparison of in vitro histologic image **(a)** and in vivo ultrasound M-mode image **(b)** of sheep esophagus. Thickness of inner circular and outer longitudinal muscle layers illustrated in histologic image correspond closely to ultrasonic images of same muscle layers (Masson's trichrome stain used for histologic sample).

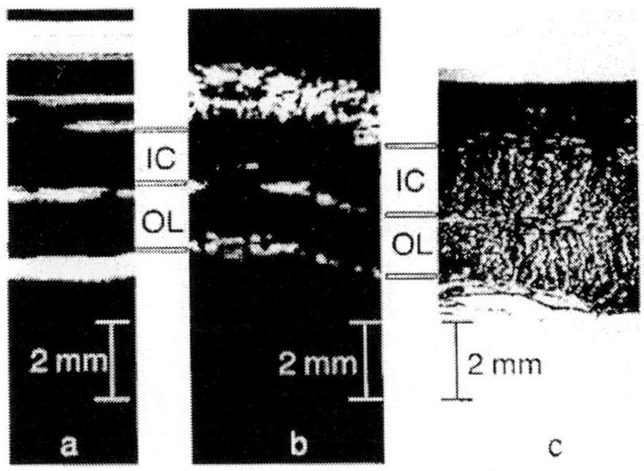


**Figure 5.** Comparison of in vivo suction M-mode **(a)** and in vitro B-mode **(b)** ultrasound image with corresponding histologic image **(c)** of sheep esophagus. The thickness of inner circular *(IC)* and outer longitudinal *(OL)* muscle layers is similar in ultrasound images and histologic image (Masson's trichrome stain).

the dog gastric mucosa by other devices including clinical nasogastric suction catheters.[10, 11] Also, the presence of the rumen in the sheep necessitated the choice of another animal model for the study of gastric mucosa.

The suction pressures used for the study were based on data obtained from measuring the perpendicular applied force necessary to displace the device from the gastrointestinal mucosa with various suction pressures. The levels of suction pressures of 710 mm Hg, 380 mm Hg, and 200 mm Hg were found in vitro to correspond with significant differences in the perpendicular force necessary for displacement. Therefore, we chose these three suction pressure levels to study in the dog model.

The levels of suction were set and maintained for the experiment by a single suction pump and three parallel, connected bleed-valve regulators. Each regulator had a separate suction gauge attached to allow monitoring of the suction pressure. Each of the three regulators had four suction ultrasound devices attached to allow the study of a total of 12 device sites for each experimental trial in the dogs.

An open laparotomy was performed after induction of halothane anesthesia. A gastrostomy was performed to allow the placement of 12 devices on the fundal mucosa. The devices were arranged in two rows of six, with each device placed next to a suture to mark the area for subsequent pathologic studies. Each row of six devices contained two devices at the 710 mm Hg, 380 mm Hg, and 200 mm Hg levels of suction pressure. The designated suction pressure was maintained for 60 minutes in all devices. After removal of the devices, each of the 12 device sites was visually examined for lesions. Subsequently, an immediate partial gastrectomy was performed to excise an area corresponding to the place where one row of six devices was located. The resected tissue was placed in Hollande's fixative for 24 hours. The gastrostomy was closed, and the animal was allowed to regain consciousness. Twenty-four hours after the procedure, the dog was sacrificed and the stomach removed. The remaining region where the other six devices had been located was identified by the suture marks. This region was resected and each device site visually inspected as before and placed in Hollande's fixative for 24 hours.

After fixation, each of the 12 device sites demarcated by the sutures was excised as an area of approximately 1.0 $cm^2$, and three histologic sections were obtained at approximately 0.3-cm intervals and then stained with hematoxylin and eosin. Control specimens were obtained from an equivalent area adjacent to each of the two rows of device sites. Three histologic sections were cut from each of the two control sites. A total of 42 histologic sections were obtained from each dog experiment (36 from device sites and 6 from control sites). Each section was graded by two examiners who were blinded to the level of suction pressure. A grading system was used to characterize the section as either normal, hemorrhagic, or necrotic. The depth of the injury was graded from 1 to 5, corresponding to involvement of the histologic layers as follows: 1, mucosa; 2, muscularis mucosa; 3, submucosa; 4, muscularis externa; 5, serosa. Conflicting results by the examiners were settled by an experienced gastrointestinal pathologist.

After completion of the two canine gastric suction experiments, we compiled a total of 24 separate visual observations of the device locations immediately after removal of the devices and 12 observations of the device sites 24 hours after removal of devices because only six device sites remained in each dog after the partial gastrectomy. A total of 84 histologic sections were reviewed including the 12 normal control sections.

## RESULTS

### M-mode and B-mode ultrasound image correlation with histology

The inner circular and outer longitudinal muscle layers in the histologic section of the sheep esophagus

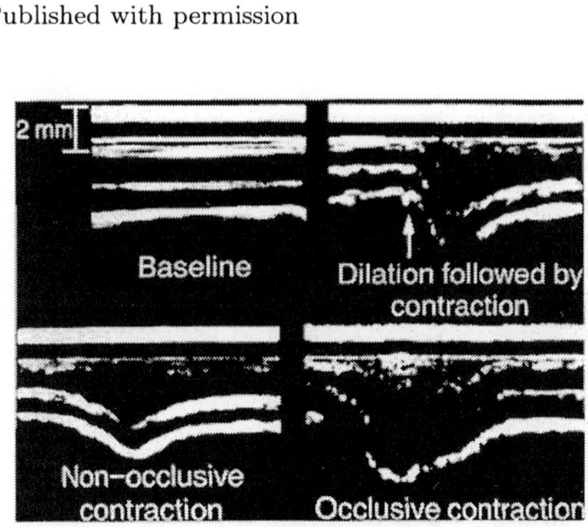


**Figure 6.** Typical examples of suction M-mode ultrasound images produced during endoscopic observation at baseline, during dilation *(arrow)* followed by contraction, non-occlusive contraction, and occlusive contraction.

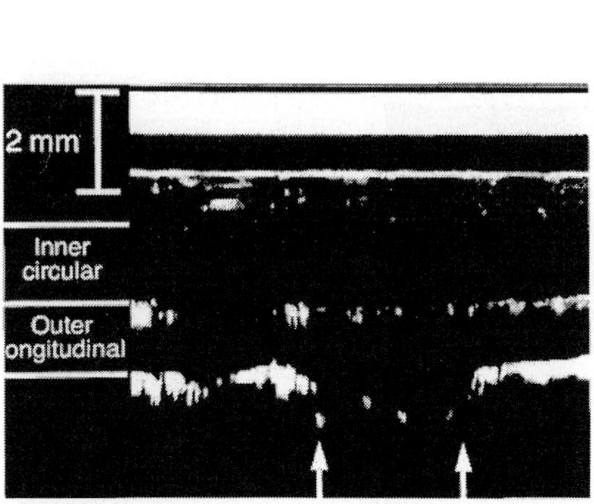


**Figure 7.** Example of suction M-mode ultrasound image possibly representing thickening of outer longitudinal muscle alone (between *arrows*). No endoscopic change in luminal diameter was noted during this event.

correlated closely with the in vivo M-mode ultrasound layers obtained with the miniature ultrasound device (Fig. 4). Also, the M-mode ultrasound layers corresponding to the inner circular and outer longitudinal muscle layers were similar in thickness to the same layers obtained with the in vitro B-mode ultrasound scan of the sheep esophagus (Fig. 5).

### Measurements of the esophageal wall layers in the unanesthetized sheep

A characteristic M-mode ultrasound image was obtained during each of the endoscopically observed luminal changes (Fig. 6). The endoscopist's description correlated directly with the ultrasound images; every change in the luminal diameter was observed as a corresponding change in the baseline ultrasound image. A total of 75 images were analyzed, and wall layer thickness was measured. Table 1 shows the mean measurements (±SD) in millimeters of the identifiable layers in the M-mode ultrasound images and the measurements of the layers during the endoscopically observed events. The mucosa and submucosa layers could not be identified as separate layers by the suction ultrasound M-mode device. Therefore, the thickness of the layers was measured together.

The mean baseline measurement (±SD) of the sheep esophagus mucosa and submucosa layers together was 1.11 ± 0.20 mm. The mean baseline measurements of the inner circular and outer longitudinal muscularis externa were 1.16 ± 0.22 mm and 1.35 ± 0.21 mm, respectively. During 20 endoscopically observed occlusive contractions the thickness of the layers increased significantly ($p < 0.01$) in the mucosa and submucosa and in the inner circular muscularis externa to 2.95 ± 0.49 mm and 2.24 ± 0.37 mm, respectively, with no change in the outer longitudinal muscularis externa. Also, during 35 endoscopically observed non-occlusive contractions the thickness increased significantly ($p < 0.01$) in the submucosa and inner circular muscularis externa to 2.04 ± 0.31 mm and 1.72 ± 0.24 mm, respectively, with no significant change in the outer longitudinal muscularis externa.

During 20 endoscopically observed dilations of the sheep esophagus, the mucosa and submucosa thickness decreased to 0.83 ± 0.11 mm and the inner circular and outer longitudinal muscularis externa measurements decreased to 0.76 ± 0.15 mm and 1.38 ± 0.14 mm, respectively; however, the changes were not statistically different ($p > 0.01$) from baseline measurements. After removal of the device at the end of the procedure, endoscopic observation revealed no evidence of mucosal damage or hemorrhage in any of the three experiments.

During one of the experiments, an isolated thickening of the outer longitudinal muscle layer was observed on the M-mode ultrasound image (Fig. 7). No change in the luminal diameter was noted by the endoscopist during the recording of this image.

### Safety of the suction device

In the safety experiments performed on the dog stomachs, visual inspection of the specimens immediately after removal of the suction devices revealed red spots on the gastric mucosa corresponding directly to the location of the suction cups for all suction devices (24 of 24 device sites inspected). During visual examination of the dog stomach specimens collected 24 hours after the removal of suction devices and initial partial gastrectomy, only 4 of 12 remaining device sites had evidence of red spots. All four sites corresponded to the 710 mm Hg level of suction pressure. No grossly visible bleeding or defects in the mucosa were seen in

Published with permission

**Table 1.**
**Mean measurements ± SD of the identifiable layers in the M-mode ultrasound images during the endoscopically observed events**

| Data | n | Full thickness (mm) | Mucosa and submucosa (mm) | Inner circular (mm) | Outer longitudinal (mm) | Muscularis externa (mm) |
|---|---|---|---|---|---|---|
| Resting baseline | 75 | 3.6 ± 0.3 | 1.1 ± 0.2 | 1.2 ± 0.2 | 1.4 ± 0.2 | 2.5 ± 0.2 |
| Occlusive contraction | 20 | 6.8 ± 0.8* | 3.0 ± 0.5* | 2.2 ± 0.4* | 1.6 ± 0.3 | 3.9 ± 0.6* |
| Non-occlusive contraction | 35 | 5.2 ± 0.5* | 2.0 ± 0.3* | 1.7 ± 0.2* | 1.4 ± 0.2 | 3.1 ± 0.3* |
| Dilation | 20 | 2.9 ± 0.3* | 0.8 ± 0.1 | 0.8 ± 0.2 | 1.4 ± 0.1 | 2.1 ± 0.3 |

n, Number of observations made.
*$p < 0.01$ compared with baseline image measurements by paired $t$ test.

the specimens resected immediately or in the specimens obtained 24 hours after the procedure.

The results of the blinded review of the 84 histologic sections demonstrated hemorrhage into the tissue in a total of 14 sections. No evidence of injury was seen in the 12 control histologic sections. The hemorrhagic injury was seen in 10 of 36 specimens taken immediately after removal of suction pressure and 4 of 36 specimens taken 24 hours after the removal of suction pressure. The depth of injury was limited to grade 1, with no extension into the muscularis mucosa or submucosa. No correlation was found between the level of suction pressure and the presence of hemorrhage in the tissue. No evidence of necrosis was found in any section.

## DISCUSSION

We have demonstrated the use of a miniature suction ultrasound device to study the sheep esophageal wall during contractions and dilations. Although the results were limited to sheep esophagus and canine stomach, our research demonstrated the efficacy and the safety of applying a miniature suction device to the intestinal mucosa to study structural changes in the intestinal wall. We found that the device could be easily introduced and attached to the esophagus of the sheep through the nasal passage. Contractions from swallowing and dilation caused by gas in the lumen could be identified on simultaneous endoscopy. These changes were correlated with ultrasound images.

The ultrasound layers of the sheep esophagus identified by the suction device are similar to those obtained with intraluminal ultrasound devices at 20 MHz in the human esophagus.[12] The typical patterns of echogenicity noted previously, which correspond to the known histologic layers, are also seen in the ultrasound device images.[13] However, the ultrasonic appearance of the mucosa and submucosa layers does not match the histologic sections of the sheep esophagus. This occurs because the direct application of the device to the mucosal surface places the electronic artifact from the receiver gain initiation near the interface of the mucosal and submucosal layers. Also, the pressure induced by suction may alter the ultrasonically measured thickness of the esophageal wall.[14]

Most previous histologic studies of suction-induced tissue injury have related to the clinical use of endotracheal or nasogastric suction.[11, 15, 16] The recorded levels of suction used in these studies were not greater than 200 mm Hg. In our study, no significant damage to the intestinal wall was detected after 1 hour of application of the device even at the maximal suction pressure of 710 mm Hg. Furthermore, endoscopic observation immediately after removal of the suction device did not reveal apparent mucosal injury or gross hemorrhage in the sheep esophagus.

The reason for the apparent lack of significant damage to the mucosa may be the small diameter and depth of the individual suction cups. The area of the mucosa subjected to the suction pressure is an important determinant of the degree of injury.[11] Nasogastric tubes and endotracheal suction tubes have a much larger diameter than the suction cups on the ultrasound device. Furthermore, the limited depth of the suction cups does not allow a large area of the mucosa to become impacted in the cups.

Several potential problems exist with the use of the miniature suction ultrasound device to study motility. The ultrasound transducer beam must maintain an orthogonal orientation with the layers of the wall to obtain accurate images of the wall layers. Departure from this orientation will affect the appearance of the various layers. For example, an oblique encounter will move the images of the two external muscle layers together until they cannot be individually distinguished. Luminal contraction or dilation may cause tilting of the transducer, altering the desired orientation to the intestinal wall and modifying the image. For example, a movement that changes the orientation of the device could produce an M-mode ultrasound image that shows the intestinal wall thickening or thinning without an actual change occurring in the dimensions of the wall. However, the observed change in the thickness of the image should demonstrate a similar change in all of the individual layers from the baseline image. Our results demonstrate non-uniform changes of thickness

Published with permission

in the various layers during swallows, which could not be completely explained by changing the orientation of the device to the wall.

We specifically designed the device to minimize the artifact created by tilting of the transducer. By locating the transducer chamber at the center of circumferentially arranged suction cups, the transducer is kept in close proximity to the intestinal wall. This should allow the device to maintain its alignment to the intestinal wall during changes in the luminal diameter.

The use of an ultrasound device to study motility offers a unique opportunity to quantitate structural changes in the gastrointestinal wall. Ultrasonography has been used to assess changes in the intestinal wall in patients with colonic tumors, achalasia, inflammatory bowel disease, and scleroderma.[17-20] We used ultrasound frequencies of 15 to 20 MHz in the sheep esophagus, which revealed that the inner circular muscle appears to thicken significantly during contractions, whereas the outer longitudinal muscle layer does not change significantly. Also, the ultrasound device demonstrated isolated thickening of the outer longitudinal muscle layer, which is unlikely to be detected by other diagnostic modalities. These types of observations may be very important in studying gastrointestinal muscle activity in the normal and diseased state.

Specifically, motility disorders that have not been well characterized by conventional methods may be better understood with use of the miniature suction ultrasound device. The use of the endoscope to observe the suction ultrasound device in our experiments may have stimulated activity in the esophagus that would not be observed under normal conditions. The presence of the endoscope in the lumen of the esophagus and the use of small amounts of air insufflation to maintain visibility could confound attempts to study normal motility. However, this device can be used in combination with other modalities that would not require the presence of the endoscope to study motility. For example, modifications to the device would allow attachment of other sensors including manometry catheters and electromyography electrodes. These types of studies would allow correlation of pressure and electric potential changes with structural changes in the gastrointestinal wall.

We conclude that the M-mode ultrasound miniature suction device provides a new modality for observing structural changes in the intestinal wall and should be evaluated for the study of human motility disorders.

## ACKNOWLEDGMENTS

We thank Andrew Proctor, John Myers, Jim Sillery, and Robert Walker for their technical assistance; Rodger Haggitt, MD, for review of histologic samples; Michael B. Kimmey, MD, and Mary Hill.

## REFERENCES

1. National Center for Health Statistics. The detailed diagnosis and procedures for patients discharged from short-stay hospitals: United States—1984. Hyattsville, MD: National Center for Health Statistics, 1984. (Vital and health statistics; series 13; no 86).
2. Richter JE, Bradley LA, Castell DO. Esophageal chest pain: current controversies in pathogenesis, diagnosis and therapy. Ann Intern Med 1989;110:66-78.
3. Davies HA. Anginal pain of esophageal origin: clinical presentation, prevalence, and prognosis. Am J Med 1992;92(suppl 5A):5S-10S.
4. Wengrower D, Zaltzman S, Karmeli F, Goldin E. Idiopathic gastroparesis in patients with unexplained nausea and vomiting. Dig Dis Sci 1991;36:1255-8.
5. Camilleri M, Prather CM. The irritable bowel syndrome: mechanisms and a practical approach to management. Ann Intern Med 1992;116:1027-8.
6. Wiley JW, Nostrant TT, Owyang C. Evaluation of gastrointestinal motility: methodologic considerations. In: Yamada T, Alpers DH, Owyang C, Powell DW, Silverstein FE, eds. Textbook of gastroenterology. Philadelphia: JB Lippincott, 1991: 2538-60.
7. Wells PN. Technical introduction to echocardiography. Br Med Bull 1989;45:829-37.
8. Martin RW, Silverstein FE, Kimmey MB. A 20-MHz ultrasound system for imaging the intestinal wall. Ultrasound Med Biol 1989;15:273-80.
9. Kimmey MB, Silverstein FE, Haggitt RC, et al. Cross-sectional imaging method: a system to compare ultrasound, computed tomography, and magnetic resonance with histologic findings. Invest Radiol 1987;22:227-31.
10. Dennis MB, Silverstein FE, Gilbert DA, People JE. Evaluation of Nd:YAG photocoagulation using a new experimental ulcer model with a single bleeding artery. Gastroenterology 1981;80: 1522-7.
11. Van Way CW III. Prevention of suction-induced gastric mucosal damage in dogs. Crit Care Med 1987;15:774-7.
12. Miller L, Liu JB, Klenn P, Dhuria M, Goldberg B, Castell DO. High frequency endoluminal sonography of the esophagus using a 20 MHz ultrasound transducer: correlation with cross-sectional histology in human autopsy specimens [Abstract]. Gastroenterology 1992;102:A486.
13. Kimmey MB, Martin RW, Haggitt RC, Wang KY, Franklin DW, Silverstein FE. Histologic correlates of gastrointestinal ultrasound images. Gastroenterology 1989;96:433-41.
14. Ødegaard S, Kimmey MB, Martin RW, Yee HC, Cheung AHS, Silverstein FE. The effects of applied pressure on the thickness, layers, and echogenicity of gastrointestinal wall ultrasound images. Gastrointest Endosc 1992;38:351-6.
15. Bailey C, Kattwinkel J, Teja K, Buckley T. Shallow versus deep endotracheal suctioning in young rabbits: pathologic effects on the tracheobronchial wall. Pediatrics 1988;82:746-51.
16. Kleiber C, Krutzfield N, Rose EF. Acute histologic changes in the tracheobronchial tree associated with different suction catheter insertion techniques. Heart Lung 1988;17:10-4.
17. Limberg B. Diagnosis and staging of colonic tumors by conventional abdominal sonography as compared with hydrocolonic sonography. N Engl J Med 1992;327:65-9.
18. Ziegler K, Sanft C, Friedrich M, Gregor M, Riecken EO. Endosonographic appearance of the esophagus in achalasia. Endoscopy 1990;22:1-4.
19. Kimmey MB, Wang KY, Haggitt RC, Mack LA, Silverstein FE. Diagnosis of inflammatory bowel disease with ultrasound: an in vitro study. Invest Radiol 1990;25:1085-90.
20. Miller L, Liu JB, Klenn P, et al. In vivo quantitative grading of the degree of severity of distal esophageal involvement in scleroderma using a high frequency ultrasound transducer compared to standard esophageal manometry [Abstract]. Gastroenterology 1992;102:A127.

CHAPTER 5

# ASSESSMENT OF THE LAYERED STRUCTURE OF THE GASTROINTESTINAL TRACT

JOO HA HWANG AND MICHAEL B. KIMMEY

## 1. Introduction

Prior to the development of endoscopic ultrasonography (EUS) imaging of the components of the wall of the gastrointestinal (GI) tract was not possible. EUS has provided gastroenterologists a valuable tool for investigating mucosal and deeper lesions of the GI wall that are identified on endoscopic examination. The ability to assess these lesions by EUS has impacted the clinical management of gastrointestinal malignancies (1–7), potentially malignant lesions such as gastrointestinal stromal tumors (GIST) (8–12) and Barrett's esophagus (13), and benign lesions such as esophageal and gastric varices (14–16), inflammatory bowel disease (17, 18), perianal fistulas and abscesses, and anal sphincter injury (19–22).

The purpose of this chapter is to present some basic ultrasound principles that establish the foundation for understanding the layered structures that are identified by EUS. The interpretation of EUS images of the layered structures and variations found in different regions of the GI tract will be reviewed. Techniques to optimize the visualization of the layered structures and indications for imaging of the GI tract wall will also be discussed.

## 2. Basic Principles of Ultrasound Imaging

In EUS, ultrasound pulses are generated by a transducer containing a piezoelectric crystal that converts an electronic pulse into an acoustic wave which then propagates into the tissue. The same transducer is then used to detect returning acoustic waves that contain information about the tissue the waves have propagated through. We will discuss some of the basic physics of ultrasound that will help to explain why the structures of the GI tract wall appear as they do on EUS imaging.

### 2.1. *Propagation of ultrasound in tissue*

The frequency of the ultrasound pulse impacts both the depth of penetration of the ultrasound pulse and the obtainable resolution. In general, as the frequency is increased, the depth of penetration decreases and the resolution increases. As ultrasound waves propagate through the tissue, the intensity of the wave becomes attenuated. Attenuation is due to effects of scattering and absorption of the ultrasound wave. The attenuation coefficient ($a$) is a function of frequency and can be determined experimentally. The only reported experimental measurements of ultrasound attenuation in the GI tract are by Dussik *et al.* (23) in measurements of the rectal wall obtained from cows (Table 1).

Table 1. Attenuation coefficients of the rectal wall.

| Frequency (MHz) | Attenuation (Np/cm) | Attenuation (dB/cm) |
|---|---|---|
| 1 | 0.07 | 0.6 |
| 3 | 0.18 | 1.6 |
| 5 | 0.28 | 2.4 |

Table 1 demonstrates the frequency dependence of the attenuation coefficient. The decrease in intensity of the ultrasound energy is given by the following equation:

$$I_x = I_0 e^{-2ax}$$

where $I_0$ is the initial intensity of the ultrasound pulse, $I_x$ is the intensity of the ultrasound pulse after it has passed a distance $x$ through tissue with an attenuation coefficient $a$ in Neper cm$^{-1}$ [Np/cm]. One can see from the above equation how intensity decreases exponentially with depth of penetration. Since the attenuation coefficient increases with frequency, intensity also decreases exponentially as frequency increases. This equation partially determines the depth of imaging since the returning ultrasound pulse from the tissue must be sufficiently intense to be detectable by the ultrasound transducer.

The velocity ($c$) of an acoustic wave in tissue is related to the bulk modulus ($K$) and density of the tissue ($\rho$). The bulk modulus is a measure of the stiffness of the tissue. The velocity of an acoustic wave in tissue is given by the following equation:

$$c = \sqrt{\frac{K}{\rho}}$$

Velocity ($c$), frequency ($f$) and wavelength ($\lambda$) are related by the well-known relationship:

$$c = \lambda f$$

The velocity of acoustic waves has been characterized for many tissues; however, it has not been characterized for independent layers of the gastrointestinal tract. From measurements of other tissues, it is believed that there is at most a 10% variation in the velocity of acoustic propagation in non-calcified solid tissue, the greatest difference being seen between fat and lean muscle (24). In fact, ultrasound imaging systems typically assume a single velocity of 1540 ms$^{-1}$ to generate the displayed images.

As an ultrasound pulse propagates through tissue, it interacts with the tissue. Potential interactions include absorption, scattering, and reflection. Absorption results in dissipation of sound energy into the tissue as heat energy. Scattering occurs when the ultrasound pulse interacts with particles that are similar or smaller in size than the wavelength of the ultrasound pulse and have different impedance values than the propagating medium. These particles are also termed non-specular reflectors. Scattering occurs in inhomogeneous media such as tissue. Tissue containing fat or collagen scatters ultrasound to a greater degree than other tissues resulting in an echogenic appearance on ultrasonography (25). Reflection occurs at the interface of large structures, relative to the wavelength, with different acoustic impedance values. These interfaces are also termed specular reflectors. The acoustic impedance ($Z$) of tissue is related to the acoustic velocity ($c$) and density ($\rho$) of the tissue by the following equation:

$$Z = \rho c$$

The concept of reflection is important to understand since this property is partially responsible for the layered appearance of the GI wall on EUS imaging. Reflection occurs when an ultrasound wave encounters an interface of two tissues with different acoustic impedance values (Fig. 1). The percent of the incident ultrasound beam that is reflected from the interface of two tissue layers with acoustic impedances of $Z_1$ and $Z_2$ is given by the following equation:

$$\%reflected = \left(\frac{Z_2 - Z_1}{Z_2 + Z_1}\right)^2 \times 100$$

It has been demonstrated that layered structures visualized on EUS imaging in general correspond to the histologic layers that include the mucosa, submucosa, muscularis propria, and serosa with subserosal fatty tissue (26–28). This is due to a combination of the echoes generated by specular reflectors that result from the acoustic impedance differences between tissue layers and the non-specular reflectors within each tissue layer creating the echogenic texture of the tissue layer. The echogenicity of the submucosa and subserosa are due to

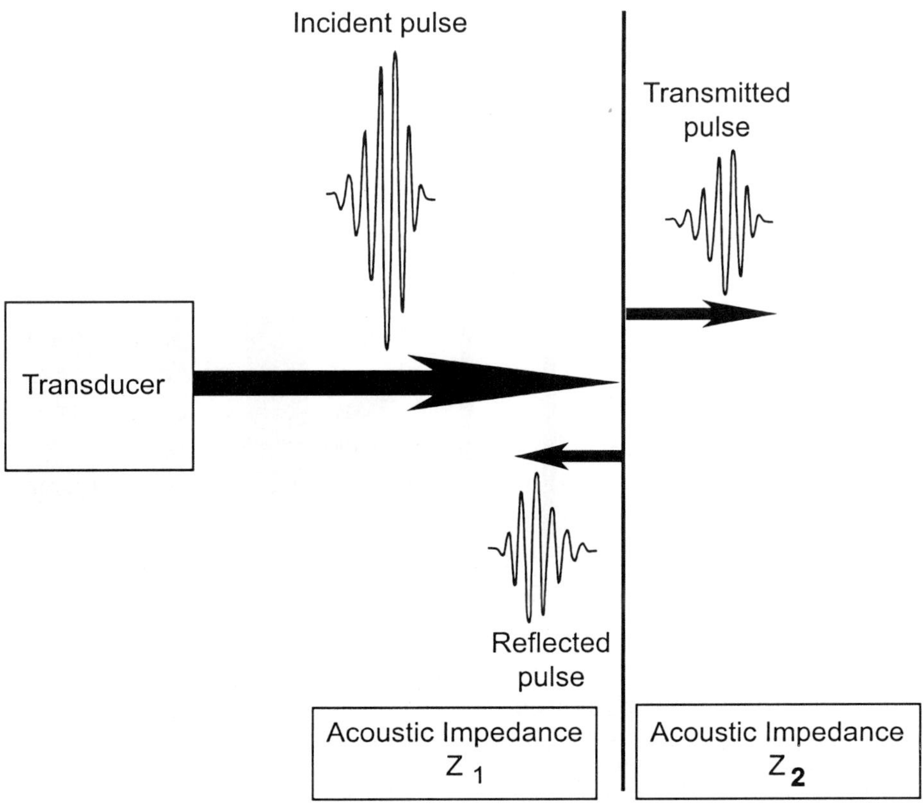


Fig. 1. An incident ultrasound pulse generated by a transducer will be partially reflected at interfaces between two tissues with different acoustic impedances. The percent reflected and transmitted is dependent on the difference in acoustic impedance between the two tissues.

speckle as a result of scattering from non-specular reflectors presumably due to the relatively high collagen content of these layers. The interpretation of the layers seen on EUS will be further detailed in the next section of this chapter.

## 3. Axial and Lateral Resolution

In ultrasound imaging one must consider both axial and lateral resolution. The axial resolution is the ability to discriminate between two distinct points along the axis of the ultrasound beam, usually corresponding to depth into the tissue (Fig. 2). The axial resolution is limited by the spatial pulse length (SPL). The SPL can be determined by the following equation:

$$SPL = \frac{c}{f} \times n$$

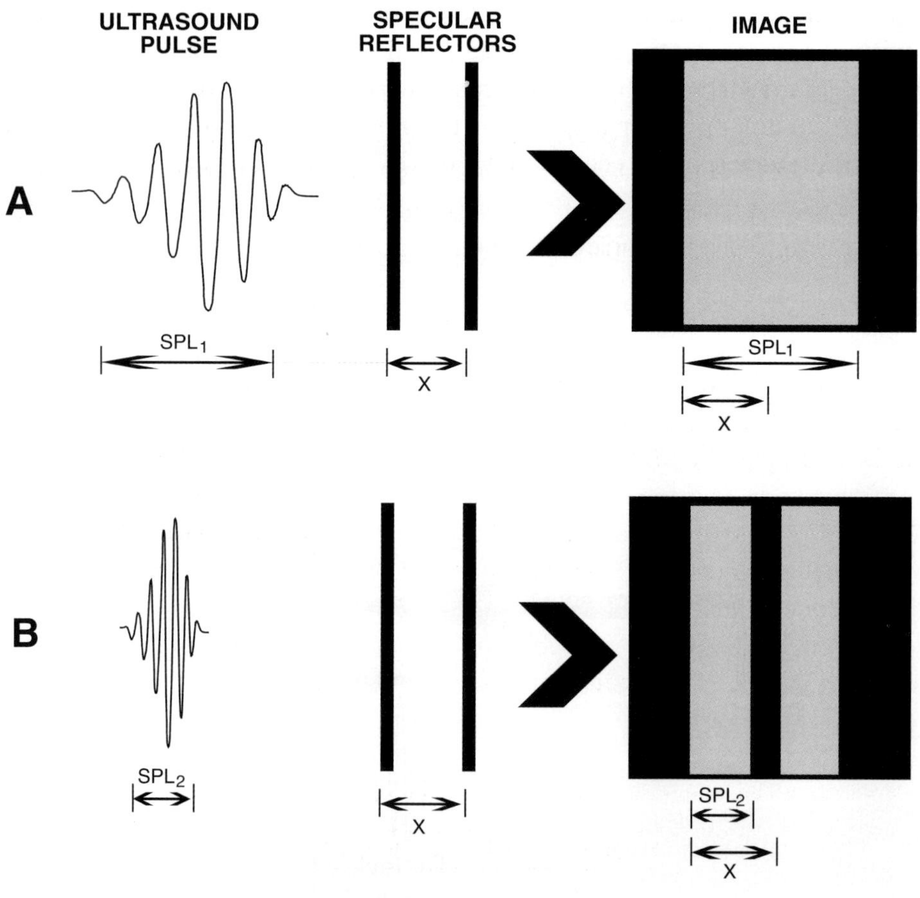


Fig. 2. Axial resolution. A pulse generated by an ultrasound transducer has a spatial pulse length (SPL) that is determined by the frequency, number of cycles, and the velocity of sound in the propagating tissue. Figure 2(A) demonstrates a lower frequency pulse that has a longer SPL. Since the SPL is greater than twice the distance between the two specular reflectors, the pulse is unable to resolve the two different reflectors and the resulting image is that of a single reflector with axial depth equal to the SPL. Figure 2(B) demonstrates a higher frequency pulse that has a shorter SPL. The SPL is less than twice the distance between the two specular reflectors, therefore, the pulse is able to resolve the two separate reflectors. The depth of each reflector on the ultrasound image is equal to the SPL of the ultrasound pulse.

where $c$ is the speed of sound in tissue (1540 $ms^{-1}$), $f$ is the frequency of the transducer, and $n$ is the number of cycles per pulse. The term $c/f$ is also equivalent to the wavelength ($\lambda$) of the ultrasound pulse in the tissue. The relationship between commonly used frequencies in EUS imaging and wavelength are illustrated in Table 2. The limit of axial resolution is equal to $SPL/2$. An ideal transducer will emit a pulse that is one cycle in duration. If the frequency of this pulse is 10 MHz then the SPL will be approximately 0.15 mm. Therefore, at best, this ideal transducer will only be able to resolve two structures that are separated by greater than 0.075 mm. Furthermore, all reflective interfaces will have a depth appearance equal to that of the SPL. In reality, the SPL is governed by the frequency and damping of the transducer. Higher frequencies and rapid damping transducers will have a shorter SPL resulting in better axial resolution. Axial resolution is the most important property in imaging the layered structures of the GI tract wall.

Lateral resolution of an imaging system is the ability to discriminate between two points that are in a plane perpendicular to the ultrasound beam. The beam width determines the lateral resolution of an ultrasound transducer and is a function of the width, frequency, and degree of focusing of the transducer. Beam formation from a transducer is a complex topic and is beyond the scope of this chapter. However, it is important to note that all transducers have a focal zone where the waist of the beam width is most narrow. For example, for an unfocused, circular disk transducer the near-field to far-field transition region is the location of the focal zone and can be determined by the following equation:

$$D = \frac{r^2}{\lambda}$$

where $D$ is the near-field to far-field transition distance from the transducer, $r$ is the radius of the transducer, and $\lambda$ is the wavelength of sound in tissue. Furthermore, the beam width at the focus is equal to the radius of the transducer (Fig. 3). The equation above also relates the frequency to the focal zone. Given a transducer of a certain radius, the focal zone will be further from the transducer for higher frequencies (Fig. 4). Therefore, the lateral resolution is a function of the transducer diameter and the frequency at which the transducer operates.

The lateral resolution will be best in the focal zone, which is determined by the transducer characteristics. The focal zone for many EUS transducers is typically 2–3 cm. This

Table 2. Relationship of frequency and wavelength in tissue ($c = 1540$ $ms^{-1}$).

| Frequency (MHz) | Wavelength (mm) |
|---|---|
| 3 | 0.513 |
| 5 | 0.308 |
| 7.5 | 0.205 |
| 10 | 0.154 |
| 12.5 | 0.123 |
| 15 | 0.103 |
| 20 | 0.077 |
| 25 | 0.062 |
| 30 | 0.051 |

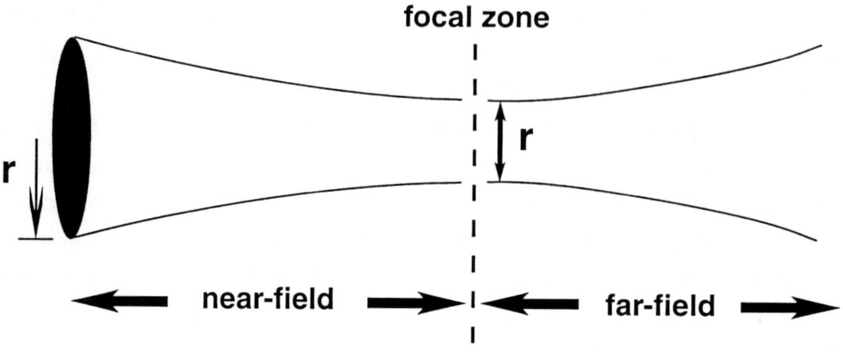


Fig. 3. Effect of transducer radius ($r$) on lateral resolution. For a non-focused, circular disk transducer, the beam width at the near-field/far-field transition is equal to the radius of the transducer. The lateral resolution in the near field is significantly influenced by the diameter of the transducer.

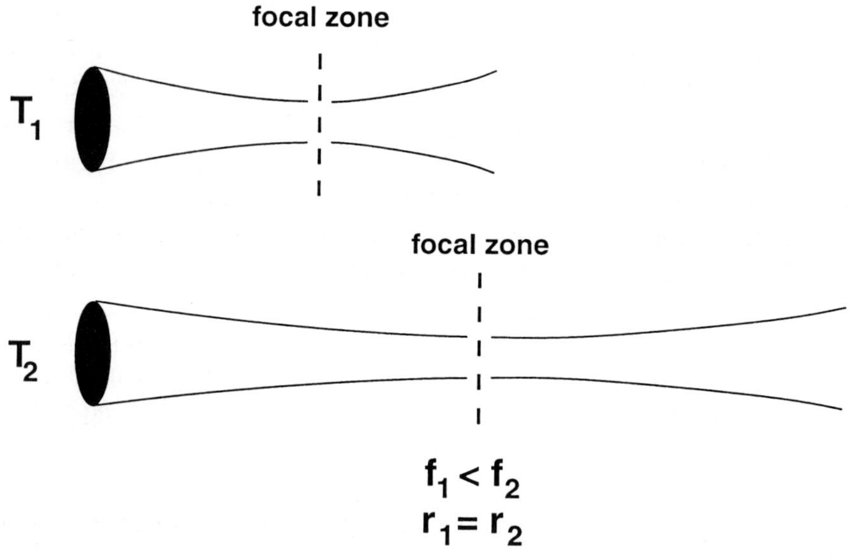


Fig. 4. The effect of transducer frequency on the distance of the focal zone from the transducer surface (depth of field). For transducers of the same radius ($r$), the focal zone is relatively closer to the transducer surface for lower frequencies ($f_1$ and $f_2$) where $f_1 < f_2$. $T_1$ will have a focal zone that is closer to the transducer surface than $T_2$, but will diverge more rapidly in the far field.

usually requires filling the GI lumen with water or filling a balloon surrounding the transducer with water in order to bring the GI wall into the focal zone. Therefore, if it is not feasible to place the GI wall in the focal zone, a transducer with a small diameter should be used since this will improve the resolution in the near-field as illustrated in Fig. 3.

## 4. The Layered Structures of the Gastrointestinal Tract Wall

EUS imaging of the GI tract wall typically exhibits 5, 7, or 9 layers depending on the region of the GI tract being examined and the frequency and operating characteristics of the transducer. Initial interpretation of the EUS images assumed direct correspondence of the layers seen on EUS to those seen on histology (29–32). The first echogenic layer was presumed to represent the mucosa, the second echolucent layer representing the muscularis mucosae, the third echogenic layer representing the submucosa, the fourth echolucent layer representing muscularis propria, and the fifth echogenic layer representing the serosa and subserosal fat. However, it was later proven that this was an incorrect interpretation of the EUS images of the GI tract wall (26). In fact, it was demonstrated that the five layers seen on EUS imaging corresponded to the following (Fig. 5): interface echo between the superficial mucosa and the acoustic coupling medium (typically water), deep mucosa, submucosa plus the acoustic interface between the submucosa and muscularis propria, muscularis propria minus the acoustic interface between the submucosa and muscularis propria, and serosa and subserosal fat. If a high-frequency (>15 MHz) transducer is used, nine layers can potentially be identified on EUS imaging (27). These nine layers corresponding to the following (Fig. 6): epithelial interface, epithelium, lamina propria plus the acoustic interface between the lamina propria and the muscularis mucosae, muscularis mucosae minus the acoustic interface between the lamina propria and muscularis mucosae, submucosa plus the acoustic interface between the submucosa and inner muscularis propria, inner muscularis propria minus interface between the submucosa and inner muscular propria, fibrous tissue band separating the inner and outer muscularis propria layers, outer muscularis propria, and serosa and subserosal fat (27, 28).

The appearance of the layered structures can be appreciated using the concepts of basic ultrasound physics that were presented earlier in this chapter. From an understanding of reflection, axial resolution, and the scattering characteristics of the different layers of the GI tract, one can understand that the layered structures seen on EUS cannot directly correspond with structures seen on histology. It is important to understand that echoes originate from interfaces between two structures with different impedances (e.g. between mucosa and submucosa). The main factor in determining the axial resolution is the spatial

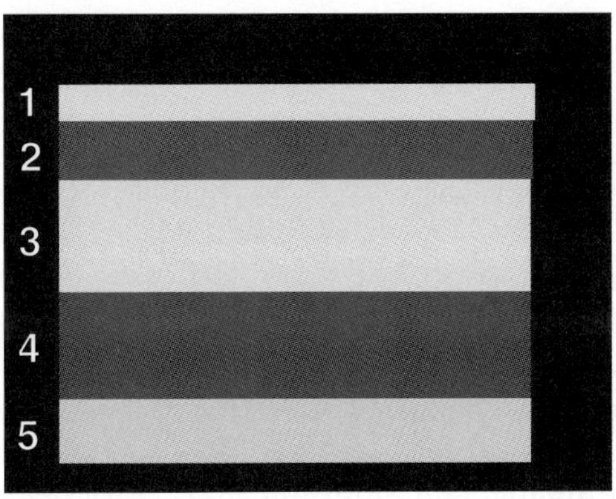


(A)

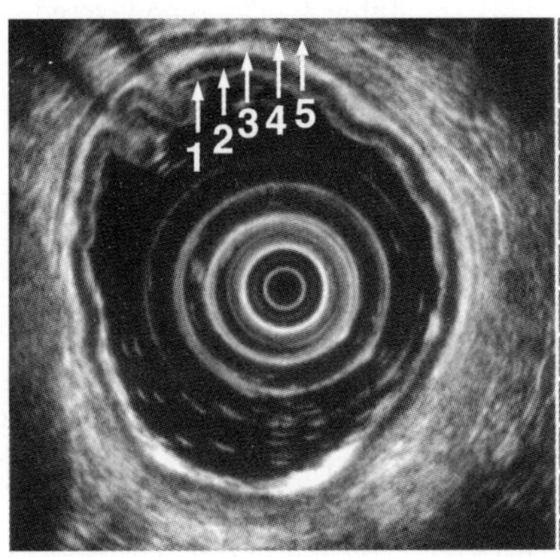


(B)

Fig. 5. The 5 layered gastrointestinal wall on EUS imaging. Figure 5(A) is a schematic of the 5 layered gastrointestinal wall and its appearance on ultrasound imaging (white is hyperechoic, dark is hypoechoic). Figure 5(B) is an actual EUS image of the gastric wall using a 12 MHz radial scanning EUS transducer. Table 3 describes the corresponding layers.

Table 3. The five layered gastrointestinal wall on EUS imaging.

| EUS layer | Corresponding histologic structure |
|---|---|
| 1 | superficial mucosa |
| 2 | deep mucosa |
| 3 | submucosa **plus** acoustic interface between submucosa and muscularis propria |
| 4 | muscularis propria **minus** acoustic interface between submucosa and muscularis propria |
| 5 | serosa and subserosal fat |

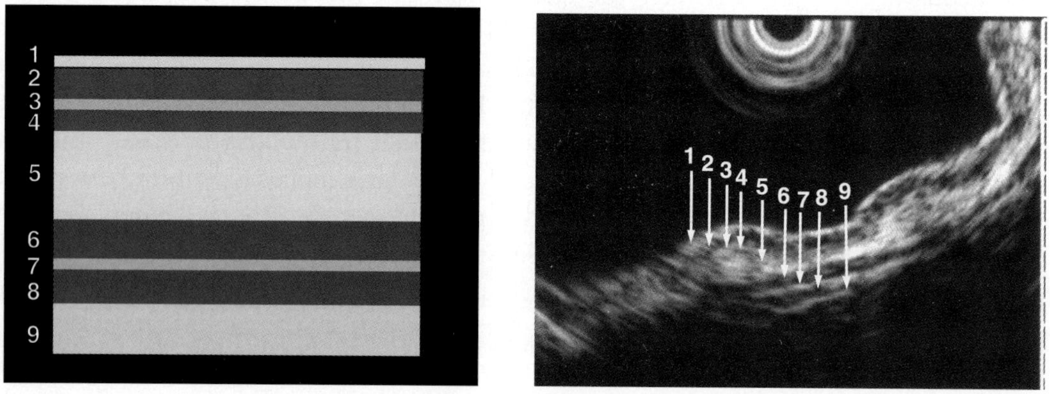


(A) (B)

Fig. 6. The 9 layered gastrointestinal wall on EUS imaging. Figure 6(A) is a schematic of the 9 layered gastrointestinal wall and its appearance on ultrasound imaging (white is hyperechoic, dark is hypoechoic). Figure 6(B) is an actual EUS image of the gastric wall using a 20 MHz catheter probe. Table 4 describes the corresponding layers.

Table 4. The nine layered gastrointestinal wall on EUS imaging.

| EUS layer | Corresponding histologic structure |
|---|---|
| 1 | epithelial interface |
| 2 | Epithelium |
| 3 | lamina propria **plus** acoustic interface between lamina propria and muscularis mucosa |
| 4 | muscularis mucosa **minus** acoustic interface between lamina propria and muscularis mucosa |
| 5 | submucosa **plus** acoustic interface between submucosa and inner muscularis propria |
| 6 | inner muscularis propria **minus** interface between submucosa and inner muscularis propria |
| 7 | fibrous tissue band separating inner and outer muscularis propria |
| 8 | outer muscularis propria |
| 9 | serosa and serosal fat |

pulse length (SPL), which is determined by the frequency and damping characteristics of the transducer. Although the interface between two tissue structures has no thickness, interface echoes will be at least the same thickness as the SPL (Fig. 2). The interface echo also appears to be thicker for irregular surfaces such as the gastric and colonic columnar epithelium with its associated pits and crypts. The finite thickness of the interface echoes can affect the apparent thickness of a structure on EUS imaging. The rationale for this is that if

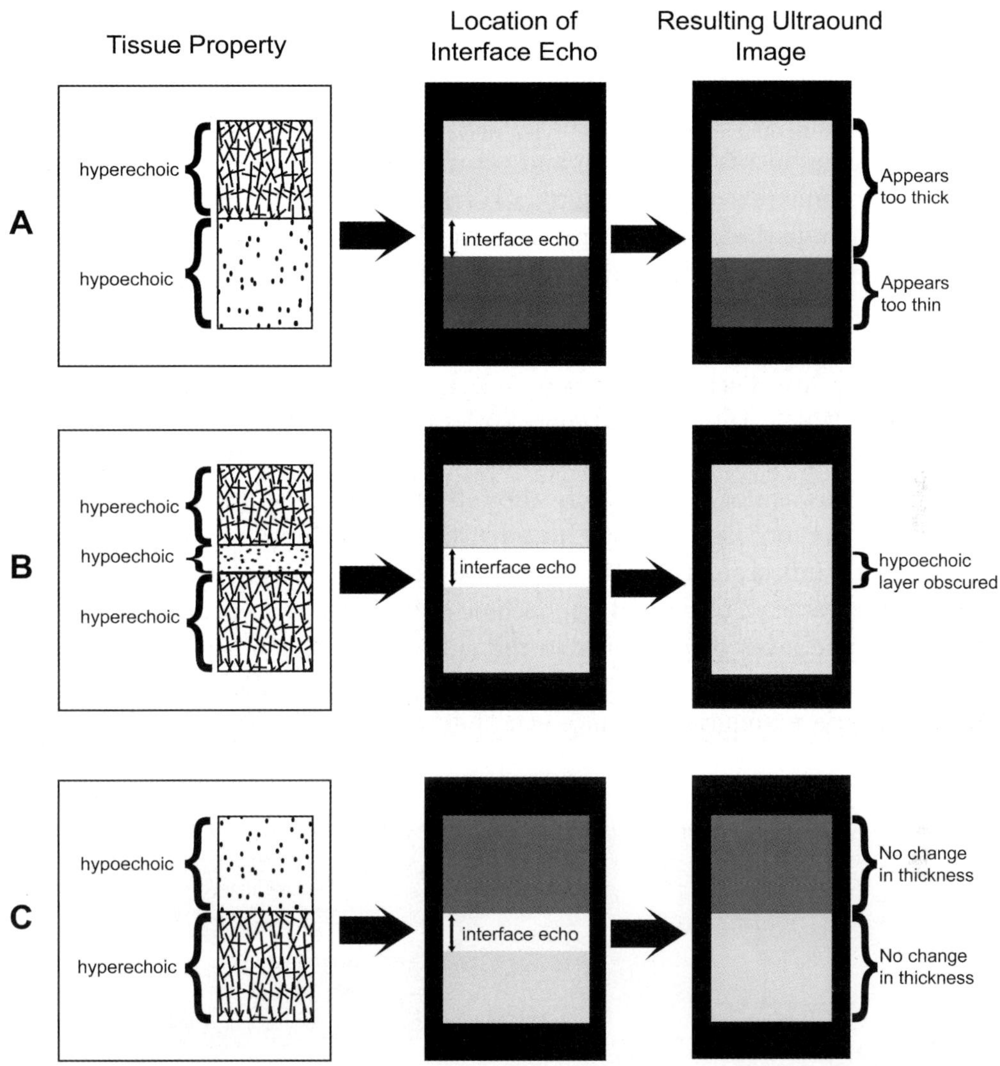


Fig. 7. The effect of interface echoes. Figure 7(A) demonstrates how the interface echo will make the superficial hyperechoic layer appear thicker than it actually is and the hypoechoic deeper layer appear thinner than it actually is. Figure 7(B) demonstrates how the interface echo can obscure a thin hypoechoic layer if the thickness of the hypoechoic layer is less than the spatial pulse length. Figure 7(C) illustrates that if the superficial layer is hypoechoic and the deeper layer is hyperechoic, the thickness of the hypoechoic layer is not changed on ultrasound imaging.

the structure beyond the interface is less echogenic than the structure superficial to the interface, the superficial layered structure will appear thicker than it actually is (Fig. 7(A)). If the structure beyond the interface is less echogenic than the structure superficial to the interface, and the structure beyond the interface is thinner than the SPL, then the structure beyond the interface will be obscured by the echo from the interface (Fig. 7(B)). If the structure beyond the interface is more echogenic than the interface, then the interface echo will blend with the echoes from the layer itself and the thickness of the structures will not change (Fig. 7(C)).

The echogenicity of a tissue structure depends on the scattering characteristics of the tissue. As was mentioned previously, scattering occurs in inhomogeneous media. Tissues with a relatively high fat, collagen, or mineral content will scatter ultrasound to a greater degree. As ultrasound waves are scattered, they interact with other structures outside the path of the original ultrasound beam and return to the transducer along different paths resulting in an echogenic texture on imaging. GI tract wall structures that appear echogenic due to scattering include the lamina propria (when it can be resolved with 20 MHz or higher frequency transducers), submucosa, and subserosal fat. All other echogenic structures are a result of reflections from interfaces.

In studies that have compared EUS images to histology (26–28), these concepts have explained why there are discrepancies between thickness of layers observed on histology and EUS imaging. When using low frequencies to image the GI tract wall, five layers are typically observed (Fig. 8). The first echogenic layer appears to be thinner than the true thickness of the mucosa since it is actually the reflection echo between the ultrasound coupling medium and the mucosal surface. Initially, the second hypoechoic layer was thought to be the muscularis mucosae. However, this layer appeared be too thick on EUS imaging to be muscularis mucosae. The second hypoechoic layer is now accepted to be deep mucosa. The third hyperechoic layer corresponds to the submucosa plus an interface echo between the submucosa and the muscularis propria. The fourth hypoechoic layer corresponds to the muscularis propria minus the interface echo between the submucosa and the muscularis

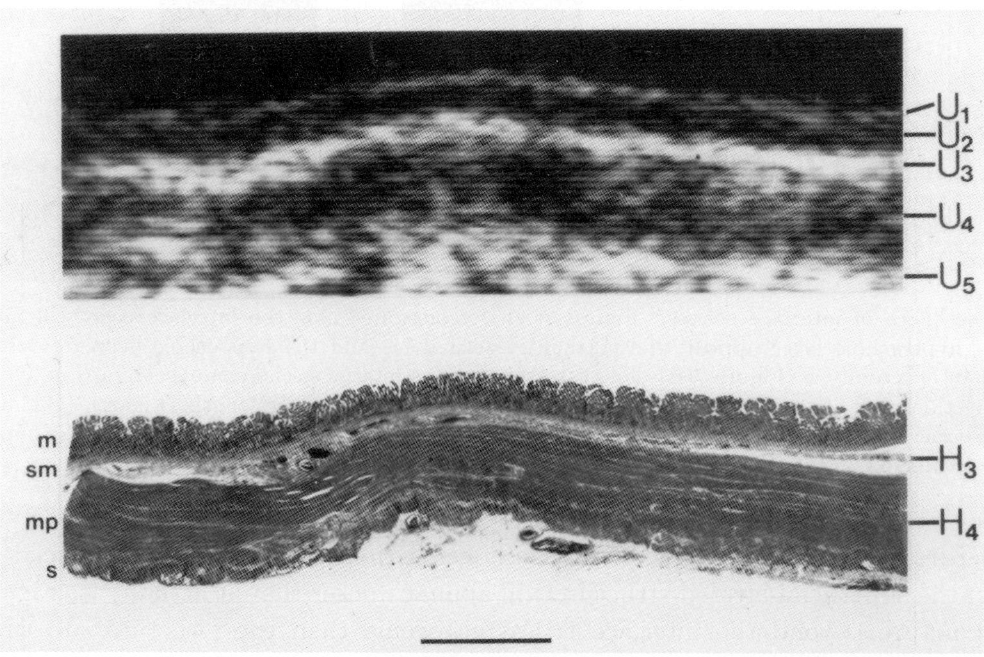


Fig. 8. The ultrasound image of a specimen of gastric antrum (top) is compared with the corresponding histologic section (bottom). The ultrasound image demonstrates 5 layers which are numbered sequentially $U_1$ through $U_5$ beginning with the mucosal surface. The submucosa (sm) is labeled $H_3$ and the muscularis propria (mp) is labeled $H_4$. The mucosa (m) and serosa (s) are also seen on the histologic section. (Reproduced from Kimmey, M. B., *et al.* Gastroenterology 1989; 96: 434, with permission WB Saunders.)

propria. The fifth hyperechoic layer corresponds to the serosa and subserosal fat. Additional discrepancies in tissue layer thickness between histologic and EUS images can be contributed to shrinkage of tissue during histologic processing and possibly variations in acoustic propagation velocities in the different tissue layers. However, these discrepancies appear to be minimal (26).

## 5. Variations in the Wall Structure

The GI tract wall maintains essentially the same layered structure from the esophagus to the rectum with some regional differences. These regional differences will be briefly reviewed.

### 5.1. *Esophagus*

The first echogenic layer in the esophagus is typically thin since the squamous epithelial lining is smooth as opposed to the rougher columnar epithelium seen in the rest of the GI tract. The mucosal and submucosal layers are quite thin in the esophagus and are difficult to resolve without using a high frequency probe and imaging through water in the lumen. These thin layers are easily compressed by the water-filled balloon surrounding the transducer on the ultrasound endoscope. The muscularis propria layer is often separated into three layers consisting of the inner circular muscle layer, an intermuscular connective tissue layer, and the outer longitudinal muscle layer. These prominent muscle layers are often especially well seen in patients with achalasia and long-standing distal esophageal obstruction. Since the esophagus does not have a serosal layer, the fifth echogenic layer is usually consisted of the adventitia and surrounding fat (33).

### 5.2. *Stomach*

The stomach has a well-developed five-layered wall structure. This is easily visualized when water is placed in the lumen. The second layer is often prominent because of the relatively thick columnar mucosa and glands. The fourth layer is often thicker in the distal stomach compared to the proximal stomach. The fifth layer generally corresponds to surrounding structures and perigastric fat as the serosa is too thin to be resolved with endoscopic ultrasound.

### 5.3. *Duodenum*

The five-layered structure is usually visible in the duodenum, although the first and second layers are also quite thin and difficult to image without the water-filled lumen technique. The muscularis propria layer is also generally thin and the separate inner circular and outer longitudinal muscle layers are rarely resolved.

### 5.4. *Colon and Rectum*

The five layers of the colonic wall are usually well developed. The muscularis propria layer is focally thickened in certain areas where the taenia coli form a well-developed outer longitudinal muscle layer.

## 6. Indications for Imaging the Wall of the GI Tract

The indications for imaging the GI wall include staging mucosal neoplasms, investigating the cause of a subepithelial mass, and imaging situations where the wall is diffusely thickened.

The TNM staging system is ideally suited for use with endoscopic ultrasound staging of GI cancer (Table 5). Malignancy confined to the mucosal or submucosal layers is a $T_1$ cancer whereas invasion of the muscularis propria represents a $T_2$ stage. When the cancer has invaded outside of the GI wall, a $T_3$ stage is present. These stages correlate very well with the EUS layer system. The influence of interface echoes on staging inaccuracy has not been fully explored, although there is a potential for these interface echoes to affect staging accuracy. For example, a malignancy that focally invades the muscularis mucosae may indent the superficial aspect of the third ultrasound layer and appear to represent submucosal invasion, when in fact, only muscularis mucosae invasion is present. Similarly, a cancer that is focally invading the muscularis propria might be obscured by the interface echo between the tumor and the muscularis propria.

EUS imaging is also useful in detecting the cause of a subepithelial mass in the GI tract. Again, the layered structure as well as the echogenecity of the lesion is useful in suggesting an etiology for the mass (Table 6). Diffuse abnormalities of the GI wall are uncommon except in the stomach. EUS can be very helpful in distinguishing the cause of a thick stomach wall by detecting which layer or layers is/are thickened (Table 7).

Table 5. TNM staging system.

| Stage | Histology | US Layer |
|---|---|---|
| $T_{1M}$ | Mucosa | 1, 2 |
| $T_{1SM}$ | Submucosa | 3 |
| $T_2$ | Muscularis propria | 4 |
| $T_3$ | Adventitia or serosa | 5 |
| $T_4$ | Adjacent organs | N/A |
| $N_0$ | No nodal involvement | N/A |
| $N_1$ | Regional lymph node involvement | N/A |
| $M_0$ | No metastasis | N/A |
| $M_1$ | Metastasis | N/A |

Table 6. Diagnosis of GI subepithelial mass.

| Layer | Anechoic | Hypoechoic | Hyperechoic |
|---|---|---|---|
| 2 | Cyst<br>Varix | Leiomyoma of the muscularis mucosae<br>Carcinoid tumor | |
| 3 | Cyst<br>Varix | Metastases<br>Granular cell tumor<br>Carcinoid tumor | Lipoma |
| 4 | | GI stromal tumor | |
| 5 | Vessel<br>Pseudocyst | Liver<br>Spleen | Bone<br>Fat |

Table 7. Differential diagnosis of gastric wall thickening.

| | |
|---|---|
| Layer 2 only | Gastrinoma<br>Menetrier's disease<br>H. pylori gastritis<br>Early MALT lymphoma |
| Diffuse (layers 1–4) thickening | Linitis plastica<br>Lymphoma<br>Metastatic cancer (esp. breast) |

## 7. Techniques for Imaging the Wall of the GI Tract

Since the gastrointestinal lumen normally contains air and since air does not readily transmit ultrasound waves, much of EUS imaging technique is devoted to removing air and providing adequate coupling for the ultrasound wave. There are several techniques available to do this. Current ultrasound endoscopes have a latex balloon surrounding the transducer that can be filled with water. This technique is useful in areas where it is difficult to keep intraluminal water in position such as the esophagus and duodenum. The best resolution of wall structure is achieved by filling the GI lumen with water and by suctioning air and is usually possible in the stomach and rectum. In the duodenum, an antiperistaltic agent such as glucagon can be administered to reduce peristaltic water movement. Keeping water within the esophageal lumen is more difficult. A number of techniques have been developed for use with the ultrasound catheter probe. These include filling the esophagus with water and preventing aspiration by placing a balloon around the shaft of the endoscope, proximal to the transducer. Another more widely available technique is to place a condom on the end of the ultrasound endoscope and fill this with water (34, 35). When the ultrasound probe is passed out the endoscope channel into the water-filled condom, imaging of the esophageal wall adjacent to the condom can be achieved.

Water is also used to keep the transducer at the optimal focal zone for resolving the GI wall structure. For most EUS transducers, this focal zone is approximately 2 cm from the transducer. It is in this focal zone that the lateral resolution is at its best and therefore the image is most clear. The water-filled lumen method and the water-filled balloon technique can be used for this purpose.

A disadvantage of the water-filled balloon technique is that the wall layers can be compressed. *In vitro* studies have shown that it is especially the superficial wall layers that are most susceptible to compression and therefore thinning on ultrasound images (36).

## 8. Conclusions

The only available *in vivo* method for examination of the GI wall, beyond the mucosal surface, is EUS. It provides gastroenterologists with a valuable diagnostic tool to assess pathology in the GI tract to help guide clinical management of the patient. The endoscopist performing EUS should understand how ultrasound images are formed in order to correctly interpret findings on EUS imaging. Selection of the correct transducer and using good technique are important in obtaining high-quality images. When imaging the wall of the GI tract, the method of acoustic coupling is critical. Without good acoustic coupling to the mucosal surface, high-quality images cannot be obtained. The highest frequency available should be used to image the wall of the GI tract since deep penetration is not necessary unless imaging a large tumor arising from the wall. Using a higher frequency transducer will result in better resolution and allow for better identification of the layers involved. Lower frequencies may be required to identify the size of a mass ($T$-staging), and to assess nodal involvement ($N$-staging). The field of EUS continues to evolve with improvements in transducer technology, signal processing, and the broadening of indications for EUS.

## References


1. Wiersema, M. J. and Harewood, G. C., Endoscopic ultrasound for rectal cancer. Gastroenterology Clinics of North America 2002; 31: 1093–1105.
2. Kelly, S., Harris, K. M., Berry, E., Hutton, J., Roderick, P., Cullingworth, J. *et al.*, A systematic review of the staging performance of endoscopic ultrasound in gastro-oesophageal carcinoma. Gut 2001; 49: 534–539.
3. Messmann, H. and Schlottmann, K., Role of endoscopy in the staging of esophageal and gastric cancer. Seminars in Surgical Oncology 2001; 20: 78–81.
4. Vickers, J., Role of endoscopic ultrasound in the preoperative assessment of patients with oesophageal cancer. Annals of the Royal College of Surgeons of England 1998; 80: 233–239.
5. Matsumoto, Y., Yanai, H., Tokiyama, H., Nishiaki, M., Higaki, S. and Okita, K., Endoscopic ultrasonography for diagnosis of submucosal invasion in early gastric cancer. Journal of Gastroenterology 2000; 35: 326–331.
6. Yanai, H., Fujimura, H., Suzumi, M., Matsuura, S., Awaya, N., Noguchi, T. *et al.*, Delineation of the gastric muscularis mucosae and assessment of depth of invasion of early gastric cancer using a 20-megahertz endoscopic ultrasound probe. Gastrointestinal Endoscopy 1993; 39: 505–512.
7. Tio, T. L., Coene, P. P., van Delden, O. M. and Tytgat, G. N., Colorectal carcinoma: Preoperative TNM classification with endosonography. Radiology 1991; 179: 165–170.
8. Kawamoto, K., Yamada, Y., Utsunomiya, T., Okamura, H., Mizuguchi, M., Motooka, M. *et al.*, Gastrointestinal submucosal tumors: Evaluation with endoscopic US. Radiology 1997; 205: 733–740.
9. Nesje, L. B., Laerum, O. D., Svanes, K. and Ødegaard, S., Subepithelial masses of the gastrointestinal tract evaluated by endoscopic ultrasonography. European Journal of Ultrasound 2002; 15: 45–54.
10. Ødegaard, S., Kimmey, M., Borkje, B. and Hausken, T., Endoscopic ultrasonographic findings in benign and malignant diseases of the stomach. European Journal of Radiology 1990; 11: 175–179.
11. Palazzo, L., Landi, B., Cellier, C., Cuillerier, E., Roseau, G. and Barbier, J. P., Endosonographic features predictive of benign and malignant gastrointestinal stromal cell tumours. Gut 2000; 46: 88–92.
12. Shen, E. F., Arnott, I. D., Plevris, J. and Penman, I. D., Endoscopic ultrasonography in the diagnosis and management of suspected upper gastrointestinal submucosal tumours. British Journal of Surgery 2002; 89: 231–235.
13. Adrain, A., Ter, H., Cassidy, M., Schiano, T., Liu, J. and Miller, L., High-resolution endoluminal sonography is a sensitive modality for the identification of Barrett's metaplasia. Gastrointestinal Endoscopy 1997; 46: 147–151.

14. Lee, Y. T., Chan, F. K., Ching, J. Y., Lai, C. W., Leung, V. K., Chung, S. C. *et al.*, Diagnosis of gastroesophageal varices and portal collateral venous abnormalities by endosonography in cirrhotic patients. Endoscopy 2002; 34: 391–398.
15. Irisawa, A., Saito, A., Obara, K., Shibukawa, G., Takagi, T., Shishido, H. *et al.*, Endoscopic recurrence of esophageal varices is associated with the specific EUS abnormalities: Severe periesophageal collateral veins and large perforating veins. Gastrointestinal Endoscopy 2001; 53: 77–84.
16. Tio, T. L., Kimmings, N., Rauws, E., Jansen, P. and Tytgat, G., Endosonography of gastroesophageal varices: Evaluation and follow-up of 76 cases. Gastrointestinal Endoscopy 1995; 42: 145–150.
17. Kimmey, M., Wang, K., Haggitt, R., Mack, L. and Silverstein, F., Diagnosis of inflammatory bowel disease with ultrasound: An *in vitro* study. Investigative Radiology 1990; 25: 1085–1090.
18. Shimizu, S., Tada, M. and Kawai, K., Endoscopic ultrasonography in inflammatory bowel diseases. Gastrointestinal Endoscopy Clinics of North America 1995; 5: 851–859.
19. Schwartz, D., Harewood, G. and Wiersema, M., EUS for rectal disease. Gastrointestinal Endoscopy 2002; 56: 100–109.
20. Bhutani, M. S. and Nadella, P., Utility of an upper echoendoscope for endoscopic ultrasonography of malignant and benign conditions of the sigmoid/left colon and the rectum. American Journal of Gastroenterology 2001; 96: 3318–3322.
21. Schwartz, D. A., Wiersema, M. J., Dudiak, K. M., Fletcher, J. G., Clain, J. E., Tremaine, W. J. *et al.*, A comparison of endoscopic ultrasound, magnetic resonance imaging, and exam under anesthesia for evaluation of crohn's perianal fistulas. Gastroenterology 2001; 121: 1064–1072.
22. Eckardt, V. F., Jung, B., Fischer, B. and Lierse, W., Anal endosonography in healthy subjects and patients with idiopathic fecal incontinence. Diseases of the Colon and Rectum 1994; 37: 235–242.
23. Dussik, K., Fritch, D., Kyriazidou, M. and Sear, R., Measurements of articular tissues with ultrasound. American Journal of Physical Medicine 1958; 37: 160–165.
24. Duck, F., Physical properties of tissue. Academic Press Ltd., London. 1990.
25. Shung, K. and Thieme, Ultrasonic scattering in biological tissues. CRC Press, Inc., Boca Raton. 1993.
26. Kimmey, M., Martin, R., Haggitt, R., Wang, K., Franklin, D. and Silverstein F., Histologic correlates of gastrointestinal ultrasound images. Gastroenterology, 1989; 96: 433–441.
27. Wiersema, M. and Wiersema, L., High-resolution 25-megahertz ultrasonography of the gastrointestinal wall: Histologic correlates. Gastrointestinal Endoscopy 1993; 39: 499–504.
28. Ødegaard, S. and Kimmey, M. B., Location of the muscularis mucosae on high frequency gastrointestinal ultrasound images. Eur J Ultrasound 1994; 1: 39–50.
29. Aibe, T., Fuji, T., Okita, K. and Takemoto, T., A fundamental study of normal layer structure of the gastrointestinal wall visualized by endoscopic ultrasonography. Scandinavian Journal of Gastroenterology 1986; 21(Suppl 123): 1–5.
30. Bolondi, L., Caletti, G., Casanova, P., Villanacci, V., Grigioni, W. and Labo, G., Problems and variations in the interpretation of the ultrasound feature of the normal upper and lower GI tract wall. Scandinavian Journal of Gastroenterology 1986; 21(Suppl 123): 12–26.
31. Silverstein, F., Kimmey, M., Martin, R., Haggitt, R., Mack, L., Moss, A. *et al.*, Ultrasound and the intestinal wall: Experimental methods. Scandinavian Journal of Gastroenterology 1986; 21(Suppl 123): 34–40.
32. Strohm, W. and Classen, M., Benign lesions of the upper GI tract by means of endoscopic ultrasonography. Scandinavian Journal of Gastroenterology 1986; 21(Suppl 123): 41–46.

33. Kimmey, M., Silverstein, F. and Martin, R., Ultrasound interaction with the intestinal wall: Esophagus, stomach, and colon, *Endoscopic Ultrasonography in Gastroenterology*, K. Kawai, Editor. Igaku-Shon Ltd; Tokyo (1988) pp. 35–43.
34. Wallacem, M., Hoffman, B., Sahai, A., Inoue, H., Van, Velse, A. and Hawes, R., Imaging of esophageal tumors with a water-filled condom and a catheter US probe. Gastrointestinal Endoscopy 2000; 51: 597–600.
35. Inoue, H., Kawano, T., Takeshita, K. and Iwai, T., Modified soft-balloon methods during ultrasonic probe examination for superficial esophageal cancer. Endoscopy 1998; 30(Suppl 1): A41–A43.
36. Ødegaard, S., Kimmey, M., Martin, R., Yee, H., Cheung, A. and Silverstein, F., The effects of applied pressure on the thickness, layers, and echogenicity of gastrointestinal wall ultrasound images. Gastrointestinal Endoscopy 1992; 38: 351–356.

Published with permission

0016-5107/92/3803-0351$03.00
GASTROINTESTINAL ENDOSCOPY


# The effects of applied pressure on the thickness, layers, and echogenicity of gastrointestinal wall ultrasound images

**S. Ødegaard, MD, M. B. Kimmey, MD**
**R. W. Martin, MD, H. C. Yee, MD**
**A. H. S. Cheung, MD, F. E. Silverstein, MD**
*Bergen, Norway and Seattle, Washington*

**Endoscopic ultrasound imaging of the gastrointestinal wall can be performed through intraluminal fluid or by direct transducer contact with the wall. We tested the hypothesis that the ultrasound appearance of the gastrointestinal wall is influenced by the amount of pressure applied when the transducer is in contact with the tissue. Fresh autopsy specimens from the porcine gastrointestinal tract were examined in vitro using an 8.5-MHz linear array ultrasound system. As transducer pressure against the wall was increased from 0 to 10 KPa, changes were seen on the images in wall thickness, tissue echogenicity, and the number of layers. The stomach and rectum were more resistant to compression than the esophagus, duodenum, and colon. Wall echogenicity increased with increasing degrees of applied pressure and some layers were obliterated by this pressure. The second ultrasound layer, or deep mucosa, appeared to be the most susceptible to compression. Endoscopic ultrasound imaging artifacts should be reduced by limiting the amount of pressure applied to the wall with the transducer. (Gastrointest Endosc 1992;38:351–356)**

Endoscopic ultrasonography provides detailed images of the gastrointestinal wall.[1,2] Ultrasound is applied to the wall and reflected echoes are received with a transducer that is part of the endoscope or that is part of an accessory device placed through the channel of the endoscope. Ultrasound is poorly conducted by air. Imaging is achieved by application of the transducer directly to the wall or by scanning through water in the gastrointestinal lumen or through a water-filled balloon surrounding the transducer.

The best images of the gastrointestinal wall are made when the transducer is not in direct contact with the mucosa and imaging is performed through luminal water. One reason for this is that the transducer can be placed at the proper distance from the wall so that the ultrasound beam is in optimal focus.

*Received May 28, 1991. For revision July 16, 1991. Accepted January 15, 1992.*
*From the Medical Department, Haukeland Hospital, University of Bergen, Bergen, Norway and Departments of Medicine, Surgery, Anesthesiology, and the Center for Bioengineering, University of Washington, Seattle, Washington. Reprint requests: Michael B. Kimmey, MD, Division of Gastroenterology, RG-24, Seattle, Washington 98195.*

Another possible reason for the better images is that pressure is not applied by the transducer, which could cause distortion of the image. However, it is not always possible to keep sufficient water in some areas of the gastrointestinal tract lumen, such as in the esophagus, duodenum, and colon. In these areas, the transducer or its surrounding water-filled balloon must be placed in contact with the wall.

The application of a balloon or transducer directly against the gastrointestinal wall can produce considerable wall pressure unless it is carefully controlled. Such pressure could potentially affect the interpretation of ultrasound images of the wall, but this phenomenon has not been well studied. We examined the effect of increasing transducer pressure applied to fresh porcine gastrointestinal tissue on the resulting ultrasound images. Images were scrutinized for changes in wall thickness, tissue echogenicity, and the normal layered appearance.

## METHODS

Tissue from three young pigs, average weight 25 kg, was studied. After sacrifice, one specimen from each of the following sections was excised: esophagus (upper and lower), stomach (body, antrum, and prepyloric area), descending duodenum, colon (cecum, ascending, transverse, descending, sigmoid), and rectum. These sections were stored in saline and studied within 5 hours.

The method used to apply a known amount of pressure to the intestinal wall is illustrated in Figure 1. A standard laboratory balance scale was used. The intestinal sample was cut open and pinned flat in a tissue chamber. A layer of paraffin was located at the bottom of the chamber to secure the needles. Above the paraffin but below the tissue was a layer of stiff or high resilience agar (Bactoagar; Difco Laboratories, Detroit, Mich.) formed by using a high concentration of agar in water (50 mg/ml). This layer provided a separation of the tissue from the paraffin, allowing all of the tissue to be seen on the ultrasound image. Without this separation, bright echoes from the paraffin would interfere with visualization of the serosa of the tissue. The paraffin and agar standoff is a method we have used previously for ultrasound imaging of tissue samples.[3] A block of high resilience agar was located between the transducer and the tissue in order to provide an acoustical standoff, and at the same time allow force to be applied to the tissue. This block of agar was held in position by a latex membrane stretched and secured to the transducer with an elastic band. Saline was then used to fill the rest of the chamber for acoustical coupling and maintenance of tissue hydration.

The measurements were conducted in the following way: weights were applied to the scale and the transducer was then moved toward the tissue to the point where the scale was balanced (0 position). At this point the ultrasound image of the tissue was recorded on video tape and hard copy media.

The beginning sequence involved applying just enough weight to counterbalance the weight of the filled tissue chamber. The agar block adjacent to the transducer (8.5-MHz, linear array, real-time equipment; Advanced Technology Laboratories, Bothell, Wash.) just touched the tissue at this point without compressing it. This was defined as the reference pressure of zero. Increasing amounts of weight were added and the transducer positioned to balance the

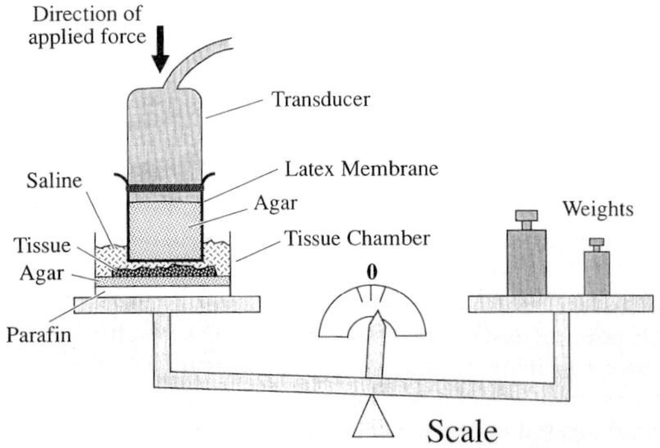


**Figure 1.** The experimental apparatus used to measure the effects of pressure on the intestinal wall is illustrated. When the transducer is pushed down to establish a balance, a force equal to the applied weight is pressed against the tissue.

scale (zero point) before recording the image for that amount of applied weight. Twelve weights ranging from 10 to 500 g were applied. The applied pressure to the tissue was then calculated by dividing the applied force, as measured by the scale, by the surface area of the agar block (1.3 cm × 3.7 cm) attached to the transducer. For example, 50 g produced a pressure of 10.4 g/cm or 1.0 kilopascals (KPa) in Standard International Units for pressure. The relative thickness of the wall as seen on the ultrasound image at each applied pressure was measured later from the hard copy recordings (Figs. 2 and 3).

The images recorded on video tape were processed with a computer to provide a measure of average wall echogenicity at each wall pressure. This processing was accomplished by "grabbing" each image from the video tape with a video frame grabber (Oculus 200; Coreco Inc., Longueuil, Quebec, Canada). The full thickness of the intestinal wall was outlined in the grabbed image using a computer pointing device (Microsoft Mouse; Microsoft Inc, Redmond, Wash.). The intensity of each pixel and the number of pixels were determined in each outlined region. The average intensity was calculated by summing all of the intensity values and dividing by the number of pixels. For each specimen the same area on the image was analyzed for all applied pressures.

The tissue layers, which could be seen on the images, were analyzed for a change in layer number and echogenicity with increasing pressure by two experienced observers.

## RESULTS

Typical examples of the effect of pressure on the images are shown in Figures 2 and 3. The results of analyzing the changes in wall thickness on the ultrasound images from different areas of the gut with increasing pressure are shown in Figures 4 to 6. The effects of pressure on echogenicity are presented in Figures 7 and 8.

A total of 36 specimens were studied to determine how well the various wall layers could be visualized with increasing pressure. A five-layer structure of the wall was considered normal. In some specimens it was difficult to identify which layer was missing with increasing pressure. However, the number of layers which could be seen on images of each specimen, and the layers which were considered missing, are listed below.

Images of four of six esophageal specimens showed a five-layer structure with pressures up to 10 KPa. One specimen had a five-layer structure up to 6 KPa, but at 10 KPa a three-layer structure was observed because layer two was missing and layer one merged with layer three. In one specimen it was only possible to see three layers at all pressures because layers three, four, and five were not distinguishable. Five layers were seen at all forces on the images from the nine gastric specimens.

Images of all three duodenal specimens had a five-layer structure when no pressure was applied. One specimen had five layers at all forces; one specimen

Published with permission

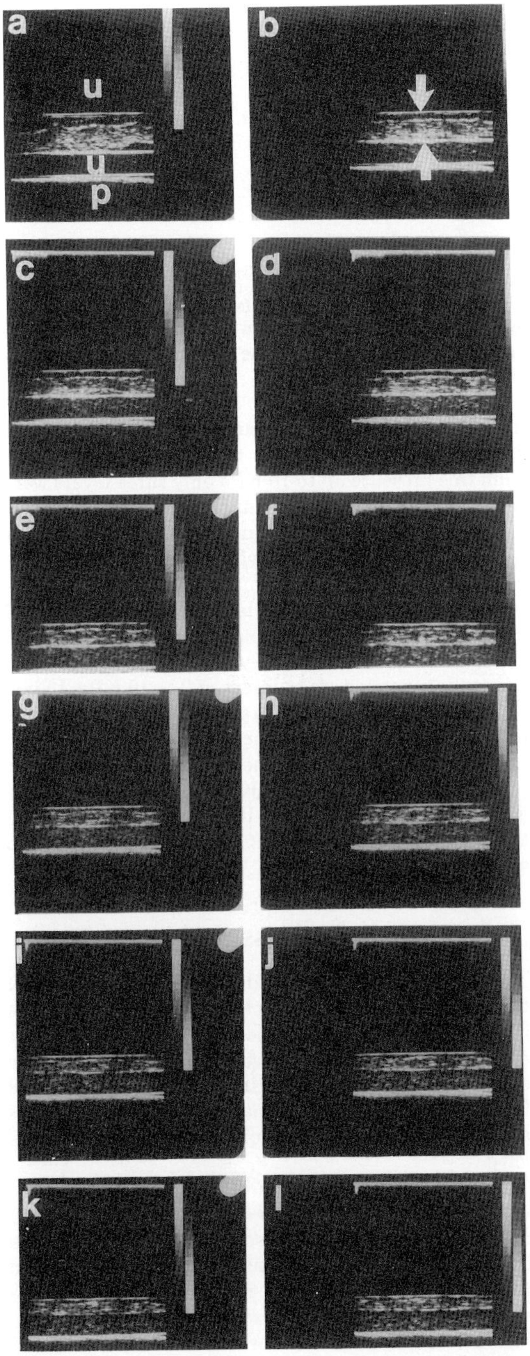


**Figure 2.** Ultrasound images of porcine gastric wall with various applied transducer pressures (in kilopascals) are shown: a, no applied pressure with agar (u) seen above and below the tissue and paraffin (p) at the bottom of the image; (b) 0.2 with the tissue shown by the arrows; (c) 0.4; (d) 0.6; (e) 1.0; (f) 1.6; (g) 2.0; (h) 2.6; (i) 3.0; (j) 4.0; (k) 6.0; and (l) 10.0.

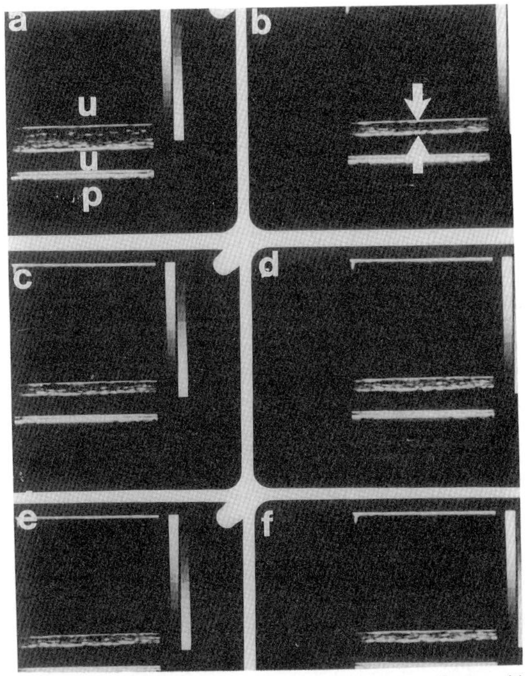


**Figure 3.** Ultrasound images of porcine colon are shown with the same pressures applied as in Figure 2. Higher pressures produced changes in the images similar to those shown for the stomach.

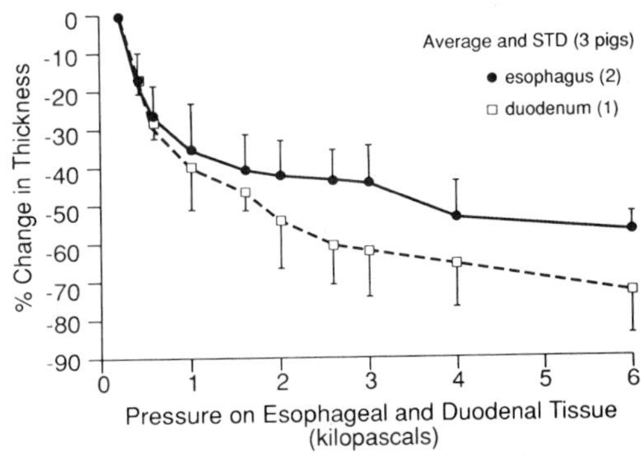


**Figure 4.** The percentage change in the wall thickness of the esophagus (dots) and the duodenum (squares) versus the applied pressure is plotted. The means and standard deviations are shown for three pigs. Esophageal wall thickness was measured in two regions for each pig and averaged because results were similar.

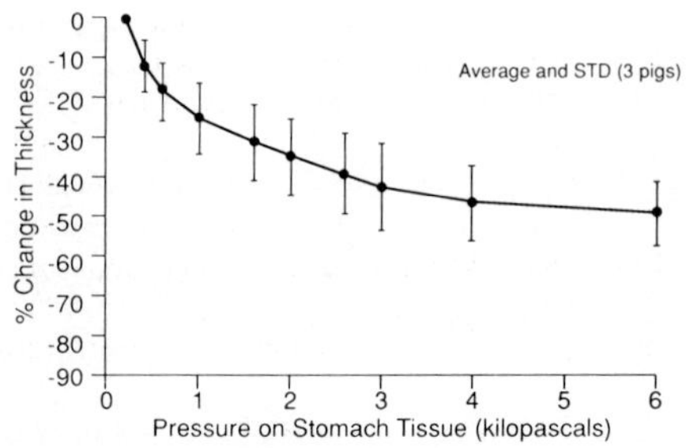


**Figure 5.** The averaged percentage change in the thickness of three regions of the stomach (body, antrum, and prepyloric antrum) versus the applied pressure is shown. The means and standard deviations are shown for three pigs.

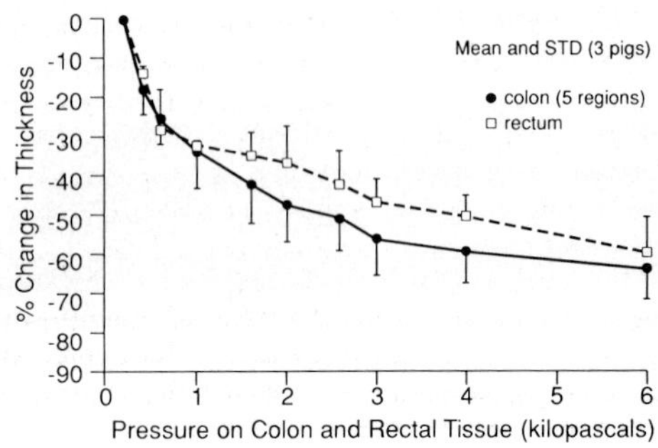


**Figure 6.** The percentage change in the colonic wall thickness (dots) and rectal wall thickness (squares) versus the applied pressure is shown. The means and standard deviations are shown for three pigs. The colon data are an average of measurements taken from five regions of the colon (cecum, ascending, transverse, descending, and sigmoid regions) because the values obtained from the various regions were similar.

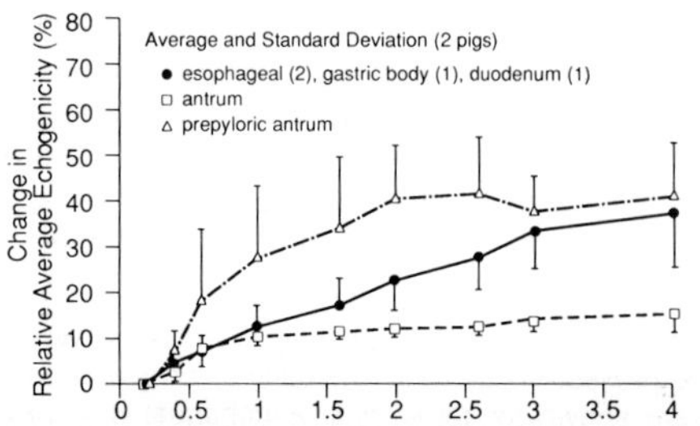


**Figure 7.** The percentage change in the echogenicity of gastrointestinal wall is plotted as a function of the applied pressure. Data from the esophagus, duodenum, and gastric body were averaged (dots) because the changes measured were very similar. The antrum (squares) and pre-pyloric antrum (triangles) are plotted separately. The means and standard deviations are shown for two pigs.

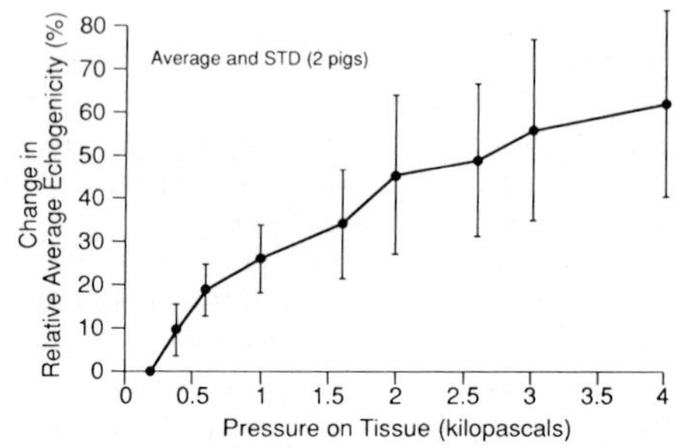


**Figure 8.** The averaged percentage change in the echogenicity of four regions of the colon and the rectum versus the applied pressure are plotted. The means and standard deviations are shown for two pigs.

missed layer two from pressures of 1 to 10 KPa. One specimen had five layers up to 0.6 KPa pressure, but from this pressure up to 10 KPa only three layers were seen because layer two was missing.

Images from the 18 colonic and rectal specimens had a five-layer structure when no pressure was applied. All three rectal specimens and 11 colonic specimens maintained this five-layered structure with all applied pressures. Four colonic specimens showed changes in the number of layers. Two specimens had a three-layer structure at forces of 2 to 10 KPa. In one of these specimens, layer three was missing and in the other specimen it was unclear which layer was missing. In one specimen, layer three was not clearly seen at pressures of 0, 0.2, and 0.4 KPa, but was better visualized at higher pressures. In one colonic specimen, three layers were seen at 10 KPa because layer two was missing.

## DISCUSSION

High frequency ultrasound gives a detailed image of the layers (mucosa, submucosa, muscularis propria) of the gastrointestinal wall. However, the layers do not correspond exactly to the histological layers due to the different imaging principles involved.[4] The ultrasound layers result from a combination of interface echoes and echoes from tissue regions with similar echogenicity.

The clarity of the layers and other details in the ultrasound images are related to a number of factors, foremost of which is the resolution of the ultrasound system. This resolution relates both to the direction the sound propagates (range resolution) and the transverse direction (lateral resolution).[5] The range resolution is related to the duration of the ultrasound pulse and the frequency of the transducer. The lateral resolution is related to the size and focusing characteristics of the transducer or an overlying lens. The most commonly used ultrasound endoscope in clinical practice (Olympus UM3; Olympus Corporation of America, Lake Success, N. Y.) is optimally focused at approximately 3 cm from the transducer.

Although these resolution principles are well known, the effect of pressure against the gastrointestinal wall on the image has not been previously studied. Experience with in vivo endoscopic ultrasound imaging has shown that structural details of the wall, its thickness, and the wall layers might be influenced by the pressure applied by the ultrasound transducer (or the balloon) to the wall. Previously it has been unclear how transducer pressure would affect ultrasound images of the gastrointestinal wall. These results indicate that transducer pressure can affect wall images, and that the degree of transducer pressure required to change the image is different for different areas of the gut. This study does not address the effect of radial forces exerted by distension of the lumen by air or water.

An important question related to these results is the magnitude of force and pressure that can be produced by an ultrasound endoscope in vivo. We used an ultrasound endoscope (Olympus UM3; Olympus Corporation of America) and simulated the curvature of an endoscopic examination. We then measured the maximum force that could be produced at the tip of the endoscope with maximum deflection of the steering wheels. Estimated pressures of 18.9, 9.5, and 6.3 KPa pressures could be applied (see Appendix). These pressures are at or above the pressures that we studied. Therefore, it seems possible that pressures in the range we studied can be produced during in vivo endoscopic ultrasound imaging.

Regional differences of wall compressibility were found within the gastrointestinal tract. The stomach was more resistant to pressure than the esophageal wall at pressures less than 2 KPa (Figs. 4 and 5). Tissue from the duodenum was less resistant to increasing pressure, reducing the wall thickness by 40% when only 1 KPa was applied (Fig. 4).

No significant differences were found in wall thickness between the different areas of the colon so the data were combined in Figure 6. The rectum was slightly more resistant to a change in thickness, especially at higher pressures. In these organs, a force of 1 to 2 KPa reduced the wall thickness by approximately 30 to 40%.

The increase in tissue echogenicity with increasing transducer pressures (Figs. 7 and 8) could cause difficulties in separating some normal and abnormal gastrointestinal tissue structures. However, the clinical importance of these observations remains to be shown. The cause of increased echogenicity of the wall when pressure is applied is uncertain, but could be due to an increase in the density of ultrasonic scatterers, leading to increased echo density.

Ideally, the actual thickness of each layer should have been measured and compared with pressure in this study. However, reliable measurements of the thickness of each layer could not be made. Therefore, the wall thickness changes reported are changes in the overall wall thickness measured on the ultrasonic images. We used 0.2 KPa as the reference pressure (instead of 0 KPa) because the tissue was not always entirely flat at zero pressure applied. After application of 0.2 KPa pressure, the intestine flattened in all cases with minimal changes observed in thickness.

When we analyzed the images visually, the influence of increasing pressure on the number of wall layers was less marked. When the pressure increased, changes in the number of wall layers were seen in only 11% of the specimens and most of these occurred with high pressures. The second ultrasound layer, or deep mucosa, appeared to be the most susceptible to compression. The stomach and rectum appeared to be less susceptible to layer changes than the esophagus, duodenum, and colon. The range resolution of the ultrasound system used may be a determining factor; worse resolution would result in the loss of more layers under pressure because the duration of the echo may cover an entire layer if it is reduced in thickness. However, we did not study the effect of pressure with different resolution imaging systems. There could also be differences between the susceptibility to pressure of swine and human gastrointestinal tissue.

These studies were performed on fresh autopsy specimens and therefore were without blood circulation. Results of in vivo examinations may differ because of different tissue types and different stiffness of the tissues surrounding the gut. Nevertheless, these in vitro results are consistent with changes that we have observed in vivo with applied probe pressure but which are difficult to study in a controlled fashion.

When high frequency ultrasound imaging of the gastrointestinal wall is performed, the force applied by the ultrasound transducer to the gastrointestinal wall should be as gentle as possible to avoid wall compression. Lighter applied pressure may yield higher quality images, better resolution of small tissue structures within or immediately adjacent to the wall, and more accurate representations of tissue and layer thickness.

## APPENDIX

A maximum force of 150 g could be generated at the transducer by deflection of the steering wheels of an ultrasound endoscope. The length of the balloon on the tip of this ultrasound endoscope is 1.5 cm and, assuming it is inflated to a radius of 1 cm, the pressure that would be delivered to a surface can be calculated. The magnitude of this pressure is dependent on how much of the balloon circumference is in contact with

Published with permission

the mucosal surface. In the cases of 30, 60, and 90 degrees of the 360-degree circumference of balloon pressing on the mucosal surface, the pressures generated by a 150-g force would be 18.9, 9.5, and 6.3 KPa, respectively.


## ACKNOWLEDGMENTS

This study was performed at the University of Washington, Seattle, Washington and was supported by grants from the National Institutes of Health (5 R 01 DK34814-06), USA, and the Norwegian Research Council for Science and the Humanities (NAVF), Oslo, Norway.


## REFERENCES


1. Tio TL. Endosonography in gastroenterology. Berlin: Springer-Verlag, 1988.
2. Kawai K. Endoscopic ultrasonography in gastroenterology. Tokyo: Igaku-Shoin Ltd., 1988.
3. Kimmey MB, Silverstein FE, Haggitt RC, et al. A system to compare ultrasound, computed tomography, and magnetic resonance with histologic findings. Invest Radiol 1987;22:227–231.
4. Kimmey MB, Martin RW, Haggitt RC, et al. Histological correlates of gastrointestinal endoscopic ultrasound images. Gastroenterology 1989;96:433–41.
5. Christensen DA. Ultrasonic bioinstrumentation. New York: John Wiley & Sons, 1988.

CHAPTER 6

# SIMULTANEOUS RECORDINGS OF GASTRIC MOTILITY BY ULTRASOUND, SCINTIGRAPHY AND MANOMETRY

KRISTIAN HVEEM AND HANS GREGERSEN

## 1. The Physiology of Gastric Emptying

Traditionally, the stomach has been looked upon as a two-compartment model in an effort to understand the mechanisms of gastric emptying (1, 2). The proximal stomach was assigned to play a dominant role for receipt and storage of food and for the control of the gastric emptying of liquids, the distal stomach to play the major role in retention, grinding and propulsion of larger-sized particles. This model, however, proved inadequate in the sense that among other factors it did not take in to account the pulsatile pattern of gastric emptying (3, 4)

The gastric motor function is complex. Both tonic and phasic contractile forces act in a complicated interplay to produce flow of intragastric content from the stomach through the pyloric region (2, 5, 6). The factors that regulate emptying differ fundamentally between nutrient and non-nutrient liquids (7). Feedback from small intestinal luminal receptors predominates in the control of emptying of nutrient-containing liquids (8) whereas gravity and intragastric volume are important determinants in emptying of isotonic liquids, which empty faster from the stomach than nutrient-containing liquids (7, 9).

Gastric and antropyloric phasic contractions control transpyloric pulsatile flow, the major mechanism of gastric emptying. Antral contractions are also responsible for mixing and grinding of a solid meal into smaller particles (<5 mm) that can pass onto the duodenum. Both the occurrence and pattern of phasic gastric contractions are modulated by intestinal feedback mechanisms with subsequent variation in gastric emptying (10). Contractions can be occlusive or non lumen-occlusive but there is no obvious relationship between the nature of the antral contraction and the volume of transpyloric flow (11). Correlation of flow and motility has in fact shown that small non-occlusive contractions appear to be important in causing high-volume pulsatile transpyloric flow (12). Intrapyloric pressure waves are particularly important in determining the outcome of antral contractions, to terminate or forward transpyloric flow (13). A considerable variation in the cycle-to-cycle stroke volumes of the stomach exists. These variations in the gastroduodenal contractions from one cycle to the next appear to be primarily determined by the intensity of small intestinal chemoreceptor and mechanoreceptor feedback produced by pulsatile emptying, the composition and volume of intragastric content and posture (14, 15). The various phases of fasting gastric motility also influence the outcome of gastric emptying (16).

## 2. The Assessment of Gastric Emptying

Imaging methods have much to offer in advancing the understanding of gastric mechanics, as they can be used to concurrently assess gastric wall motion and luminal diameter and, in some cases, the movement of luminal contents (17, 18). Fluoroscopic imaging has been used since the turn of the century for this purpose, but its application in humans is severely constrained by radiation exposure limits. Other techniques such as magnetic resonance imaging (MRI) and ultrasound imaging are attractive options since they permit prolonged observation of the human stomach without exposure to radiation. Real time gastric MRI has special appeal but as yet, its full potential has not been realized because of its cost and technical complexity (18, 19).

### 2.1. *Scintigraphy*

Scintigraphy is at present the "gold standard" for clinical measurement of gastric emptying. Scintigraphy provides quantitative information about total stomach emptying and intragastric meal distribution of both solid and liquid meals (20). With the use of a gamma camera the rate of gastric emptying of a standardized test meal marked with a radioisotope can be calculated. Scintigraphy requires expensive equipment that is often not readily available, is associated with a radiation burden, and cannot detect individual episodes of transpyloric flow.

In evaluating gastric emptying, a single isotope test which measures total, proximal and distal stomach emptying has been applied (8). Test meals may vary and various amounts of $^{99m}$Tc-sulphur colloid may be added to the meal. Radionuclide data are acquired at different frame rates until at least 90% of the meal has emptied or for a maximum period of 180 min. Data are corrected for subject movement and radionuclide decay using previously described methods (2, 8). Correction for gamma ray attenuation is performed using factors derived from a lateral image of the stomach (1) or automatically if using a dual-head camera.

A region-of-interest (ROI) is defined around the total stomach, which is subsequently divided into proximal and distal regions — the proximal region corresponding to the gastric fundus and proximal corpus and the distal region representing the gastric antrum and distal corpus. Gastric emptying curves for the total, proximal and distal stomach (representing % retention over time) are derived. Several parameters are obtained from the curves for subsequent statistical analysis. For the total stomach, the lag phase before any liquid has left the stomach and the 50% emptying time ($T_{50}$) can be calculated.

The lag phase (the delay before emptying commences) is determined visually by the frame preceding that in which activity is first seen in the proximal small intestine (1).

### 2.2. *Ultrasound*

Ultrasound imaging is rather inexpensive and widely available. Ultrasound has been used by several groups to evaluate gastric emptying, patterns of gastric wall motion and luminal flow (4, 21–25). These studies have revealed substantial variability in the wall motion and complex, pulsatile episodes of flow within and from the stomach.

Ultrasound imaging of gastroduodenal motility has mainly been performed with a transabdominal approach and until recently mainly as 2D-ultrasonography (22, 23, 25–27). Three-dimensional ultrasound has so far only been applied as an investigational tool in scientific studies due to the complex and time-demanding procedure of image recording and processing (28, 29). Due to its high availability, modest costs and lack of radiation hazard, 2D-real time ultrasonography has found its place in clinical diagnostic practice and not only as an experimental tool. The subjects are studied in a seated position, with a 3, 5 –5 MHz transducer placed on the abdomen to visualize the antrum either in a standardized manner or longitudinally as previously described. Images are videotaped and stored for later analysis.

Studies of the antropyloroduodenal region are performed with the ultrasound probe positioned at the level of the transpyloric plane, and the antrum, the pylorus and the proximal duodenum visualized simultaneously (30, 31). In gastric emptying studies, either the proximal stomach or the antrum has been visualized in standardized sections. Ultrasound imaging of the antrum has been achieved by placing the transducer in a vertical section so the aorta and the superior mesenteric vein are presented longitudinally (Fig. 1).

## 2.3. *Interobserver agreement*

Interobserver agreement is critical in studies where data are partly based on a visual interpretation of the ultrasound image as well as the interpretation of pressure events where there is no lower limit of the magnitude of the pressure rise.

Evaluation of interobserver variability has only been performed in one concurrent study (30). There was a mean variability in the judgment of the two observers of the time of arrival of the contraction at the metal marker of 0.45 s (SE, 0.18 s) and a 90% concordance

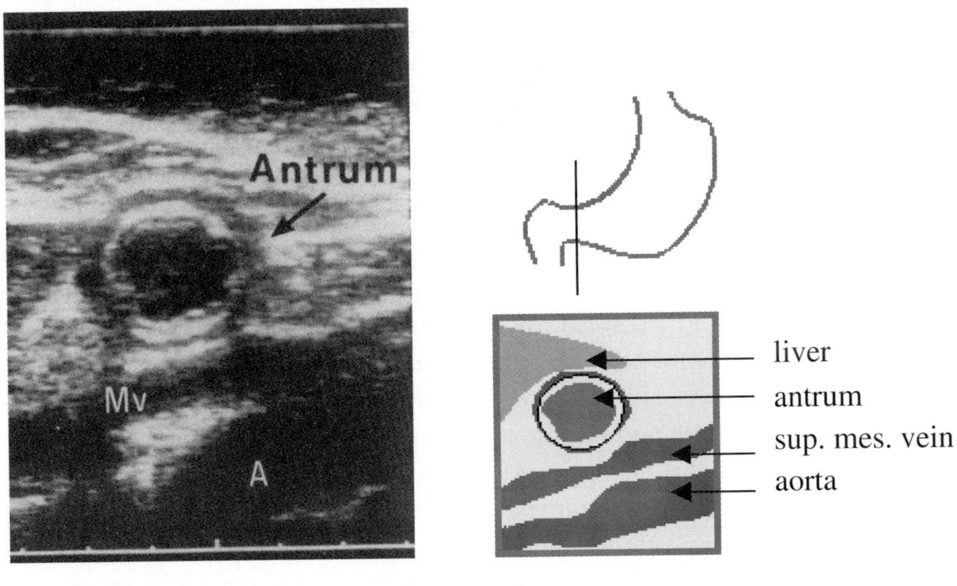


Fig. 1. The Ultrasonographic (left) and schematic (right) vertical scan through the antrum, superior mesenteric vein (Mv) and aorta (A).

between the two observers for the first independent analysis of whether the contractions were lumen occlusive.

### 2.4. *Definitions and terminology relevant to motor events*

In published studies, it appears to be a general agreement on some basic definitions as:

(i) *Antral contraction*: an indentation of the gastric wall greater than one antral wall thickness, which is not due to respiration, pulsation transmitted from the aorta or heart, or to movements of adjacent intestine.

(ii) *A lumen-occlusive contraction*: a contraction in which the ultrasound image shows the gastric walls to come into apposition at some point along the imaged antrum.

(iii) *A propagated contraction*: a gastric contraction seen to progress aborally along the entire length of the imaged antrum.

(iv) *A pressure event*: a phasic rise in pressure in a single manometric recording channel.

(v) *A pressure event sequence*: a group of pressure events recorded in different manometric channels that are established as being related by specific spatiotemporal criteria.

### 2.5. *Synchronization of ultrasound images with manometric data*

A purpose-designed time-coding system has been developed to record and synchronize both the manometric data and the videotaped ultrasound image (30). Correlation of the time code between the display of manometric data on the computer screen and the number recorded on the video image allows accurate synchronization of data to within 100 ms. Manometric and image data are initially analyzed separately to avoid any possibility of observer bias before being correlated. Later, both the ultrasound image and the pressure recording can be digitized to appear on the computer screen simultaneously (31).

### 2.6. *Manometry*

Manometry is by far the most widely used method for measuring gastric motility (32, 33). Manometric studies have demonstrated that the patterns of luminal pressure waves are complex in both the fasting and fed states (34). However, information about the relationship between the luminal pressure and gastric wall motion has until recently been very limited. In order to investigate this relationship, techniques with high spatial and temporal resolution such as manometry and electromagnetic flow meters have been combined in animal models (4, 35, 36). Later, high-resolution antropyloric manometry combined with simultaneous ultrasound imaging and/or flow duplex ultrasonography of gastric wall motion has provided insight into the understanding of these mechanisms in humans (30, 31). Combination of similar techniques have also been used to assess motility and pressure in other parts of the gastrointestinal tract, such as the esophagus (37, 38) and the distal colon (39). However, these organs will not be dealt with specifically in this chapter.

Motor events play a key role in the understanding of upper gastrointestinal physiology and have been studied by a number of investigators using manometry (33, 40–42). Computer analysis of pressure events is now established (43, 44).

Pressure-sensitive systems generally comprise a pressure transducer, an amplifier and a recorder. The first manometric recordings of motor activity were obtained by flaccid balloons in the 1940s. Techniques initially designed to study esophageal motor activity (45) were later introduced for studies of gastric motility. With the perfused sleeve sensor continuous motor activity could be measured along whole lengths in the distal esophageal sphincter and the antroduodenal region (32).

Measurement of antropyloric pressures has been used in a number of previous studies (5, 13, 34, 40), performed with a multi-lumen perfused manometric assembly. This may incorporate a 4–4.5 cm sleeve sensor in parallel with a chain of antral, pyloric and duodenal side holes spaced at about 1.5 cm intervals which straddles the pyloric region (Fig. 2). Opening at each end of the sleeve are used to measure transmucosal potential difference (TMPD) as well as pressure and referred to as the antral and duodenal TMPD side holes. Manometric channels other than those used to record TMPD are perfused with degassed distilled water at 0.3 ml minute$^{-1}$ with a low compliance manometric infusion pump. TMPD channels are perfused with normal saline from separate reservoirs. Signals from the pressure transducers are amplified and digitized before further processing and storage in a personal computer.

Following an overnight fast, the manometric assembly is introduced transnasally and positioned in the antropyloroduodenal region either by the guidance of the TMPD or using fluoroscopy. The positioning of the catheter is monitored during the test using measurement of the TMPD between two side holes located in the distal antrum and proximal duodenum. Established criteria (antral TMPD $< -40$ mV, duodenal TMPD $>0$ mV, minimal difference

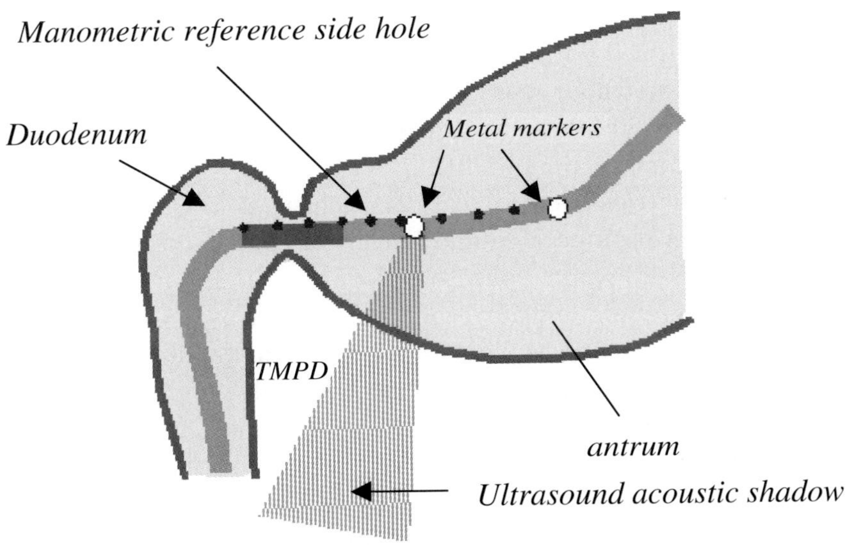


Fig. 2. A manometric assembly with metal markers for ultrasound identification of the position of the catheter (modified from Hveem *et al.*, AJP 2001).

between the two, 15 mV) are generally used to define the position of the proximal side holes positioned in the gastric antrum and more distally in the duodenum. Once the catheter is in the correct position the subjects are placed in a comfortable chair leaning slightly backwards.

Evaluation of interobserver variability of pressure events has also been performed (30). The interobserver agreement for scoring of pressure events $<5$ mmHg, between 5 and 10 mmHg, and $>10$ mmHg was 85%, 97%, and 100%, respectively. Eighty-nine percent of the onset times of pressure events were in agreement within 1 second and 95% within 2 seconds.

## 3. Concurrent Ultrasound and Scintigraphy

In order to establish ultrasound as an acceptable or even preferred method in assessing gastric emptying, studies have been conducted to compare ultrasound with scintigraphy. Even though gastric emptying studies have been performed with both liquid and solid meal, the image quality and the lag face creates a certain obstacle in the interpretation of emptying of a solid meal. Thus, studies with concurrent ultrasound and manometry have so far only been performed with a liquid test meal. The test meal has been a low caloric meal (less than 20 kcal), usually a commercially available meat soup (46). The soup (300–500 ml) is prewarmed to 37°C and gradually ingested during a few min. Fat, proteins and carbohydrates are all soluble in water. The emptying curve follows an exponential curve, with the greater part of the emptying occurring initially and 50% of the meal emptying after approximately 22 minutes (24).

Ultrasound and scintigraphy has been performed simultaneously in order to investigate gastric emptying of various liquids, and the limits of agreements between the two methods. In order to do so, the subjects are usually seated with their back against the gamma camera and the ultrasound transducer was positioned at the region of the umbilicus. The first measurement is performed within 1 min after the meal ingestion, followed by images at 5 min intervals for the first hour and 10 min intervals thereafter, until 90% has left the stomach for a maximum of 180 min. Ultrasound $T_{50}$ is defined as the time when the antral area has decreased to half its maximum (19).

With a high-and low-nutrient liquid meal (24), scintigraphic and ultrasonographic 50% emptying times ($T_{50}$'s) were comparable and longer for dextrose than for meat soup (dextrose $107 \pm 16$ min vs $108 \pm 18$ min, soup $24 \pm 4$ min vs $23 \pm 5$ min). A close correlation was found between scintigraphic and ultrasound $T_{50}$ (dextrose $r = 0.94$, $p < 0.005$, soup $r = 0.97$, $p < 0.001$) and between the time at which the distal stomach content decreased from its maximum value by 50% (measured scintigraphically) and the ultrasound $T_{50}$ (dextrose $r = 0.95$, $p < 0.005$, soup $r = 0.99$, $p < 0.0001$). In contrast, a significant relationship was not found between the distal stomach content when expressed as a percentage of the maximum content of the total stomach and the ultrasound $T_{50}$.

For the $T_{50}$ the limits of agreement were $+5.7$ min (24%) and $-7.9$ min ($-41$%) for the soup (mean difference $-1.1$ min) and $+32.5$ min (30%) and $-30.7$ min ($-31$%) for dextrose (mean difference 0.9 min). The limits of agreement were less than $\pm 15$% for 11 of the 14 tests. Other studies have reached the same conclusion that ultrasound measurements of gastric emptying are of comparable sensitivity to scintigraphy in quantifying emptying of both low and high nutrient liquids (27, 47).

A number of motility studies have now established ultrasound as a valuable method of studying both the proximal (48) and the distal stomach (23, 49–51), as well as transpyloric flow (4, 52–54). Using ultrasound, gastric emptying has typically been assessed by changes in either the antral cross-sectional area or diameter (23, 27). It is, however, uncertain why the rate of gastric emptying of liquids could be related to changes in the antral area. The width of the antrum is determined by the interplay of both passive and active forces favoring distension, including intragastric volume, gravity and fundic tone, and resistance to distension occurring as a result of the antral muscular contractions. It is therefore potentially both a determinant of, and determined by, the content of the distal stomach. While the observed relationship between ultrasound measurements of antral area and gastric emptying suggests that the distal stomach, and in particular the antral "tone", plays a role in regulating gastric emptying of liquids (27) emptying of liquids is known to correlate with content of the proximal stomach and not that of the distal stomach measured scintigraphically. The proximal stomach usually "empties" in parallel with the total stomach, whereas the distal stomach content initially increases and subsequently decreases (20). However, a possible relationship between emptying from the total stomach and the rate at which the antral content decreases, i.e. antral content (expressed as a percentage of its maximum), rather than the maximum content of the total stomach, has not been evaluated.

The validity of using changes in antral "size" in assessing gastric emptying of liquids has been in studies of normal subjects (24). This is accounted for by the close relationship between the total stomach emptying and the content of the distal stomach when the latter is expressed as a percentage of its maximum, and by the changes in the antral area measured ultrasonographically and the content of the distal stomach measured scintigraphically. The validity of using measurements of the antral diameter to evaluate gastric emptying is consistent with the concept that the antral tone plays a major role in regulating gastric emptying of liquids in concert with other factors including the tone of the proximal stomach, antral phasic contractions, pyloric resistance and proximal small intestinal motility (7). When considering the potential clinical use of ultrasound it should be recognized that ultrasonographic measurement of gastric emptying of solids is technically more complicated and can have substantial limitations (50).

### 3.1. *Limits of agreements*

In considering the potential use of ultrasound as opposed to scintigraphy, for measurement of gastric emptying for clinical and research purposes, the limits of agreement between the two techniques must be acceptable. Previous studies have demonstrated a close relationship between rates of gastric emptying of liquids measured by the two modalities (23, 27, 47), implying that ultrasound has the capacity to measure gastric emptying precisely. The use of regression analysis and correlation coefficients, however, may not provide accurate information about the concordance between two methods because the correlation coefficient $r$ measures the strength of the association, not the agreement (55). It would be surprising if methods designed to measure the same quantity were not correlated. The range of values substantially influences the correlation, but not the agreement.

Comparative studies between ultrasound and scintigraphic measurements of gastric emptying have shown a very close relationship between the two methods (24, 27, 47). Estimations of limits of agreement were only performed in one study (24) with approximately ±30% for the overall group but less than ±15% in 11 of the 14 tests. As previously demonstrated (8) the intraindividual variation in gastric emptying of liquids in normal subjects is relatively large (8, 24) with ranges for gastric emptying (50% emptying time) of 13–44 min for meat soup and 37–177 min for a drink of dextrose. As the limits of agreement for dextrose were about four times greater, the precision of measurement of emptying of low and high nutrient liquids was similar. This indicates that the ultrasonographic method has the capacity, at least in normal subjects, to discriminate between fast and slow emptying of both low and high nutrient liquids.

## 4. Concurrent Ultrasound and Manometry

A sector transducer (3.5–5 MHz) is positioned on the abdomen to image the antrum and manometric assembly in a longitudinal section. A metal marker attached to the manometric assembly provides a hyperechoic signal to ensure a proper surveillance of the position of the catheter so that wall motion can be related to pressure events at specific side holes (Fig. 1). The orientation of the transducer has to be optimized to ensure clear images of the ultrasound (metal) marker, related to the manometric reference channel. The side hole closest to the marker is best suited as the manometric data reference channel for analysis.

In the study by Hausken *et al.* (31), 84% of contraction observed by ultrasound in the fasting state were detected by manometry. One antral contraction was seen by manometry only. In the pre- and postprandial period, a total of 44% of antral contractions were not detected by manometry, and only 1/5 of non-occluding contractions.

In the study by Hveem *et al.* (30), only 53% of antral contractions seen ultrasonographically, had a temporally associated pressure event in the manometric reference channel. However, in two-thirds of the 47% of contractions for which no pressure event could be detected in the manometric reference channel, temporally associated pressure events were found in other antropyloric recording channels (i.e. within 10 s of the contraction reaching the metal marker). Therefore, in total, 86% of all contractions had a temporally related pressure event somewhere in the antrum. The lumen-occlusive contractions had in 69% an associated pressure event. Of the non-lumen-occlusive contractions, only 20% were associated with a pressure event ($P < 0.01$).

The median amplitude of the pressure events in the manometric reference channel was 16 mmHg (range 4–98 mmHg) for lumen-occlusive and 7 mmHg (range 4–23 mmHg) for non-lumen-occlusive contractions ($P < 0.01$). However, a substantial overlap exists between the two categories of contraction, with 23% of lumen-occlusive contractions being associated with a pressure event <10 mmHg and 25% of non-lumen-occlusive contractions being associated with a pressure event >10 mmHg.

So far, only two studies assessing concurrent ultrasound and high-resolution manometry have been published (30, 31). A major challenge in the first study was to determine the position of the pressure recording point of the manometric assembly in the ultrasound image (Fig. 1). Initially, a metal marker was placed within the center lumen of the catheter, but the ultrasound signals from the markers could not adequately be distinguished from the acoustic shadow of the catheter itself. However, when the metal marker was positioned around the manometric assembly, a sufficiently sharp and distinct acoustic shadow was seen. Since the distal marker was positioned close to the manometric reference side hole and manometric and image data were synchronized, the spatial/temporal relationships between pressure events and gastric wall motion could be examined.

In the study by Hausken *et al.*, this problem was overcome by simply image- digitizing all the ultrasound data along with the pressure recordings, allowing both modalities to be simultaneously displayed on the same PC-monitor. Coded timing information during recording also ensured correct synchronizing, even during playback analysis.

### 4.1. *Detection of antral contractions*

In about 50% of antral contractions observed by ultrasound, the corresponding pressure events are not identified in the manometric reference channel (30). This more than indicates that the knowledge of gastric mechanics based solely on manometry is at the least inadequate, missing almost half of the information given by ultrasound with regard to antral contractions. Lumen-occlusive contractions are more likely to be associated with a pressure event. This pressure event is also more likely to be of higher amplitude than when associated with a non lumen-occlusive contraction. These observations, along with the observation that the onset of pressure events and arrival of the antral contraction waves at the ultrasound marker correlated closely in time, indicate that pressure events associated with contractions are usually a relatively localized phenomena, with significant elevations in pressure extending perhaps only a few mm from the edge of the antral contraction.

Traditionally, a lumen-occlusive contraction has been defined as a pressure wave with an amplitude >10 mmHg. The basis for this rather arbitrary definition is questioned (30) — finding a substantial overlap where approximately 25% of lumen-occlusive contractions were associated with a pressure event sequence <10 mmHg, and a similar proportion of non lumen-occlusive contractions being associated with a pressure event sequence >10 mmHg. Detailed analysis of gastric wall motion as imaged by ultrasound and intraluminal pressures suggests that the maximum amplitude of pressure waves can only be used as an approximate predictor of the occurrence of lumen-occlusion.

The characteristics of the antral contractions observed (i.e. lumen-occlusive or not and propagated or not) are not predictive of the overall pattern of the pressure event sequence as determined by manometry. This may reflect the limitations of the ultrasound image in terms of spatial resolution and the fact that only a single plane could be visualized. Three-dimensional ultrasound imaging of the antrum would provide more spatial information than the technique currently employed, but at the cost of considerably poorer temporal resolution.

## 5. Two New Methods for Assessment of Antral Function

Strain of the muscle layers within the gastric wall can be measured by transabdominal strain rate imaging (SRI), a novel Doppler ultrasound (US) method. Both grey-scale and Doppler US data can be acquired with a 5–8 MHz linear transducer in cineloops of 97 to

256 frames. Rapid stepwise inflation with volumes up to 60 ml of an intragastric bag is carried out and bag pressure and SRI are measured simultaneously. SRI enables detailed studies of layers within the gastric wall in all subjects. Using this technique, it has been found that the radial strain is higher in the circular than in the longitudinal muscle layer. Strains derived from SRI correlate well with strains obtained with B-mode measurements and during balloon distension, an inverse correlation is found between pressure and radial strain. SRI data are shown elsewhere in this book.

Gastric antral geometry and stress-strain properties can be evaluated by using transabdominal ultrasound scanning during volume-controlled distensions in the human gastric antrum. The subjects undergo stepwise inflation of a bag located in the antrum with

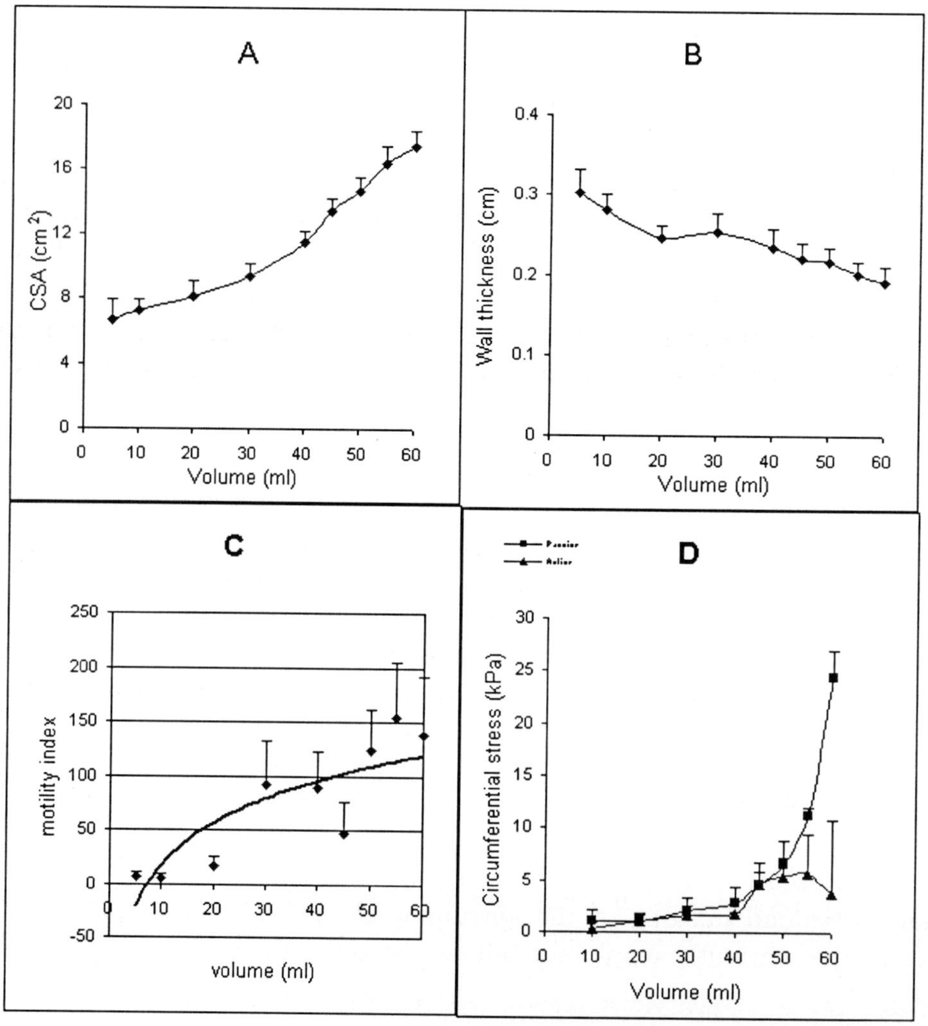


Fig. 3. Balloon distension of the antrum with up to 60 ml. The top figures show the cross-sectional area and the wall thickness as measured using ultrasound. The left bottom Fig. 3(c) shows the antral motility index (number of contractions multiplied by the contraction amplitude) and an exponential trendline. Figure 3(d) shows the active and passive tensions computed from the pressure and geometric data under various drug effects (modified from Gregersen *et al.*, AJP 2002).

volumes up to 60 ml. The stretch ratio and Cauchy stress and strain can be calculated from measurements of pressure, luminal cross-sectional area, diameter, and wall thickness [Figs. 3(a) and 3(b)]. The motility index can also be studied during the distension (Fig. 3(c)). The distension can be performed without and with the influence of drugs. Analysis of stretch ratios demonstrates positive strain in the circumferential direction, negative strain in the radial direction, and no strain in the longitudinal direction. The stress-strain relation is exponential. The wall stress can be decomposed into its active and passive components (Fig. 3(d)) and the well-known length-tension diagram from *in vitro* studies of smooth muscle strips can be reproduced.

## 6. Is There a Single Preferable Method?

Stereotyped pattern of aboral propagation along the antrum are likely to have significantly different mechanical outcomes such as pro- and retropulsion within the stomach and/or transpyloric flow. At present, far too little information is available on the relationships between transpyloric flow, contraction patterns and spatial-temporal patterns of pressure wave sequences in humans, in spite of extensive research with almost any of the following modalities such as fluoroscopy, manometry, ultrasound, regular and dynamic scintigraphy, MRI, barostat and other modalities to evaluate antral distension (17, 19, 27, 36, 56–62) and in various combinations. Actually there is no single method that has the potential to resolve all these questions and give us the answers. Currently, and in the near future, our best option is still to combine the various techniques in an effort to explain the simple but crucial challenge — *what determines gastric emptying*?

## References

1. Collins, P. J., Horowitz, M., Cook, D. J., Harding, P. E. and Shearman, D. J., Gastric emptying in normal subjects — A reproducible technique using a single scintillation camera and computer system. Gut 1983; 24(12): 1117–1125.
2. Collins, P. J., Houghton, L. A., Read, N. W., Horowitz, M., Chatterton, B. E., Heddle, R. *et al.*, Role of the proximal and distal stomach in mixed solid and liquid meal emptying. Gut 1991; 32(6): 615–619.
3. King, P. M., Adam, R. D., Pryde, A., McDicken, W. N. and Heading, R. C., Relationships of human antroduodenal motility and transpyloric fluid movement: Non-invasive observations with real-time ultrasound. Gut 1984; 25(12): 1384–1391.
4. Hausken, T., Ødegaard, S., Matre, K. and Berstad, A., Antroduodenal motility and movements of luminal contents studied by duplex sonography. Gastroenterology 1992; 102(5): 1583–1590.
5. Houghton, L. A., Read, N. W., Heddle, R., Horowitz, M., Collins, P. J., Chatterton, B. *et al.*, Relationship of the motor activity of the antrum, pylorus, and duodenum to gastric emptying of a solid-liquid mixed meal. Gastroenterology 1988; 94(6): 1285–1291.
6. Azpiroz, F., Control of gastric emptying by gastric tone. Dig Dis Sci 1994; 39(12 Suppl): 18S–19S.
7. Horowitz, M. and Dent, J., Disordered gastric emptying: mechanical basis, assessment and treatment. Baillieres Clin Gastroenterol 1991; 5(2): 371–407.

8. Horowitz, M., Edelbroek, M. A., Wishart, J. M. and Straathof, J. W., Relationship between oral glucose tolerance and gastric emptying in normal healthy subjects. Diabetologia 1993; 36(9): 857–862.
9. Horowitz, M., Jones, K., Edelbroek, M. A., Smout, A. J. and Read, N. W., The effect of posture on gastric emptying and intragastric distribution of oil and aqueous meal components and appetite. Gastroenterology 1993; 105(2): 382–390.
10. Dent, J., Sun, W. M. and Anvari, M., Modulation of pumping function of gastric body and antropyloric contractions. Dig Dis Sci 1994; 39(12 Suppl): 28S–31S.
11. Horowitz, M. and Dent, J., The study of gastric mechanics and flow: a Mad Hatter's tea party starting to make sense? [editorial; comment]. Gastroenterology 1994; 107(1): 302–306.
12. Anvari, M., Dent, J., Malbert, C. and Jamieson, G. G., Mechanics of pulsatile transpyloric flow in the pig [published erratum appears in J Physiol (Lond) 1996 Aug 1; 494(Pt 3): 907]. J Physiol (Lond) 1995; 488(Pt 1): 193–202.
13. Heddle, R., Fone, D., Dent, J. and Horowitz, M., Stimulation of pyloric motility by intraduodenal dextrose in normal subjects. Gut 1988; 29(10): 1349–1357.
14. Heddle, R., Collins, P. J., Dent, J., Horowitz, M., Read, N. W., Chatterton, B. *et al.*, Motor mechanisms associated with slowing of the gastric emptying of a solid meal by an intraduodenal lipid infusion. J Gastroenterol Hepatol 1989; 4(5): 437–447.
15. Hunt, J. N., Smith, J. L. and Jiang, C. L., Effect of meal volume and energy density on the gastric emptying of carbohydrates. Gastroenterology 1985; 89(6): 1326–1330.
16. Medhus, A., Sandstad, O., Bredesen, J. and Husebye, E., The migrating motor complex modulates intestinal motility response and rate of gastric emptying of caloric meals. Neurogastroenterol Motil 1995; 7(1): 1–8.
17. Ehrlein, H. J., A new technique for simultaneous radiography and recording of gastrointestinal motility in unanesthetized dogs. Lab Anim Sci 1980; 30(5): 879–884.
18. Code, C. F., The interdigestive housekeeper of the gastrointestinal tract. Perspect Biol Med 1979; 22(2 Pt 2): S49–S55.
19. Schwizer, W., Maecke, H. and Fried, M., Measurement of gastric emptying by magnetic resonance imaging in humans. Gastroenterology 1992; 103(2): 369–376.
20. Collins, P. J., Horowitz, M. and Chatterton, B. E., Proximal, distal and total stomach emptying of a digestible solid meal in normal subjects. Br J Radiol 1988; 61(721): 12–18.
21. King, P. M., Adam, R. D., Pryde, A., McDicken, W. N. and Heading, R. C., Relationships of human antroduodenal motility and transpyloric fluid movement: Non-invasive observations with real-time ultrasound. Gut 1984; 25(12): 1384–1391.
22. Holt, S., McDicken, W. N., Anderson, T., Stewart, I. C. and Heading, R. C., Dynamic imaging of the stomach by real-time ultrasound — A method for the study of gastric motility. Gut 1980; 21(7): 597–601.
23. Bolondi, L., Bortolotti, M., Santi, V., Calletti, T., Gaiani, S. and Labo, G., Measurement of gastric emptying time by real-time ultrasonography. Gastroenterology 1985; 89(4): 752–759.
24. Hveem, K., Jones, K. L., Chatterton, B. E. and Horowitz, M., Scintigraphic measurement of gastric emptying and ultrasonographic assessment of antral area: relation to appetite. Gut 1996; 38(6): 816–821.
25. Bateman, D. N. and Whittingham, T. A., Measurement of gastric emptying by real-time ultrasound. Gut 1982; 23(6): 524–527.
26. King, P. M., Pryde, A. and Heading, R. C., Transpyloric fluid movement and antroduodenal motility in patients with gastro-oesophageal reflux. Gut 1987; 28(5): 545–548.

27. Holt, S., Cervantes, J., Wilkinson, A. A. and Wallace, J. H., Measurement of gastric emptying rate in humans by real-time ultrasound. Gastroenterology 1986; 90(4): 918–923.
28. Gilja, O. H., Detmer, P. R., Jong, J. M., Leotta, D. F., Li, X. N., Beach, K. W. *et al.*, Intragastric distribution and gastric emptying assessed by three-dimensional ultrasonography. Gastroenterology 1997; 113(1): 38–49.
29. Berstad, A., Hausken, T., Gilja, O. H., Thune, N., Matre, K. and Odegaard, S., Volume measurements of gastric antrum by 3-D ultrasonography and flow measurements through the pylorus by duplex technique. Dig Dis Sci 1994; 39(12 Suppl): 97S–100S.
30. Hveem, K., Sun, W. M., Hebbard, G., Horowitz, M., Doran, S. and Dent, J., Relationship between ultrasonically detected phasic antral contractions and antral pressure. Am J Physiol–Gastrointest Liver Physiol 2001; 281(1): G95–G101.
31. Hausken, T., Mundt, M. and Samsom, M., Low antroduodenal pressure gradients are responsible for gastric emptying of a low-caloric liquid meal in humans. Neurogastroenterology and Motility 2002; 14(1): 97–105.
32. Dent, J., A new technique for continuous sphincter pressure measurement. Gastroenterology 1976; 71(2): 263–267.
33. Malagelada, J. R. and Stanghellini, V., Manometric evaluation of functional upper gut symptoms. Gastroenterology 1985; 88(5 Pt 1): 1223–1231.
34. Sun, W. M., Hebbard, G. S., Malbert, C. H., Jones, K. L., Doran, S., Horowitz, M. *et al.*, Spatial patterns of fasting and fed antropyloric pressure waves in humans. J Physiol-London 1997; 503(2): 455–462.
35. Malbert, C. H. and Ruckebusch, Y., Relationships between pressure and flow across the gastroduodenal junction in dogs. Am J Physiol 1991; 260(4 Pt 1): G653–G657.
36. Malbert, C. H. and Mathis, C., Antropyloric modulation of transpyloric flow of liquids in pigs. Gastroenterology 1994; 107(1): 37–46.
37. Liu, J. M., Parashar, V. K. and Mittal, R. K., Asymmetry of lower esophageal sphincter pressure: Is it related to the muscle thickness or its shape? Am J Physiol–Gastrointest Liver Physiol 1997; 35(6): G1509–G1517.
38. Pehlivanov, N., Liu, J. M., Kassab, G. S., Puckett, J. L. and Mittal, R. K., Relationship between esophageal muscle thickness and intraluminal pressure: An ultrasonographic study. Am J Physiol–Gastrointest and Liver Physiol 2001; 280(6): G1093–G1098.
39. Pittman, J. S., Benson, J. T. and Sumners, J. E., Physiological evaluation of the anorectum — A new ultrasound technique. Diseases Colon Rectum 1990; 33(6): 476–478.
40. Heddle, R., Dent, J., Read, N. W., Houghton, L. A., Toouli, J., Horowitz, M. *et al.*, Antropyloroduodenal motor responses to intraduodenal lipid infusion in healthy volunteers. Am J Physiol 1988; 254 (5 Pt 1): G671–G679.
41. Rees, W. D., Miller, L. J. and Malagelada, J. R., Dyspepsia, antral motor dysfunction, and gastric stasis of solids. Gastroenterology 1980; 78(2): 360–365.
42. Husebye, E., The patterns of small bowel motility: Physiology and implications in organic disease and functional disorders. Neurogastroenterol Motility 1999; 11(3): 141–161.
43. Ehrlein, H. J. and Hiesinger, E., Computer-analysis of mechanical-activity of gastroduodenal junction in unanesthetized dogs. Q J Exp Physiol Cognate Med Sci 1982; 67(1): 17–29.
44. Husebye, E., Skar, V., Aalen, O. O. and Osnes, M., Digital ambulatory manometry of the small-intestine in healthy-adults — Estimates of variation within and between individuals and statistical management of incomplete Mmc periods. Dig Dis Sci 1990; 35(9): 1057–1065.
45. Arndorfer, R. C., Stef, J. J., Dodds, W. J., Linehan, J. H. and Hogan, W. J., Improved infusion system for intraluminal esophageal manometry. Gastroenterology 1977; 73(1): 23–27.

46. Frislid, K., Berstad, A. and Guldvog, I., Simulated meal test. A new method for estimation of parietal and non-parietal secretion in response to food. Scand J Gastroenterol 1985; 20(1): 115–122.
47. Marzio, L., Giacobbe, A., Conoscitore, P., Facciorusso, D., Frusciante, V. and Modoni, S., Evaluation of the use of ultrasonography in the study of liquid gastric emptying. Am J Gastroenterol 1989; 84(5): 496–500.
48. Gilja, O. H., Hausken, T., Odegaard, S. and Berstad, A., Monitoring postprandial size of the proximal stomach by ultrasonography. J Ultrasound Med 1995; 14(2): 81–89.
49. Hausken, T. and Berstad, A., Wide gastric antrum in patients with non-ulcer dyspepsia. Effect of cisapride. Scand J Gastroenterol 1992; 27(5): 427–432.
50. Ricci, R., Bontempo, I., Corazziari, E., La, Bella, A. and Torsoli, A., Real time ultrasonography of the gastric antrum. Gut 1993; 34(2): 173–176.
51. Undeland, K. A., Hausken, T., Aanderud, S. and Berstad, A., Lower postprandial gastric volume response in diabetic patients with vagal neuropathy. Neurogastroenterol Motil 1997; 9(1): 19–24.
52. Hausken, T., Gilja, O. H., Odegaard, S. and Berstad, A., Flow across the human pylorus soon after ingestion of food, studied with duplex sonography. Effect of glyceryl trinitrate. Scand J Gastroenterol 1998; 33(5): 484–490.
53. King, P. M., Pryde, A. and Heading, R. C., Transpyloric fluid movement and antroduodenal motility in patients with gastro-oesophageal reflux. Gut 1987; 28(5): 545–548.
54. Kawagishi, T., Nishizawa, Y., Okuno, Y., Shimada, H., Inaba, M., Konishi, T. *et al.*, Antroduodenal motility and transpyloric fluid movement in patients with diabetes studied using duplex sonography [see comments]. Gastroenterology 1994; 107(2): 403–409.
55. Bland, J. M. and Altman, D. G., Statistical methods for assessing agreement between two methods of clinical measurement. Lancet 1986; 1(8476): 307–310.
56. Jones, K., Edelbroek, M., Horowitz, M., Sun, W. M., Dent, J., Roelofs, J. *et al.*, Evaluation of antral motility in humans using manometry and scintigraphy. Gut 1995; 37(5): 643–648.
57. Parkman, H. P., Trate, D. M., Knight, L. C., Brown, K. L., Maurer, A. H. and Fisher, R. S., Cholinergic effects on human gastric motility. Gut 1999; 45(3): 346–354.
58. Fraser, R., Schwizer, W., Borovicka, J., Asal, K. and Fried, M., Gastric motility measurement by MRI. Dig Dis Sci 1994; 39(12 Suppl): 20S–23S.
59. Kunz, P., Feinle, C., Schwizer, W., Fried, M. and Boesiger, P., Assessment of gastric motor function during the emptying of solid and liquid meals in humans by MRI. J Magn Reson Imaging 1999; 9(1): 75–80.
60. Feinle, C., Kunz, P., Boesiger, P., Fried, M. and Schwizer, W., Scintigraphic validation of a magnetic resonance imaging method to study gastric emptying of a solid meal in humans. Gut 1999; 44(1): 106–111.
61. Undeland, K. A., Hausken, T., Gilja, O. H., Aanderud, S. and Berstad, A., Gastric meal accommodation studied by ultrasound in diabetes. Relation to vagal tone. Scand J Gastroenterol 1998; 33(3): 236–241.
62. Gregersen, H., Gilja, O. H., Hausken, T., Heimdal, A., Gao, C., Matre, K. *et al.*, Mechanical properties in the human gastric antrum using B-mode ultrasonography and antral distension. Am J Physiol–Gastrointest Liver Physiology 2002; 283(2): G368–G375.

Published with permission

*Am J Physiol Gastrointest Liver Physiol*
281: G95–G101, 2001.

# Relationship between ultrasonically detected phasic antral contractions and antral pressure

K. HVEEM,[1] W. M. SUN,[2] G. HEBBARD,[3] M. HOROWITZ,[2] S. DORAN,[2] AND J. DENT[2]
[1]*Innherred Hospital, Levanger 7600, Norway;* [2]*Departments of Gastrointestinal Medicine and Medicine, Royal Adelaide Hospital, and* [3]*Division of Medicine, Repatriation General Hospital, Adelaide, South Australia 5000, Australia*

Received 16 May 2000; accepted in final form 6 March 2001

**Hveem, K., W. M. Sun, G. Hebbard, M. Horowitz, S. Doran, and J. Dent.** Relationship between ultrasonically detected phasic antral contractions and antral pressure. *Am J Physiol Gastrointest Liver Physiol* 281: G95–G101, 2001.—The relationships between gastric wall motion and intraluminal pressure are believed to be major determinants of flows within and from the stomach. Gastric antral wall motion and intraluminal pressures were monitored in five healthy subjects by concurrent antropyloroduodenal manometry and transabdominal ultrasound for 60 min after subjects drank 500 ml of clear soup. We found that 99% of antral contractions detected by ultrasound were propagated aborally, and 68% of contractions became lumen occlusive at the site of the ultrasound marker. Of the 203 contractions detected by ultrasound, 53% were associated with pressure events in the manometric reference channel; 86% of contractions had corresponding pressure events detectable somewhere in the antrum. Contractions that occluded the lumen were more likely to be associated with a pressure event in the manometric reference channel ($P < 0.01$) and to be of greater amplitude ($P < 0.01$) than non-lumen-occlusive contractions. We conclude that heterogeneous pressure event patterns in the antrum occur despite a stereotyped pattern of contraction propagation seen on ultrasound. Lumen occlusion is more likely to be associated with higher peak antral pressure events.

gastric emptying

IMAGING METHODS HAVE MUCH to offer in advancing the understanding of gastric mechanics, because they can be used to assess gastric wall motion, luminal diameter, and, in some cases, the movement of luminal contents (8). Fluoroscopic imaging has been used since the turn of the century for this purpose (2), but its application in humans is severely constrained by radiation exposure limits. Imaging with magnetic resonance and ultrasound are attractive options, because they permit prolonged observation of the human stomach without exposure to radiation. Real-time gastric magnetic resonance imaging (10) has special appeal, but as yet, its full potential has not been realized because of its cost and technical complexity. In contrast, ultrasound imaging is relatively inexpensive and widely available. Ultrasound has been used in several studies to evaluate patterns of gastric wall motion and intraluminal flow (5, 8, 9). These studies have revealed substantial variability in the patterning of wall motion and complex patterns of pulsatile flow episodes within and from the stomach.

Luminal manometry is the most widely used method for measuring gastric motility (6). We (11) have demonstrated that the patterns of intraluminal pressure are complex in both the fasting and fed states. Although information about the relationship between intraluminal pressure and gastric wall motion is very limited, it is clear that phasic and tonic contractions of the gastric wall provide the major forces favoring gastric emptying. The mechanisms by which gastric wall motion leads to changes in intraluminal pressure and the associations of movement of gastric contents with wall motion, however, are unclear. In this study, to investigate the relationship between wall motion and luminal pressures, we have combined antropyloric manometry with simultaneous ultrasound imaging of gastric wall motion in healthy human volunteers.

## MATERIALS AND METHODS

### *Subjects*

Nine healthy volunteers participated in the study. For technical reasons, ultrasound images and manometric data were considered to be of adequate quality for analysis in only five of the subjects (3 males and 2 females). None of the subjects had any history of clinically significant dyspeptic symptoms. The median age of the subjects was 21 yr (range 18–24 yr), and the median body mass index was 21 (range 17.7–22.7).

### *Protocol*

Subjects fasted overnight before studies, which were conducted in the seated position. A multilumen sleeve/side hole manometric assembly (Fig. 1) was introduced through an anesthetized nostril and positioned across the pylorus, based on manometric and dual point transmucosal potential difference (TMPD) criteria as previously described (6). The positions of the manometric side holes 3 and 6 cm above the

Address for reprint requests and other correspondence: K. Hveem, Innherred Hospital, Levanger 7600, Norway (E-mail: hveem @innherred-sykehus.no).

The costs of publication of this article were defrayed in part by the payment of page charges. The article must therefore be hereby marked "*advertisement*" in accordance with 18 U.S.C. Section 1734 solely to indicate this fact.

  

Published with permission



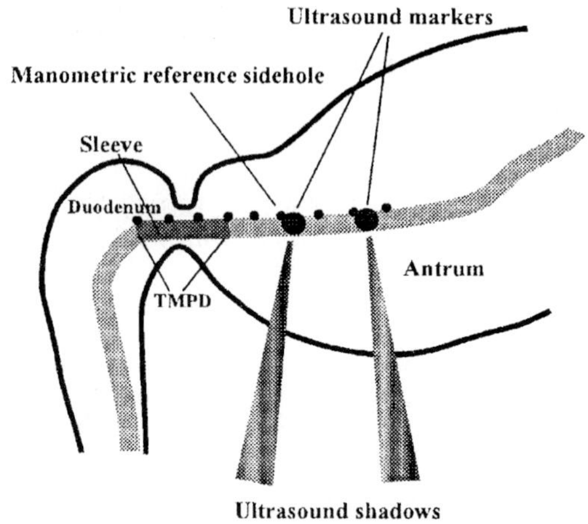


Fig. 1. Positioning of the manometric assembly and marker within the antropyloroduodenal region. TMPD, transmucosal potential difference.

proximal sleeve margin were monitored by observation of the acoustic shadows of two metal markers (Fig. 1) and by continuous observation of TMPD (see *Measurement of Antropyloric Pressures*). Subjects drank 500 ml of clear meat soup (20 kcal, 1 g fat, TORO, Rieber & Søn, Bergen, Norway), and simultaneous recordings of antral wall motion and intraluminal pressure were made for 60 min.

*Measurement of Antropyloric Pressures*

The manometric technique used was similar to that described in previous studies (11). Pressures were measured with a 10-lumen perfused manometric assembly. This incorporated a 4.5-cm sleeve sensor in parallel with a chain of nine side holes spaced at 1.5-cm intervals that straddled the pyloric region (Fig. 1). Side holes positioned at each end of the sleeve were used to measure TMPD as well as pressure (6).

Manometric channels other than those used to record TMPD were perfused with degassed distilled water at 0.3 ml/min with a low compliance manometric infusion pump. TMPD channels were perfused with degassed normal saline from separate reservoirs. Signals from pressure transducers were amplified by a 16-channel Polygraf (Medtronic, Copenhagen, Denmark) and digitized at 10 Hz using an A-D card (NB-MI016, National Instruments Corporation, Austin, TX). Signals were then processed and stored in a personal computer (Apple Computer, Cupertino, CA) with purpose-designed software (MAD 16, Medtronic/Royal Adelaide Hospital/C. H. Malbert) based on LabVIEW (National Instruments).

*Ultrasound imaging*

A 5-MHz sector transducer was positioned on the abdomen to image the antrum and manometric assembly in longitudinal section. The orientation of the transducer was optimized to ensure clear images of the distal ultrasound marker, as this was where the manometric reference channel was located. Because of the orientation of the distal stomach, these images did not reliably include the most distal antrum, pylorus, or duodenum. The metal markers provided a hyperechoic signal that allowed them to be accurately located on the image (Fig. 1). The side hole closest to the distal marker was used as the manometric data reference channel for analysis. In the first two subjects, a marker in the center lumen of the manometric assembly was situated 2 mm aboral to the reference channel (*assembly A*). In the last three subjects, a revised assembly design was used to obtain improved marker definition. In this assembly, the marker was external to the assembly and situated 2 mm oral to the reference side hole (*assembly B*).

*Synchronization of Ultrasound Images with Manometric Data*

A purpose-designed time-coding system was used. This recorded a time code both with the manometric data and on the videotaped ultrasound image. Correlation of the time code between the display of manometric data on the computer screen and the number recorded on the video image allowed accurate synchronization of data to within 100 ms. Manometric and image data were initially analyzed separately to avoid any possibility of observer bias (see *Interobserver Agreement*) before being correlated. Because of the minor differences between assemblies in the relative positions of recording side holes and markers, data used to examine the detailed temporal relationships between ultrasonographically visible contraction waves and manometric pressure events were drawn from the three studies in which *assembly B* was used (see Fig. 5). All other data were analyzed for both assemblies.

*Data Analysis*

*Definitions and terminology relevant to motor events.* A contraction was defined as an indentation of the gastric wall greater than one antral mucosal thickness, which was not due to respiration, pulsation transmitted from the aorta or the heart, or to movements of adjacent intestine, and was observed to propagate for some distance in space and time. Accordingly, for this study, contraction refers specifically to events observed by ultrasound imaging.

A lumen-occlusive contraction was defined as a contraction in which the ultrasound image showed the gastric walls to come into apposition at some point along the imaged antrum (Fig. 2). A propagated contraction was defined as a gastric contraction seen to progress aborally along the entire length of the imaged antrum. A phasic rise in pressure in a single manometric recording channel was referred to as a pressure event. When a group of pressure events recorded in different manometric channels was established as being related by specific spatiotemporal criteria (see *Analysis of pressure event sequences*), each of these grouped events was defined as a pressure event sequence. A contraction was defined as having an associated pressure event when a pressure event was recorded in the manometric reference channel within

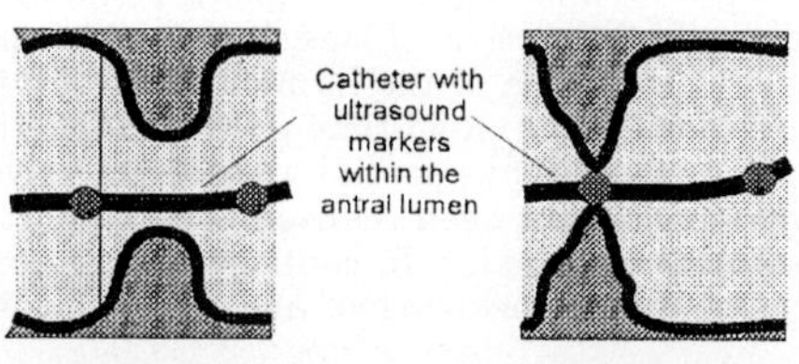


Fig. 2. Timing of contractions reaching the ultrasound marker. *Left*: the time of arrival of the leading edge of the contraction at the marker. *Right*: the timing of lumen occlusion at the marker.

10 s of the timing of the contraction first reaching the level of the ultrasound marker on imaging (see *Analysis of pressure event sequences*).

*Analysis of pressure event sequences.* Manometric recordings were analyzed only when the ultrasound images confirmed that the distal ultrasound marker was positioned in the distal antrum and TMPD recordings confirmed that the manometric assembly was correctly positioned across the pylorus (see *Protocol*). The position of the distal ultrasound marker (and manometric reference channel) was therefore maintained between 3 and 7.5 cm above the pylorus.

The space-time organization of pressure event sequences was evaluated by the following five steps, which were based on a technique previously described in detail (11). *1)* Any resolvable pressure event that was <20 s in duration was scored, provided it was not attributable to respiration, straining, or change in posture. *2)* The time of onset of pressure events was measured in each individual recording channel. *3)* Pressure events in individual channels were then examined for temporal association with events recorded in other channels. Two events were considered to be related if the event in the more distal channel occurred between 5 s before to 10 s after the event in the more proximal channel. An extra second was added to these values for each intervening channel that was "skipped." To define a pressure event sequence, this process was repeated until the channel at or immediately above the pylorus (11) was reached. *4)* The space-time pattern of a pressure event sequence was then classified. If the difference in onset time between pressure events recorded in adjacent channels was ≤1 s, the spatial relationship was defined as synchronous (*s*); if this difference was >1 s, the relationship was defined as antegrade (*a*) or retrograde (*r*), according to the relative position of the recording points. If no other pressure event was present within the time window above, an event was defined as isolated (*i*). The space-time patterning of pressure event sequences was then summarized. For example, a sequence of events recorded over five side holes could be scored *aaaa*, *aasa*, *assr*, and so on, with each lower case letter denoting the relationship between events at a pair of side holes. *5)* Pressure event sequence patterns were then grouped in two ways. First, they were grouped by the aboral evolution of propagation patterns within the sequence (i.e., *aaaa* became *A*, *aasr* became *ASR*, *saar* became *SAR*, and so on). Second, sequences were grouped by the propagation pattern of the most aboral pair of side holes of the pressure event sequence. Pressure event sequences terminating with a synchronous or retrograde component were grouped together and compared with those with a terminal antegrade pattern or with isolated pressure events.

*Definitions and terminology relevant to ultrasound images.* The time of onset of the contraction was defined as the time at which the leading edge of the contraction reached the acoustic reflection of the distal metal ring (Fig. 2). In contractions classified as lumen occlusive, the time at which the occluding contraction wave merged with the acoustic shadow of the marker was taken as the time of lumen occlusion (Fig. 2).

*Interobserver Agreement*

The timing of the onset of pressure events and of the characteristics of antral contractions was analyzed independently by two investigators (Hveem and Sun). Both scored the amplitude and time of appearance of pressure events in the manometric data as well as the timing and character (i.e., whether lumen occlusive and whether propagated) of wall motion on the ultrasound image. Events for which there was a discrepancy were reviewed, and a mutually agreed decision was arrived at before further analysis.

*Statistical Analysis*

Nonparametric statistics were calculated using the Wilcoxon rank sum test and the one-sample sign test. Categorical data were analyzed using a chi square test. All tests were two tailed; $P < 0.05$ was used as the criterion of statistical significance.

**RESULTS**

*Interobserver Agreement*

*Ultrasound data.* There was a mean variability in the judgment of the two observers of the time of arrival of the contraction at the marker of 0.45 s (SE, 0.18 s) and a 90% concordance between the two observers for the first independent analysis of whether contractions were lumen occlusive.

*Manometric data.* The interobserver agreement for scoring of pressure events <5 mmHg, between 5 and 10 mmHg, and >10 mmHg was 85%, 97%, and 100%, respectively. Eighty-nine percent of the onset times of pressure events were in agreement within 1 s and 95% within 2 s.

*Ultrasound Imaging of Distal Antrum*

A longitudinal ultrasound image of ~10 cm of the antrum and clear definition of at least the distal metal marker was achieved in the five subjects in whom imaging was considered adequate for data evaluation. The manometric assembly was seen to lie approximately parallel to the gastric wall (Fig. 1). Satisfactory images were obtained for 72 min with a median duration of 11.5 min/subject (range 10.5 to 27 min, Fig. 3).

Of the 203 antral contractions detected by ultrasound, 99% ($n = 201$) were propagated along the length of the imaged antrum. At the level of the manometric assembly ultrasound marker, 68% ($n = 138$) of contractions were judged to be lumen occlusive.

*Manometric Recordings*

During the periods when ultrasound images were judged to be adequate (72 min), 174 pressure event sequences or isolated pressure events were detected. The frequencies of the different space-time patterns of these sequences are shown in Fig. 4. Antegrade pressure event sequences were the most numerous (40%,

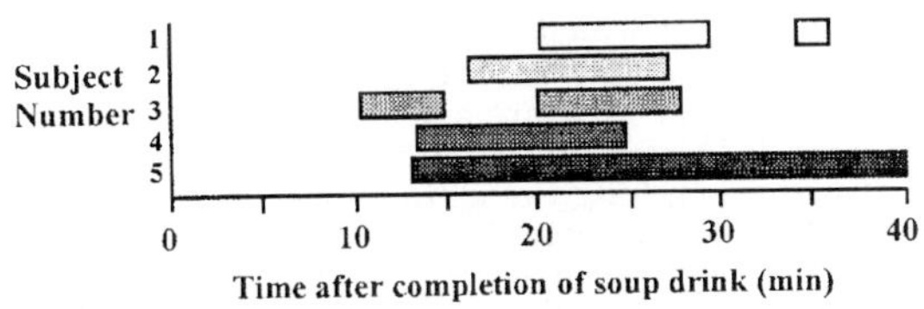


Fig. 3. Recording periods for each subject during which ultrasound images and manometry were considered to be adequate for reliable analysis.

Published with permission



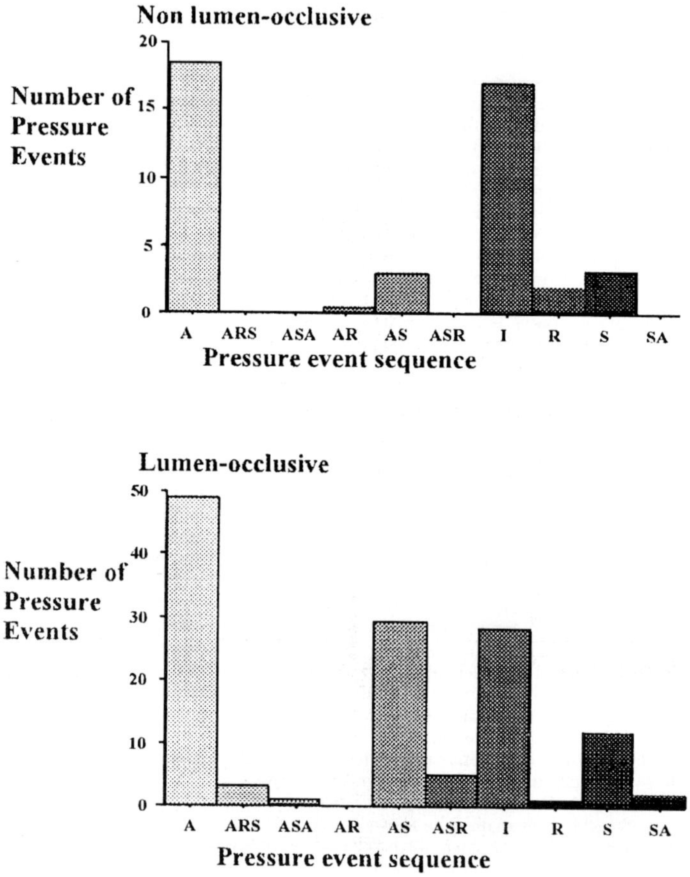


Fig. 4. Relative frequencies of different patterns of pressure events for lumen-occlusive and non-lumen-occlusive contractions. See MATERIALS AND METHODS (*Analysis of pressure event sequences*) for coding of pressure event sequences.

$n$ = 59) followed by isolated pressure waves (25%, $n$ = 37) and then initially antegrade pressure event sequences with a terminal synchronous component (20%, $n$ = 30).

*Relationship Between Contractions and Pressure Events*

*Sensitivity of pressure events for detection of antral contractions.* Of the 203 antral contractions detected by ultrasound, 53% ($n$ = 108) had a temporally associated pressure event in the manometric reference channel. In two-thirds (67%, $n$ = 66) of the 47% ($n$ = 95) of contractions for which no pressure event could be detected in the manometric reference channel, temporally associated pressure events were found in other antropyloric recording channels (i.e., within 10 s of the contraction reaching the metal marker). Therefore, in total, 86% of all contractions had a temporally related pressure event somewhere in the antrum.

*Relative timing of pressure events and antral contractions.* There was a nonsignificant trend for the time of arrival of the leading edge of the contraction wave at the marker to precede the onset of the pressure wave in the manometric reference channel (mean, 0.6 s; $P$ = 0.07; Fig. 5). For lumen-occlusive pressure waves, the time of lumen occlusion at the marker (assessed with ultrasound ) was not significantly different to the time of onset of the pressure event in the manometric reference channel ($P > 0.5$, Fig. 5).

*Relationship between lumen occlusion and detection of pressure events.* There was a significant association between contractions that were judged by ultrasound to have occluded the lumen at the level of the metal marker and the occurrence of a pressure event in the manometric reference channel; 69% ($n$ = 95) of 138 lumen-occlusive contractions had an associated pressure event detected in the manometric reference channel. In contrast, of the 65 non-lumen-occlusive contractions, only 20% ($n$ = 13) were associated with a pressure event ($P < 0.01$).

The median amplitude of the pressure events in the manometric reference channel was 16 mmHg (range 4–98) for lumen-occlusive and 7 mmHg (range 4–23) for non-lumen-occlusive contractions ($P < 0.01$). There

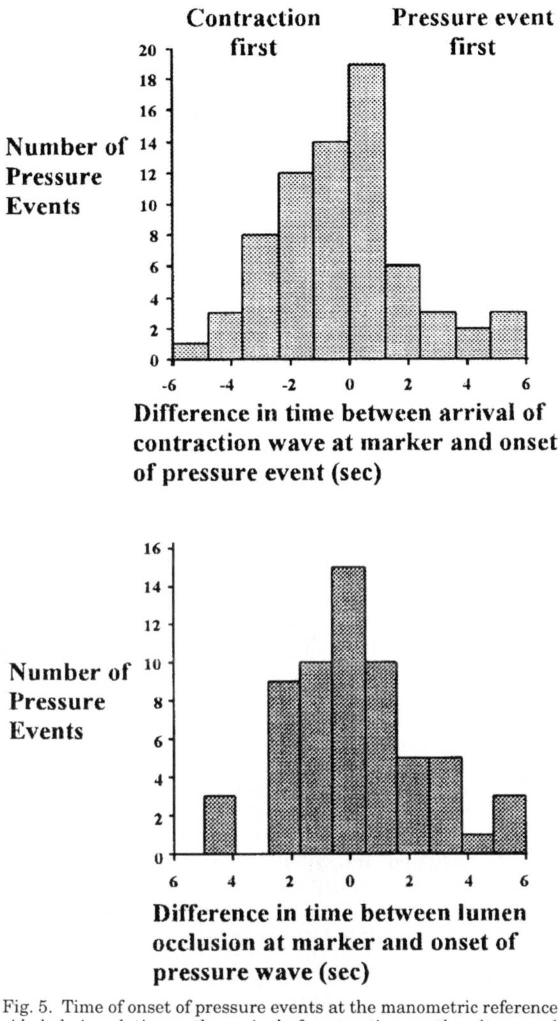


Fig. 5. Time of onset of pressure events at the manometric reference side hole in relation to the arrival of contractions at the ultrasound marker and time of lumen occlusion. A positive value means that the pressure event occurred before the contractile event [arrival of the contraction at the marker or occlusion of the lumen at the marker (Fig. 2)].

was, however, a substantial overlap between the two categories of contraction, with 23% of lumen-occlusive contractions being associated with a pressure event <10 mmHg and 25% of non-lumen-occlusive contractions being associated with a pressure event >10 mmHg (Fig. 6).

*Relationship between lumen occlusion and pressure event sequence.* There was no significant relationship between lumen occlusion and the spatial patterns of pressure event sequences ($P > 0.2$; Fig. 4). However, 54% of pressure event sequences temporally related to lumen-occlusive contractions had a terminal synchronous or retrograde component, compared with 22% of pressure event sequences temporally related to non-lumen-occlusive contractions ($P < 0.05$).

## DISCUSSION

This study adds substantially to knowledge about antral mechanics by providing objective data on the relationships between time-space patterns of intraluminal pressure and antral wall motion and apposition in humans after ingestion of a low-nutrient liquid. Such data are remarkably scanty, especially in humans, but central to the understanding of how the antropyloric region varies the mechanical outcomes of individual contraction sequences. These outcomes vary from retropulsive mixing to pulsatile ejection of gastric content into the duodenum over a wide range of pulse volumes. Our major findings are as follows: *1*) despite a very stereotyped and regular aboral progression of antral contraction to the pylorus, the simultaneously observed patterning of intraluminal pressure and antral wall apposition is variable; *2*) in 86% of ultrasonically detected antral contractions, there is a temporally associated pressure wave somewhere in the

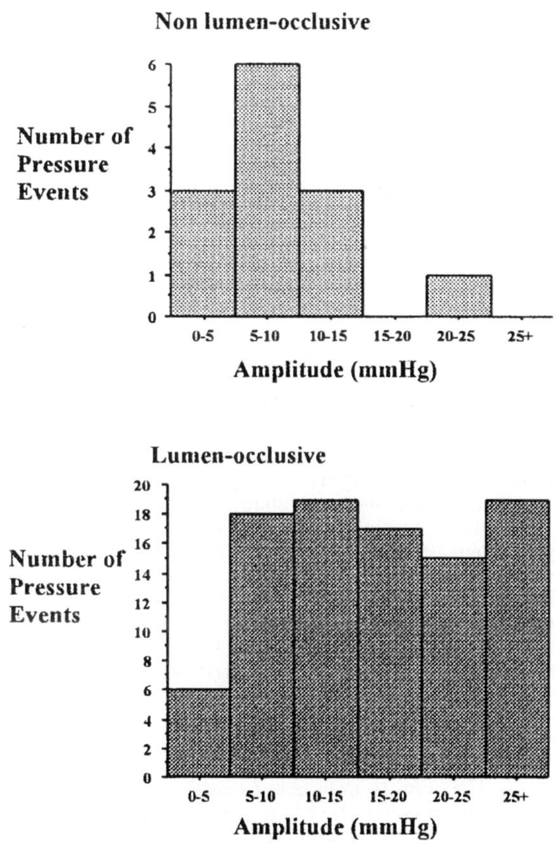


Fig. 6. Amplitudes of pressure events associated with lumen-occlusive and non-lumen-occlusive contractions.

Published with permission



antropyloric region; and *3*) there is a relationship between pressure wave amplitude, occurrence of lumen occlusion, and synchronous or retrograde onset times of terminal antral/pyloric pressure waves.

The scantiness of information about the relationships among antral contractions, contraction-induced antral luminal apposition, and intraluminal pressures reflects the technical challenge of studying these relationships, rather than indicating that they are not physiologically or clinically important. This importance is evident from the predominantly pulsatile pattern of emptying of gastric contents into the duodenum, which is timed with individual antropyloric contraction sequences. The mechanics of individual antropyloric contraction sequences are not stereotyped, as they produce widely differing outcomes with regard to flow, varying from relatively high-volume pulses to forcible retropulsion of the antral content with no forward transpyloric flow. In a previous study (11) in healthy subjects, we found a great diversity of spatial patterning of antral pressure wave onset times among individual contraction sequences, especially in the distal antrum. The observed diversity of antropyloric pressure patterns led us to propose that these spatial variations in antral pressures reflect the relatively subtle variations of antropyloric mechanics that account for the differing observed outcome of luminal flows associated with episodes of antropyloric contractions. Thus far, though, spatial-temporal patterns of pressure have not been well correlated with other changes of antropyloric geometry associated with individual antropyloric contractions or with simultaneous flow patterns. In the present study, we have followed through on our (11) previous observation that there is substantial spatiotemporal diversity of antral pressures, by making ultrasonic observations of antral wall motion concurrently with multipoint antropyloric manometry.

A major challenge in this study was to determine the position of the pressure recording point on the manometric assembly in the ultrasound image. Initially, a metal marker was placed within the center lumen of the manometric assembly, but the ultrasound signals from the markers could not be distinguished consistently from the acoustic shadow of the manometric assembly. However, when the metal markers were positioned around the manometric assembly, a sufficiently sharp and distinct acoustic shadow was seen. Because the distal marker was positioned close to the manometric reference side hole and manometric and image data were synchronized, the relationships between pressure events and gastric wall motion were able to be examined in both space and time.

In contrast to some previous studies (3, 4), we have found that the vast majority (86%) of antral contractions were associated with some form of pressure event, although in only about two-thirds of these was the pressure event identified in the manometric reference channel. This high detection rate of contractions by manometry may be due partly to the closeness of the manometric side holes and partly because we set a low threshold for detection of pressure events. Other factors such as the position of the manometric assembly within the antrum and the volume and composition of the meal probably also influence the relationship between the number of antral contractions and pressure events by changing the relative proportions of lumen-occlusive and non-lumen-occlusive contractions, especially under conditions of more substantial rates of nutrient delivery to the duodenum than was the case in the present setting. With regard to the differences between lumen-occlusive and non-lumen-occlusive contractions, we found that lumen-occlusive contractions were more likely to be associated with a pressure wave in the manometric reference channel, and these pressure waves were likely to be of higher amplitude than those associated with non-lumen-occlusive contractions. These observations, along with the observation that the onset of pressure events and arrival of the antral contraction waves at the ultrasound marker correlated closely in time, indicate that pressure events associated with contractions are usually relatively localized phenomena, with significant elevations in pressure extending perhaps only a few millimeters from the edge of the antral contraction. On the basis of physical principles, the spatial extent of the pressure waves would be expected to vary with the rate of propagation of the antral contraction, the degree of lumen occlusion, and the viscosity of the antral content. Contractions have also been noted (1) to result in a generalized rise in the luminal pressure of the stomach, the "common cavity" pressure. However, we did not identify this in the current study, probably because of the relatively modest volume within the stomach.

The characteristics of the antral contractions that we were able to observe using ultrasound (i.e., whether lumen occlusive and whether propagated) were not predictive of the overall pattern of the pressure event sequence as determined by manometry. This may reflect the limitations of the ultrasound image in terms of spatial resolution and the fact that only a single plane could be visualized. Three-dimensional ultrasound imaging of the antrum would provide better spatial information than the technique we employed, but at the cost of poorer temporal resolution.

These data indicate that complex patterns of pressure event sequences can be generated by contractions that have a stereotyped pattern of aboral propagation along the antrum. These patterns are likely to have significantly different mechanical outcomes, such as retropulsion within the stomach and/or transpyloric flow. However, currently there are no reliable data on the relationships between transpyloric flow, contraction patterns, and spatiotemporal patterning of pressure wave sequences in humans.

We observed that the presence and amplitude of pressure events in the manometric reference channel and the presence of a terminal synchronous or retrograde component of the pressure event sequence were all associated with lumen occlusion at the level of the metal marker. We believe that all of these factors probably reflect increased vigor of those contractions

Published with permission



with a terminal retrograde component, or a synchronous component in some pressure wave sequences probably correlates with the "terminal antral contraction" observed fluoroscopically.

Our analysis of gastric wall motion and intraluminal pressures suggests that the maximum amplitude of pressure waves can only be used as an approximate predictor of the occurrence of lumen occlusion, with approximately one-quarter of lumen-occlusive contractions being associated with a pressure event sequence <10 mmHg, and a similar proportion of non-lumen-occlusive contractions being associated with a pressure event sequence >10 mmHg. Above a pressure of 25 mmHg, however, all pressure waves were associated with lumen-occlusive contractions, probably reflecting mucosal "contact pressure."

One significant limitation of this and many other studies of gastric motor function is that the mechanical significance of the contractions and manometrically recorded pressures could not be determined. The patterns of intragastric pressure and wall motion associated with transpyloric flow have not been defined and await simultaneous measurement of these and other relevant parameters, such as pyloric resistance and the transpyloric pressure gradient (7).

### REFERENCES


1. **Anvari M, Dent J, Malbert C, and Jamieson GG.** Mechanics of pulsatile transpyloric flow in the pig. *J Physiol (Lond)* 488: 193–202, 1995. [Corrigenda. *J Physiol (Lond)* 494: August, 1996, p. 907.]
2. **Cannon WB.** The movements of the stomach, studied by means of the Röntgen rays. *Am J Physiol* 1: 359–382, 1898.
3. **Edelbroek M, Schuurkes J, de Ridder W, Horowitz M, Dent J, and Akkermans L.** Pyloric motility. Sleeve sensor versus strain gauge transducer. *Dig Dis Sci* 39: 577–586, 1994.
4. **Fone DR, Akkermans LM, Dent J, Horowitz M, and van der Schee EJ.** Evaluation of patterns of human antral and pyloric motility with an antral wall motion detector. *Am J Physiol Gastrointest Liver Physiol* 258: G616–G623, 1990.
5. **Hausken T, Odegaard S, Matre K, and Berstad A.** Antroduodenal motility and movements of luminal contents studied by duplex sonography. *Gastroenterology* 102: 1583–1590, 1992.
6. **Heddle R, Dent J, Toouli J, and Read NW.** Topography and measurement of pyloric pressure waves and tone in humans. *Am J Physiol Gastrointest Liver Physiol* 255: G490–G497, 1988.
7. **Horowitz M and Dent J.** The study of gastric mechanics and flow: a Mad Hatter's tea party starting to make sense? *Gastroenterology* 107: 302–306, 1994.
8. **King PM, Adam RD, Pryde A, McDicken WN, and Heading RC.** Relationships of human antroduodenal motility and transpyloric fluid movement: non-invasive observations with real-time ultrasound. *Gut* 25: 1384–1391, 1984.
9. **Pallotta N, Cicala M, Frandina C, and Corazziari E.** Antropyloric contractile patterns and transpyloric flow after meal ingestion in humans. *Am J Gastroenterol* 93: 2513–2522, 1998.
10. **Schwizer W, Fraser R, Borovicka J, Asal K, Crelier G, Kunz P, Boesiger P, and Fried M.** Measurement of proximal and distal gastric motility with magnetic resonance imaging. *Am J Physiol Gastrointest Liver Physiol* 271: G217–G222, 1996.
11. **Sun WM, Hebbard GS, Malbert CH, Jones KL, Doran S, Horowitz M, and Dent J.** Spatial patterns of fasting and fed antropyloric pressure waves in humans. *J Physiol (Lond)* 503: 455–462, 1997.

CHAPTER 7

# THERAPEUTIC POTENTIAL AND CONSIDERATION OF HIGH INTENSITY ULTRASOUND IN GASTROENTEROLOGY

ROY W. MARTIN AND JOO HA HWANG

## 1. Introduction

Diagnostic ultrasound is widely employed in gastroenterology as discussed in this text. However, the question arises: Can ultrasound also be used in therapy for gastrointestinal (GI) disease? This may be a startling question to those only familiar with the low levels of ultrasound used in diagnosis. At much higher intensities, is it possible to evoke tissue changes that are beneficial?

As early as 1954, Lindstrom (1) and Fry *et al.* (2) investigated this possibility for the purposes of treating neurologic disorders. They produced these elevated intensities by using focusing methods (Fig. 1) in a manner analogous to the way a magnifying glass can be used to focus light from the sun onto a spot size on a surface. In the case of the magnifying glass, enough heat can be generated at the focus that combustion of wood or paper can be rapidly initiated. The larger the lens and the sharper the focusing, the more rapidly such heating occurs. In contrast, ultrasound can be focused not only on a surface, but at some depth below the surface and deliver enough energy to rapidly evoke heating of tissue to high temperatures in a few seconds. An example of this is given in Fig. 2, where a gel phantom is used to demonstrate the focal area that heat is generated. This creates the possibility of producing necrosis of tissue at a selected point at some depth. This was the potential that Fry and his colleagues tried to utilize in the brain for the treatment of Parkinson's disease and other hyperkinetic disorders of the central nervous system. The technical difficulties at that time and development of various alternative treatments negated acceptance of this approach. Nevertheless, in the 1970's ultrasound was again investigated but at lower intensities and for the purpose of treating tumors (3). The new concept was to induce hyperthermia (elevation of tissue temperature to $\sim$43°C) within the entire tumor volume and then maintain the tumor at that temperature for an extended time period. Unfortunately, this strategy was unsuccessful largely due to lack of a noninvasive temperature measuring method to use in feedback control of the delivered acoustic power to the tumor. This inability resulted in the lack of uniform heating and maintenance of the entire tumor volume at the hyperthermic range. The next innovation arose in the 1980's with the development of an extracorporeal shock wave lithotrispy (ESWL) (4). The use of ESWL as a method for treating kidney stones was approved in 1984 by the US Federal Drug Administration. It has represented the first clinical application of high intensity ultrasound. This has continued to be a viable treatment and has been extended by some to

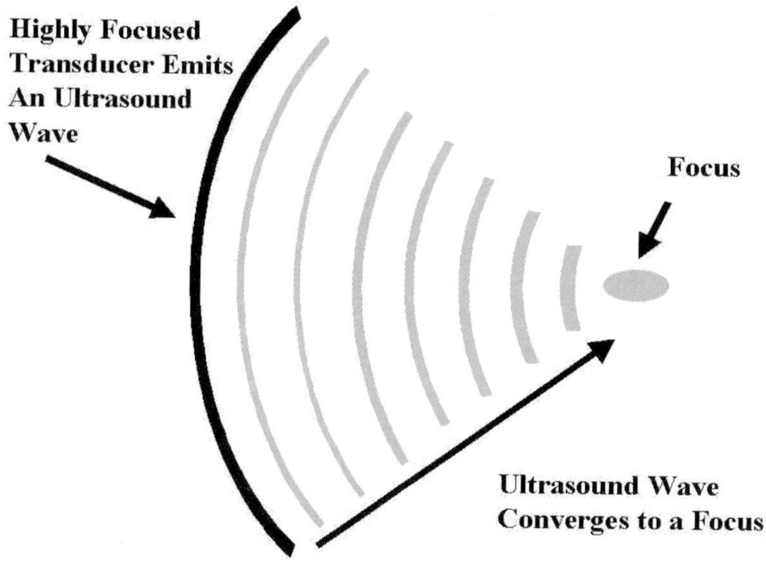


Fig. 1. A schematic of high intensity focused ultrasound. Ultrasound waves are emitted from a spherically curved transducer resulting in convergence of ultrasound energy at the focus. Due to this focusing effect, intervening structures between the focus and transducer surface are exposed to significantly lower ultrasound intensities.

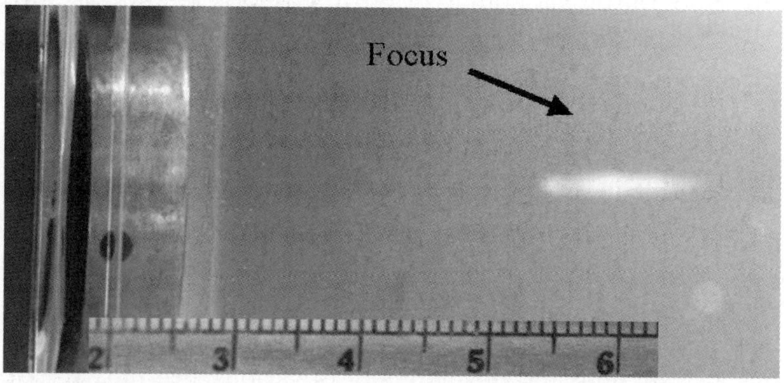


Fig. 2. An example of a spherically curved transducer creating a thermal lesion in a gel phantom. The phantom is made of a 7% polyacrylamide gel with 3% bovine serum albumin. The transducer is a 23 mm diameter, spherically curved, single-element piezoelectric transducer (PZT-4), with a radius of curvature of 35 mm (Sonic Concepts, Woodinville, WA).

treating gallstones as well (5). A "rediscovery" of high intensity focused ultrasound (HIFU) occurred in the 1990's with the refinement of modern technology being applied to tranducer development and the ability to monitor the therapy with advanced imaging techniques such as MRI. Further, the realization that it can produce almost instantaneous cell death to very selected regions of tissue has made it a candidate for direct and rapid treatment of tumors (6–16). Investigations and early clinical utilization are currently underway. Finally, not only has tumor treatment been targeted, but it has been demonstrated in animal experiments that HIFU can also be used to produce hemostasis (17–24).

The thrust of this chapter is to look to the future and address the question of whether ultrasound can also be used in therapy for gastrointestinal (GI) disease or for other diseases that can be treated via the endoscopic route? In order to do this, first, a brief discussion is given regarding high intensity ultrasound, some of the phenomena associated with it that are not so prevalent at the lower diagnostic levels, and some of the bioeffects that can occur as a result of it. Next, the current evidence is reviewed of the effectiveness of high intensity ultrasound in treating diseased tissue. Several specific investigations are then discussed that have been reported using high intensity ultrasound in the GI tract. Fourthly, the engineering and physics considerations of delivering such energy to the gastrointestinal lumen wall or adjacent tissue will be presented. Finally, the concluding discussion analyzes the technical details of ultrasound therapy techniques that have been reported involving the use of HIFU by an intraluminal delivery method.

## 2. High Intensity Ultrasound and Related Phenomena

The primary difference between high intensity ultrasound and diagnostic ultrasound is the time averaged intensity. Typical diagnostic ultrasound transducers deliver ultrasound with intensities on the order of 0.1–100 mWcm$^{-2}$ or 0.001–3 MPa depending on the mode of imaging (B-mode, pulsed Doppler, or continuous wave Doppler) (25). In contrast, high intensity focused ultrasound transducers deliver ultrasound with intensities in the range of 100–4,000 Wcm$^{-2}$ to the focal region, which is several orders of magnitude greater. Furthermore, with the exception of continuous wave Doppler, diagnostic transducers deliver a short pulse of ultrasound, whereas high intensity applications usually deliver continuous wave ultrasound.

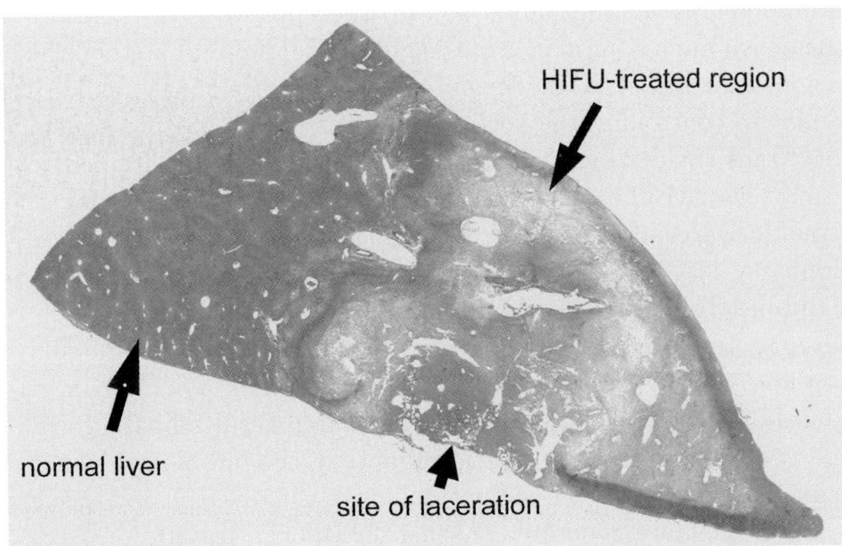


Fig. 3. A lacerated rabbit liver 3 days after treatment with HIFU. This photograph demonstrates the clear demarcation between treated and untreated liver tissue. The HIFU-treated liver tissue has undergone coagulative necrosis. A rim of ischemic necrosis borders the region between normal liver tissue and HIFU-treated tissue.

The major effect of this elevated intensity in tissue is that considerable heat is generated due to the absorption of a portion of the energy. The heat raises the temperature rapidly to 60°C or higher in the tissue causing coagulative necrosis within a few seconds (Fig. 3). The absorption rate as with diagnostic ultrasound is highly frequency dependent with higher frequencies being more rapidly absorbed. Further, as mentioned earlier focusing has been most often used to achieve the high intensities at a specific location and over only a small volume (e.g. a 1 mm diameter and 9 mm length). This focusing avoids damaging tissue located between the transducer and the focal point as the intensities are much lower there (see Fig. 1). Thus, very importantly, focusing confines tissue damage to a precise region. This region can be moved once the desired tissue temperature is reached in order to treat a larger volume with fairly good precision.

There are mechanical phenomena in addition to the thermal effects that are associated at high intensities. These are not prevalent or present at lower intensities. Foremost, is the possibility that cavitation may occur. Also of importance are radiation forces that result from the change in the momentum of the propagating waves due to absorption or reflection of the wave. In tissue, this force can generate pressure on the focal region and, if fluid is present, can produce streaming. Finally, nonlinear effects may occur. The major effect is that a wave can become distorted as it propagates. This distortion is from a sinusoidal wave towards a saw tooth shape which has the effect of converting energy from the fundamental frequency to higher harmonics,[a] which in turn are more quickly absorbed.

Cavitation is the generation of gas and/or vapor-filled bubbles in a liquid through the action of ultrasound. Bioeffects can result from cavitation and depend to a considerable extent on the nature of the cavitation. Historically, cavitation has been classified as either stable or inertial. Although these two terms have varied in meaning over the past years, the current rigorous definition relates to the controlling factors of the bubble's oscillation, i.e. the growth and collapse of the bubble due to the applied ultrasound. If the bubble is controlled by the density and compliance of the gas inside the bubble, then this is referred to as stable cavitation. In contrast, if the density and compliance of the media surrounding the bubble is dominant in controlling the action, then this is referred to as inertial cavitation. An earlier term "transient cavitation" now is more appropriately applied to the duration that a bubble may last. Bubble oscillation occurs by expansion during the rarefaction phase of an acoustic wave and contraction during the compressional phase of the wave. Stable cavitation may lead to a phenomenon called microstreaming (rapid movement of fluid near the bubble due to its oscillating motion). Microstreaming can produce high shear forces close to the bubble that can disrupt cell membranes and may play a role in ultrasound-enhanced drug delivery. Inertial cavitation is associated with the violent collapse of bubbles due to the ultrasound field and often results in the formation of high-speed liquid jets created from an asymmetric collapse of the bubbles. These liquid jets, and the shock waves emanating from the violent collapse can tear cells or tissue apart due to the high shear forces that are generated. Generally, inertial cavitation is associated with the conversion of liquid to vapor and vice versa. During the rarefaction portion of the acoustic wave the reduced pressure promotes liquid to vapor conversion at temperatures

[a]Harmonics in this case are frequencies higher than the fundamental frequency (e.g. twice, three, or four times higher in frequency).

less than the boiling temperature. Inertial cavitation thus has frequency dependence in that the lower frequencies provide more time for liquid evaporation and thus more time for bubble growth, which in turn results in larger bubbles. These larger bubbles collapse more violently. Thus, lower frequencies usually result in more violent inertial cavitation. On the other hand, higher ultrasonic frequencies are more readily absorbed in tissue, resulting in increased tissue temperature. If the tissue temperature is increased very rapidly, the liquid is unable to contain the same amount of absorbed gas, and cavitation is nucleated at lower intensities. To summarize, lower frequencies result in more violent cavitation and lower tissue absorption. Higher frequencies result in less violent cavitation, but increased tissue heating. If the temperature increase occurs very rapidly, then cavitation thresholds are reduced due to the inability of the higher-temperature liquids to contain the dissolved gas. Thus, the generation of cavitation in tissues exposed to high intensity focused ultrasound is a very complicated problem.

Cavitation has been reported to appear in two types of forms during *in vivo* HIFU treatment. Sanghvi *et al.* report on what they call the "popcorn" and "cloud" action, and we have observed these activities in our studies as well (26). The "popcorn" action is the occurrence, sometimes randomly, of an audible "pop" sound that occurs while HIFU energy is being applied similar to exploding and spurting grease when frying meat at a high temperature. Sanghvi *et al.* reported finding a cavity formed in the prostate when this "popcorn" action occurred. This action only occasionally occurred in the treatment of patients when the intensities at the focus were kept under 1,700 $\mathrm{Wcm}^{-2}$ at 4 MHz. However, it could be consistently produced in dog prostates at peak intensities ranging from 2,200 $\mathrm{Wcm}^{-2}$ to 3,400 $\mathrm{Wcm}^{-2}$. The "cloud" action was the formation of a bright echo in the image when both ultrasonic imaging and treatment were used. This bright echo forms at the focal point and then increases in size and grows towards the HIFU transducer if the energy application is continued. The higher the intensity, to a point, the more rapidly the echo forms and grows toward the transducer. Lesions formed by this process are generally more irregular than if the "cloud" does not appear (27, 28). Both the "popcorn" and the "cloud" action are thought to be due to cavitation.

Radiation forces are developed when a wave is either absorbed or reflected. Complete reflection produces twice the force that complete absorption does. These forces are constant if the amplitude of a wave is steady and the absorption and/or reflection is constant. If the reflecting or absorbing media is tissue or other solid material, the force presses against the media producing a pressure, termed *radiation pressure.* If the media is liquid and can move under pressure, then streaming results. The magnitude of radiation pressure and streaming can be quite high at intensities of 2,000 $\mathrm{Wcm}^{-2}$ for example. We have observed that the blood ejecting from an artery as a result of a needle puncture could be completely stopped by this phenomena if the acoustic wave impinged on the blood in a direction opposite to its exit direction. As a further example, a fountain of water can shoot a meter or so above the surface of a water tank if a HIFU transducer is held underwater such that the focus is at the surface. In this situation, atomization[b] of water can also occur depending on where the focal point of the transducer is positioned with respect to the surface. These examples are given to illustrate that there is a powerful mechanical force present at high intensities.

[b] Atomization is the formation of fine water droplets in the air.

## 3. Biologic Effects Of High Intensity Ultrasound

Diagnostic ultrasound has an excellent safety profile without any clinically significant deleterious biologic effects being reported using current diagnostic equipment. However, at high intensities, ultrasound can result in tissue heating and necrosis, cell apoptosis, and cell lysis. Mechanisms involved in HIFU induced biologic effects are primarily due to thermal and cavitational mechanisms as previously discussed.

### 3.1. *Thermal mechanisms*

#### 3.1.1. *Coagulative necrosis*

Coagulative necrosis occurs in tissue exposed to high intensity ultrasound when the temperature of the tissue is elevated. The temperature required to induce coagulative necrosis is time dependent. Tissue temperature raised to over 60°C for one second will generally lead to instantaneous cell death via coagulative necrosis in most tissues. This is the primary mechanism for tumor cell destruction in HIFU therapy. In a study performed by Wu *et al.* (15) the pathologic changes in malignant tumors that were initially treated with HIFU then surgical resected 1–14 days following HIFU therapy were reported. Tissue evaluated 1–7 days following HIFU therapy demonstrated homogeneous areas of coagulative necrosis without any evidence of residual viable tumor cells. Seven to 14 days following HIFU therapy granulation tissue began to replace the necrotic tissue and the boundary area between treated and untreated tissue was replaced by fibrous tissue. Figure 3 demonstrates a typical HIFU induced lesion of coagulative necrosis in liver tissue.

#### 3.1.2. *Apoptosis*

Although the majority of the initial cell death within a high intensity ultrasound field is due to cell necrosis from thermal injury, high intensity ultrasound can also induce apoptosis. In apoptotic cells, the nucleus of the cell self-destructs with rapid degradation of DNA by endonucleases. It has been demonstrated that the primary mechanism of cell death by hyperthermia is due to apoptosis (29). Apoptosis has also been demonstrated in leukemic cells exposed to low intensity ultrasound (30), and in leukemic cells exposed to ultrasound-induced cavitation (31).

### 3.2. *Cavitation-related effects*

Ultrasound-induced cavitation has been previously described in this chapter. Many of the bioeffects resulting from high intensity ultrasound that cannot be attributed to necrosis is usually believed to be a result of cavitation. The recent introduction of gas-filled microspheres (diameter 2–5 $\mu$m) as a contrast agent in ultrasound imaging has created increased interest in the role of cavitation on ultrasound induced bioeffects.

#### 3.2.1. *Capillary disruption*

Miller and Quddus (32) as well as Skyba *et al.* (33) have demonstrated that, in the presence of contrast agents,capillaries exposed to ultrasound of sufficient intensity can rupture. This bioeffect can actually be observed at ultrasound intensities that are used for diagnostic ultrasound. There is some controversy as to the mechanism that is involved in the rupture of the capillaries. One theory is that capillary rupture occurs during the expansion phase of the microsphere. This action occurs while the microsphere is exposed to negative pressure (rarefaction portion of the ultrasound wave) allowing it to expand (34). Another possible mechanism is that due to inertial cavitation of the microsphere, a significant force is exerted against the capillary wall, thus, causing damage.

### 3.2.2. *Platelet activation*

Poliachik *et al.* demonstrated that HIFU induced cavitation could lead to activation and aggregation of platelets (35). Regression analysis demonstrated that there was a weak correlation between the ultrasound intensity and platelet aggregation, but a strong correlation existed between cavitation activity and platelet aggregation. The mechanism is believed to be cavitation-induced platelet damage leading to a release of prothrombotic mediators from the platelets causing further activation and aggregation of platelets.

### 3.2.3. *Cell membrane disruption*

Ultrasound-mediated cell membrane disruption is an active area of research due to its potential in drug and gene delivery applications. Tachibana *et al.* have published electron micrographs demonstrating pores in cell membranes after ultrasound exposure (continuous wave mode, 255 kHz, 0.4 Wcm$^{-2}$, 30 second exposure) in the presence of a photosensitive drug (merocyanine 540) (36). We have also demonstrated that endothelial cells can become damaged with pore formation on the endothelial surface of arteries infused with gas-filled microbubbles and exposed to pulsed ultrasound (37). Others have also demonstrated the disruption of cell monolayers in culture when exposed to ultrasound in the presence of gas-filled microbubbles (38–40). It is widely believed that inertial cavitation is the mechanism leading to this form of cell membrane disruption.

Several studies examining the impact of ultrasound contrast agents erythrocytes have also been published (41–47). These studies demonstrate that hemolysis occurs when whole blood containing ultrasound contrast agent is exposed to ultrasound. This body of literature clearly demonstrates that cavitation is involved in cell lysis.

## 4. Clinical Applications of High Intensity Ultrasound

Currently, several clinically trials involving high intensity ultrasound are ongoing in the USA, Europe, and Asia. Several centers in China are treating patients with extracorporeal HIFU, with commercially available HIFU therapy machines, primarily for solid tumors that have not responded to conventional therapies. A review of the current clinical applications that are most relevant to the purpose of this chapter is presented.

### 4.1. *The response of tumors to HIFU therapy*

The greatest interest in HIFU therapy is its potential application in the treatment of tumors. Several clinical trials are ongoing in investigating its role in the management of cholangiocarcinoma, hepatocellular carcinoma, metastatic liver disease, pancreatic cancer, prostate cancer, breast cancer, renal cell carcinoma, osteosarcoma, and other various solid tumors. The primary mechanism used to treat these tumors is thermally induced coagulative necrosis. These studies are presented below to demonstrate the potential for treating tumors endoscopically.

#### 4.1.1. *Prostate cancer and benign prostatic hyperplasia*

Several groups in Europe, Japan, and the United States are investigating the use of transrectal HIFU probes for treating prostate cancer and benign prostatic hyperplasia (BPH). The significance of these studies to gastroenterology is obvious: if a HIFU transducer can be used to treat the prostate via a transrectal probe, then a transducer capable of treating other peri-luminal structures should be feasible.

The most recent published clinical study out of Japan reports results from a Phase I trial in 20 patients with biopsy-proven localized prostate cancer (Stage 1b to Stage 2b) (48). In this treatment, the entire prostate volume received therapy. The size of the lesion created by the HIFU probes varied from $2 \times 2 \times 10$ mm$^3$ to $3 \times 3 \times 10$ mm$^3$ depending on the probe used, with focal lengths ranging from 2.5 to 4.5 cm, and a focal intensity of 1,680 Wcm$^{-2}$ that resulted in tissue temperature elevations to over 80°C in less than 1 second. The treatment time ranged from 55 minutes to 5 hours, 56 minutes (mean 2 hours, 49 minutes). They demonstrated a complete response in 100% of patients who underwent therapy with transrectal HIFU, as evidenced by negative post-therapy biopsies and no elevation of the serum prostate-specific antigen (PSA) following the treatment. Complications of the procedure included a rectourethral fistula in one patient and urethral stricture formation in two patients. Mean follow-up time in this study was 13.5 months with a range of 6–31 months.

Early studies examining the use of HIFU for the treatment of BPH (49) demonstrated an initial response to transrectal HIFU therapy; however, the response was not durable, with many patients requiring transurethral resection of the prostate (TURP) to relive their symptoms. However, recent data from Japan (50) suggests that treatment of BPH using a transrectal HIFU probe improves peak urinary flow rates and patients' quality of life which were maintained over a 3–4 year period.

These studies and others similar to it (7, 10, 26, 51–60) demonstrate the feasibility of applying HIFU to tissue up to 4.5 cm distance from the rectal lumen. The duration of HIFU therapy is a concern as demonstrated by the prostate cancer studies. Endoscopic HIFU therapy that exceeds 2 hours will likely require intubation of the patient.

#### 4.1.2. *Cholangiocarcinoma*

Prat *et al.* have published results of a phase I trial of an intraductal high intensity ultrasound probe used for the palliative treatment of cholangiocarcinoma (61). The instrument that they have constructed consists of a probe that can be advanced through the accessory channel of a therapeutic side-viewing duodenoscope (62–65). The probe can be inserted into the common bile duct over a guide wire. Prior to placement of the high intensity ultrasound probe, cholangiography is performed identifying the location of the cholangiocarcinoma, which has previously been diagnosed with histology or cytology demonstrating malignancy. Radio-opaque markers are placed on the abdomen to assist in positioning of the ultrasound probe. Once the ultrasound probe is placed in the common bile duct, with the transducer positioned at the level of the cholangiocarcinoma, the high intensity ultrasound (10 MHz, 14 $Wcm^{-2}$) is applied for 10 seconds at a time. After each 10-second treatment the probe is rotated 18° and treated for another 10 seconds. This is repeated until the probe has been rotated a full 360° resulting in treatment of the entire circumference of the bile duct (66). Prat *et al.* report promising results with this therapy. Treated segments of strictures did not progress. Some patients no longer required stent placement at 3 months of follow-up. Progression of tumors did occur either upstream or downstream of the treated segment, which is thought to be due to inadequate treatment of the entire length of the tumor. Intraductal ultrasound imaging or cholangioscopy was not used to characterize the length or depth of involvement of the tumors that might have improved localization of the tumor. This therapy was not effective in the treatment of ampullary carcinomas.

#### 4.1.3. *Liver tumors*

Liver tumors are an obvious potential target for HIFU therapy. Ablative therapy using radio-frequency energy, ethanol, and chemoembolization are currently being utilized in the treatment of liver tumors such as hepatocellular carcinoma (HCC). Since HIFU is a noninvasive method of thermally ablative therapy, its application in the treatment of liver tumors is ideal. It has benefits over the other currently used methods since the volume and distribution of therapy can be precisely controlled if image guidance is used. One of the difficulties in the current application of HIFU for the treatment of liver tumors is the acoustic window required to target hepatic lesions. Most of the liver is obscured by the overlying ribs that do not allow penetration of ultrasound energy. In an attempt to overcome this, a group in Chongqing, China, has performed partial rib resections to obtain an adequate acoustic window to treat liver tumors with HIFU (67). This approach is not ideal and research is being performed to develop transducer arrays that could potentially be used such that rib resection would not be required to treat liver tumors transcutaneously. Another potential approach is via the endoscopic or laparoscopic route. Although these approaches are more invasive than treating transcutaneously, it is certainly better than having to surgically resect ribs.

Initial studies examining the use of HIFU in treating liver tumors demonstrate that it is well tolerated by patients, does not appear to cause significant pain, and can be performed without sedation (68, 69). A preliminary study performed in China of 50 patients with advanced-stage HCC compared treatment with transcatheter arterial chemoembolization (TACE) alone versus TACE plus HIFU (70). Median survival ratios at 6 and 12 months were reported to be significantly higher in the TACE plus HIFU group. These results may be due to more complete destruction of the tumor with HIFU therapy. The same group reported findings from 6 patients that had resectable HCC that underwent surgical resection of their tumors 2–3 weeks following HIFU treatment alone with pathology of these resected specimens demonstrating complete necrosis of the treated lesion (67).

### 4.1.4. *Pancreatic cancer*

The use of high intensity ultrasound for the palliative treatment of pancreatic cancer may be useful in patients that develop symptoms that would benefit from tumor volume reduction. Some preliminary results in 251 patients with advanced pancreatic cancer (TNM stage II–IV), again from China, suggest that HIFU treatment can reduce the size of pancreatic tumors without causing pancreatitis, and prolong survival (71). An interesting finding was that 84% of patients with pain due to pancreatic cancer obtained significant relief of their pain after treatment with HIFU. In another study, all 11 patients with pain related to pancreatic cancer treated with HIFU obtained relief of pain immediately following the ablative therapy with only one patient developing recurrent pain after one week post-therapy; however, the duration of follow-up was not reported (72). Potential mechanisms include relief of pancreatic or bile duct obstructions by decreasing the size of the tumor and the destruction of parenchymal pain fibers.

## 5. Hemostasis and Vessel Occlusion

Previous studies have demonstrated the ability of HIFU to induce hemostasis in lacerated vessels of large animals (17, 22, 23). Depending on the intensity and duration of HIFU application, HIFU can result in occlusive or non-occlusive hemostasis in punctured femoral arteries and veins of large animals. HIFU has also been demonstrated to effectively stop bleeding in lacerated liver and spleen (20, 21). The primary mechanism for this is believed to be thermal coagulation; however, HIFU also has mechanical effects such as acoustic streaming and radiation pressure that may exert a tamponade-like effect on the actively bleeding vessel. We have investigated the possible use of HIFU for the treatment of GI bleeding using the rabbit auricular vein to simulate a vessel that would be of similar caliber to that found in the GI tract (24). A 2 mm length laceration of the auricular vein was treated with HIFU at an intensity of 750 $\mathrm{Wcm}^{-2}$ in 5-second intervals. The median time to hemostasis was 10 seconds (range 5–25 seconds). Animals were followed for 28 days to see the evolution of the treated vessel. No vessels exhibited evidence of re-bleeding. Histology demonstrated the formation of an occlusive thrombus, and by day 28, the treated vessel was replaced by fibrous scar without significant residual inflammation.

HIFU has potential benefits over current methods of hemostasis. It potentially could be incorporated with ultrasound imaging or Doppler ultrasound to identify and then occlude bleeding vessels. This could be beneficial in situations such as massive GI bleeding or bleeding from submucosal lesions where the bleeding vessel cannot be identified endoscopically. It has been demonstrated that the use of Doppler guidance, when treating punctured vessels with HIFU, decreases the time of treatment presumably due to improved targeting of the HIFU (23).

Current thinking in endoscopic hemostasis is that pressure to the vessel must be applied in order to achieve coaptive welding of the vessel when applying thermal therapy such as electrocautery. Pressure may also be required in order to treat the entire circumference of the bleeding vessel since blood flowing through the vessel will serve as a heat sink and may prohibit thermal injury of the opposing vessel wall; therefore, pressure must be applied to the vessel in order to deliver thermal energy to the opposing vessel wall. HIFU, however, has the ability to transmit energy through blood to the opposing vessel wall. Thermal injury to a vessel results in contraction of collagen surrounding the vessel leading to circumferential constriction of the vessel. Decreased blood flow and circumferential endothelial injury leads to thrombus formation. Thermal injury also results in the an inflammatory response that causes the thrombus to evolve, eventually leading to fibrous scar and neovascularization. Further studies are necessary to determine if HIFU induced hemostasis has a role in GI bleeding.

## 6. Drug and Gene Delivery

Cavitation-mediated drug and gene delivery offers a potentially new, noninvasive, or minimally invasive method for targeted therapy. Given the concerns regarding the safety of viral-mediated gene delivery (73), interest in cavitation-mediated gene delivery has grown. Microbubbles can be loaded with drug or genes that can be released within a specific target volume determined by the activating ultrasound beam (74). When microbubbles, loaded with the drug or gene, are exposed to an ultrasound field of sufficient intensity, they undergo inertial cavitation resulting in release of the drug or gene. Although the exact mechanism has yet to be elucidated, inertial cavitation and microstreaming may lead to increased membrane permeability, allowing the locally released drug or gene to penetrate into the cell or into the perivascular tissue. Taniyama *et al.* have demonstrated enhanced transfection of a p53 plasmid into *in vivo* rat carotid arteries (75), and Miao *et al.* have recently demonstrated that gene delivery of naked human factor IX plasmid could be enhanced into *in vivo* rat livers with the aid of ultrasound contrast agent and ultrasound (76). Therefore, targeted gene and drug delivery using focused ultrasound appears to be promising.

## 7. Engineering and Physics Considerations

The potential of HIFU has been described, but what are the considerations in developing high intensity ultrasound applicators that can be employed via an endoscope? Several key areas related to engineering and physics will be addressed in the following sections.

### 7.1. *Generating thermal effects*

A number of investigators have found that the following relationship involving ultrasound energy (UE) fairly well approximates the threshold dose needed for the formation of lesion:

$$UE = IT^{0.5} = C \tag{1}$$

where $C$ has units of $(\mathrm{Wcm}^{-2}) \cdot \mathrm{sec}^{0.5}$, $I$ = intensity $(\mathrm{Wcm}^{-2})$ and $T$ = the time (seconds) of exposure. For cat brain and liver, $C$ has been reported to be approximately 200 $(\mathrm{Wcm}^{-2}) \cdot \mathrm{sec}^{0.5}$ and 470 $(\mathrm{Wcm}^{-2}) \cdot \mathrm{sec}^{0.5}$ (77), respectively. Further, the constant for rabbit liver is the essentially the same as the value above for cat liver (78). Finally, Sanghvi *et al.* (26) reported $C = 1,150$ $(\mathrm{Wcm}^{-2}) \cdot \mathrm{sec}^{0.5}$ for dog prostate and this latter relationship is plotted in Fig. 4.

The challenges facing the investigator are how to develop applicators that will allow delivering ultrasound energy to or through the luminal wall of the GI tract to the specific

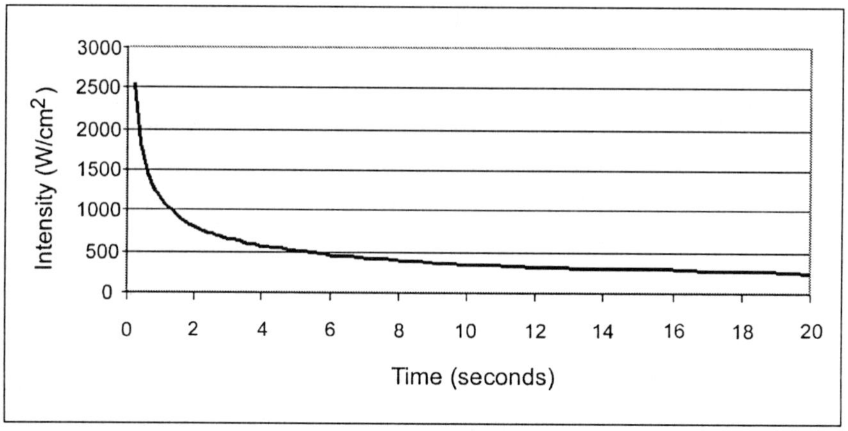


Fig. 4. A plot of the intensity versus time for a lesion threshold in dog prostate based on the Eq. (1) with $C = 1150\ \text{Wcm}^{-2} \cdot \text{sec}^{0.5}$.

tissue to be treated. Mathematical models have been developed for calculating the field patterns of various apertures (79–83) and these are very useful for designing transducers for specific needs. Further, as ultrasound propagates through tissue, it is attenuated as given by the following equation:

$$I_z = I_0 e^{-2\alpha z} \tag{2}$$

where $I_o$ = the initial intensity ($\text{Wcm}^{-2}$), $I_z$ = the intensity at some distance, $z$, from the initial position, and $\alpha$ = the attenuation coefficient. This equation allows estimating the intensity that will be present at a particular distance. Additionally, the attenuation is due to both absorption of energy and scattering of energy. Thus, the attenuation coefficient relates to the absorption coefficient ($\alpha_a$) in the following way:

$$\alpha = \alpha_a + \alpha_s \tag{3}$$

where $\alpha_s$ = the scattering coefficient. The absorption coefficient is less than the attenuation coefficient and is mostly likely greater than 70% of the attenuation coefficient in most tissue (84). Both the attenuation and absorption are frequency dependent and are represented by the following equation in many cases:

$$\alpha = af^b \tag{4}$$

where $f$ = frequency, a is often expressed in $\text{Npcm}^{-1}\ \text{MHz}^{-1}$ and $b$ tends to range from 1–1.5, but for some fits to measured data it is less than 1. One also must be careful if attempting to use this equation for frequencies beyond the frequency range for which specific tissue coefficients were measured at. Unfortunately, most reported measurements are only over a limited frequency range. Measurement of the absorption coefficient is difficult and consequently the attenuation coefficient has been more widely measured and an excellent compilation can be found in Duck (84). However, measurements associated with the gastrointestinal system are lacking, as are measurements on in vivo tissue. In Tables 1 and 2 some values are given which have some pertinence but illustrate the sorry state of information currently. Consequently, a nominal value of 0.05 $\text{Npcm}^{-1}\ \text{MHz}^{-1}$ for both attenuation

Table 1. Absorption Coefficient $\alpha_a = af^b$.

| Tissue | Species | Temp. (°C) | Freq. Range (MHz) | Coefficient $a$ ($\mathrm{Npcm^{-1}\ MHz^{-1}}$) | Coefficient $b$ | Ref. |
|---|---|---|---|---|---|---|
| Kidney | Cat, Cow | 37 | 0.7–7 | 0.028 | 1.02 | (86) |
| Liver | Pig | 37 | 1–7 | 0.026 | 1.17 | (86) |
| Cardiac Muscle | Cat | 37 | 0.7–7 | 0.028 | 1.04 | (86) |
| Testis | Mouse, horse | 37 | 0.5–7 | 0.015 | 1.11 | (86) |

Table 2. Attenuation Coefficient $\alpha = af^b$.

| Tissue | Species | Temp. (°C) | Freq. Range (MHz) | Coefficient $a$ ($\mathrm{Npcm^{-1}\ MHz^{-1}}$) | Coefficient $b$ | Ref. |
|---|---|---|---|---|---|---|
| Rumen | Sheep | 37 | 15–20 | $0.014 \pm 0.01$ | $1.65 \pm 0.51$ | (87) |
| Omental fat | Sheep | 37 | 15–20 | $0.158 \pm 0.07$ | $1.1 \pm 0.15$ | (87) |
| Pancreas | Cow | 24 | 1.4–9.8 | 0.119 | 0.780 | (88) |
| Rectum | Cow | NR | 1–5 | 0.06 | 0.957 | (89) |
| Liver (normal) | Pig | *In vivo* | 1–5 | 0.041 | 0.82 | (90) |
| Liver (HIFU lesion) | Pig | *In vivo* | 1–5 | 0.99 | 1 | (90) |
| Myometrium | Human | 22 | 1–3 | 0.056 | 1.085 | (91) |
| HIFU Myometrium | Human | 22 | 1–3 | 0.19 | 0.59 | (91) |
| Fibroid | Human | 22 | 1–3 | 0.11 | 0.78 | (91) |
| HIFU Fibroid | Human | 22 | 1–3 | 0.21 | 0.65 | (91) |

and absorption have been used for calculations by others (85) and will also be used here to provide some insight. (It is worth noting that Sanghvi *et al.* (26) have used a higher value (0.1 $\mathrm{Npcm^{-1}\ MHz^{-1}}$) for simulation of prostate treatment.)

The ultrasound energy produces heat at a rate of heat production per unit volume ($q_v$) which is related to the intensity and the absorption coefficient:

$$q_v = 2\alpha_a I \tag{5}$$

The resulting temperature rise ($\Delta T$) that occurs in a tissue, due to applied heat, depends on the heat capacity per unit volume ($c_v$), the thermal diffusivity ($\kappa$), and the perfusion to the tissue ($\tau$ = time constant for perfusion). A mathematical relationship called the bio-heat transfer equation has been given:

$$\frac{\partial T}{\partial t} = \kappa \left[\frac{\partial^2 T}{\partial x^2} + \frac{\partial^2 T}{\partial y^2} + \frac{\partial^2 T}{\partial z^2}\right] - \frac{\Delta T}{\tau} + \frac{q_v}{c_v} \tag{6}$$

where $x$, $y$, and $z$ are the Cartesian coordinates, and $t$ = time. The solution to this equation for many points in a radiation field of a transducer can be quite complex. Some approximations will be used to provide insight into how various variables contribute.

The solution to the equation, if the perfusion and the diffusivity are zero, reduces to:

$$T = \frac{2\alpha_a I t}{c_v} + T_0 \tag{7}$$

where $T$ is the temperature of the tissue after exposure to ultrasound, $\alpha_a$ is the absorption coefficient of the tissue [$\mathrm{Npcm^{-2}\ MHz}$], I is the intensity of the ultrasound [$\mathrm{Wcm^{-2}}$], $t$ is the time of exposure in seconds, $c_v$ is the specific heat/unit volume [$\mathrm{Jcm^{-3}{}^\circ C}$], and $T_0$ is the initial temperature of the tissue. For high levels of applied ultrasound, the perfusion does not affect the temperature much, but ignoring the diffusivity results in temperatures that are much higher than they would be unless one is considering a point within a uniform field that extends on each side of the point for some distance. Nevertheless, manipulating Eq. (7) allows it to be put in the following form:

$$I = \left[\frac{\Delta T c_v}{2\alpha_a t}\right] = \left[\frac{\Delta T c_v}{2af^b t}\right] \tag{8}$$

with the latter form using the relationship $\alpha_a = af^b$. Figure 5 shows the results of some calculations with this equation which clearly illustrate how much less intensity is needed at higher frequencies. However, the attenuation at higher frequencies also rapidly reduces the intensity at increasing distance from the transducer. This is apparent in Figs. 7 and 8, which will be discussed later.

### 7.2. *Transducer considerations*

The design of an applicator that can be used in the intestinal lumen poses a number of difficult considerations. The level of sophistication needed is even greater for an applicator

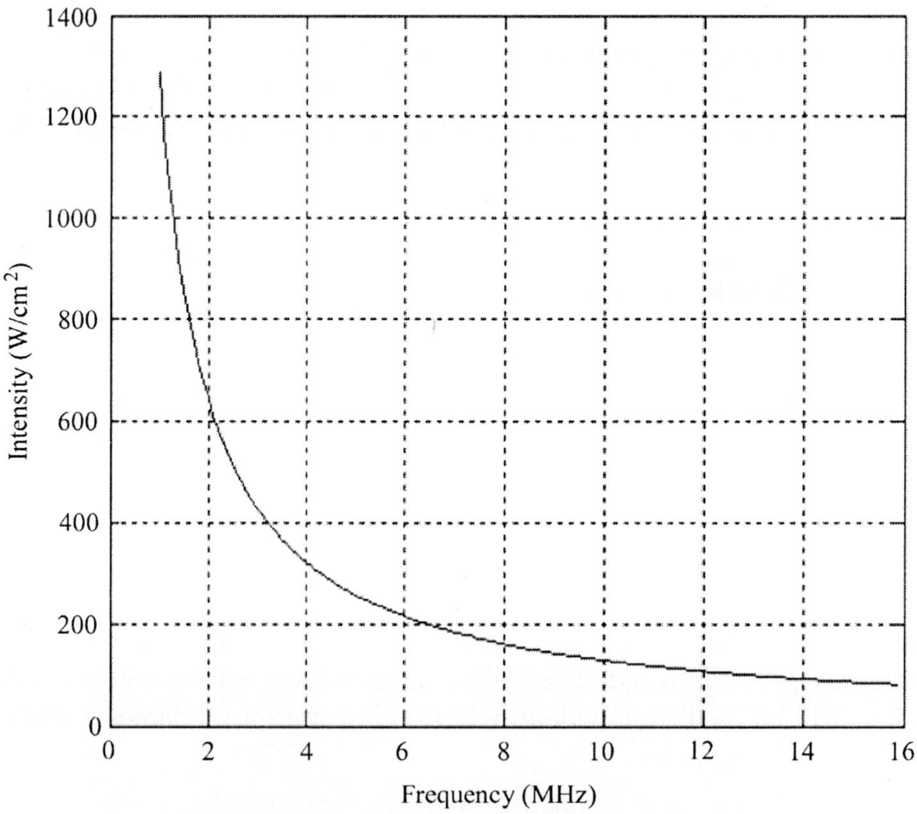


Fig. 5. The necessary intensity at various frequencies to raise tissue with absorption coefficient of 0.05 $\text{Npcm}^{-1}\ \text{MHz}^{-1}$ from 37°C to 70°C in 1 second at various ultrasound frequencies, if there was no cooling from perfusion or heat dispersion from conduction [Eq. (8)]. The specific heat was assumed to be 3.9 $\text{Jcm}^{-3}$°C for this calculation.

that is to be passed into the common bile duct from the duodenum. One of the foremost considerations is the aperture size and type that is practical to insert into the lumen and to couple to endoscopes for guidance. Transducers may be composed of a single element disk, a single element spherically focused disk, a rectangular element, a disk that is truncated on two opposite sides approximating a rectangle, an array of small rectangular elements, or an annular element array (Fig. 6). The advantages of single elements are their simplicity, but the disadvantage, if designed to focus at a specific distance, is how to vary the distance to the focus for various tissue treatment requirements. In contrast, the array devices allow for electronic control of the depth of focus but add considerable complexity to an applicator.

Understanding of the design tradeoffs of ultrasound frequency, size of an aperture, and physical configuration (flat versus focused) are easily obtained from simulations with equations available in the literature. Combining the nominal attenuation for tissue, mentioned above, with equations for the intensity along the axis of either a disk (79, 81) or a spherically focused disk (80), have been conducted and results are presented in Figs. 7 and 8. The flat disk axial intensities shown in Fig. 7 show numerous maximums-to-zero excursions and a tapering off of the peak amplitudes with distance due to the attenuation. The normalized values are all less than 1. In contrast, with spherical focusing (Fig. 8) the peaks at focus are much greater than 1, and although there are maximums-to-zero excursions between the transducer and the focal point, the maximums are of values much less than at the focus. It is possible to obtain considerable gain (peak intensity value at focus/intensity at the transducer face) in intensity at the focus over what is applied at the surface of the transducer with focusing. Further, one can see from the figures that when the radius of curvature is

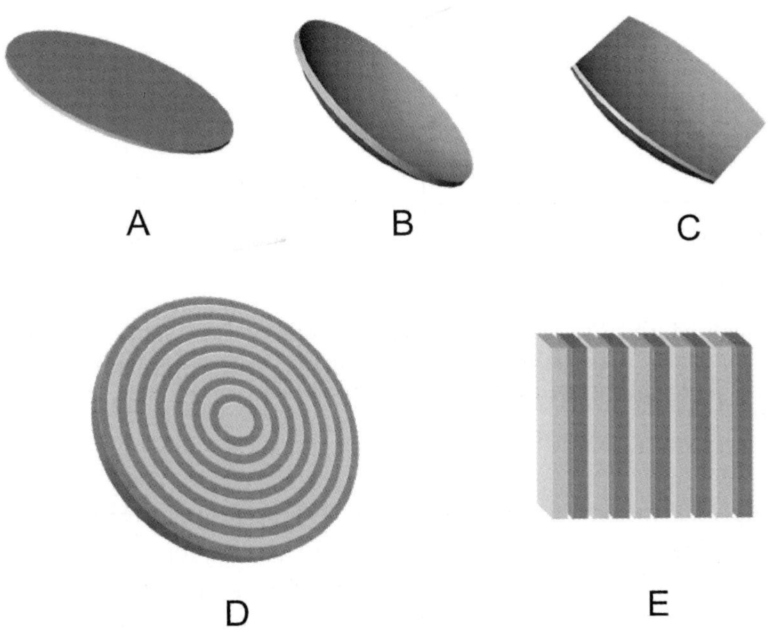


Fig. 6. Transducer configurations: (A) Flat circular disk. (B) Spherically curved disk. (C) Truncated, spherically curved disk resulting in a rectangular shaped aperture. (D) Annular array of circular ring elements. (E) Linear array of rectangular elements. (*Illustration by Arthur Chan.*)

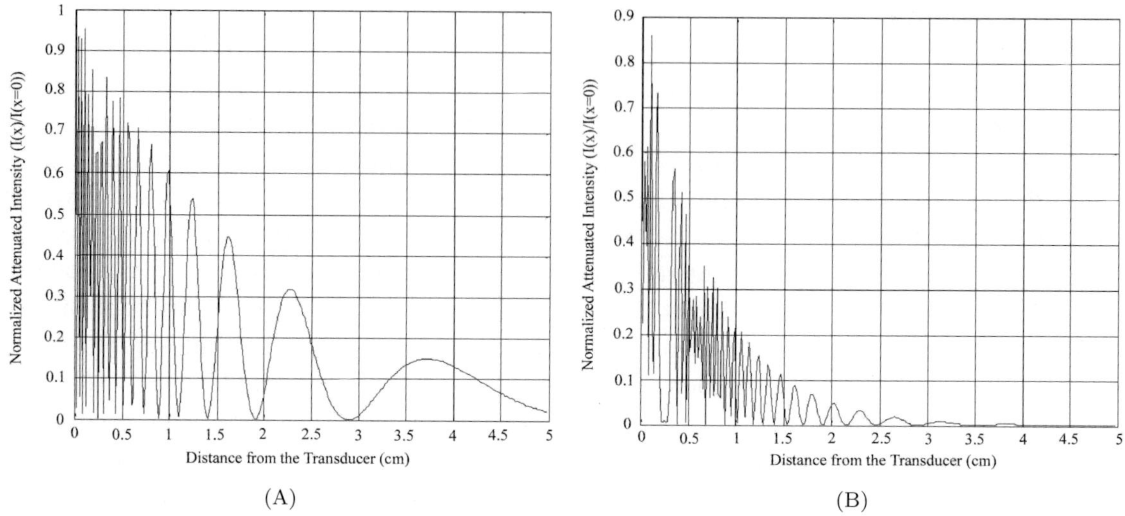


Fig. 7. Simulation of the normalized intensity (gain) along the axis for two disk 12 mm diameter apertures with attenuation included. Figure 7(A) is for a frequency of 5 MHz, with an attenuation coefficient of 0.25 NPcm$^{-1}$ while Fig. 7(B) is for 15 MHz with an attenuation coefficient of 0.75 NPcm$^{-1}$.

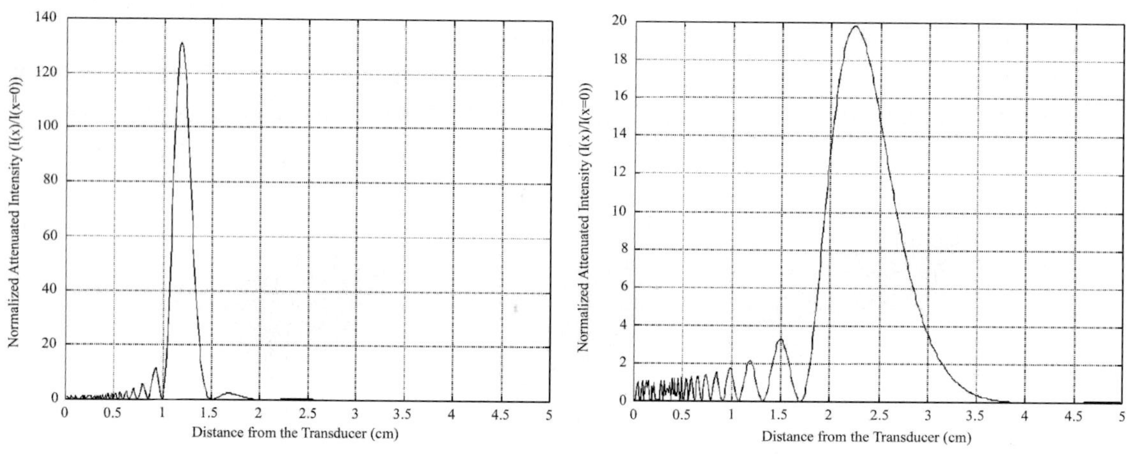


Fig. 8. The axial normalized intensity with attenuation is plotted for two spherically curved apertures (see reference 80 for axial equation). The radius of curvature for Fig. 8(A) is 1.2 cm whereas for Fig. 8(B) it is 2.4 cm. The frequency was 5 MHz and the attenuation coefficient equation $\alpha_a = af^b$ with $a = 0.05$ and $b = 1$ which gave 0.25 NPcm$^{-1}$.

1.2 ($f_{\#} = 1$)[c] compared to 2.4 ($f_{\#} = 2$) the gain is respectively, 135 to 19.8. Computing similar curves by varying the radius of curvature and the frequency and determine the peak value at focus for each curve, one can construct curves as shown in Fig. 9. These curves determine the gain for various frequency and curvatures for the 1.2 cm diameter transducer. Similar curves can be generated for other aperture diameters and frequencies.

[c]The $f_{\#}$ is defined as the distance from the transducer aperture to the focus divided by the diameter of the aperture.

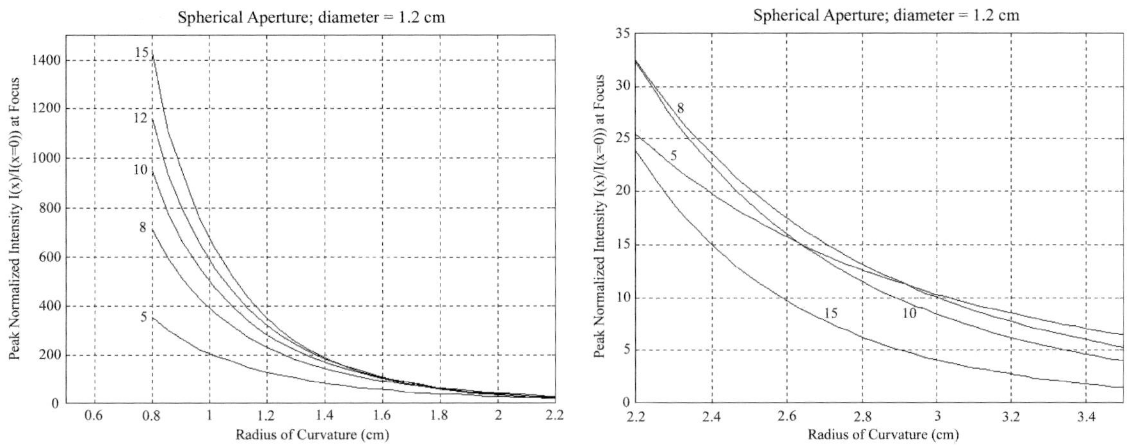


(A) (B)

Fig. 9. The normalized peak attenuated intensity is plotted for spherical disks with a diameter of 12 mm for frequencies (5, 8, 10, 12 and 15 MHz) with the radius curvatures of the disk varied. Each point on a line represents the peak value at focus in curves similar to Fig. 6.8. Figure 9(A) shows the effect of the radius of curvature varied from 0.8 cm to 2.2 cm while Fig. 9(B) shows the effect of varying the radius of curvature from 2.2 to 3.5.

Consider, apertures of diameter 1.2 cm and frequencies 5 and 12 MHz. One can obtain an estimate of the intensity needed at these two frequencies to raise tissue to 70°C in 1 second (Fig. 5), based on all the assumption used in producing that graph. (The estimate is respectively, 280 and 100 $\mathrm{Wcm}^{-2}$). If a flat transducer is used one can see that the intensity at the transducer would have to be over 280 at 5 MHz and 100 $\mathrm{Wcm}^{-2}$ at 12 MHz to achieve 70°C in one second (Fig. 7) at close proximity to the transducer. The transducer intensity would have to be even greater to treat at a further distance from the transducer. As will be discussed later, such transducer surface intensities are beyond what currently can be produced without damaging the transducer. Of course, one might apply the intensity for longer time and then less intensity would be required to produce necrosis. In contrast, for a focusing transducer, intensities one can see at the focus (for a specific radius of curvature) are much higher than intensities that are needed on the surface of the transducer due to the gain that results from focusing (e.g. for a $f_{\#} = 1$, radius of curvature of 1.2, the intensities needed are respectively, 0.77 and 0.87 $\mathrm{Wcm}^{-2}$). Some rapid estimates of what is required in a specific tissue treatment problem can be obtained by looking at Fig. 9.

The transducers that have been used for high intensity are piezoelectric material with low dielectric loss such as PZT4 or PZT8 or equivalent. The material is usually air-backed so all the emitted ultrasound radiates in the forward direction to increase efficiency of electrical to ultrasound conversion. Some transducers employ matching layers or layer on the front face to increase the efficiency of transfer and to widen the frequency range over which a transducer will transmit (92). Composite material is also being employed where piezoelectric pillars are embedded in a non-piezoelectric material (e.g. epoxy) (93). These can offer flexibility in manufacturing various shaped transducers and also tend to be broader bandwidth than the solid transducers if no matching is used.

A very useful parameter to know is what maximum intensity can be generated at the surface of a transducer without it deteriorating or failing. This is a function of a number of variables: the maximum voltage that can be applied without depoling the material, the maximum stress that can be produced without fracturing the ceramic material, and the maximum temperature the material can tolerate before deterioration. The electrical to ultrasound conversion efficiency of transducers that have been reported tend to vary between 50% to 60%, with some front face matched devices up to 80–90%. This means that in the first case, 50% to 40% of the applied electrical power is converted into heat in the device. If the transducer is not designed to remove the heat (e.g. by air or water cooling) the temperature can quickly build up to an excessive value and ruin the device. This is less of a problem in treating tumors as one can apply a short burst of excitation (e.g. 3 seconds) and then wait (e.g. 15 seconds) before applying the next excitation. That reduces the operating duty cycle and provides cooling to the transducer and adjacent tissue. However, for hemostasis, we generally must apply excitation continuously for a longer time and scan the transducer over a region (20, 21, 93). We have applied net power levels of up to 31 $Wcm^{-2}$ across the transducer for an intraoperative applicator that is water-cooled (94). Some of the power loss is in the solid cone for coupling the ultrasound energy from the transducer to the tissue. So, at 51% efficiency, the ultrasound power on the transducer itself is higher than 15 $Wcm^{-2}$, the value computed using the 51% transfer efficiency. A manufacturer of ultrasound HIFU transducer [Imasonic, Besancon, France] specify 5–10 $Wcm^{-2}$ for one type of their composite transducers and up to 30 $Wcm^{-2}$ for their newer type.

Some of the other major concerns are how to direct the applicator so that the ultrasound energy is aimed at the target tissue and how to scan it over a volume of tissue to be treated. Mucosal lesions may be treated by direct endoscopic visualization. The applicator needs to be designed for this case so it is in the view of the endoscope. If the tissue is beyond the wall, then it would be necessary to combine the applicator with some other imaging method such as endoscopic ultrasound (EUS). Combined ultrasound imaging and therapy in one device is desired in many applications. The use of arrays that are electronically controlled has proven to be the best for most ultrasound imaging applications and so would also electronically controlled focusing and perhaps even steering be the best for therapy. Combining imaging and therapy in arrays, or perhaps using the same array for both imaging and therapy, approaches the ideal but will require much future development. Undoubtedly, different applicators will be needed for treating different disease problems.

## 8. Analysis of Ultrasound Therapy Techniques via the Intestinal Lumen

It is useful to consider some of the applicators that have been reported for intralumenal use. First, Lafon *et al.* reported in 1998 on experiments with an interstitial applicator using flat 3 × 10 mm transducers (62, 63). One applicator operated at 5.1 MHz and the other at 10.7 MHz. Efficiency measurements showed these to be initially ~75% efficient but they were reported to deteriorate with use possibly due to the high powers applied to them. They were air backed and water-cooled at the front face. *In vivo* studies with

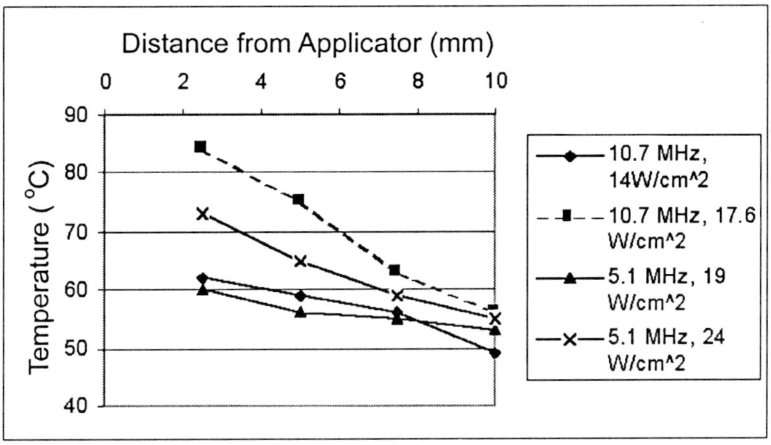


Fig. 10. The mean of the measured temperature values versus distance obtained *in vivo* in liver using 3 mm × 10 mm transducer elements, two frequencies, and each excited at two levels. Each point was obtained after 20 seconds of exposure. The plotted data were taken from Lafon *et al.*, 1998 (63) and plotted here by adding a base tissue temperature of 36°C to allow it to be compared to the other figures in this chapter.

pig liver showed more intensity was required than *ex vivo* liver. *In vivo* acquired data given in the paper have been plotted in Fig. 10 with an assumed base liver temperature of 36°C. It is interesting to note that 14 $\text{Wcm}^{-2}$ for the 10.7 MHz element gave almost the same result as 19 $\text{Wcm}^{-2}$ gave at 5.1 MHz. The high intensity ultrasound was applied for 20 seconds in each case at each datum. They discuss that for the 10.7 MHz they anticipated larger temperature increases for the 17.6 $\text{Wcm}^{-2}$ excitation in contrast to the 14 $\text{Wcm}^{-2}$. They believed that near the transducer at some point during the 20 seconds of excitation, temperatures approached boiling for the higher excitation level and when that occurred it blocked transmission at further distances and thus limited the temperatures that could be reached distal to that site. This illustrates some of the advantages of focusing as it allows achieving higher temperatures at the distal focus without producing highly elevated temperatures near the transducer. In more recent work, Lafon *et al.* report on a new applicator with slight focusing (focusing at 22 mm) (95). They have produced necrosis with this device at a depth of 15 mm in contrast to a limited depth of 10 mm previously.

Melo de Lima *et al.* have reported on investigating a partial cylindrical array consisting of 16 elements each 15 mm in length and placed 70 $\mu$m apart around part of the surface of a 10.6 mm diameter cylinder (96). Each element operated at 4.55 MHz. The front and back of the transducer was cooled with circulating water at a flow rate of 210 ml $\text{min}^{-1}$, which avoided the elements rising above 45°C during excitation. A group of eight elements were excited with appropriate phasing to represent a planar wave propagating away from the array. With the probe inserted in a water filled hole cut in *ex vivo* liver, three different groups of elements were excited to produce lesions extending from the applicator 22.4° apart. An excitation level of 17 $\text{Wcm}^{-2}$ was used for 20 seconds to produce well-defined liver lesions. This test applicator was located in a 15 mm diameter housing which allowed a 65 $\mu$m thick latex balloon to be used as a cover over the ultrasound active region and thus contain the cooling water. A more recent report (93) shows a picture of a 64 element array built as discussed but having the complete surface of the cylinder covered with array elements for 360° treatment arc. The transducer is built with a composite piezoelectric material. This design appears to be promising for intraluminal therapy.

The definitive investigations of the treatment of the prostate via the rectum (26) provide useful information if considering treatment of organs adjacent to the stomach, for example. Over a long series of studies their work evolved to the use of a 4 MHz, spherically curved circular transducer truncated in a manner to provide a rectangular aperture that was 22 mm × 30 mm. The truncation allowed a practical device to be made so it could be passed into the rectum. The 4 MHz transducer curvature was 2.5 cm to 4 cm in focal length depending on the studies. They report a treatment exposure that involved the application of 1,700 $\mathrm{Wcm}^{-2}$ with an "on" time of 4 sec and "off" time of 12 sec before the next exposure. Note UE is much higher than the threshold predicted from Fig. 4 for 4 seconds on. The off time promoted tissue and transducer cooling. The unit was scanned both longitudinally and in an arc with respect to the axis of the rectal wall with presumably scanning movement applied during the "off" time.

## Summary

The exciting work that is emerging in applying high intensity ultrasound to the treatment of difficult disease processes is most promising. Many of these pathological conditions are extremely difficult to manage with current methods. Side effects are prominent and cures elusive. A marked advantage of ultrasound therapy is that it can be repeated as often as necessary without accumulative effects as such is found with radiation therapy or chemotherapy. It can be used to deliver directed thermal and/or mechanical therapy with the aid of image guidance. With high intensity ultrasound cell death can be initiated almost instantly. Many of the initial clinical studies using high intensity ultrasound in the treatment of tumors have provided promising early results. Although much of the focus has been on the response of tumors to high intensity ultrasound therapy, some of the most promising, and possibly most clinically applicable results have to do with palliation. For example, the work by He *et al.* (71) and Zhang *et al.* (72) suggest that treatment of advanced pancreatic tumors with HIFU may relieve symptoms of pain. The work of Prat *et al.* (61) on the intraductal high intensity ultrasound probe to treat cholangiocarcinoma lesions is especially exciting for the gastroenterologist as it may lead to a viable therapy to palliate and potentially improve survival in patients with cholangiocarcinoma.

Current studies have concentrated on the extracorporeal application of HIFU, particularly in the treatment of solid tumors. However, many structures within the body are not easily accessible to transcutaneously applied ultrasound. The ribs pose a significant barrier to transcutaneous HIFU treatment of the liver and ultrasound penetration into intra-abdominal structures can be limited by overlying bowel gas. The application of HIFU endoscopically follows similar logic to that of endoscopic ultrasound imaging. Perigastric organs such as the pancreas and liver are more readily accessible via the endoscopic route. The primary limitations and challenges of endoscopic high intensity ultrasound therapy are the size of the transducer that can be inserted into the lumen of the GI tract, image guidance of therapy delivered by such a device, and duration necessary to deliver the therapy to a large tumor. These are challenges we believe will be met in the early years of the new century.

## References


1. Lindstrom, P. A., Prefrontal ultrasonic irradiation — A substitute for lobotomy. Arch Neurol Psych, 1954; 72: 399–425.
2. Fry, W. J., Meyers, R., Fry, F. J., Schultz, D. F., Dreyer, L. L. and Noyes, R. F., Topical differentia of pathogenetic mechanisms underlying Parkinsonial tremor and rigidity as indicated by ultrasonic irradiation of the human brain, In: Trans Am Neurol Assoc. William Byrd Press; Richmond, VA. 1958, 16–24.
3. Hynynen, K. and Lulu, B. A., Hyperthermia in cancer treatment. Invest Radiol, 1990; 25: 824–34.
4. Chaussy, C., Schmiedt, E., Jocham, D., Brendel, W., Forssmann, B. and Walther, V., First clinical experience with extracorporeally induced destruction of kidney stones by shock waves. 1981. J Urol, 2002; 167: 1957–60.
5. Ferrucci, J. T., Gallstone ESWL — The first 175 patients. AJR Am J Roentgenol, 1988; 150: 1231–3.
6. Adams, J. B., Moore, R. G., Anderson, J. H., Strandberg, J. D., Marshall, F. F. and Davoussi, L. R., High-intensity focused ultrasound ablation of rabbit kidney tumors. J Endourol, 1996; 10: 71–5.
7. Chaussy, C. and Thuroff, S., High-intensity focused ultrasound in prostate cancer: Results after 3 years. Mol Urol, 2000; 4: 179–82.
8. Chen, L., ter. Haar, G., Robertson, D., Bensted, J. P. and Hill, C. R., Histological study of normal and tumor-bearing liver treated with focused ultrasound. Ultrasound Med Biol, 1999; 25: 847–56.
9. Cline, H. E., Hynynen, K., Watkins, R. D., Adams, W. J., Schenck, J. F., Ettinger, R. H. *et al.*, Focused US system for MR imaging-guided tumor ablation. Radiology, 1995; 194: 731–7.
10. Madersbacher, S., Pedevilla, M., Vingers, L., Susani, M. and Marberger, M., Effect of high-intensity focused ultrasound on human prostate cancer *in vivo.* Cancer Res, 1995; 55: 3346–51.
11. Prat, F., Centarti, M., Sibille, A., Abou, el. Fadil, F. A., Henry, L., Chapelon, J. Y. *et al.*, Extracorporeal high-intensity focused ultrasound for VX2 liver tumors in the rabbit. Hepatology, 1995; 21: 832–6.
12. Sibille, A., Prat, F., Chapelon, J. Y., abou, el. Fadil, F., Henry, L., Theilliere, Y. *et al.*, Characterization of extracorporeal ablation of normal and tumor-bearing liver tissue by high intensity focused ultrasound. Ultrasound Med Biol, 1993; 19: 803–13.
13. ter. Haar, G. R., High intensity focused ultrasound for the treatment of tumors. Echocardiography, 2001; 18: 317–22.
14. Vaezy, S., Fujimoto, V. Y., Walker, C., Martin, R. W., Chi, E. Y. and Crum, L. A., Treatment of uterine fibroid tumors in a nude mouse model using high-intensity focused ultrasound. Am J Obstet Gynecol, 2000; 183: 6–11.
15. Wu, F., Chen, W. Z., Bai, J., Zou, J. Z., Wang, Z. L. and Zhu, H. *et al.*, Pathological changes in human malignant carcinoma treated with high-intensity focused ultrasound. Ultrasound Med Biol, 2001; 27: 1099–106.
16. Yang, R., Reilly, C. R., Rescorla, F. J., Faught, P. R., Sanghvi, N. T., Fry, F. J. *et al.*, High-intensity focused ultrasound in the treatment of experimental liver cancer. Arch Surg, 1991; 126: 1002–9; discussion 1009–10.

17. Vaezy, S., Martin, R., Kaczkowski, P., Keilman, G., Goldman, B., Yaziji. H. *et al.*, Use of high-intensity focused ultrasound to control bleeding. J Vasc Surg, 1999; 29: 533–42.
18. Vaezy, S., Martin, R., Mourad, P. and Crum, L., Hemostasis using high intensity focused ultrasound. Eur J Ultrasound, 1999; 9: 79–87.
19. Vaezy, S., Martin, R. and Crum, L., High intensity focused ultrasound: A method of hemostasis. Echocardiography, 2001; 18: 309–15.
20. Vaezy, S., Martin, R., Keilman, G., Kaczkowski, P., Chi, E., Yazaji, E. *et al.*, Control of splenic bleeding by using high intensity ultrasound. J Trauma, 1999; 47: 521–5.
21. Vaezy, S., Martin, R., Schmiedl, U., Caps, M., Taylor, S., Beach, K. *et al.*, Liver hemostasis using high-intensity focused ultrasound. Ultrasound Med Biol, 1997; 23: 1413–20.
22. Vaezy, S., Martin, R., Yaziji, H., Kaczkowski, P., Keilman, G., Carter, S. *et al.*, Hemostasis of punctured blood vessels using high-intensity focused ultrasound. Ultrasound Med Biol, 1998; 24: 903–10.
23. Martin, R. W., Vaezy, S., Kaczkowski, P., Keilman, G., Carter, S., Caps, M. *et al.*, Hemostasis of punctured vessels using Doppler-guided high-intensity ultrasound. Ultrasound Med Biol, 1999; 25: 985–90.
24. Hwang, J. H., Vaezy, S., Martin, R. W., Cho, M. Y., Noble, M. L., Crum, L. A. *et al.*, High-intensity focused ultrasound: A potential new treatment for gastrointestinal bleeding. Gastrointest Endosc, 2003; 58: 111–115.
25. Hedrick, W. R., Hykes, D. L. and Starchman, D. E., Ultrasound Physics and Instrumentation. Third ed. 1995, St. Louis, Mosby.
26. Sanghvi, N. T., Fry, F. J., Bihrle, R., Foster, R. S., Phillips, M. H., Syrus, J. *et al.*, Noninvasive surgery of prostate tissue by high-intensity focused ultrasound. IEEE Trans Ultrason Ferroelec Freq Contr, 1996; 43: 1099–1110.
27. Chen, W. S., Lafon, C., Matula, T. J., Vaezy, S., Brayman, A. A. and Crum, L. A., Mechanisms of lesion formation in high intensity focused ultrasound therapy. 2nd International Symposium on Therapeutic Ultrasound: Conference Proceedings, 2002; 400–409.
28. Bailey, M. R., Couret, L. N., Sapozhnikov, O. A., Khokhlova, V. A., ter. Haar, G., Vaezy, S. *et al.*, Use of overpressure to assess the role of bubbles in focused ultrasound lesion shape *in vitro*. Ultrasound Med Biol, 2001; 27: 695–708.
29. Vykhodtseva, N., McDannold, N., Martin, H., Bronson, R. T. and Hynynen, K., Apoptosis in ultrasound-produced threshold lesions in the rabbit brain. Ultrasound Med Biol, 2001; 27: 111–7.
30. Lagneaux, L., de. Meulenaer, E. C., Delforge, A., Dejeneffe, M., Massy, M., Moerman, C. *et al.*, Ultrasonic low-energy treatment: a novel approach to induce apoptosis in human leukemic cells. Exp Hematol, 2002; 30: 1293–301.
31. Ashush, H., Rozenszajn, L. A., Blass, M., Barda-Saad, M., Azimov, D., Radnay, J. *et al.*, Apoptosis induction of human myeloid leukemic cells by ultrasound exposure. Cancer Res, 2000; 60: 1014–20.
32. Miller, D. L. and Quddus, J., Diagnostic ultrasound activation of contrast agent gas bodies induces capillary rupture in mice. Proc Natl Acad Sci USA, 2000; 97: 10179–84.
33. Skyba, D. M., Price, R. J., Linka, A. Z., Skalak, T. C. and Kaul, S., Direct *in vivo* visualization of intravascular destruction of microbubbles by ultrasound and its local effects on tissue. Circulation, 1998; 98: 290–3.
34. Zhong, P., Zhou, Y. and Zhu, S., Dynamics of bubble oscillation in constrained media and mechanisms of vessel rupture in SWL. Ultrasound Med Biol, 2001; 27: 119–34.

35. Poliachik, S. L., Chandler, W. L., Mourad, P. D., Ollos, R. J. and Crum, L. A., Activation, aggregation and adhesion of platelets exposed to high- intensity focused ultrasound. Ultrasound Med Biol, 2001; 27: 1567–1576.
36. Tachibana, K., Uchida, T., Ogawa, K., Yamashita, N. and Tamura, K., Induction of cell-membrane porosity by ultrasound. Lancet, 1999; 353: 1409.
37. Hwang, J. H., Brayman, A. A. and Vaezy, S., Pulsed high-intensity focused ultrasound-induced endothelial cell injury in vessels infused with ultrasound contrast agent. 2nd International Symposium on Therapeutic Ultrasound: Conference Proceedings, 2003; 63–70.
38. Miller, D. L. and Quddus, J., Lysis and sonoporation of epidermoid and phagocytic monolayer cells by diagnostic ultrasound activation of contrast agent gas bodies. Ultrasound Med Biol, 2001; 27: 1107–13.
39. Miller, D. L. and Quddus, J., Sonoporation of monolayer cells by diagnostic ultrasound activation of contrast-agent gas bodies. Ultrasound Med Biol, 2000; 26: 661–7.
40. Brayman, A. A., Lizotte, L. M. and Miller, M. W., Erosion of artificial endothelia *in vitro* by pulsed ultrasound: Acoustic pressure, frequency, membrane orientation and microbubble contrast agent dependence. Ultrasound Med Biol, 1999; 25: 1305–20.
41. Miller, D. L. and Thomas, R. M., Contrast-agent gas bodies enhance hemolysis induced by lithotripter shock waves and high-intensity focused ultrasound in whole blood. Ultrasound Med Biol, 1996; 22: 1089–95.
42. Dalecki, D., Raeman, C. H., Child, S. Z., Cox, C., Francis, C. W., Meltzer, R. S. *et al.*, Hemolysis in vivo from exposure to pulsed ultrasound. Ultrasound Med Biol, 1997; 23: 307–13.
43. Everbach, E. C., Makin, I. R., Azadniv, M. and Meltzer, R. S., Correlation of ultrasound-induced hemolysis with cavitation detector output in vitro. Ultrasound Med Biol, 1997; 23: 619–24.
44. Brayman, A. A., Strickler, P. L., Luan, H., Barned, S. L., Raeman, C. H., Cox, C. *et al.*, Hemolysis of 40% hematocrit, Albunex-supplemented human erythrocytes by pulsed ultrasound: frequency, acoustic pressure and pulse length dependence. Ultrasound Med Biol, 1997; 23: 1237–50.
45. Miller, M. W., Everbach, E. C., Cox, C., Knapp, R. R., Brayman, A. A. and Sherman, T. A., A comparison of the hemolytic potential of Optison and Albunex in whole human blood *in vitro*: Acoustic pressure, ultrasound frequency, donor and passive cavitation detection considerations. Ultrasound Med Biol, 2001; 27: 709–21.
46. Poliachik, S. L., Chandler, W. L., Mourad, P. D., Bailey, M. R., Bloch, S., Cleveland, R. O. *et al.*, Effect of high-intensity focused ultrasound on whole blood with and without microbubble contrast agent. Ultrasound Med Biol, 1999; 25: 991–8.
47. Miller, D. L. and Gies, R. A., Enhancement of ultrasonically-induced hemolysis by perfluorocarbon-based compared to air-based echo-contrast agents. Ultrasound Med Biol, 1998; 24: 285–92.
48. Uchida, T., Sanghvi, N. T., Gardner, T. A., Koch, M. O., Ishii, D., Minei, S. *et al.*, Transrectal high-intensity focused ultrasound for treatment of patients with stage T1b-2n0m0 localized prostate cancer: A preliminary report. Urology, 2002; 59: 394–8; discussion 398–9.
49. Madersbacher, S., Schatzl, G., Djavan, B., Stulnig, T. and Marberger, M., Long-term outcome of transrectal high-intensity focused ultrasound therapy for benign prostatic hyperplasia. Eur Urol, 2000; 37: 687–94.
50. Sanghvi, N. T., Gardner, T. A., Uchida, T. and Koch, M. O., Treatment of BPH and prostate cancer using ultrasound image guided high intensity focused ultrasound. Workshop on MRI-Guided Focused Ultrasound Surgery, 2002. Cambridge, MA.

51. Chaussy, C. G. and Thuroff, S., High-intensive focused ultrasound in localized prostate cancer. J Endourol, 2000; 14: 293–9.
52. Chaussy, C. and Thuroff, S., Results and side effects of high-intensity focused ultrasound in localized prostate cancer. J Endourol, 2001; 15: 437–40; discussion 447–8.
53. Chaussy, C. and Thuroff, S., HIFU and localized prostate cancer: Efficacy results from the European multicentric study. 2nd International Symposium on Therapeutic Ultrasound: Conference Proceedings, 2002; 1–7.
54. Foster, R. S., Bihrle, R., Sanghvi, N. T., Fry, F. J. and Donohue, J. P., High-intensity focused ultrasound in the treatment of prostatic disease. Eur Urol, 1993; 23 Suppl 1: 29–33.
55. Gelet, A., Chapelon, J. Y., Margonari, J., Theillere, Y., Gorry, F., Cathignol, D. *et al.*, Prostatic tissue destruction by high-intensity focused ultrasound: Experimentation on canine prostate. J Endourol, 1993; 7: 249–53.
56. Gelet, A., Chapelon, J. Y., Margonari, J., Theillere, Y., Gorry, F., Souchon, R. *et al.*, High-intensity focused ultrasound experimentation on human benign prostatic hypertrophy. Eur Urol, 1993; 23 Suppl 1: 44–7.
57. Gelet, A., Chapelon, J. Y., Bouvier, R., Souchon, R., Pangaud, C., Abdelrahim, A. F. *et al.*, Treatment of prostate cancer with transrectal focused ultrasound: Early clinical experience. Eur Urol, 1996; 29: 174–83.
58. Gelet, A., Chapelon, J. Y., Bouvier, R., Rouviere, O., Lasne, Y., Lyonnet, D. *et al.*, Transrectal high-intensity focused ultrasound: Minimally invasive therapy of localized prostate cancer. [erratum appears in J Endourol 2000 Oct; 14(8): 697]. J Endourol, 2000; 14: 519–28.
59. Gelet, A., Chapelon, J. Y., Bouvier, R., Rouviere, O., Lyonnet, D. and Dubernard, J. M., Transrectal high intensity focused ultrasound for the treatment of localized prostate cancer: Factors influencing the outcome. Eur Urol, 2001; 40: 124–9.
60. Hegarty, N. J. and Fitzpatrick, J. M., High intensity focused ultrasound in benign prostatic hyperplasia. Eur J Ultrasound, 1999; 9: 55–60.
61. Prat, F., Lafon, C., De. Lima, D. M., Theilliere, Y., Fritsch, J., Pelletier, G. *et al.*, Endoscopic treatment of cholangiocarcinoma and carcinoma of the duodenal papilla by intraductal high-intensity US: Results of a pilot study. Gastrointest Endosc, 2002; 56: 909–15.
62. Lafon, C., Chapelon, J. Y., Prat, F., Gorry, F., Theillere, Y. and Cathignol, D., Design and *in vitro* results of a high intensity ultrasound interstitial applicator. Ultrasonics, 1998; 36: 683–7.
63. Lafon, C., Chapelon, J. Y., Prat, F., Gorry, F., Margonari, J., Theillere, Y. *et al.*, Design and preliminary results of an ultrasound applicator for interstitial thermal coagulation. Ultrasound Med Biol, 1998; 24: 113–22.
64. Prat, F., Lafon, C., Margonari, J., Gorry, F., Theillere, Y., Chapelon, J. Y. *et al.*, A high-intensity US probe designed for intraductal tumor destruction: experimental results. Gastrointest Endosc, 1999; 50: 388–92.
65. Lafon, C., Theillere, Y., Prat, F., Arefiev, A., Chapelon, J. Y. and Cathignol, D., Development of an interstitial ultrasound applicator for endoscopic procedures: Animal experimentation. Ultrasound Med Biol, 2000; 26: 669–75.
66. Prat, F., Lafon, C., Theilliere, J. Y., Fritsch, J., Choury, A. D., Lorand, I. *et al.*, Destruction of a bile duct carcinoma by intraductal high intensity ultrasound during ERCP. Gastrointest Endosc, 2001; 53: 797–800.
67. Wu, F., Wang, Z. B., Chen, W. Z., Zou, J. Z., Bai, J., Zhu, H. *et al.*, High intensity focused ultrasound for extracorporeal treatment of solid carcinomas: Four-year Chinese clinical experience. 2nd International Symposium on Therapeutic Ultrasound: Conference Proceedings, 2002; 34–43.

68. Rivens, I. H., Allen, M. A., Visioili, A., Cunningham, D. C., Horwich, A., Huddart, R. A. *et al.*, Ultrasound guided clinical focused ultrasound surgery: Patient response to tumor treatments in different organs. 2nd International Symposium on Therapeutic Ultrasound: Conference Proceedings, 2002; 57–62.
69. Allen, M. A., Rivens, I., Visioili, A. and ter. Haar, G., Focused ultrasound surgery (FUS): A noninvasive technique for the thermal ablation of liver metastases. 2nd International Symposium on Therapeutic Ultrasound: Conference Proceedings, 2002; 17–25.
70. Wang, W., Zhou, J., Liu, W., Bai, L., Ye, H., Gai, L. *et al.*, Treatment of hepatocellular carcinoma with high-intensity focused ultrasound combined with transarterial oily chemoembolization: Preliminary clinical outcomes. 2nd International Symposium on Therapeutic Ultraound: Conference Proceedings, 2002; 44–50.
71. He, S. X. and Wang, G. M., The noninvasive treatment of 251 cases of advanced pancreatic cancer with focused ultrasound surgery. 2nd International Symposium on Therapeutic Ultrasound: Conference Proceedings, 2002; 51–56.
72. Zhang, M., Li, W. and Bai, X., The application of high intensity focused ultrasound in the treatment of advanced pancreatic cancer: A preliminary report of 13 cases. 2nd International Symposium on Therapeutic Ultrasound: Conference Proceedings, 2002; 76–80.
73. Marshall, E., Gene therapy death prompts review of adenovirus vector. Science, 1999; 286: 2244–5.
74. Unger, E. C., Hersh, E., Vannan, M., Matsunaga, T. O. and McCreery, T., Local drug and gene delivery through microbubbles. Prog Cardiovasc Dis, 2001; 44: 45–54.
75. Taniyma, Y., Tachibana, K., Hiraoka, K., Namba, T., Yamasaki, K., Hashiya, N. *et al.*, Local delivery of plasmid DNA into rat carotid artery using ultrasound. Circulation, 2002; 105: 1233–1239.
76. Miao, C. H., Brayman, A. A., Ye, P., Mourad, P. and Crum, L. A., Enhancement of gene delivery of naked human factor IX plasmid into mouse livers by ultrasound exposure. 2nd International Symposium on Therapeutic Ultrasound: Conference Proceedings, 2002; 71–75.
77. Frizzell, L. A., Threshold dosages for damage to mammalian liver by high intensity focused ultrasound. IEEE Trans Ultrason Ferroelec Freq Contr, 1988; 35: 578–581.
78. Frizzell, L. A., Linke, E. L., Carstensen, E. L. and Fridd, C. W., Thresholds for focal ultrasonic lesions in rabbit kidney, liver and testicle. IEEE Trans Biomed Eng, 1977; 24: 393–396.
79. Kinsler, L. E., Frey, A. R., Coppens, A. B. and Sanders, J. V., Fundamentals of Acoustics. 1982, John Wiley & Sons, New York.
80. Kossoff, G., Analysis of focusing action of spherically curved transducers. Ultrasound Med Biol, 1979; 5: 359–65.
81. Wells, P. N. T., Biomedical Ultrasonics. 1977, Academic Press, London.
82. Weyns, A., Radiation field calculations of pulsed ultrasonic transducers. Part 1: Planar circular, square and annular transducers. Ultrasonics, 1980; 18: 183–188.
83. Weyns, A., Radiation field calculations of pulsed ultrasonic transducers: Part 2: Spherical disc and ring shaped transducers. Ultrasonics, 1980; 18: 219–223.
84. Duck, F. A., Physical Properties of Tissue: A Comprehensive Reference Book. 1990, Academic Press, London.
85. Exposure criteria for medical diagnostic ultrasound: I. Criteria based on thermal mechanisms. 1992, National Council on Radiation Protection and Measurements: Bethesda, MD.
86. Goss, S. A., Frizzell, L. A. and Dunn, F., Ultrasonic absorption and attenuation in mammalian tissues. Ultrasound Med Biol, 1979; 5: 181–6.

87. Taniguchi, D. K., Martin, R. W., Myers, J. and Silverstein, F. E., Measurement of the ultrasonic attenuation of fat at high frequency. Acad Radiol, 1994; 1: 114–20.
88. Segal, L. A. and O'Brien, W. D., Frequency dependent ultrasonic attenuation coefficient assessment in fresh tissue. IEEE Ultrasonics Symp Proc, 1983: 797–799.
89. Dussik, K. T., Fritch, D. J., Kyriazidou, M. and Sear, R. S., Measurements of articular tissue with ultrasound. Am J Phys Med, 1958; 37: 160–165.
90. Zderic, V., Keshavarzi, A., Andrew, M. A., Vaezy, S. and Martin, R. W., Attenuation of porcine tissues *in vivo* after high intensity ultrasound treatment, Ultrasound Med Biol, 2004; 30: 61–66.
91. Keshavarzi, A., Vaezy, S., Kaczkowski, P. J., Keilman, G., Martin, R., Chi, E. Y. *et al.*, Attenuation coefficient and sound speed in human myometrium and uterine fibroid tumors. J Ultrasound Med, 2001; 20: 473–80.
92. Keilman, G., 2002. Bothell, WA.
93. Fleury, G., Melo, de. Lima, D., Hynynen, K., Berriet, R., Le. Baron, O. and Hugenin, B., New piezocomposite transducers for therapeutic ultrasound. SPIE Biomedical Optics Symposium, 2003. San Jose, CA.
94. Martin, R. W., Vaezy, S., Cornejo, C. and Jurkovich, J., Water cooled intraoperative HIFU applicators with frequency tracking. 2nd International Symposium on Therapeutic Ultrasound: Conference Proceedings, 2002; 359–365.
95. Lafon, C., de. L., Theillere, Y., Prat, F., Chapelon, J. Y. and Cathignol, D., Optimizing the shape of ultrasound transducers for interstitial thermal ablation. Med Phys, 2002; 29: 290–7.
96. Melo, de., Lima, D., Lafon, C., Prat, F., Theillere, Y., Birer, A. and Cathignol, D., Cylindrical array for intraductal thermal ablation. 2nd International Symposium on Therapeutic Ultrasound: Conference Proceedings, 2002; 366–373.

Published with permission

Ultrasound in Med. & Biol., Vol. 25, No. 6, pp. 985–990, 1999

0301-5629/99/$–see front matter

ELSEVIER

PII S0301-5629(99)00027-7

● *Original Contribution*

# HEMOSTASIS OF PUNCTURED VESSELS USING DOPPLER-GUIDED HIGH-INTENSITY ULTRASOUND

Roy W. Martin,[†‡] Shahram Vaezy,[†] Peter Kaczkowski,[||] George Keilman,[¶] Steve Carter,[*] Michael Caps,[§] Kirk Beach,[†§] Melani Plett[†] and Lawrence Crum[†||]

Departments of [†]Bioengineering, [‡]Anesthesiology, *Radiology, [§]Surgery and [||]Applied Physics Laboratory, University of Washington, Seattle, WA, USA; and [¶]Sonic Concepts, Woodinville, WA, USA

(*Received* 5 *October* 1998; *in final form* 18 *February* 1999)

Abstract—**The use of Doppler ultrasound was investigated to determine if it would aid in guiding the application of high-intensity focused ultrasound (HIFU) to stop bleeding from punctured vessels. Major vessels (abdominal aorta, illiac, carotid, common femoral and superficial femoral arteries and the jugular vein) were surgically exposed, punctured and treated in anesthetized pigs. Treatment was applied when the Doppler sounds indicated the focus coincided with the bleeding site. In 89 treatment trials, the average time to achieve major hemostasis (a point where bleeding was reduced to a level of only oozing) was 8 s, and for complete hemostasis was 13 s. These times were significantly shorter than those of an identical former study in which only visual guidance was used. In that study, the average times for major and complete hemostasis were 40 and 62 s, respectively. The advantage of Doppler guidance in applying HIFU in treating bleeding vessels was demonstrated. © 1999 World Federation for Ultrasound in Medicine & Biology.**

*Key Words:* **Doppler, Ultrasound, Doppler guidance, High-intensity focused ultrasound, HIFU, Acoustic hemostasis, Blood vessel.**

## INTRODUCTION

We have demonstrated the potential of high-intensity focused ultrasound (HIFU) in producing hemostasis in cut livers (Vaezy et al. 1997) and punctured blood vessels (Vaezy et al. 1998). In both cases, we encountered situations where it took several minutes of HIFU application to suppress the bleeding and obtain complete hemostasis. In other circumstances, we had achieved hemostasis in 10 or less seconds. Our general impression was that the large range of times was due to variability in aiming the HIFU energy at the bleeding site properly, when first applying the energy. Hemostasis could be achieved rapidly when the HIFU was initially targeted on the bleeding site precisely, but a long exposure was needed when HIFU was not targeted correctly. Moreover, there was sometimes a point of diminishing returns. If bleeding was not stopped after a short HIFU exposure, continuing treatment might begin to overexpose the vessel. Overexposure appeared to make the wall of the vessel hard and, thus, difficult to close. Thus, if overexposed, it became even more difficult to stop the bleeding. In this paper, we report on utilizing Doppler interrogation to aid us in targeting the bleeding site accurately. Our purpose was to develop a method to achieve hemostasis in a short time, avoid overexposure and minimize blood loss.

## METHODS

Three anesthetized pigs, each weighing 20–30 kg and 2–3 months old, were studied. An intramuscular injection was used initially to sedate them, using a mixture of ketamine and Acepromazine at a dose of 22 mg/kg and 1 mg/kg body weight, respectively. Next, they were anesthetized using a ketamine/Xylazine, 8:1 ratio, at a dose of 3.5–4 mL given intravenously. Intubation followed and then positive pressure ventilation was used with oxygen and halothane to maintain the animals ventilated and anesthetized. We heparinized the animal with a dosage of 5000 units (~200 units/kg) about every 3 h of the experiment to test our ability to achieve hemostasis without the help of the natural clotting system. The

Address correspondence to: Roy W. Martin, Ph.D., University of Washington, Departments of Anesthesiology and Bioengineering, Box 356540, Seattle, WA 98195 USA. E-mail: rmartin @u.washington.edu

Published with permission

986 Ultrasound in Medicine and Biology Volume 25, Number 6, 1998

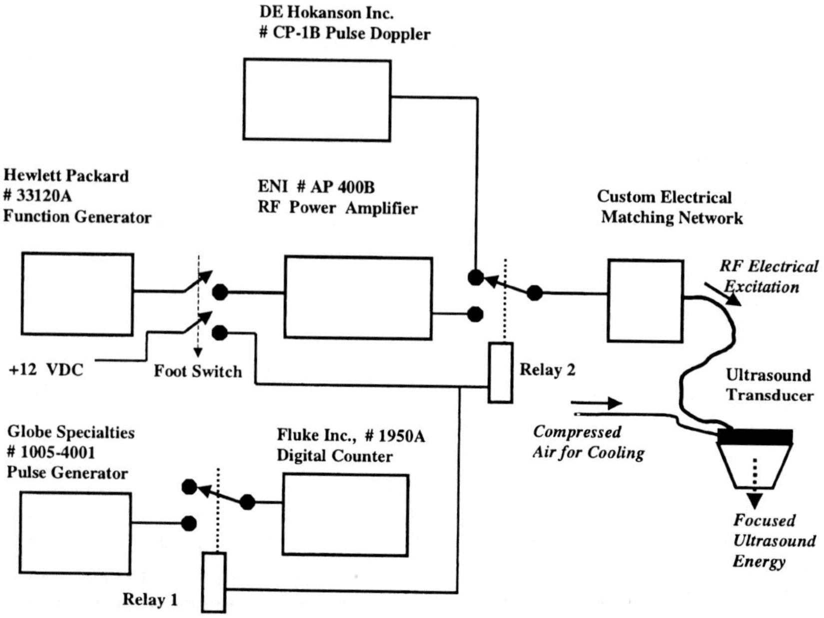


Fig. 1. System used for Doppler-guided HIFU treatment.

University of Washington Animal Care Committee approved the experiments conducted.

We surgically exposed each blood vessel of interest (superficial femoral, common femoral, illiac, and carotid arteries, the abdominal aorta and the jugular vein) shortly before we punctured and treated it. Eighteen-gauge needles were used for the superficial femoral arteries (smaller vessels) and 14-gauge needles for the rest. These punctures produced moderate to profuse bleeding, as we have demonstrated before (Vaezy et al. 1998). Also, in the former studies with these types of punctures, we had determined that the bleeding would not stop by itself during a time period much longer than our treatment times. Therefore, no control bleeds were produced in this study because that would have diminished the number of treatment trials we could have performed in each animal. A total of 92 trials were conducted. At the end of the experiments, each animal was euthanized with an overdose of the same anesthetic mixture, followed within 2 min by 2 mL of KCl-saturated solution.

The system used for the study is shown in Fig. 1. The transducer and electrical matching network were produced by Sonic Concepts, Woodinville, WA. The transducer was a 3.5-MHz spherically-focused transducer with an aperture of 35-mm diameter, a radius of curvature of 55 mm (F number of 1.6). The transducer was attached to a water-filled conical chamber that was truncated before the conical apex, as illustrated in Fig. 1 and described previously (Vaezy et al. 1998). The truncated region was covered with a 12.7 $\mu$m polyethylene membrane held in place with a rubber O-ring. This truncated region with the membrane provided an acoustic window. The height of the chamber was chosen so the acoustic focus was centered about 5 mm outside of the chamber. Therefore, when the surface of the truncated chamber was near the vessel wall, the energy was focused in the wall region. A function generator (Hewlett Packard, Palo Alto, CA) was used to produce the ultrasound frequency. The output of it was coupled through a foot switch to a RF power amplifier (ENI, Rochester, NY) that, in turn, was coupled to the transducer through a RF relay (Relay 2, Magnecraft Inc, Northfield, IL) to the transducer. A second contact on the foot switch routed 12 v/dc to both Relay 1 and Relay 2 in a way that allowed Relay 2 to apply the RF power to the matching network and, in turn, the RF energy to the transducer. The transducer was excited in continuous mode while this relay was activated. Relay 1 coupled the output of the pulse generator (Globe Specialties, New Haven, CT) to the digital counter (Fluke Inc., Seattle, WA) whenever the foot switch was depressed. The pulse generator was set to produce a repeated pulse at a repetition rate of 1 kHz. The digital counter then recorded the number of ms that the foot switch was closed and, consequently, the

Published with permission



Table 1. Data from the Doppler-guided treatment

| Punctured vessel | Number of trials | Major hemostasis time (s) range (mean ± SD) | Complete hemostasis time (s) range (mean ± SD) |
|---|---|---|---|
| *c Abdominal aorta | 7 | 4–49 (20.6 ± 14.4) | 6–65 (26.0 ± 18.9) |
| *c Iliac artery | 6 | 9–40 (19.8 ± 12.2) | 12–49 (26.0 ± 15.5) |
| *c Common femoral artery | 8 | 4–30 (12.6 ± 10.9) | 5–59 (12.5 ± 20.7) |
| *Carotid artery | 17 | 2–16 (6.2 ± 4.8) | 2–23 (8.4 ± 6.4) |
| *Superficial femoral artery | 26 | 1–10 (4.9 ± 3.5) | 1–29 (9.8 ± 7.5) |
| *Jugular vein | 25 | 1–12 (5.2 ± 3.6) | 3–21 (9.6 ± 5.7) |
| All vessels | 89 | 1–49 (8.2 ± 8.5) | 1–65 (13.1 ± 12.3) |

*c These three vessels were combined for statistical comparison of hemostasis times to the times of the individual vessels with the *. SD = standard deviation.

time the ultrasound transducer was excited with the high-level excitation. This count was used to measure the exposure time necessary to achieve the various levels of hemostasis (major and complete). The control of Relay 2 was such that, when the foot switch was not activated, the pulsed Doppler unit was connected to the transducer.

Utilizing this system, the treatment proceeded as follows. After a blood vessel was punctured, the transducer was brought in close proximity to the bleeding site and the Doppler sound was listened to while moving the transducer around the general area. No stand-off was used between the water-filled cone and the tissue. The blood between the vessel wall and the cone provided coupling. The pulsed Doppler window depth was set at the transducer's focus. The cue to begin treatment was detection of a Doppler sound indicative of a jet of blood from the vessel (see Discussion for more details). At that point, the foot switch and relays were activated, disconnecting the Doppler unit from, and connecting the power amplifier to, the transducer; thus, applying HIFU energy continuously until the foot switch was released. The temporal peak spatial average was 2000 W/cm$^2$, a value determined in the same manner as previously reported (Vaezy et al. 1998). The digital counter began counting HIFU exposure time at the same time. After a few s of exposure, the HIFU was stopped and the Doppler was again applied; visual inspection was used as well to determine if bleeding was continuing. If jet flow was persisting, then the Doppler was used to guide further application of the HIFU energy to suppress it. At the completion of treatment, the Doppler was positioned distal to the treatment site to learn if the vessel was still patent.

In several trials, the quadrature output of the Doppler unit was also digitized and recorded on a digital oscilloscope (Model 9350 AL, Lecroy Corp., Chestnut Ridge, NY). Off-line spectral analysis was performed using a general mathematical computation package (Matlab™, The Mathworks Inc., Natick, MA).

## RESULTS

Major hemostasis was achieved in all 92 puncture and treatment trials. However, in three trials, complete hemostasis was not obtained: at 1 femoral artery and 2 jugular vein sites. In 1 vein, poor access and targeting interfered with obtaining complete hemostasis. In the other jugular vein and the femoral artery, difficulty was ascribed to "overtreatment" in trying to achieve complete hemostasis. Applying a high intensity for too long a time (overexposure), we believe, not only denatures the tissue but raises the temperature to a point where it starts to become dehydrated due to vaporization and perhaps other mechanisms (*e.g.*, atomization or fluid movement from radiation pressure). Dehydrated and denatured tissue can become hard and sometimes fragile. In these 2 cases, the vessels had became fragile and the puncture was further enlarged, in the case of the vein, by the continuing application of energy. In the case of the artery, it was actually torn apart by the additional energy. The results for the remaining 89 trials are given in Table 1 as ranges, means and standard deviations (SD) of times required to reach major and complete hemostasis. The mean times for the 89 trials were 8.2 and 13.1 s for major and complete hemostasis, respectively. All of these vessels were found to be patent after the completion of the treatment. Further, hemostasis was achieved with a high level of anticoagulant present in the blood. The hemostasis times for the abdominal aorta, iliac artery and the common femoral artery were combined for statistical analysis, because of the small number of each and their larger size compared to the other arteries. The combined (*c) times compared against the hemostasis times of the carotid artery were found to be highly statistically different at the $p = 0.0008$ and $p = 0.0005$ levels, for major and complete hemostasis, respectively (Table 1). Similarly, the superficial femoral artery and the jugular vein times individually were statistically different from the combined data of the abdominal aorta, illiac and common femoral arteries.

Published with permission

988 Ultrasound in Medicine and Biology Volume 25, Number 6, 1998

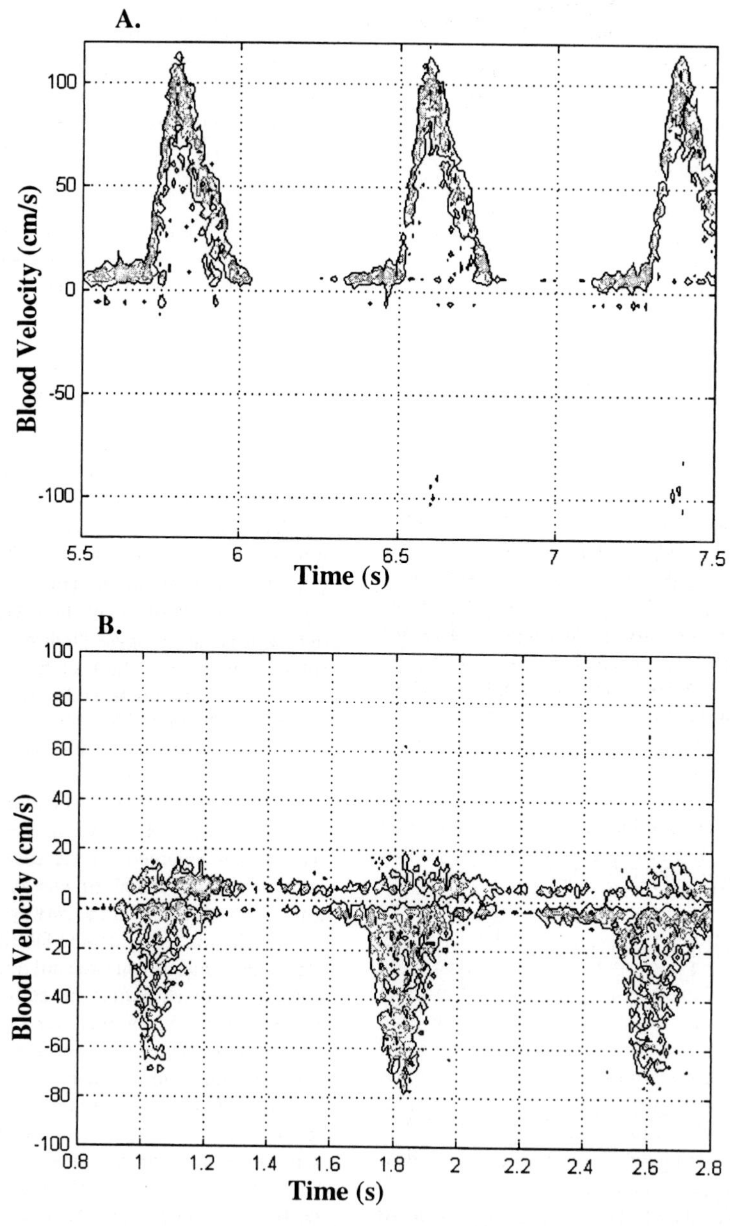


Fig. 2. Example spectograms of the Doppler signals obtained: (A) An intact blood vessel with the transducer tilted at a 45° angle to the axis of the vessel and with the blood flow direction away from the transducer. (B) A punctured blood vessel, with the transducer tilted at 90° to the vessel axis. The signal is from the jet of blood exiting through the puncture.

The Doppler signal that was used to indicate if the transducer was correctly positioned over a hemorrhaging arterial site was generally pulsatile in nature (Fig. 2). The main characteristics were similar to the arterial signal obtained when the probe was held at an angle of 45° to the axis of an intact artery (Fig. 2). However, there was considerable variation in this pattern due to a variety of considerations that will be discussed later. The probe was

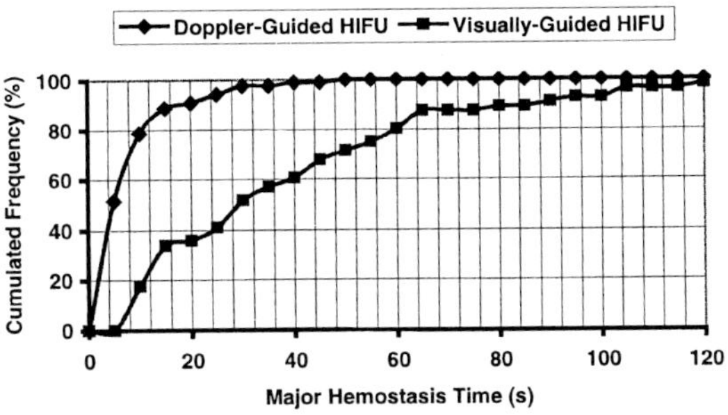


Fig. 3. The cumulated frequency of the major hemostasis times for the Doppler-guided treatment in this study and a similar puncture treatment, but with only visual guidance, previously reported (Vaezy et al. 1998).

generally held at about 90° to the axis of the vessel when searching for the hemorrhaging site. This angle gave little to no Doppler signal in an intact vessel. However, when positioned on a punctured artery with a jet, it gave a strong signal. In the case of punctured jugular veins, Doppler signals were not very distinct with the specific Doppler unit we used. Part of this lack in distinction we believe was due to our failure to remove wall filters when treating venous bleeds. As a consequence of this shortcoming in this study, our venous treatments were mostly governed by visual guidance.

## DISCUSSION

A comparison was made between this study and a prior study of our group. The results of this comparison are presented in Figs. 3 and 4. In the former study, blood vessels were punctured in an identical manner to that in this investigation, but they were treated without the aid of Doppler guidance; only visual guidance was used (Vaezy et al. 1998). The advantage of utilizing Doppler to aid in directing the application of the HIFU is clearly apparent from these graphs, with regard to the marked reduction of the time necessary to achieve hemostasis. Major hemostasis was achieved in 90% of all treatments within 16 s with Doppler guidance and within 80 s with visual guidance. Complete hemostasis was reached in 90% of all treatments within 25 s with Doppler guidance and within 125 s with visual guidance. The overall average major and complete hemostasis times for Doppler-guided HIFU were 8 and 13 s, whereas those of the visually-guided method were very significantly higher at 42 and 62 s, respectively (Table 1). The improvement achieved in treatment times demonstrates to us the advantages of an accurate means of guiding the HIFU. We ponder if it may even be possible further to reduce the treatment time, with a Doppler system that is specifically optimized for HIFU guidance.

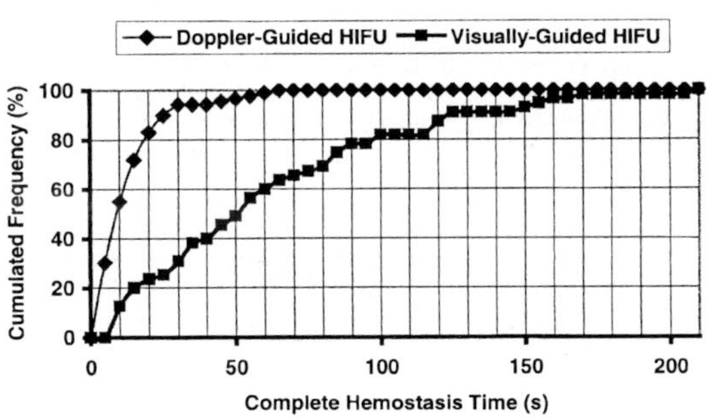


Fig. 4. The cumulated frequency of the complete hemostasis times for the Doppler-guided treatment in this study and a similar puncture treatment, but with only visual guidance, previously reported (Vaezy et al. 1998).

The Doppler technique we employed was pulsed Doppler, the same transducer was used for both Doppler and HIFU and the pulse Doppler interrogation window was set at the focal point of the HIFU transducer. This setting was accomplished by first adjusting the time delay according to settings on the instrument so it would occur at the focal point, and then optimizing the setting slightly to obtain the best Doppler signal when interrogating an intact blood vessel. The sample window had a time duration equivalent to a spatial length of about 1 mm. Placement of this Doppler window at the point on the vessel wall where the blood was exiting required spatially moving the probe along the punctured region while listening to the Doppler sound. Proper placement was usually fairly rapid (requiring only a few s) when blood was not pooling around the vessel. However, in the case of blood welling up and forming a pool, visual clues were lost and it became necessary to search not only laterally, but axially as well. When one considers that the beam width is about 1 mm in diameter at the focus and the window length is 1 mm, it can be difficult to place this small spatial window right on the jet with no visual clues to guide the operator. Therefore, it would be advantageous to have a Doppler method such as color Doppler or a multigate Doppler to aid in the initial searching to locate the flow jet. After identification, the transducer could then be positioned to place the HIFU focus at the point where the jet is exiting from the vessel, the best treatment point.

The nature of a Doppler signal varied and, of course, would vary depending on the type of jet and where the Doppler window is placed. For example, differences occur depending on whether: 1. a high pressure artery or a low pressure vein is bleeding, 2. the pulsed Doppler window placement is directly in the center of

Published with permission



the jet axis or to one side, and 3. the Doppler is aligned or misaligned with the axis of the jet. Another consideration is the jet orifice itself (*e.g.*, its size, shape and wall thickness). Finally, in the case of an arterial bleed, one can easily visualize the variations that can occur in the pulsatility and pulse duration of the flow during the cardiac cycle. Blood will flow out of the puncture as long as it is open and there is a positive pressure gradient from the inside of the vessel to the outside, but it will stop or reverse direction when the gradient goes to zero or becomes negative, respectively.

The use of Doppler ultrasound in detecting bleeding seems to be as yet an undeveloped method. Very few citations were found in searching the world's literature. Only one report discusses specifically the use of color Doppler for assessing bleeding; in this case, after renal biopsy (Nakamura et al. 1998). Four citations were found utilizing ultrasound to study vessel trauma; two animal studies (Panetta et al. 1992a, 1992b) and two human investigations (Montalvo et al. 1996, Demetriades et al. 1997). Doppler ultrasound has been used for some time in detecting arteriovenous malformations (AVM) (Black et al. 1988) and, recently, a report appeared of its use in emergency management of a hematoma resulting from cerebral AVM (Kitazawa et al. 1998). The value of ultrasound imaging in assessing the presence of free fluid (*e.g.*, blood) in the abdomen after blunt abdominal trauma has become clear in numerous studies (Melanson and Heller 1998; McKenney et al. 1998); however, it appears that Doppler methods have not been employed to try to locate a hemorrhaging site in this situation. Whether the logistics of acute trauma treatment and diagnosis have prevented such Doppler exploration, the ultrasound users were not trained in Doppler techniques, and/or the application of Doppler here has not been fruitful, is open to speculation at this point. We anticipate Doppler methods will be explored in this arena and its potential in acute trauma will be identified.

In conclusion, the use of the Doppler technique greatly aided the treatment of arterial bleeds in our study. The time to achieve hemostasis was reduced by a factor of 5 on the average. We credit this improvement to the enhancement in accuracy of targeting the bleeding site. This reduction is important for several reasons. First, we have found that the overall success in using HIFU for hemostasis is improved if only a short duration of exposure is necessary. A short treatment avoids overexposure of the vessel, a condition detrimental for hemostasis. Second, less damage to the vessel wall will occur with minimum exposure. Third, the amount of blood loss can be reduced with a faster, successful treatment time. Last, in many cases, such as surgery, rapid hemostasis of various bleeding sites is necessary for a method to be practical. The primary motivation for this study is the potential capability of a Doppler-guided HIFU treatment to achieve hemostasis in conditions where the bleeding site is not visible. For example, a long-term objective is to develop transcutaneous methods of treating internal bleeding in emergency situations. Doppler guidance in these circumstances may be valuable, but that is yet to be proven.

*Acknowledgments*—We thank Frank Starr, Sherry Stemen, Bryan Goldman, and Marla Paun for their aid with the animal experimentation. This work was supported by a grant from the Defense Advanced Research Programs Administration (DARPA) under its MURI program, Number N00014-96-0630, supervised by Dr. Wallace A. Smith.

## REFERENCES

Black KL, Rubin JM, Chandler WF, McGillicuddy JE. Intraoperative use of real-time ultrasonography in neurosurgery. J Neurosurg 1988;68:635–639.

Demetriades D, Theodorou D, Cornwell E, Berne TV, Asensio J, Belzberg H, Velmahos G, Weaver F, Yellin A. Evaluation of penetrating injuries of the neck: prospective study of 223 patients. World J Surg 1997;21(1):41–48.

Kitazawa K, Nitta J, Okudera H, Kobayashi S. Color Doppler ultrasound imaging in emergency management of an intracerebral hematoma caused by cerebral arteriovenous malformations: Technical case report. Neurosurgery 1998;42(2):405–407.

Melanson SWM, Heller H. The emerging role of bedside ultrasonography in trauma care. Emerg Med Clin North Am 1998;16(1):165–189.

McKenney KL, Nunez DB Jr, McKenney MG, Asher J, Zelnick K, Shipshak D. Sonography as the primary screening technique for blunt abdominal trauma: experience with 899 patients. AJR Am J Roentgenol 1998;170(4):979–985.

Montalvo BM, LeBlang SD, Nunez DB Jr, Ginzburg E, Klose KJ, Becerra JL, Kochan JP. Color Doppler sonography in penetrating injuries of the neck. Am J Neuroradiol 1996;17(5):943–951.

Nakamjura M, Taniguchi N, Kawai F, Itoh K.Color Doppler imaging for detection of bleeding immediately following renal biopsy. Clin Nephrol 1998;49(2):132.

Panetta TF, Hunt JP, Buechter KJ, Pottmeyer A, Batti JS. Duplex ultrasonography versus arteriography in the diagnosis of arterial injury: an experimental study. J Trauma 1992;33(4):627–636.

Panetta TF, Sales CM, Marin ML, Schwartz ML, Jones AM, Berdejo GL, Wengerter KR, Veith FJ. Natural history, duplex characteristics, and histopathologic correlation of arterial injuries in a canine. J Vasc Surg 1992;16(6):867–876.

Vaezy S, Martin R, Schmiedl U, Caps M, Taylor S, Beach K, Carter S, Kaczkowski P, Keilman G, Helton S, Chandler W, Mourad P, Rice M, Roy R, Crum L. Liver hemostasis using high intensity focused ultrasound. Ultrasound Med Biol 1997;23(9):1413–1420.

Vaezy S, Martin RW, Yaziju H, Kaczkowski P, Keilman G, Carter S, Caps M, Crum LA. Hemostasis of punctured blood vessels using high intensity focused ultrasound. Ultrasound Med Biol 1998; 24(6):903–910.

CHAPTER 8

# STRAIN RATE IMAGING — A NEW TOOL FOR STUDYING THE GI TRACT

ANDREAS HEIMDAL AND ODD HELGE GILJA

## 1. Introduction

Strain rate imaging is a recently introduced technique to measure deformation of biological tissue. The technique is based on tissue velocity imaging, which is an ultrasound technique that provides quantitative information on the velocity of the tissue. Even though pulsed wave Doppler methods were used to detect cardiac motion already in 1961 (1), it is only recent that the method has gained widespread use. By color-coded tissue velocity imaging, velocity samples from the whole field of view are available simultaneously (2). This allows for extraction of other parameters through spatial and temporal processing of the velocity data. Strain rate and strain are examples of such parameters. The methods have primarily been used in echocardiography, but other uses have also been reported. These include measurements of arterial pulse wave velocities (3), skeletal muscle contractions (4), and measurements of gastric motor function (5).

Elastography, a method calculating the strain directly from the radio frequency (RF) ultrasound signal, may be an alternative to estimating the strain from tissue velocities (6).

Since it forms a basis for strain rate imaging, this chapter starts by describing the technical aspects of tissue velocity imaging, including the acquisition technique, how the velocity is estimated and how it may be presented and analyzed. Furthermore, the chapter defines the parameters strain and strain rate and explains how they can be derived from the tissue velocity data. Finally, our experience with the use of strain rate imaging for studying the gastric antrum is reviewed. Throughout the chapter, examples and illustrations are mainly from the gastric antrum, but illustrations from echocardiography are used in some cases.

## 2. Tissue Velocity Imaging

Tissue velocity imaging (TVI) is a technique where the velocity of the tissue towards or away from the transducer is measured and displayed. The velocities can be calculated and displayed as a pulsed wave (PW) spectrogram or as a color-coding of the image. The two methods both calculate the velocity based on the echoes of several ultrasound pulses fired in the same direction. The pulses are fired at a certain pulse repetition frequency (PRF). Each echo is sampled at a fixed depth, and the samples are collected into a new signal representing a certain position in the image. This signal is called the *Doppler signal*. The frequency of the Doppler signal is related to the velocity of the tissue in the sample region through the Doppler equation:

$$f_d = \frac{2f_0 v}{c} \tag{1}$$

In this equation, $f_0$ is the central frequency of the transmitted ultrasound pulse, $c$ is the speed of sound, and $v$ is the tissue velocity component in the ultrasound beam direction.[a]

A consequence of using pulsed imaging is that there is a limit on the maximum velocity that can be measured. This limit is called the Nyquist velocity:

$$v_{Nyq} = \frac{c \cdot PRF}{4f_0} \tag{2}$$

If the actual velocity is higher than this limit, there will be frequency aliasing, resulting in the misrepresentation of the velocity. The Nyquist velocity can be adjusted by changing the PRF or the ultrasound frequency $f_0$.

The frequency, pulse length and beam width that gives the optimal Doppler acquisition is not the same that gives a good grayscale image quality. Typically lower frequencies, longer pulses and wider beams are used for the Doppler acquisition. Therefore, the grayscale image and the Doppler data are usually based on different acquisitions, and may have different frame rates and spatial resolutions.

### 2.1. *Pulsed wave TVI*

In PW TVI, the Doppler signal from only one sample region is collected. In the basic type of processing, the signal is first split into overlapping segments, and the frequency content of each signal segment is calculated next using the Fourier transform. Other, more advanced processing methods involving data from several sample regions may also be used. The result is a signal spectrum for each segment, representing the frequency content at a certain time, as illustrated in Fig. 1.

Note that the peak in the spectrum corresponds to the mean Doppler frequency $f_d$ in the Doppler equation, and that the mean tissue velocity thus can be derived from the same equation. Also note that the bandwidth of the peak is inversely related to the duration of the signal segments. To make accurate estimates of the velocity, a narrow peak is desired, but to get this, the signal segment must have a long duration. The accuracy of the velocity estimation is therefore inversely related to the temporal resolution. The bandwidth is also influenced by the acceleration in the tissue and acoustical noise.

The signal spectra are next collected in a spectrogram, with Doppler frequency on the vertical axis and time on the horizontal axis. The Doppler frequency is directly related to the tissue velocity, so the vertical axis can also be a velocity axis. The spectral intensity is coded as gray scale intensity in the PW TVI display. An example of the PW TVI from the mid part of a normal interventricular septum is shown in Fig. 2. Note that the spectrum bandwidth is represented as the vertical thickness of the spectrogram signal. The peak of each spectrum, representing the mean velocity, is therefore found in the *middle* of the spectrogram signal, as indicated by the black trace in Fig. 2.

[a]If second harmonic Doppler imaging is used, $2f_0$ must be used instead of $f_0$ in the Doppler equation.

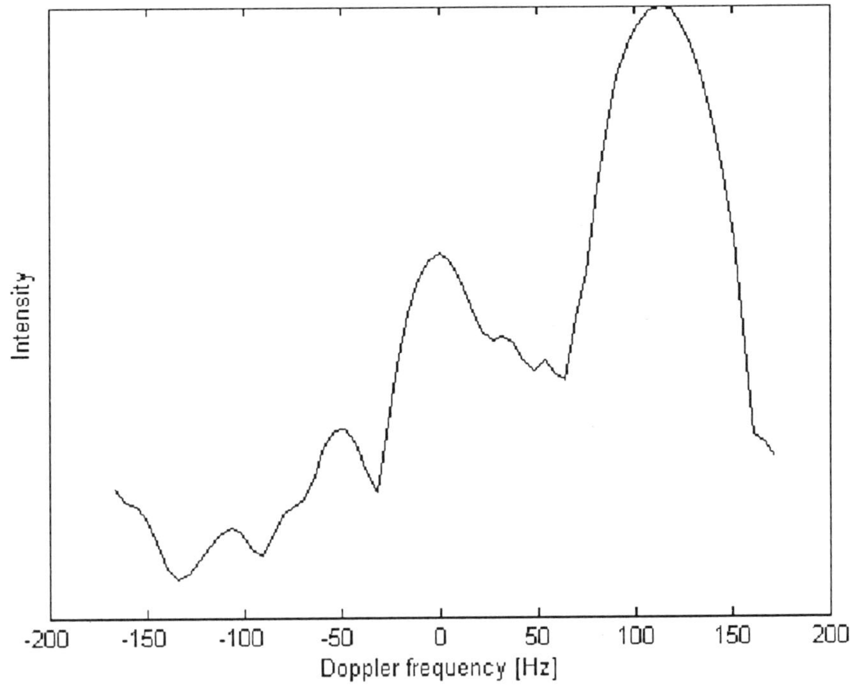


Fig. 1. Tissue Doppler spectrum from mid level of a healthy heart wall at 0.25 s after onset of QRS. The peak in the spectrum at approximately 115 Hz corresponds to a velocity of approximately 2.5 $\text{cms}^{-1}$ (assuming an ultrasound frequency of 3.5 MHz and a speed of sound of 1540 $\text{ms}^{-1}$). Stationary reverberations cause the smaller peak at zero Doppler frequency.

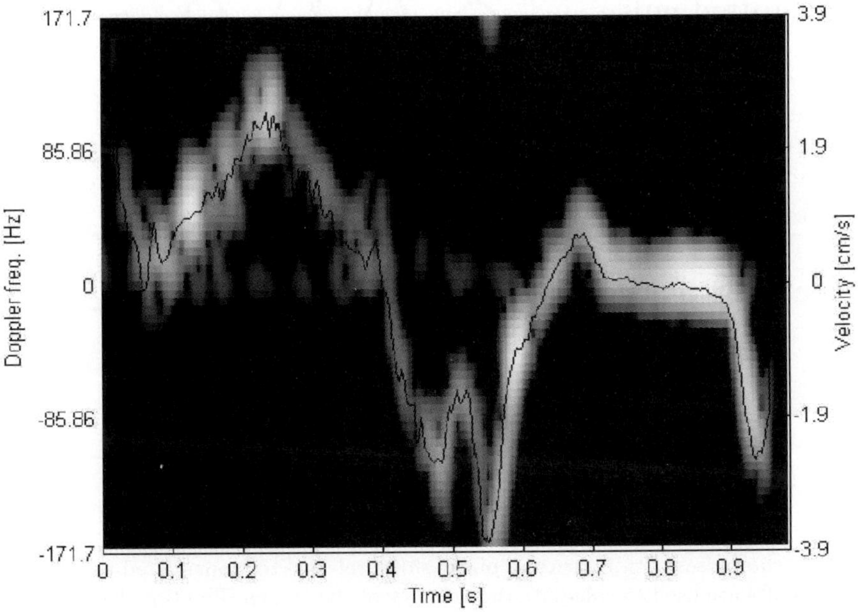


Fig. 2. Pulsed wave (PW) TVI from mid level of a healthy heart wall. The left vertical axis is the Doppler frequency, while the right vertical axis is the corresponding velocity found through the Doppler equation. The spectrum in Fig. 1 can be found at 0.25 s, with intensity in grayscale.

## 2.2. *Color TVI*

In color TVI, a Doppler signal is collected for each depth and each ultrasound beam. This normally requires more time, so each Doppler signal consists of fewer samples per time unit than in the PW case. This normally limits the ability to calculate full signal spectra for each position in the image. Instead, only the mean Doppler frequency is estimated for each position.

The most common way to estimate this mean frequency is to calculate the phase shift relative to the transmitted ultrasound pulse for each sample in the Doppler signals. If the tissue is not moving, the phase shift is the same for all the samples. If the tissue is moving relative to the transducer, the phase shift increases or decreases from sample to sample according to the velocity of the tissue, as illustrated in Fig. 3. The difference in phase shift from sample to sample in the Doppler signal can thus be used to calculate the mean velocity.

When the mean velocity has been estimated for all parts of the ultrasound image, each pixel is color coded according to the velocity. As mentioned earlier, the Doppler acquisition is usually separated from the image acquisition, so for each grayscale image there is at least one corresponding velocity image. The velocity image may have a lower resolution than the grayscale image, but is normally interpolated to match the resolution of the grayscale image. This means that neighboring pixels in the color-coded image may represent identical velocity values.

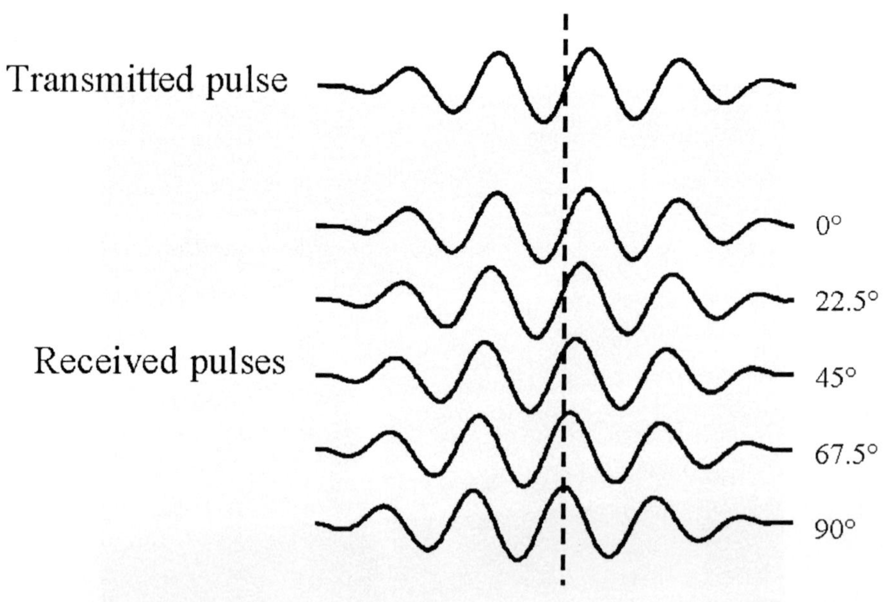


Fig. 3. Illustration of echo pulses with increasing phase shifts relative to transmitted pulse. In the color TVI method, these phase shifts are used to calculate the velocity of the tissue. The time between each echo pulse is given by the pulse repetition frequency (PRF). If the PRF is too high, the phase shift between the pulses becomes too small to detect reliably, and if the PRF is too low the phase shift may exceed 180°, making the velocity estimate ambiguous. The latter phenomenon is termed aliasing.

The color code is normally ranging from dark red for low velocities to bright yellow for high velocities towards the transducer, and from dark blue for low velocities to bright cyan for high velocities away from the transducer.

## 3. Concepts of Strain and Strain Rate

Strain and strain rate are characteristics of changes in shape, i.e. deformations. The strain and strain rate can be defined and measured in various ways as will be described in the following sections.

### 3.1. *Definition of strain*

Strain is a mechanical characteristic that describes the deformation of objects. There are several different ways to measure strain. For one-dimensional deformations, i.e. shortening or lengthening, perhaps the simplest measurement is the so-called *conventional strain.*[b] It describes the relative change in length between two configurations. For an object of initial length $L_0$ that is being stretched or compressed to a new length $L$, the conventionsl strain is defined as (7):

$$\varepsilon = \frac{L - L_0}{L_0} \tag{3}$$

The Greek letter *epsilon* ($\varepsilon$) is commonly used as a symbol for the conventional strain. The strain value is unit-less, and can be presented as a fractional number or as a percentage (by multiplying with 100). For instance, a fractional strain of −0.2 corresponds to a percentage strain of −20%. The strain is positive if $L$ is larger than $L_0$, meaning that the object has increased in length, and negative if $L$ is smaller than $L_0$, meaning that the object has decreased in length. If $L$ equals $L_0$, there has been no change in length, and the strain is zero.

Other measurements of one-dimensional strain include *logarithmic strain,*[c] which is defined as

$$\varepsilon' = \ln\left(\frac{L}{L_0}\right) \tag{4}$$

The name reflects the use of the *natural logarithm* function, ln. The logarithmic strain has the same properties as the conventional strain regarding the sign: it is positive for lengthening, negative for shortening and zero for no change in length. The actual strain value, however, is slightly different. Compared to the conventional strain, the logarithmic strain value is compressed for positive strains, and expanded for negative strains. For instance, a conventional strain of 10% corresponds to a logarithmic strain of 9.5%, while a conventional strain of −10% corresponds to a logarithmic strain of −10.5%. The strain traces in Fig. 6 illustrate the difference between conventional and logarithmic strain for an actual measurement.

[b] Conventional strain is sometimes termed "lagrangian strain" in the literature.
[c] Logarithmic strain is sometimes termed "natural strain" in the literature.

The conventional and logarithmic strains have a fixed nonlinear relationship given by

$$\begin{aligned} \varepsilon' &= \ln(\varepsilon + 1) \\ \varepsilon &= \exp(\varepsilon') - 1 \end{aligned} \tag{5}$$

Note that in these formulas, the strains are represented as fractional numbers. For percentage strains, the corresponding formulas are:

$$\begin{aligned} \varepsilon'_{\%} &= 100 \ln\left(\frac{\varepsilon_{\%}}{100} + 1\right) \\ \varepsilon_{\%} &= 100\left(\exp\left(\frac{\varepsilon'_{\%}}{100}\right) - 1\right) \end{aligned} \tag{6}$$

When reporting strain values, it should be specified whether conventional or logarithmic strain is used. In addition, both the initial and the final reference states should be specified, for example: "At peak contraction, the conventional strain was −20% relative to the reference state". When measuring one-dimensional strains in a two- or three-dimensional object, it is also important to specify in what direction the one-dimensional strains were measured.

### 3.1.1. *Two- or three-dimensional strain*

For two- or three-dimensional deformations the concept of strain becomes more complex. In the given coordinate system, one can use the one-dimensional strain in each of the coordinate directions using the same definitions as presented earlier in this section. This type of strain is termed *normal strain*, since the deformation is normal to the surfaces defined by the coordinate system. In addition, there might be *shear strains*, indicating changes in angle, as illustrated in Fig. 4. The maximal and minimal strains might not occur in any of the coordinate directions, therefore it is common to specify the directions and magnitudes of the maximal and minimal strains. These are termed the *principal strains*, and *principal*

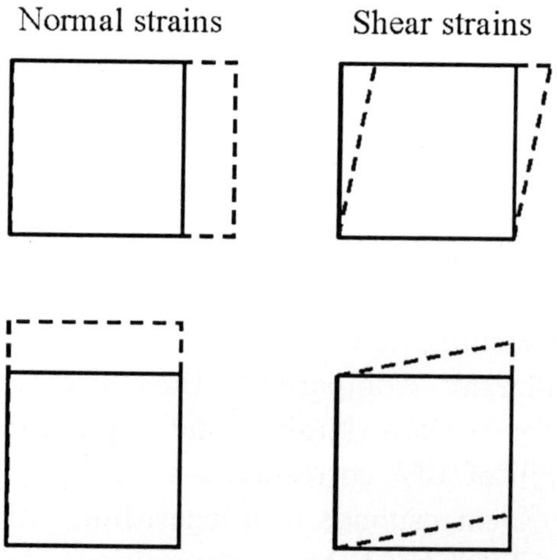


Fig. 4. Illustration of the two types of strains possible in a two-dimensional object. The left column shows *normal strains*, where the deformation is normal to either of the edges, while the right columns shows *shear strains*, where the deformation causes a change in angle.

*strain directions*. If the principal strain directions coincide with the axis directions of the coordinate system, there are no shear strains.

### 3.2. *Definition of strain rate*

The *strain rate* is the temporal derivative of the strain:

$$\dot{\varepsilon} = \frac{d\varepsilon}{dt} \tag{7}$$

This means that while the strain indicates the extent of deformation, strain rate indicates the rate of the deformation. The relation between strain rate and strain can be compared to the relation between velocity and displacement. Assuming that the velocity is constant, displacement equals time multiplied with velocity. Similarly, assuming the strain rate is constant, strain equals time multiplied with strain rate. A positive strain rate means that the length of the object is increasing, while a negative strain rate means that the length is decreasing. If the length is constant, the strain rate is zero.

The notation for strain rate is an epsilon with a dot above it, indicating the temporal derivative. Since this notation is cumbersome in many occasions, the acronym SR is commonly used to represent the strain rate. The unit of the strain rate is normally /s or $s^{-1}$, which might be read as "per second".[d] In other applications, the unit Hertz (Hz) is used for $s^{-1}$, but this is not recommended for strain rate. Hertz means number of cycles per second, while for strain rate it is more correct to speak of the extent of deformation per second. A strain rate of $-2\ s^{-1}$ applied over one second would result in a relative strain of $-2$ or corresponding percentage strain of $-200\%$.

Note that while the strain is a measurement of deformation relative to a reference state, the strain rate is an instantaneous measurement. There is no need to specify a reference state for strain rate, for example: "The peak strain rate was $-1.0\ s^{-1}$".

Since there are several definitions of strain, there are a corresponding number of similar definitions for strain rate. In particular the *logarithmic strain rate* is defined as[e]

$$\dot{\varepsilon}' = \frac{d\varepsilon'}{dt} = \frac{1}{L}\frac{dL}{dt} \tag{8}$$

## 4. Estimation of Strain Rate and Strain from Ultrasound Data

One way to measure strain is by M-mode through a muscle wall. By measuring the wall thickness before ($L_0$) and after ($L$) contraction, the wall thickening Lagrangian strain can be calculated as

$$\varepsilon = \frac{L - L_0}{L_0} \tag{9}$$

This is a cumbersome method that might not be applicable to all muscle walls. A faster method is to use tissue velocity imaging and calculate the strain rate and strain from the velocity data.

[d]In rare occasions, the notation %/s is seen for strain rate, meaning that the strain rate is multiplied with 100. A strain rate of $-1\ s^{-1}$ corresponds to $-100\%$/s.
[e]The formulation arises from the fact that the derivative of $\ln(u)$ is $(du/dt)/u$.

### 4.1. *Strain rate and velocity gradient*

Under certain assumptions, the one-dimensional logarithmic strain rate in an object is equivalent to the spatial velocity gradient.

$$\dot{\varepsilon}' = \frac{dv}{dx}$$

This relation can be illustrated by considering the small object in Fig. 5, which is being deformed. The instantaneous length is defined by the positions of the end-points as $L = x_b - x_a$. Since the temporal derivative of spatial position is velocity, the logarithmic strain rate of the object can be written:

$$\dot{\varepsilon}' = \frac{1}{L}\frac{dL}{dt} = \frac{1}{L}\left(\frac{dx_b}{dt} - \frac{dx_a}{dt}\right) = \frac{v_b - v_a}{L} = \frac{dv}{dx} \tag{10}$$

Here, $v_a$ and $v_b$ are the instantaneous velocities of the end-points of the segment. The last equation is correct if the spatial velocity distribution within the segment is assumed to be linear.

In practice, it is rarely feasible to accurately track the end-points of such a segment, and a fixed "strain length" $\Delta x$ may be used instead. As long as the velocities are linearly increasing or decreasing within the region, this method will give exactly the same answer.

The velocity gradient may be estimated only using the two velocity estimates $v_1$ and $v_2$ from the end-points of the estimation area as:

$$\dot{\varepsilon}' = \frac{v_2 - v_1}{\Delta x} \tag{11}$$

or a linear regression of all the velocity samples within the area may be performed.[f]

Note that this estimation is performed separately for each frame in a cineloop, and that the region of interest may be moved from frame to frame to follow the motion of the tissue, as explained earlier.

For 2D and M-mode, the color-coding of strain rate is typically ranging from yellow for low negative strain rates to red for high negative strain rates, and from light cyan for low

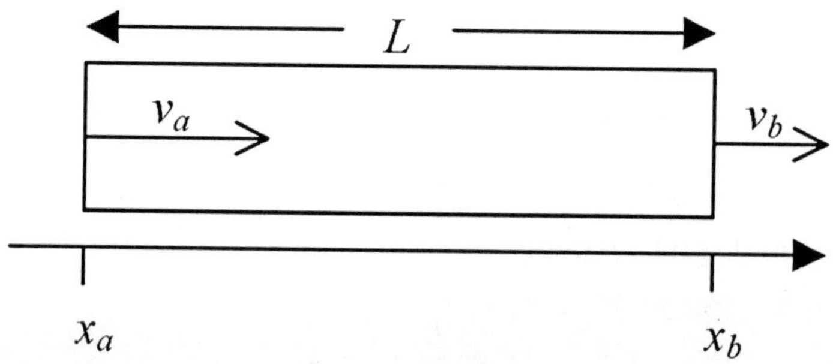


Fig. 5. Illustration of a small tissue segment of instantaneous length $L$ that is being deformed. If the velocities $v_a$ and $v_b$ of the two ends $x_a$ and $x_b$ of the segment are different, there is a strain rate different from zero, and the length $L$ is either increasing or decreasing.

[f] In ultrasound, velocities are defined positive for motion towards the transducer, while in the equations here, the velocities have for simplicity been defined positive for increasing depth.

positive strain rates to dark blue for high negative strain rates. A green color is sometimes used for the near zero strain rates.

### 4.2. *Integrating strain rate to get strain*

When the strain rate has been calculated for each time point during the deformation, the strain can be found as the temporal integral of the strain rate:

$$\varepsilon' = \int_{T_0}^{T} \dot{\varepsilon}'(t)dt\,. \tag{12}$$

Here $T_0$ and $T$ are the time points of the start and end of the deformation. Note that it is the logarithmic strain that is found through this integral. To find the more commonly used conventional strain, one might use the conversion formula

$$\varepsilon = \exp(\varepsilon') - 1\,. \tag{13}$$

Note also that in commercially available post-processing tools, this is normally performed automatically, so that it is the conventional strain that is presented to the user.

The color-coding for strain is typically red/yellow for negative strain and blue/cyan for positive strain.

## 5. Quantitative Analysis

One of the major advantages of TVI and strain rate imaging is that it allows quantitative analysis of the motion pattern of the tissue. In PW TVI, accurate timing and velocity measurements may be performed from the spectrogram. In the color modes, each pixel in the image represents a measurement, and the quantitative value can be presented in various ways, as described in the following sections.

### 5.1. *Time-traces*

By picking one region of interest (ROI) in each frame of a color mode cineloop, the corresponding values can be presented as a time-trace as illustrated in Fig. 6. The top panel shows the radial strain rate in the anterior wall of the stomach during a contraction. The bottom panel shows the strain calculated from the strain rate. As seen, the strain increases over time when the strain rate is positive, and decreases when the strain rate is negative. When the strain rate is close to zero, there is little change in strain.

For TVI, the time-trace represents the velocity pattern of the tissue within the ROI, similar to PW TVI. The difference is that the PW TVI can only be acquired from one position at a time while with color TVI multiple time-traces from various regions can be generated from a single cineloop.

The ROI used to generate the time-trace can be fixed to the same position in all the frames, or it can be manually moved to follow a certain anatomical structure. To avoid having to adjust the position of the ROI in every single frame, it is recommended to reposition the ROI only in the extreme positions, and let the software perform a linear translation between these positions for the intervening frames.

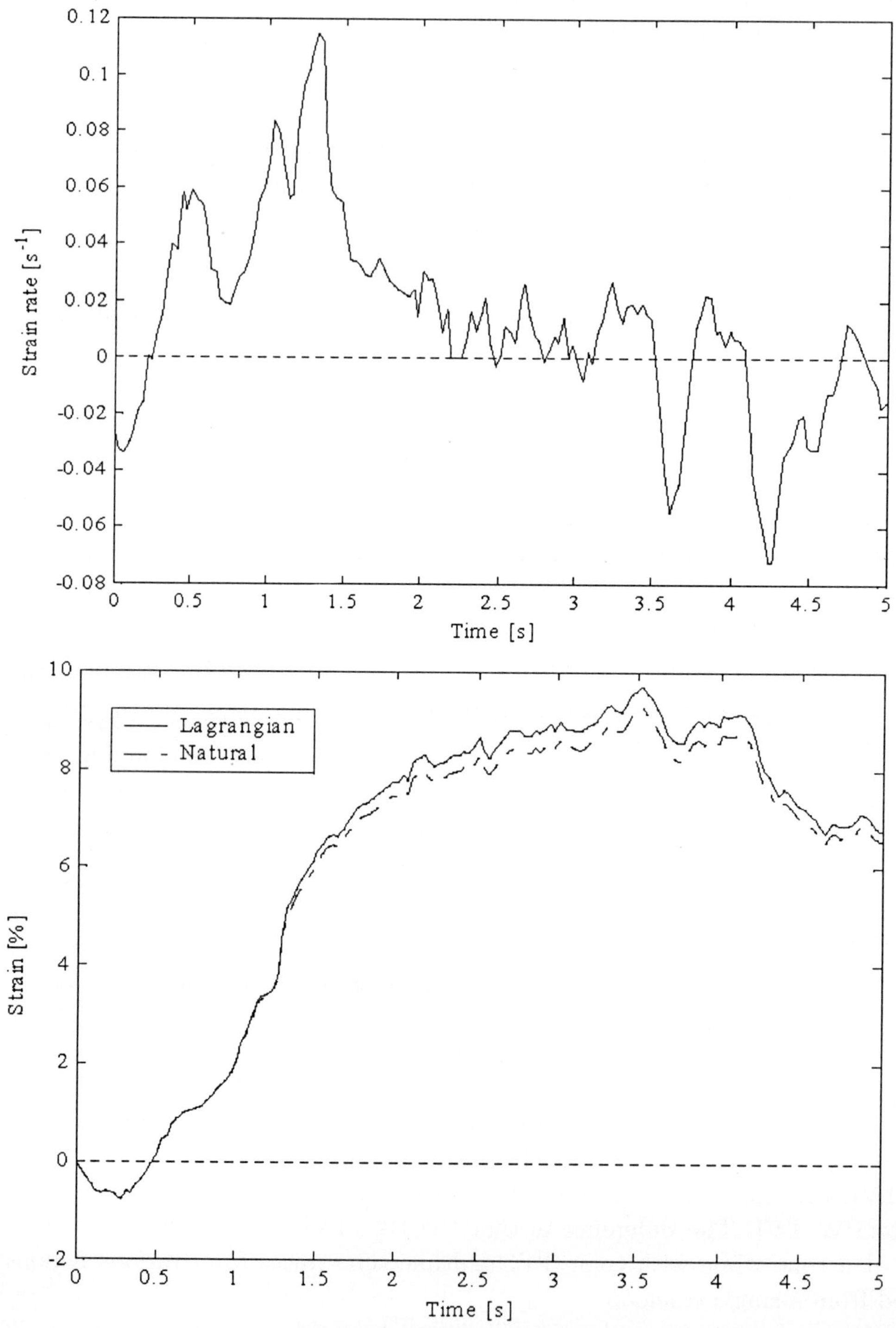


Fig. 6. Radial strain rate (top) and strain (bottom) traces from the anterior wall of the stomach during a contraction. When the strain rate is positive, the strain is increasing, and when it is negative the strain is decreasing. The measurement shows that the anterior wall thickened by almost 10% is this example. The peak contraction strain rate was approximately 0.12 $s^{-1}$.

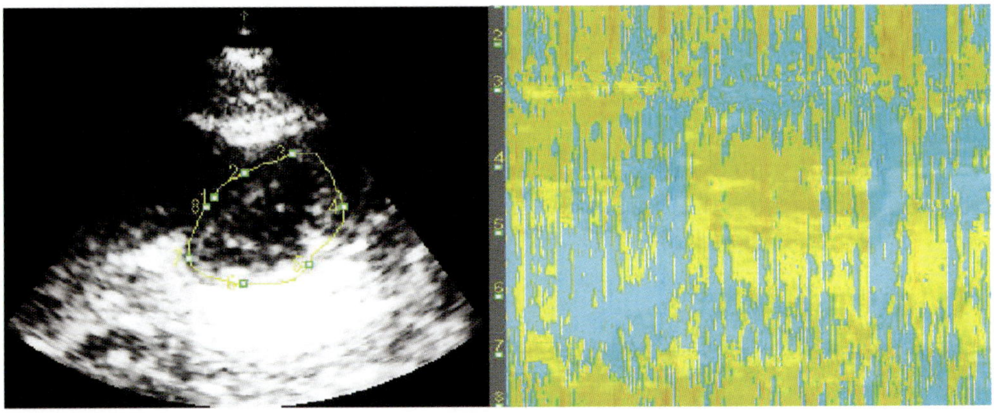

Fig. 7. Illustration of a curved anatomic M-mode (CAMM) of a healthy stomach wall during a 4 second contraction. The numbers on the vertical axis correspond to the marked positions on the CAMM curve in the left panel. Since the angle between the ultrasound beams and the muscle varies, care must be taken when analyzing the data. At markers 3 and 6 the beams are perpendicular to the muscle, and the blue colors indicate wall thickening. At markers 4 and 8, the beams are parallel to the muscle, so the yellow colors indicate circumferential contraction.

### 5.2. *Curved anatomical M-mode*

Another way to visualize the color TVI data is to make an anatomical M-mode (AMM). The M-mode line may be a straight line in any direction through the 2D image. Alternatively, a curve may be manually drawn to an arbitrary shape, usually along a muscle. The resulting image is then called a Curved anatomical M-mode (CAMM).

The CAMM curve may be drawn separately in either of the visible walls, or, as illustrated in Fig. 7, the curve may be drawn through all the walls in one operation. The latter method produces a still CAMM image that represents the acquired data from all the segments in all the 2D frames. In the example in Fig. 7, it can be seen by the blue colors at markers 3 and 6 how the posterior and anterior walls thickens, while the yellow colors at markers 4 and 8 indicate circumferential contraction in the lateral walls.

## 6. Strain Rate Imaging of the Gastric Antrum

Dyspepsia is one of the most frequent complaints encountered by physicians in the western countries (8). The prevalence of dyspepsia in population-based studies carried out in the Scandinavian countries varies from 12% to 54% with an average of 30% (9–15). Of those referred to gastroscopy, 71% were found to have non-organic dyspepsia in Norway (16). With such a high incidence and prevalence of dyspepsia, there is a considerable economic impact of this condition, as reported in a Swedish study (17).

Functional dyspepsia (FD) has been studied using a variety of methods, most commonly being gastroscopy, 2D and 3D ultrasonography (18–22), manometry, radionuclide methods and balloon distension. However, many of these are invasive, e.g. the barostat and manometry, thus disturbing the motility of the stomach (23, 24). In this regard, ultrasound has proven to be a valuable tool for studying gastric motility since it leaves the organ undisturbed. The application of Strain Rate Imaging on the distal stomach was investigated by Gilja *et al.* in a pilot study (5, see also attached paper).

High-frequency real-time ultrasonography and Strain Rate Imaging enabled detailed studies of layers within the gastric wall. The anterior part of the gastric antrum was most accessible for SRI as visualized in Fig. 8, where CAMM is applied to study strain during a contraction. Interestingly, radial strain was significantly higher in the circular muscle layer compared to the longitudinal layer (Fig. 9).

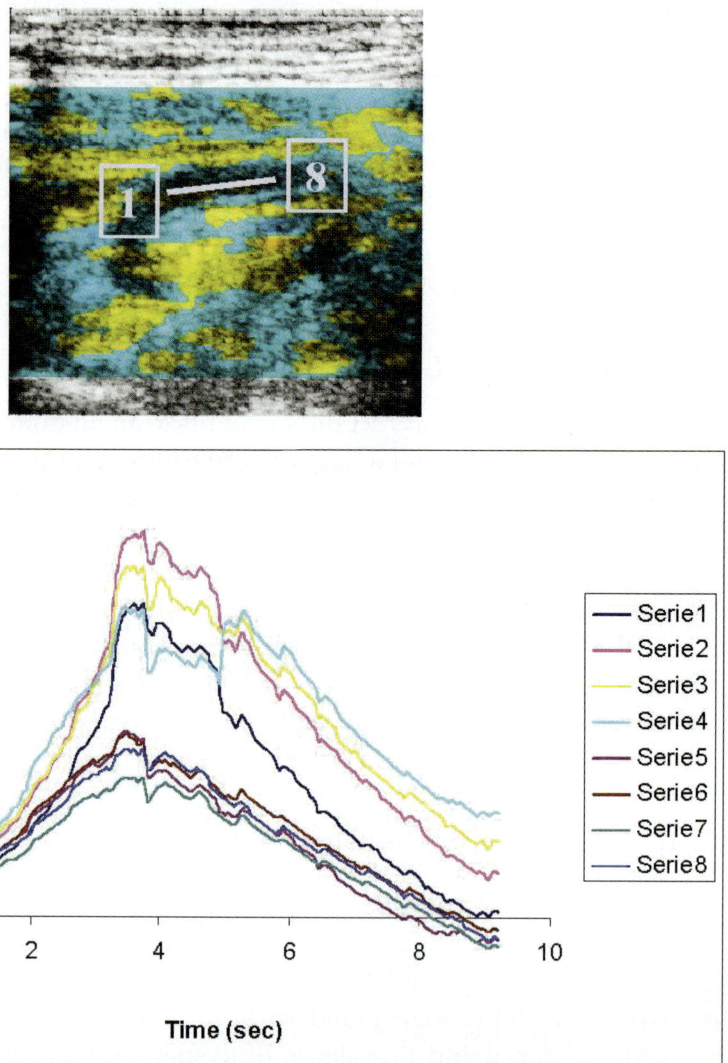


Fig. 8. Curved M-mode analysis of relative strain estimation in the antral muscle layer by using Strain Rate Imaging, a novel Doppler ultrasound method, is shown. A line consisting of 8 measurement points is drawn within and in parallel to the main muscle layer of the anterior part of the human antrum. In this contraction-relaxation cycle lasting 9 sec, a detailed mapping of strain distributions was enabled using Strain Rate Imaging. In the lower panel, relative strain curves for each of the 8 measurement points are shown. One may appreciate that there is a difference in the time periods for the contraction versus the relaxation phase.

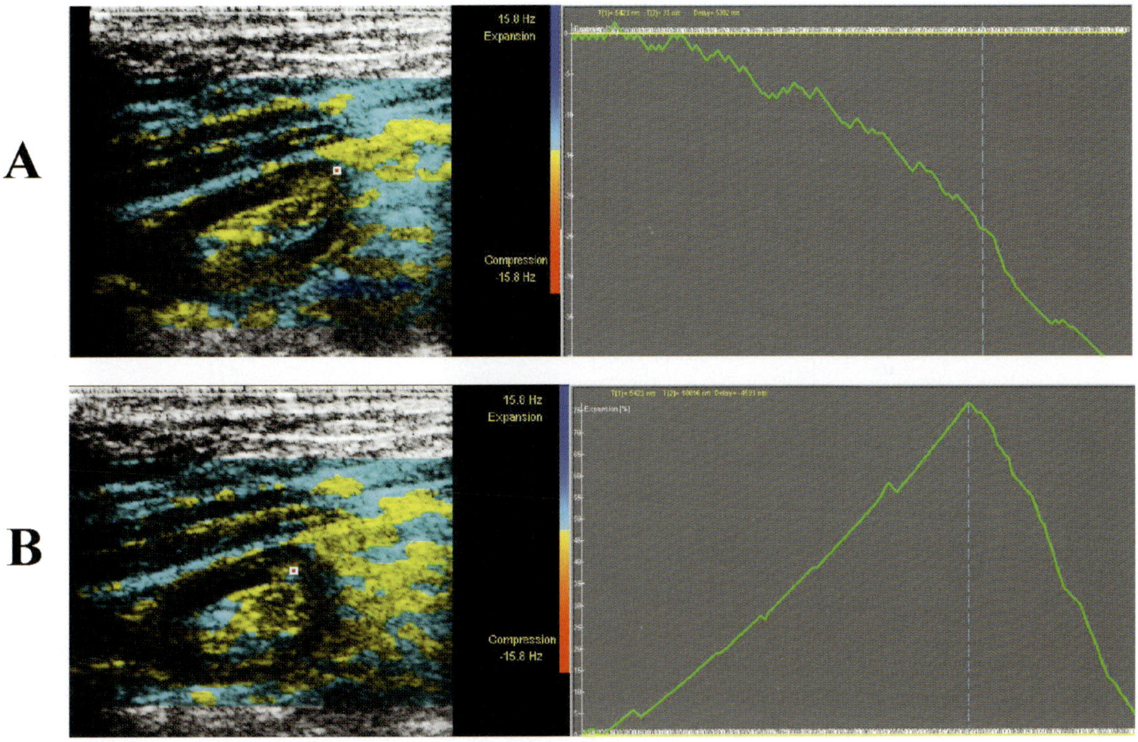


Fig. 9. This graph shows how Strain Rate Imaging can be used to separate the two layers of muscularis propria of the gastric wall; the inner circular versus the outer longitudinal muscle layer. The sampling points in the gastric wall are denoted with a dot in the ultrasonograms. In panel A, the strain curve of the outer layer is shown. The lower panel B demonstrates the high positive strain (elongation) of the circular (inner) muscle layer, illustrating the separate biomechanical events occurring in the two portions of the main muscle layer. All data were obtained by scanning the gastric wall in a radial direction.

We designed a distension probe with a polyesterurethane bag that could be inflated with fluid through an infusion channel. The probe contained a metal clip in the middle of the bag as a marker for ultrasound. The middle of the balloon was placed approximately 3 cm proximal to the pylorus and visualized by ultrasonography. The fluid volume of the bag was changed intermittently with volumes ranging from 5 to 60 ml for one-minute-periods using a hand-held syringe. The distensions were separated by 2-min resting periods, i.e. the volume was withdrawn from the bag and the bag pressure was kept slightly negative during these periods to ensure complete emptying of the bag. SRI was performed simultaneously with the infusion of water into the balloon. We found that the volume of the intragastric bag and strain was negatively correlated ($r = -0.97$; $p < 0.01$; Fig. 10). A typical pattern of strain during distension is shown in Fig. 11.

The regular distension pattern was negative radial strain in the proper muscle layer of the anterior wall in response to sudden pressure increments. However, other distinct patterns were also noted during careful post-processing of image data; distension on contraction (the balloon was inflated when a barely visible contraction had already started) or contraction on distension, see Fig. 12 (the gastric wall was compressing the balloon undergoing inflation).

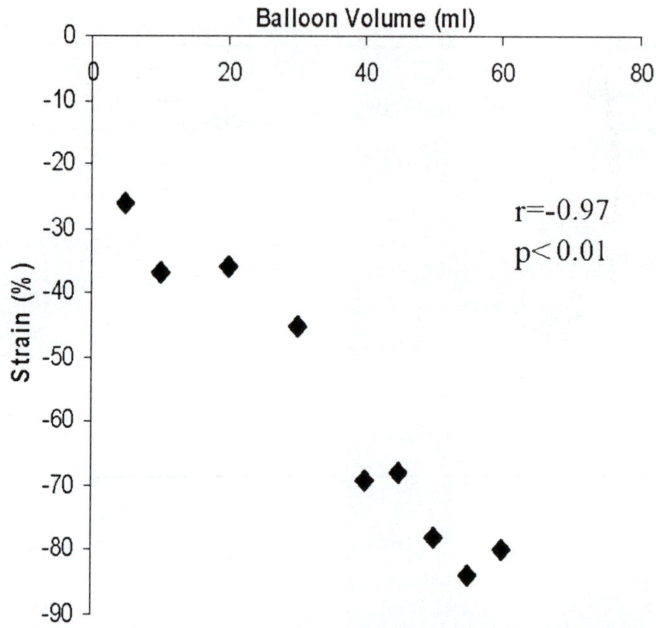


Fig. 10. This scatterplot is demonstrating the association between strain estimation using Strain Rate Imaging and volume infusion into an intragastric balloon distending the antrum. A significant negative correlation is depicted, showing that as increasing volume is distending the antrum, increasing negative strain (shortening) is measured radially in the anterior proper muscle layer of the wall.

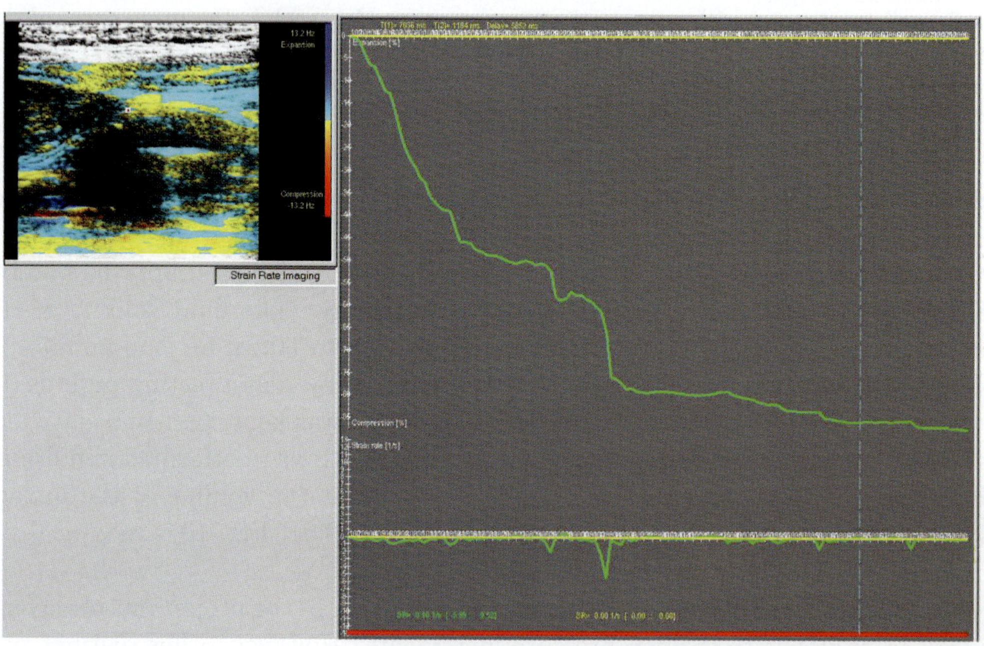


Fig. 11. The image in the upper left corner shows a B-mode ultrasonogram and Strain Rate Imaging while a balloon is distending the gastric antrum. The hyperechoic line in the gastric lumen is the catheter centered in the balloon. The curve to the right depicts the negative strain strain as the balloon during distension is compressing the muscle layer of the gastric wall.

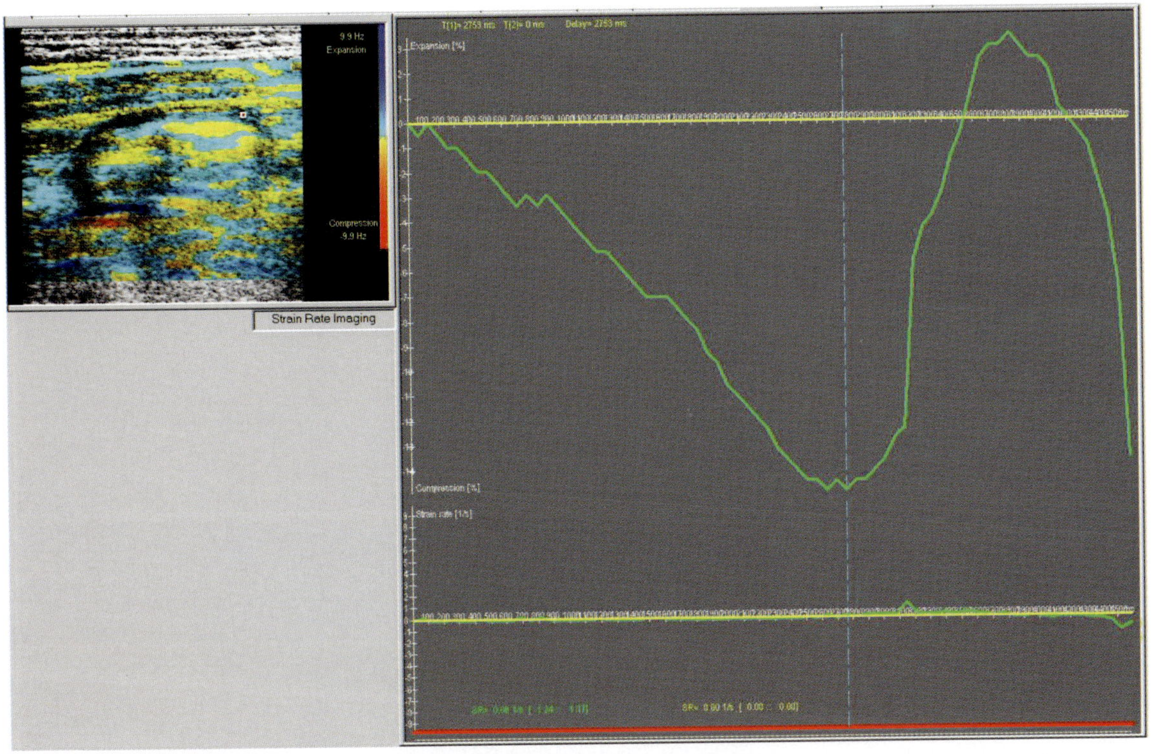


Fig. 12. The image in the upper left corner shows a B-mode ultrasonogram and Strain Rate Imaging while a balloon is distending the gastric antrum. In the first phase of distension, a compression (negative strain) of the muscle layer is taking place. After 4–5 sec strain rises and becomes positive, reflecting a wave of contraction superimposing the distension enforced by the pressure of the balloon.

The influence of aortic pulsatility on the antral wall could often be observed as spikes superimposed onto the strain curves (Fig. 13). This illustrates another possible application of Strain Rate Imaging; the study of pressure induction and the resulting changes in compliance and strain on tissue *in vivo*. A clinical application could be the variation in elasticity of hepatic tumors compared to healthy liver tissue measured by Strain Rate Imaging.

Strain Rate Imaging was applicable on the human antrum but the variance in the measured strain in normal patients was relatively large. Therefore, an *in vitro* study was performed to optimize the method for slow contractions and to reduce this variance (25). We found that the variance of strain was substantial if single samples were used, especially for a small strain sample size (0.8 mm). Increasing the strain sample size to 1.9 mm removed some of the underestimation. Our results showed low inter and intraobserver variation. This *in vitro* study indicates that for the SRI method to give accurate estimates of strain, strain sample size should be in the region of 2 mm.

## 7. Artifacts and Methods to Improve Signal Quality

As all ultrasound modalities, the tissue velocity and strain rate imaging methods are also affected by noise components like random thermal noise and reverberations. These noise

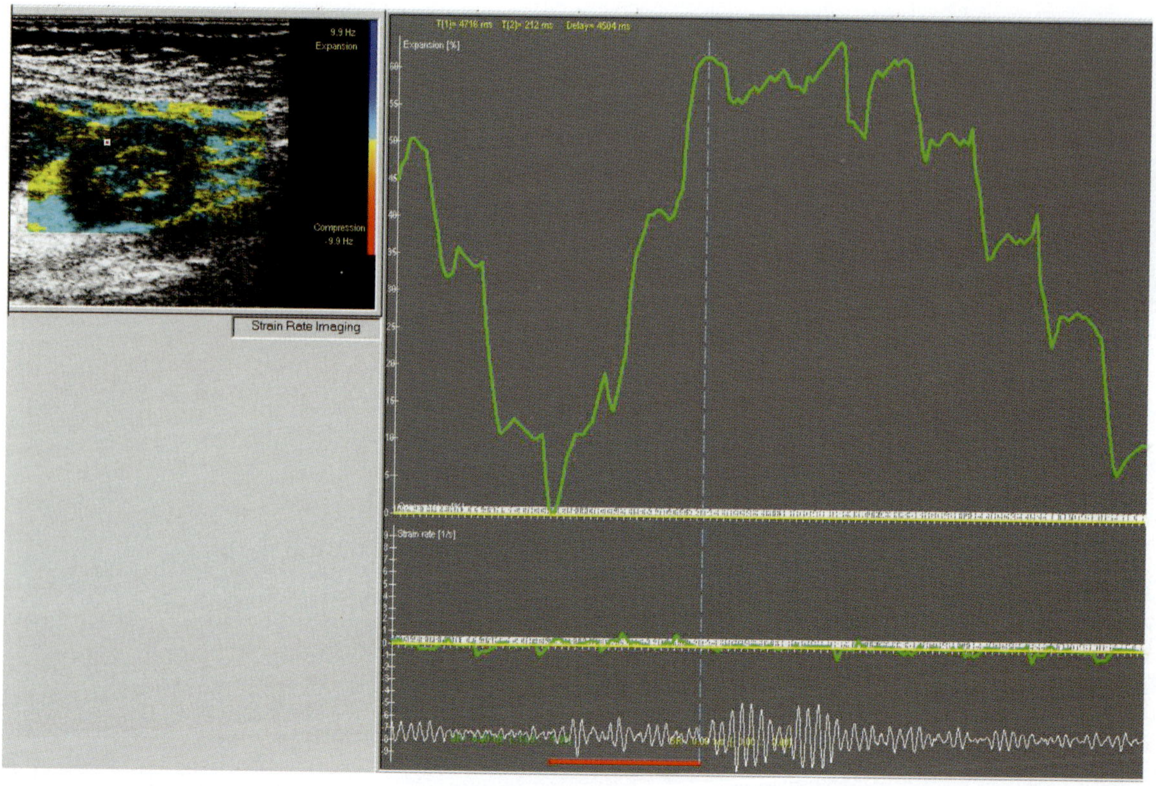


Fig. 13. The image in the upper left corner shows Strain Rate Imaging of a sagittal view of the antrum. The graph depicts how the aortic pulsation influences on the muscle layer of the antrum visualized as spikes on the strain curve. This phenomenon can be utilized to study compliance of tissue in the vicinity of the aorta.

components may degrade the quality of the velocity and strain rate measurements. In addition, angle mismatches between the ultrasound beams and the examined structure may cause errors.

### 7.1. *Reverberation artifacts*

Reverberations are false echoes resulting from multiple reflections within the body. In the grayscale image they are seen as false echoes. The reverberations are often caused by tissue layers close to the body surface. These layers are relatively motionless, and the reverberation artifacts are therefore often seen as immobile structures mixed with the true signal.

In PW TVI, reverberations can be seen as an increased intensity at zero velocity, as shown in Fig. 14. In many cases, it is still relatively easy to identify the true velocity signal. PW TVI may therefore be a preferred method for velocity measurements in patients with poor acoustic windows.

For color TVI, the reverberations may cause a bias in the mean velocity estimate, as shown by the trace in Fig. 14. Typically the bias is towards zero velocity. The amount of bias depends on the intensity of the reverberation signal relative to the tissue velocity signal. Still, the sign of the velocity is seldom affected, so it might be difficult to detect reverberations from the color display, as illustrated in the central part of Fig. 15.

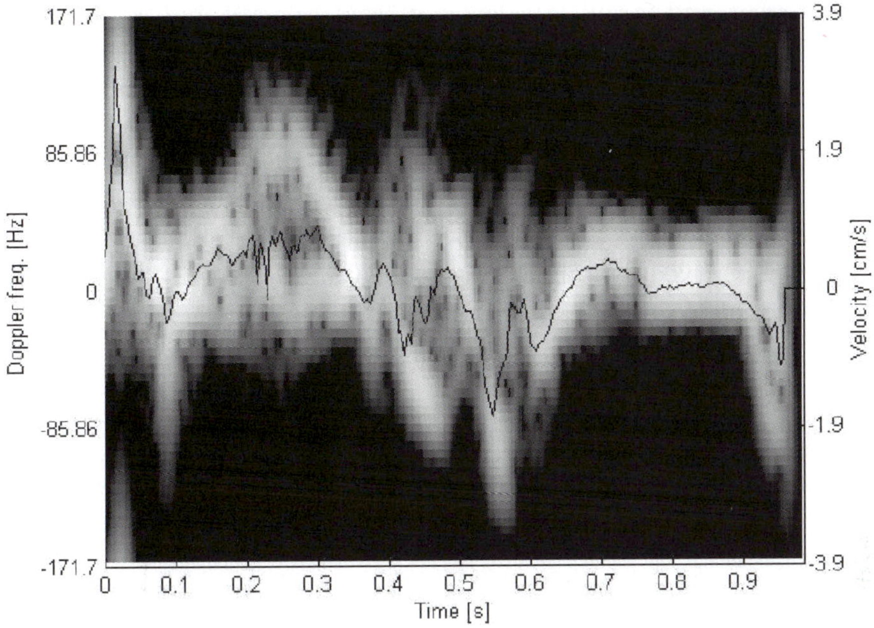


Fig. 14. PW TVI from a region with strong reverberations in a cardiac wall. The reverberations are seen as an increased intensity around zero Doppler frequency. The black trace shows the corresponding TVI trace based on color TVI. Notice how this velocity estimate is biased towards zero by the reverberations.

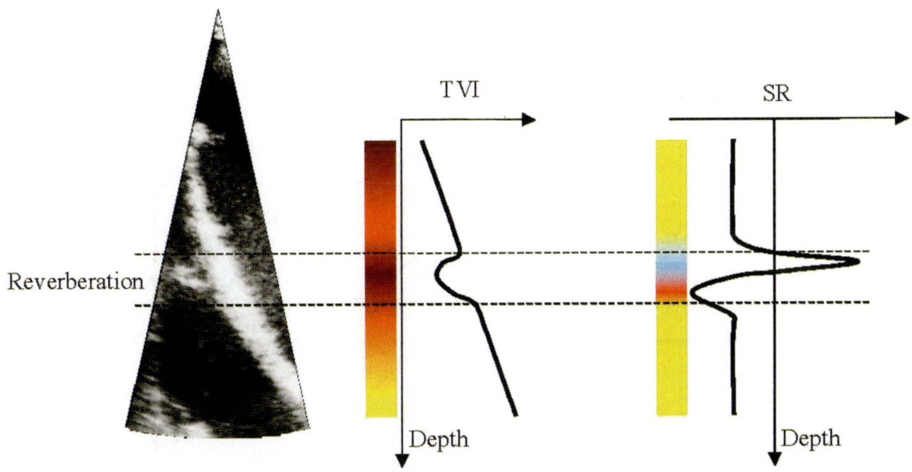


Fig. 15. Illustration of effect of a local reverberation on the longitudinal tissue velocity and strain rate. The color bars indicate the coloring of the cardiac muscle, while the plots show the actual velocities and strain rates at different depths along the muscle. The horizontal dashed lines indicate the region affected by the reverberation. In the velocity data, the reverberations cause a slight bias towards zero, while in the strain rate data, the effect is much worse.

In strain rate imaging, reverberations may cause large errors, as illustrated in Fig. 15. A small local bias in the velocity will cause large changes in the spatial velocity gradient and thus the strain rate. A typical reverberation artifact in strain rate is a strong blue and red stripe next to each other.

Since displacement and strain is calculated from velocity and strain rate, reverberation errors in velocity and strain rate will also cause errors in displacement and strain. Since strain rate is most affected by reverberation errors, strain will be more affected than displacement.

Unfortunately, there is little the user can do when there is reverberation noise, other than trying to get the best scanning window when performing the imaging. When analyzing the strain rate data, it is important to recognize the reverberation artifacts, and to avoid the regions affected. Curved anatomical M-mode (CAMM) may be a good tool to get an overview of the amount of reverberation artifacts in the strain rate, and may be used prior to detailed analysis.

### 7.2. *Angle dependence*

All Doppler methods are angle dependent. It is only the velocity component in the ultrasound beam direction that is picked up. If the true velocity direction is known, the true velocity may be calculated by dividing the measured velocity component by $\cos(\theta)$, where $\theta$ is the angle between the ultrasound beam and the true velocity direction. This means that as the angle increases, the measured velocity component decreases from 100 percent of the true velocity at zero angle to zero at ninety degrees' angle, as illustrated in Fig. 16.

For strain rate, the angle dependence is more complicated. Assuming, for simplicity, that the beam is perpendicular to the longitudinal direction, which usually is the case for short axis views, a relation can be formulated. Assuming also no shear, the measured strain

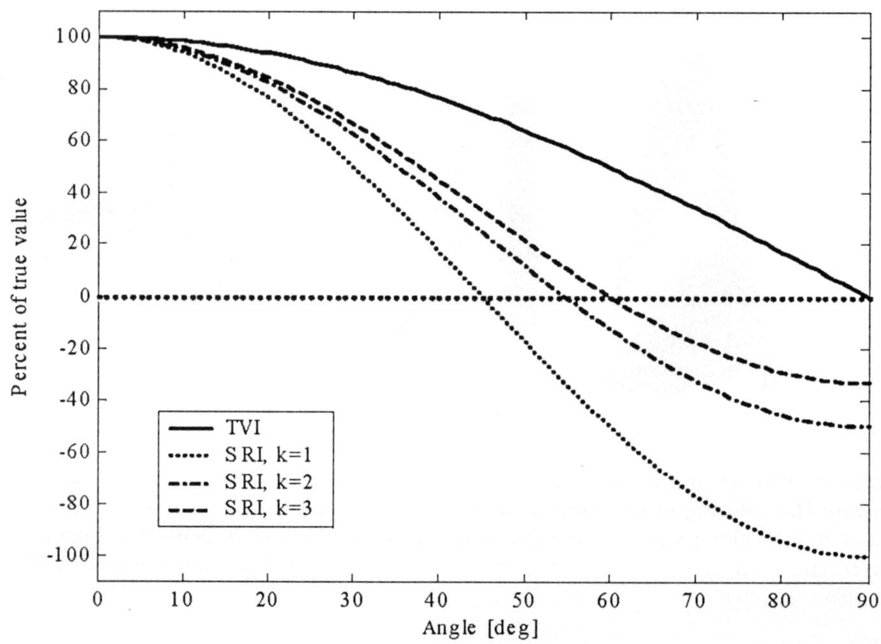


Fig. 16. Angle dependence of tissue velocity imaging (TVI) and strain rate imaging (SRI) for three different assumptions of radial-circumferential relationship ($k$). When the angle increases from zero, the circumferential shortening is picked up in addition to the radial thickening, and depending on the assumed of $k$, the two signals cancel out each other at between 45 and 60°.

rate is a component of both the circumferential ($c$) and the radial ($r$) strain rates (26):

$$\dot{\varepsilon} = \dot{\varepsilon}_c \cos^2 \theta + \dot{\varepsilon}_r \sin^2 \theta$$

Figure 16 shows the angle dependence of the measured strain rate as the percentage of the circumferential strain rate for various values of the assumed linear relation

$$k = \frac{\dot{\varepsilon}_r}{\dot{\varepsilon}_c}$$

Since the value of $k$ is generally unknown, it is not possible to angle correct the measured strain rate. Also, the assumptions of no shear and linear relation between radial and circumferential strain rates are in general not fulfilled, so the model is somewhat inaccurate. Still, the model may give some indications of the angle dependence of the estimate.

Note that strain rate is more angle dependent than tissue velocity. For example, assuming $k = 1$, the measured strain rate is reduced to 50 percent of the true value already at 30 degrees, while the measured tissue velocity is 87 percent of the true value at the same angle. It is therefore important to align the ultrasound beam exactly perpendicular to the muscle when measuring radial strains and strain rates. Similarly, it is important to align the beam parallel to the muscle when measuring circumferential or longitudinal strains and strain rates. To be able to do this, it might be necessary to image the different walls and segments of the stomach with different probe positions.

### 7.3. *Noise reduction by averaging*

Spatial and temporal averaging may be helpful to reduce random noise. Note that reverberation artifacts and errors caused by angle mismatch are generally not of random nature, so averaging will generally not improve these artifacts.

All averaging techniques may be performed using a "sliding window" technique as illustrated in Fig. 17. Every sample in the averaged data is based on a set of samples in the original data. The set can be a collection of spatial and/or temporal samples. Spatial averaging is usually performed along the ultrasound beams (axial averaging), perpendicular to them (lateral averaging) or a combination. Temporal averaging may be performed by combining data from a set of frames.

Note that the sample resolution in the averaged data is the same as in the original data, but that neighboring samples in the averaged data will be correlated. This means

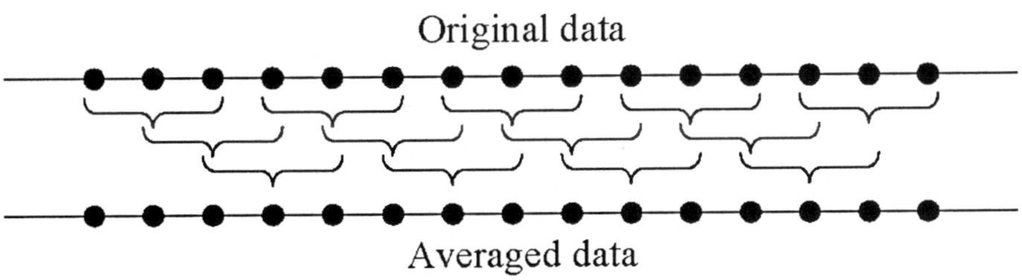


Fig. 17. Illustration of the "sliding window" technique when averaging data to obtain noise reduction. The averaged data has the same data resolution as the original data, but neighboring samples will be correlated since they are partly based on the same data.

that averaging should not be performed in the directions where the user wants to measure differences. For example, if the user wants to study differences in strain rate between various layers of the muscle, no averaging should be performed in the direction parallel to the layers.

## References


1. Yoshida, T., Mori, M., Nimura, Y. *et al.*, Analysis of heart motion with ultrasonic Doppler methods and its clinical applications, Am Heart J, 1961; 61: 61–75.
2. McDicken, W. M., Sutherland, G. R., Moran, C. M. and Gordon, L. N., Colour Doppler velocity imaging of the myocardium, Ultrasound Med Biol, 1992; 18: 651–4.
3. Eriksson, A., Greiff, E., Loupas, T., Persson, M. and Pesque, P., Arterial pulse wave velocity with tissue Doppler imaging, Ultrasound Med Biol. 2002; 28(5): 571–80.
4. Grubb, N. R., Fleming, A., Sutherland, G. R. and Fox, K. A., Skeletal muscle contraction in healthy volunteers: Assessment with Doppler tissue imaging. Radiology 1995; 194(3): 837–842.
5. Gilja, O. H., Heimdal, A., Hausken, T., Gregersen, H., Matre, K., Ødegaard, S. and Berstad, A., Strain during gastric contractions can be measured using Doppler ultrasonography. Ultrasound Med Biol 2002; 28: 1457–1465.
6. Ophir, J., Cespedes, I., Ponnekanti, H., Yazdi, Y. and Li, X., Elastography: A quantitative method for imaging the elasticity of biological tissues. Ultrason Imaging 1991; 13: 111–134.
7. Malvern, L. E., Introduction to the mechanics of a continuous medium. Prentice Hall, Inc., Englewood Cliffs, New Jersey, 1969.
8. Switz, D. M., What the gastroenterologist does all day. A survey of a state society's practice. Gastroenterology 1976; 70(6): 1048–1050.
9. Tibblin, G., Introduction to the epidemiology of dyspepsia. Scand J Gastroenterol Suppl 1985; 109: 29–33.
10. Jones, R. and Lydeard, S., Prevalence of symptoms of dyspepsia in the community. BMJ 1989; 298: 30–32.
11. Krag, E., Non-ulcer dyspepsia introduction: epidemiological data. Scand J Gastroenterol Suppl 1982; 79: 6–8.
12. Holtmann, G., Goebell, H. and Talley, N. J., Dyspepsia in consulters and non-consulters: Prevalence, health-care seeking behaviour and risk factors. Eur J Gastroenterol Hepatol 1994; 6: 917–924.
13. Jones, R. H., Lydeard, S. E., Hobbs, F. D., Kenkre, J. E., Williams, E. I., Jones, S. J. *et al.*, Dyspepsia in England and Scotland. Gut 1990; 31: 401–405.
14. Kay, L. and Jorgensen, T., Epidemiology of upper dyspepsia in a random population. Prevalence, incidence, natural history, and risk factors. Scand J Gastroenterol 1994; 29: 2–6.
15. Knill Jones R. P., Geographical differences in the prevalence of dyspepsia. Scand J Gastroenterol Suppl 1991; 182: 17–24.
16. Johnsen, R., Straume, B. and Forde, O. H., Peptic ulcer and non-ulcer dyspepsia — A disease and a disorder. Scand J Prim Health Care 1988; 6: 239–243.
17. Nyren, O., Adami, H. O., Gustavsson, S., Loof, L. and Nyberg, A., Social and economic effects of non-ulcer dyspepsia. Scand J Gastroenterol Suppl 1985; 109: 41–47.
18. Gilja, O. H., Hausken, T., Odegaard, S. and Berstad, A., Monitoring postprandial size of the proximal stomach by ultrasonography. J Ultrasound Med 1995; 14(2): 81–89.
19. Gilja, O. H., Smievoll, A. I., Thune, N., Matre, K., Hausken, T., Odegaard, S. *et al.*, *In vivo* comparison of 3D ultrasonography and magnetic resonance imaging in volume estimation of human kidneys. Ultrasound Med Biol 1995; 21: 25–32.

20. Gilja, O. H., Hausken, T., Odegaard, S. and Berstad, A., Three-dimensional ultrasonography of the gastric antrum in patients with functional dyspepsia. Scand J Gastroenterol 1996; 31: 847–855.
21. Gilja, O. H., Detmer, P. R., Jong, J. M., Leotta, D. F., Li, X.-N., Beach, K. W., Martin, R. and Strandness, D. E., Intragastric distribution and gastric emptying assessed by three-dimensional ultrasonography. Gastroenterology 1997; 113: 38–49.
22. Gilja, O. H., Hausken, T., Olafsson, S., Matre, K. and Odegaard, S., *In vitro* evaluation of three-dimensional ultrasonography based on magnetic scanhead tracking. Ultrasound Med Biol 1998; 24(8): 1161–1167.
23. Stadaas, J. and Aune, S., Intragastric pressure-volume relationship before and after vagotomy. Acta Chir Scand 1970; 136: 611–615.
24. Moragas, G., Azpiroz, F., Pavia, J. and Malagelada, J. R., Relations among intragastric pressure, postcibal perception, and gastric emptying. Am J Physiol 1993; 264: G1112–7.
25. Matre, K., Ahmed, A. B., Gregersen, H., Heimdal, A., Ødegaard, S. and Gilja, O. H., *In vitro* evaluation of ultrasound Doppler strain rate imaging. Modification for measurement in a slowly moving tissue phantom. Ultrasound Med Biol. 2003; 29: 1725–1734.
26. Heimdal, A., Doppler based ultrasound imaging method for noninvasive assessment of tissue viability, Ph.D. thesis, Norwegian University of Science and Technology, Trondheim, 1999.

Published with permission

Ultrasound in Med. & Biol., Vol. 28, Nos. 11/12, pp. 1457–1465, 2002

0301-5629/02/$–see front matter

ELSEVIER

PII: S0301-5629(02)00614-2

● *Original Contribution*

# STRAIN DURING GASTRIC CONTRACTIONS CAN BE MEASURED USING DOPPLER ULTRASONOGRAPHY

Odd Helge Gilja,* Andreas Heimdal,† Trygve Hausken,* Hans Gregersen,‡
Knut Matre,* Arnold Berstad* and Svein Ødegaard*
*Institute of Medicine, Haukeland Hospital, University of Bergen, Bergen, Norway; †Dept. of Informatics, University of Oslo, Oslo, Norway; and ‡Department of Surgical Gastroenterology A, Aalborg Hospital and Center for Sensory-motor Interaction, Aalborg University, Aalborg, Denmark

(*Received* 6 *February* 2002; *in final form* 26 *July* 2002)

**Abstract—This study was undertaken to explore if strain of the muscle layers within the gastric wall could be measured by transabdominal strain rate imaging (SRI), a novel Doppler ultrasound (US) method. A total of 9 healthy fasting subjects (8 women, 1 man; ages 22 to 55 years) were studied and both grey-scale and Doppler US data were acquired with a 5- to 8-MHz linear transducer in cineloops of 97 to 256 frames. Rapid stepwise inflation (5 to 60 mL) of an intragastric bag was carried out and bag pressure and SRI were measured simultaneously. SRI enabled detailed studies of layers within the gastric wall in all subjects. Great variations in strain distribution of the muscle layers were found. Radial strain was much higher in the circular than in the longitudinal muscle layer. Strains derived from SRI correlated well with strains obtained with B-mode measurements (r = 0.98, $p < 0.05$). During balloon distension, we found an inverse correlation between pressure and radial strain (r = −0.87, $p < 0.05$). Intraobserver correlation of strain estimation was r = 0.98 ($p < 0.05$) and intraobserver agreement was 0.2% ± 18.6% (mean difference ± 2SD, % strain). Interobserver correlation was r = 0.84 ($p < 0.05$) and interobserver agreement was 6.9% ± 56.8%. SRI enables detailed mapping of radial strain distribution of the gastric wall and correlates well with B-mode measurements and pressure increments. (E-mail: Odd.Gilja@med.uib.no) © 2002 World Federation for Ultrasound in Medicine & Biology.**

*Key Words:* **Strain rate imaging, Ultrasonography, Gastric motility, Stomach, Doppler, Strain.**

## INTRODUCTION

Distal gastric motor function has been investigated using several methods carried out to study motility and patients with gastroparesis and functional dyspepsia. Antral hypomotility with either decreased frequency or decreased amplitude of postprandial phasic pressure waves has been reported (Malagelada and Stanghellini1985; Camilleri et al. 1986; Kerlin 1989). A wide gastric antrum was observed, both during fasting and postprandially in these patients using ultrasonography (Hausken and Berstad 1992; Hausken et al. 1993), a finding also indicated in an earlier study on gastric emptying (Bolondi et al. 1985).

Transabdominal ultrasonography is a noninvasive and radiation-free method that has proven applicable in the study of antral motility, partly due to the fact that it leaves gastric motility undisturbed (Gilja et al. 1996). Hausken and colleagues have developed duplex Doppler methods using both color and pulsed Doppler for the study of transpyloric flow (Hausken et al. 1992, 1998b, 1998a,2001). Tissue Doppler imaging (TDI) enables mapping of local tissue velocities; thus, providing information about moving walls (Uematsu et al. 1997; Bach et al. 1996; Grubb et al. 1995). In color mapping, particularly in M-mode, TDI can accurately delineate the phases of the contractions with high temporal resolution. However, the point velocity of tissue does not differentiate between actively contracting and passively following tissue. Therefore, a novel method based on strain rate imaging (SRI) and estimation of strain has been developed to enable this differentiation.

In general terms, strain is a measure of tissue deformation due to an imposed force (stress) (Gregersen and Kassab 1996; Gregersen et al. 2000; Gregersen 2000). It represents the fractional change from the original or unstressed dimension (Lagrangian strain), includes both

Address correspondence to: Odd Helge Gilja, M.D., Ph.D., Institute of Medicine, Haukeland University Hospital, N-5021 Bergen, Norway. E-mail: Odd.Gilja@med.uib.no lengthening, or expansion (positive strains), and shortening, or compression (negative strains). Strain is a dimensionless quantity, such as the Cauchy strain (Gregersen et al. 1999a, 2000; Gregersen 2000). Because zero stress lengths are impossible to measure *in vivo*, $L_0$ is replaced by the initial muscle length or the precontractile state of the antrum. Strain can alternatively be expressed as natural strain, defined as $\ln(L/L_0)$, where ln is the natural logarithm. The temporal derivative of natural strain (*i.e.*, the strain rate) is a measure of the rate of deformation. This measure is equivalent to the spatial derivative of the velocity of contraction.

Ophir and colleagues have developed ultrasonic methods for quantitative imaging of strain and elastic modulus distributions in soft tissues (Ophir et al. 1991, 2000). This method is not based on the Doppler method, but on external tissue compression with subsequent computation of the strain profile along the transducer axis. The purpose of our study was to explore the applicability of a novel ultrasound (US) Doppler method (SRI) for the measurement of Cauchy's strain in the wall of the contracting gastric antrum.

## MATERIALS AND METHODS

### *Subjects*

A total of 9 healthy volunteers, 8 women and 1 man, 22 to 55 years old (median: 24 years), entered the study. Mean body mass index was 21.9 ± 2.8 kg/m$^2$. The criteria of exclusion from the study were previous surgery of the upper GI tract, present or previous peptic ulcer, alcoholism, and pregnant or lactating women.

### *Definitions*

Strain in our context means relative strain. Strain is a measure of tissue deformation. Cauchy's strain is defined as $e = (L - L_0)/L_0$, where $L_0$ is the reference length and $L$ is the instantaneous length during loading. The reference for relative strain is the precontractile state, which constitutes a resting level; however, not necessarily zero strain.

Strain rate (SR) is defined as the temporal derivative of strain, and is a measure of the rate of deformation. See Appendix 1 for more details. Negative strain rate means that the tissue segment is becoming shorter (or thinner), and positive strain rate means that the segment is becoming longer (or thicker).

The sample size of strain is analogous to sample volume in ordinary pulsed Doppler. Sample size denotes the distance between the two measurement points along the US beam used when estimating the velocity gradient.

Phase 1 of the interdigestive motor pattern cycle is the period without any contractions seen on ultrasonography. Phase 2 denotes sporadic contractions and phase 3 is the short period of regular contractions with a frequency of 3/min, before phase 1 is restored. Fed state means the postprandial motor pattern consisting of regular contractions of 3/min, lasting much longer than the phase 3 interdigestive pattern.

### *Experimental procedure*

The protocol consisted of two different acquisition series: one of fasting contractile activity and one of responses to intragastric rapid volume distensions. The volunteers were fasting for a minimum of 8 h. They were scanned while sitting in a chair, leaning slightly backwards, with the transducer positioned in the epigastrium. US images were obtained using a digital scanner (System Five, GE Vingmed Ultrasound, Horten, Norway). We used a B-mode transducer frequency of 8 MHz during most acquisitions and a Doppler frequency of 5.7 MHz. To minimize the noise level and to decrease the Doppler sample size, the pulse repetition frequency (PRF) was set to 250 Hz. The average Doppler sample size, defined as the spatial distance between the two measurement points along the US beam, was 2.0 ± 0.6 mm (SD). The range of frames in the cine-loops was 97 to 256, with a mean of 168 frames recorded at a speed of 45 to 72 ms/frame. A typical sonogram of the antrum including the color Doppler data is shown in Fig. 1. The average maximum depth of scanning was 6 cm. All selected US cineloops were scanned while the subjects held their breath, and the data were temporarily stored on the scanner before transfer through the ethernet to a PC workstation (Dell Optiplex, Austin, TX). The workstation had a 500-MHz Pentium III processor and 250 MB of RAM. A prototype software application (tvi.exe) was used to calculate strain values from the Doppler data.

### *The strain-rate imaging method*

The velocity component $v$ of every point in the muscle is available from tissue Doppler data, so the spatial gradient can be estimated from two points along the US beam. This estimate can be performed in real-time as a small extension of the tissue Doppler data processing, and this method was termed strain rate imaging (SRI) (Heimdal et al. 1998; Stoylen et al. 1999). Because only the velocity component along the US beam is available, only the strain rate in the beam direction is estimated (Fig. 2). Subsequently, the strain rate was mapped in segments of the gastric antrum wall.

A color scheme using a transition from yellow to red for increasingly more negative strain rate (*i.e.*, shortening) and a transition from cyan to blue for increasingly more positive strain rate (*i.e.*, elongation) was chosen for 2-D and M-mode displays, see Fig. 1. In addition, strain rates near zero were colored green to facilitate the definition of areas and periods of low strain rates. This is

Published with permission



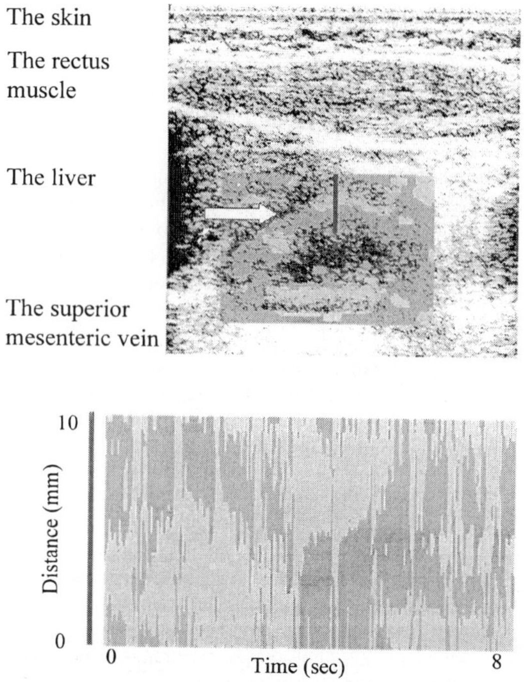


Fig. 1. (top) Photograph showing the human gastric antrum in a sagittal section with a superimposed color Doppler region for SRI. The image was acquired with a linear-array transducer at 8 MHz B-mode frequency. Different wall layers can be observed in the antrum and the main muscle layer is outlined by a white arrow. The skin, the rectus muscle, the liver and the superior mesenteric vein are also visualized. A red line depicts the distance that is viewed in anatomical M-mode. (bottom) A typical anatomical M-mode registration of SRI is shown, where blue denotes expansion and green denotes compression of tissue. The spikes on the graph correspond to the aortic pulsation.

different from tissue Doppler imaging, where there is a sharp color discontinuity around zero velocity.

In a prototype computer postprocessing program, tissue velocities and strain rate values from multiple points along an M-mode cursor line were extracted. In this software, the images showing the velocity of tissue motion were superimposed on the 2-D ultrasonic images for real-time display in color. The velocities and strain rates were also available as numerical values for quantitative analysis.

*The strain measurements*

In the postprocessing of data, we averaged our measurements over three samples in the lateral direction to the beam and of five samples in the radial beam direction, corresponding to 1.2 mm in the lateral direction and 1.0 mm in the radial direction. Gain, color rejection and tissue priority were all optimized before strain estimation started. The speed of the cineloop could be varied, adjusted to improve characterization of details. The strain calculations were done relative to the starting point of the cineloop, defined as the beginning of the contraction, as assessed visually by ultrasonography. Two main options for strain calculations existed; one (strain/motion) based on the application of a single spatial point of measurement onto the image. The other was based on curved M-mode analysis, where a line consisting of up to eight measurement points was drawn along a region-of-interest (ROI). Subsequently, time integrals were calculated either based on the labeled values or the mean or median values between the neighboring points. Ordinary B-mode images of the antrum were also analyzed with respect to measurement of the width of the proper muscle layer in a relaxed and contracted state. Based on these measurements, strain values were computed and compared to SRI data for validation purposes.

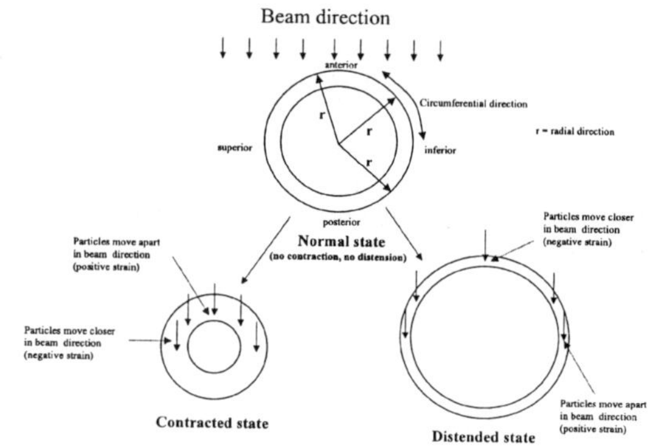


Fig. 2. The schematic drawing shows how the US beams traverse through the gastric wall. The beam direction is depicted in a normal, contracted and relaxed state of the gastric antrum and its relation to circumferential and radial strain directions.

The antral wall changes position in the image frame during a contraction; thus, inducing a potential error in strain estimation. The software inherits a built-in compensation for such movements because the intended point of measurement can be moved to track the position of the anatomical focus of interest. One SRI analysis of a single cineloop took approximately 1 min. One cineloop was traced 3 times and then the average value was recorded.

*Distension protocol*

A specially designed distension probe was constructed. The probe was 120-cm long and contained a

Published with permission



30-$\mu$m thick polyesterurethane bag 10 cm from the tip of the probe. The cylindrical bag was 5-cm long and could be inflated with fluid through an infusion channel of 3.5 mm to a diameter of 40 mm without stretching the bag wall. The probe contained a metal clip in the middle of the bag as a marker for US. Two side-holes for pressure measurements were placed in the middle of the bag and 2-cm proximal to the bag. The lumens and side-holes both had diameters of 0.5 mm. The perfusion rate for the pressure channels was 0.1 mL $min^{-1}$. The pressure was measured by a low compliance perfusion system connected to external transducers (Medex, Denmark). The pressure data were amplified and analog-to-digital converted at a sampling rate of 10 Hz using a motility data-acquisition system (Gatehouse Ltd., Nørresundby, Denmark). The digitized data were stored on a PC for later analysis in the same software.

After calibrating the measurement system, the tube was passed into the stomach *via* the nostrils. A manometric investigation was carried out to evaluate the position of the catheter and to confirm that the contractile pattern was consistent with phase 1. The middle of the balloon was then placed approximately 3 cm proximal to the pylorus. The position of the catheter was also visualized by ultrasonography. In one subject, fluoroscopic guidance was necessary to ensure correct position of the balloon. The zero pressure level for the distension series was determined before the distension protocol was performed as a volume-controlled series. The fluid volume of the bag was changed intermittently with volumes ranging from 5 to 60 mL for 1-min periods using a hand-held syringe. The volume infusions were done manually as fast as it was possible to empty the syringe volume. The distensions were separated by 2-min resting periods (*i.e.,* the volume was withdrawn from the bag and the bag pressure was kept slightly negative during these periods to ensure complete emptying of the bag). SRI was performed simultaneously with the infusion of water into the balloon. A mark on the skin, as well as the localization of the metal marker on the probe, ensured that the same area was scanned each time.

*Variability experiments*

Two independent observers (O. H. Gilja and T. Hausken) estimated intra- and interobserver variabilities of the strain calculations. A total of 14 data sets were analyzed twice by each observer using the dedicated software program, and the mean result was recorded. Some data sets were utilized more than once and traced at different portions of the gastric wall. Because of relatively high strain variations in the different portions of the wall (see results), the two observers had to agree on which part of the antrum to measure before the actual tracing was performed.

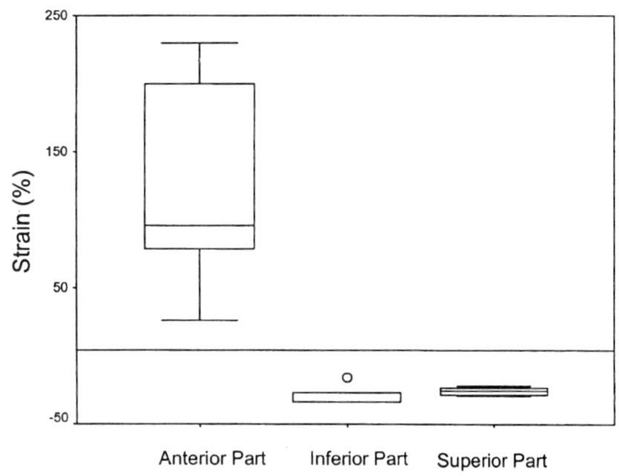


Fig. 3. The box plot shows the magnitude and the differences in strain (%) of the anterior, inferior and superior part of the muscularis propria in a sagittal section of the gastric antrum. Data were acquired in a radial direction by SRI using Doppler ultrasonography.

*Statistical analysis*

Median values and interquartile ranges were calculated and reported, if not otherwise specifically noted. Coefficient of correlation was computed for intra- and interobserver analysis. Limits of agreement were determined as suggested by Bland and Altmann (1986) to evaluate intra- and interobserver agreement. The level of statistical significance was $p < 0.05$. All statistical calculations and graphic designs were performed using commercially available software.

*Ethical aspects*

The study was approved by the regional ethic committee and was conducted in accordance with the revised Declaration of Helsinki. All volunteers gave written, informed consent to participate in the trial.

## RESULTS

High-frequency real-time ultrasonography and SRI enabled detailed studies of layers within the gastric wall in all subjects. Most of the antral contractions were obtained in phase II according to ultrasonographic evaluation, but one of the contractions was of phase III origin. The anterior part of the gastric antrum was more accessible for SRI than the other parts of the antral circumference. A high positive radial strain was found in the anterior part of the gastric wall (96%); 163% (median values; interquartile range) during contraction. Negative strain was found in the inferior part (−33%, 23%) and in the superior part (−25%, 6%) (circumferential strain), see Fig. 3. The posterior part of the antral circumference

Published with permission



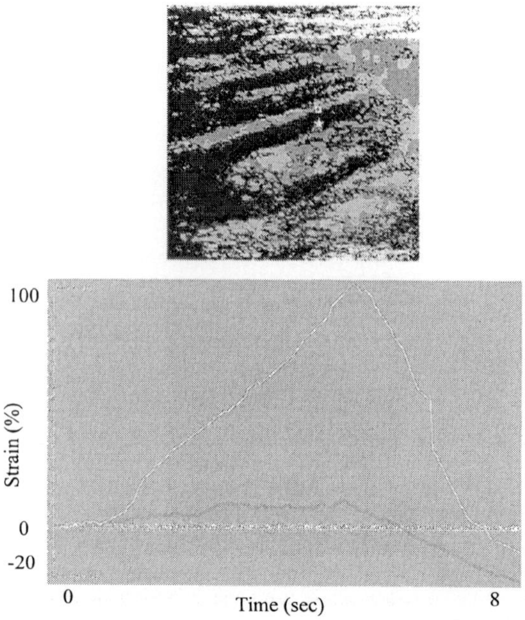


Fig. 4. These graphics outline the difference in strain of the circular vs. the longitudinal muscle layer of the antral wall. (top) The exact sampling points in the gastric wall are denoted with a square and an asterix in the ultrasonogram. Blue denotes expansion and green denotes compression of tissue. (bottom) The difference between the high positive strain (elongation) of the circular (inner) muscle layer and the low strain of the longitudinal (outer) muscle layer, illustrates the separate biomechanical events in the two portions of the main muscle layer. The green line corresponds to the red square and the yellow line corresponds to the white asterisk (inner circular muscle layer). The data were obtained in a radial direction.

was frequently difficult to image adequately for SRI analysis due to movement of luminal particles and the long distance from the scan head.

Local mapping of radial strain distributions of the anterior part of the muscle layers was enabled with this Doppler-based method. In three individuals, it was possible, due to a combination of high resolution and a slim body habitus, to distinguish between strain in the longitudinal and circular muscle layers. During contractions, radial strain was significantly higher in the circular muscle layer compared to the longitudinal layer, where radial strain was closer to zero (*e.g.*, 105% vs. 10%, see Fig. 4). Measurements of the proper muscle diameters on the B-mode ultrasonograms showed good correlation with SRI measurements ($r = 0.98, p < 0.05$), as visualized in Fig. 5. The mean difference was 0.8% and the limits of agreement were −28.6% to 30.2%.

The intraobserver correlation between two observers calculating radial strain using the designed software was

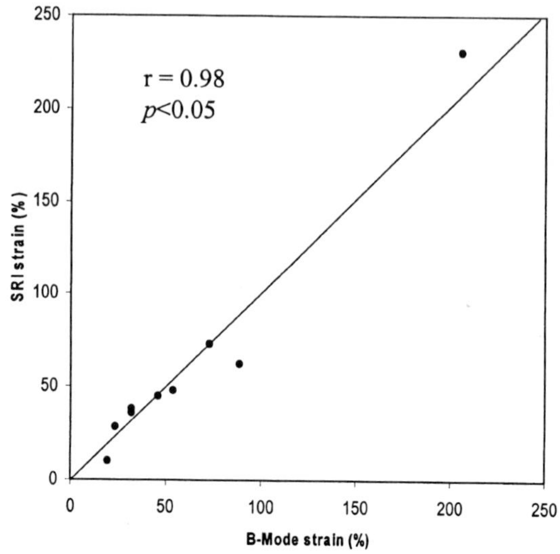


Fig. 5. This scatter plot shows the association between strain measured by Doppler ultrasonography and deformation calculated by radial measurements on the ordinary B-mode images. The line of identity is drawn.

$r = 0.98$ ($p < 0.01$) (Fig. 6) and the intraobserver agreement was 0.2% ± 18.6% (mean difference ± 2 SD, % strain) (Fig. 7). The interobserver correlation was $r = 0.84$ (Fig. 8) and the interobserver agreement was 6.9% ± 56.8% (Fig. 9). However, as observed in Fig. 8, there

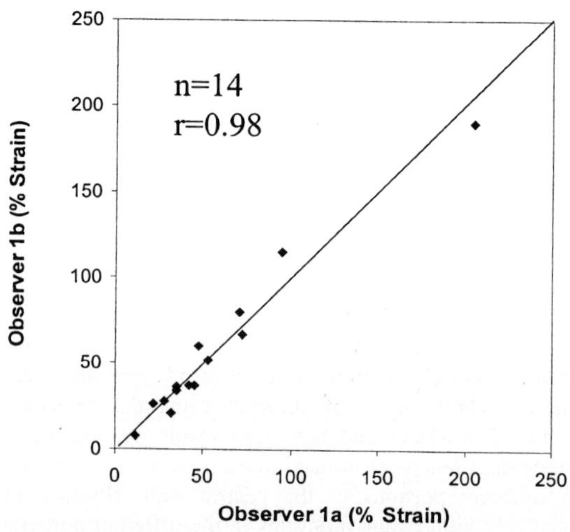


Fig. 6. Scatter plot showing the intraobserver correlation of strain in the antral muscle layer using SRI. The line of identity is drawn.

Published with permission



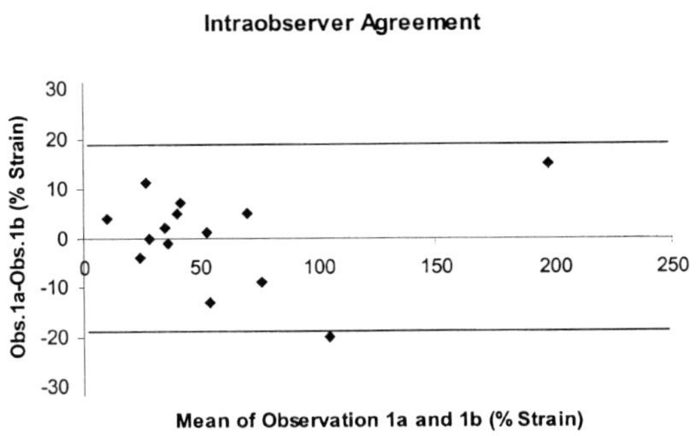


Fig. 7. Plot displaying the intraobserver agreement of strain calculation in antral wall muscle using SRI. The difference between the two observations (Obs 1a – Obs 1b) is depicted on the y-axis. The average of the two observations is plotted along the x-axis. The intraobserver agreement was 0.2% ± 18.6% (mean difference ± 2 SD, % strain), displaying no proportional error effect.

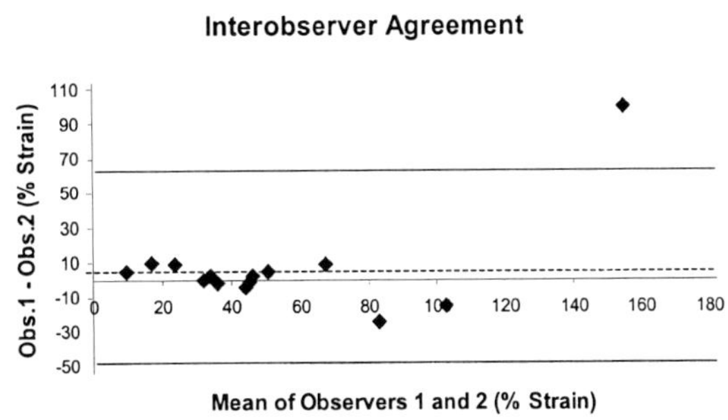


Fig. 9. Interobserver agreement of strain calculation in antral wall muscle using SRI. The difference between the 2 observers (Obs 1 – Obs 2) is depicted on the y-axis. Mean of the two observers is plotted along the x-axis. The interobserver agreement was 6.9% ± 56.8% (mean difference ± 2 SD, % strain). However, if the outlier was excluded, interobserver agreement was −0.3% ± 19.6%.

is an obvious outlier in the data, representing the only phase 3 measurement in this study. A phase 3 contraction has much more complex and dynamic movements compared to phase 2 contractions. If we exclude the outlier of the phase 3 contraction, the correlation coefficient is 0.95 and limits of agreement are −0.3% ± 19.6% for the interobserver variation

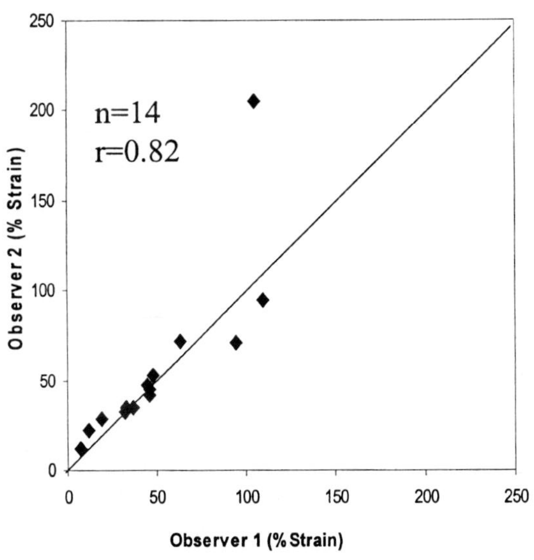


Fig. 8. Scatter plot showing the interobserver correlation of strain in the antral muscle layer by using SRI. The line of identity is drawn.

During distensions, we observed that SRI could discriminate between active and passive deformation of the gastric muscle layer. The regular distension pattern was negative radial strain in the anterior wall in response to sudden pressure increments. However, two other distinct patterns were noted during careful postprocessing of image data; distension on contraction (the balloon was inflated when a barely visible contraction had already started) or contraction on distension (the gastric wall was compressing the balloon undergoing inflation). Accordingly, SRI was able to discriminate between active and passive deformation of the wall, not observed during ordinary 2-D scanning. We found an inverse significant relationship between radial strain estimated by SRI and maximum intraballoon pressure ($r = -0.87$, $p < 0.05$) during distension (Fig. 10).

## DISCUSSION

For the first time, a noninvasive method based on Doppler ultrasonography was applied to estimate strain in moving gastrointestinal tissue in humans. In this pilot study, SRI demonstrated high spatial and temporal resolution facilitating detailed analysis of contracting gastric smooth muscle. Using SRI, it was possible to discern biomechanical events in the inner circular vs. the outer longitudinal muscle layer of the antral wall, a phenomenon not observed during ordinary 2-D scanning. Furthermore, SRI enabled mapping of local strain distribution within a muscle layer showing the existence of significant strain variations within small areas.

Gastrointestinal strain is a measure of regional deformation and, by definition, negative strain means shortening and positive strain elongation. SRI is an extension

Published with permission



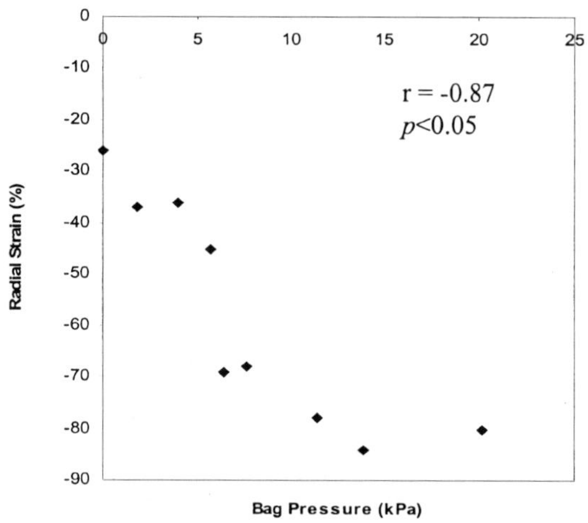


Fig. 10. Scatter plot demonstrating the association between radial strain estimated using SRI and volume infusion into a balloon distending the antrum. A significant negative correlation is depicted, showing that, as increasing volume is distending the antrum, an increasing negative strain (shortening) is measured radially in the anterior proper muscle layer of the wall.

of existing tissue Doppler methods and makes measurement of deformation possible (Sutherland et al. 1999). Recently, SRI was used to quantify myocardial movement (Voigt et al. 2000; Stoylen et al. 1999) and to assess coronary artery disease (Stoylen et al. 2000; Belohlavek et al. 2001). In a study in anesthetized dogs, SRI was validated against sonomicrometry as a reference method (Urheim et al. 2000). The authors found that, after placing longitudinal ultrasonic segment-length crystals in contracting tissue, strain by Doppler correlated well with strain by sonomicrometry. They concluded that strain estimation by this novel Doppler ultrasonography represented a powerful method for quantifying regional muscle function, and was less influenced by tethering effects than ordinary Doppler tissue imaging. In our study, we found a significant association between SRI measurements and strain calculated on the basis of metric data obtained directly from the B-mode images. Furthermore, intra- and interobserver variabilities of the strain measurements made by SRI were acceptable. SRI correlated well with pressure increments following distension of the antrum by a balloon, showing that strain measured by the SRI method is associated to the pressure force generated by the antral muscle.

Interestingly, we found that the outer longitudinal muscle layer of the antral wall had different strain levels than the inner circular muscle layer during a contraction. When radial strain was measured, the longitudinal layer exhibited a relatively low negative strain (shortening) and the circular muscle layer had higher positive strain (elongation) (Gregersen et al. 1999b). Previously, the separation of the inner and outer muscle layer has been demonstrated with endoluminal ultrasonography with increasing transducer frequencies (Taniguchi et al. 1993, 1995). In these studies, a miniaturized US device attached to the gastrointestinal mucosa by suction has been used to examine motility of esophageal wall layers using M-mode. In that study, an average of 83% thickening of the inner circular muscle layer was observed during contractions. In the present study, a typical reading is shown in Fig. 4, where the positive strain of the circular layer was 105% and strain of the longitudinal layer was approximately 10%. Accordingly, this study shows that the inner circular layer constitutes the driving force during contraction and that the outer layer passively follows the movements during this sequence of phase II contractile activity of the antral wall muscle.

To be able to distinguish between the outer and inner muscle layer of muscularis propria of the antral wall, the scanner was preset to a very small strain sample size (average 2 mm), which determines the spatial resolution of the strain estimates. We also took care in not applying too much manual force with the scan head to avoid pressure effects on the gastric wall (Odegaard et al. 1992). However, when a small sample size was used for calculating the strain rate, the random noise became relatively larger. The demand for high spatial resolution was compromised by lower SNR. To reduce the noise, multiple samples from a longer segment along the M-mode beam were averaged during analysis using dedicated software. Furthermore, by the integration procedure from SR to strain the random noise was considerably reduced, and we obtained relatively smooth strain curves.

Generally, SRI is limited by the same factors that hamper routine ultrasonography, namely, bowel gas and excessive abdominal fat. However, for ultrasonography of the fasting gastric antrum, gas is seldom a problem for image quality. In our study, the volunteers had normal body habitus and luminal gas was not a significant problem. Another limitation of SRI is marked angle-dependency, more so than for other Doppler modalities. This is due to the fundamental difference between measurement of fluid velocities where particles move freely, and tissue velocities in solid structures where deformation in one direction is always associated with deformation in other directions to keep the volume of the structure constant. To minimize this problem, we took care in aligning the US beams as perpendicular to the anterior part of the muscle as possible; thus, measuring only the axial strain component. While evaluating intra- and interobserver agreement, we observed relatively large variations in our

Published with permission



strain estimates. This was due partly to the need for selecting a very small strain sample to be able to distinguish the inner and outer muscle layers. Furthermore, we studied a variety of gastric contractions ranging from early phase 2 to phase 3 and, in future studies, variability can probably be reduced by omitting outliers originating from other phases of the interdigestive motor cycle. The data provided by the SRI technique can likely be used for further mechanical analysis, such as to compute longitudinal strains using incompressibility assumptions and to derive mechanical parameters from pressure-strain relationships.

In conclusion, we found that Doppler examination based on SRI and dedicated software can be used to noninvasively obtain biomechanical information of the contracting gastric antrum. Fasting antral contractions have different strain distributions within the muscle layers and the circular and longitudinal muscle layers show different strain levels. Moreover, SRI enables discrimination between active and passive deformation of the gastric muscle layer during distension. The high temporal and spatial resolutions inherent in SRI offer very detailed transabdominal imaging, but further studies are needed to establish the precise role of this method, improve the technique to reduce variance in the recorded strain and to investigate possible clinical applications.

*Acknowledgments*—This study was supported by grants from Innovest Strategic Research Programme, Haukeland University Hospital, Bergen, Norway; the Karen Elise Jensens Foundation; the Scandinavian Association for Gastrointestinal Motility (SAGIM); and the Danish Technical Research Council. The authors are grateful for the technical support from GE Vingmed Ultrasound, Horten, Norway.

## REFERENCES

Bach DS, Armstrong WF, Donovan CL, Muller DW. Quantitative Doppler tissue imaging for assessment of regional myocardial velocities during transient ischemia and reperfusion. Am Heart J 1996;132:721–725.

Belohlavek M, Pislaru C, Bae RY, Greenleaf JF, Seward JB. Real-time strain rate echocardiographic imaging: Temporal and spatial analysis of postsystolic compression in acutely ischemic myocardium. J Am Soc Echocardiogr 2001;14:360–369.

Bland JM, Altmann DG. Statistical methods for assessing agreement between two methods of clinical measurements. Lancet 1986;1: 307–310.

Bolondi L, Bortolotti M, Santi V, et al. Measurement of gastric emptying time by real-time ultrasonography. Gastroenterology 1985; 89:752–759.

Camilleri M, Malagelada JR, Kao PC, Zinsmeister AR. Gastric and autonomic responses to stress in functional dyspepsia. Dig Dis Sci 1986;31:1169–1177.

Gilja OH, Hausken T, Odegaard S, Berstad A. Three-dimensional ultrasonography of the gastric antrum in patients with functional dyspepsia. Scand J Gastroenterol 1996;31:847–855.

Gregersen H. Residual strain in the gastrointestinal tract: A new concept. Neurogastroenterol Motil 2000;12:411–414.

Gregersen H, Barlow J, Thompson D. Development of a computer-controlled tensiometer for real-time measurements of tension in tubular organs. Neurogastroenterol Motil 1999a;11:109–118.

Gregersen H, Kassab GS. Biomechanics of the gastrointestinal tract. Neurogastroenterol Motil 1996;8:77–97.

Gregersen H, Kassab GS, Fung YC. The zero-stress state of the gastrointestinal tract: Biomechanical and functional implications. Dig Dis Sci 2000;45:2271–2281.

Gregersen H, Lee TC, Chien S, Skalak R, Fung YC. Strain distribution in the layered wall of the esophagus. J Biomech Eng 1999b;121: 442–448.

Grubb NR, Fleming A, Sutherland GR, Fox KA. Skeletal muscle contraction in healthy volunteers: Assessment with Doppler tissue imaging. Radiology 1995;194:837–842.

Hausken T, Berstad A. Wide gastric antrum in patients with non-ulcer dyspepsia. Effect of cisapride. Scand J Gastroenterol 1992;27:427–432.

Hausken T, Gilja OH, Odegaard S, Berstad A. Flow across the human pylorus soon after ingestion of food, studied with duplex sonography. Effect of glyceryl trinitrate. Scand J Gastroenterol 1998a;33: 484–490.

Hausken T, Gilja OH, Undeland KA, Berstad A. Timing of postprandial dyspeptic symptoms and transpyloric passage of gastric contents. Scand J Gastroenterol 1998b;33:822–827.

Hausken T, Goldman B, Leotta DF, Odegaard S, Martin RW, Quantification of gastric emptying and duodenogastric reflux stroke volumes using three-dimensional guided digital color Doppler imaging. Eur J Ultrasound 2001(in press).

Hausken T, Odegaard S, Matre K, Berstad A. Antroduodenal motility and movements of luminal contents studied by duplex sonography. Gastroenterology 1992;102:1583–1590.

Hausken T, Svebak S, Wilhelmsen I, et al. Low vagal tone and antral dysmotility in patients with functional dyspepsia. Psychosom Med 1993;55:12–22.

Heimdal A, Stoylen A, Torp H, Skjaerpe T. Real-time strain rate imaging of the left ventricle by ultrasound. J Am Soc Echocardiogr 1998;11:1013–1019.

Kerlin P. Postprandial antral hypomotility in patients with idiopathic nausea and vomiting. Gut 1989;30:54–59.

Malagelada JR, Stanghellini V. Manometric evaluation of functional upper gut symptoms. Gastroenterology 1985;88:1223–1231.

Odegaard S, Kimmey MB, Martin RW, et al. The effects of applied pressure on the thickness, layers, and echogenicity of gastrointestinal wall ultrasound images. Gastrointest Endosc 1992;38:351–356.

Ophir J, Cespedes I, Ponnekanti H, Yazdi Y, Li X. Elastography: A quantitative method for imaging the elasticity of biological tissues. Ultrason Imaging 1991;13:111–134.

Ophir J, Garra B, Kallel F, et al. Elastographic imaging. Ultrasound Med Biol 2000;26(Suppl. 1):S23–S29.

Stoylen A, Heimdal A, Bjornstad K, Torp HG, Skjaerpe T. Strain rate imaging by ultrasound in the diagnosis of regional dysfunction of the left ventricle. Echocardiography 1999;16:321–329.

Stoylen A, Heimdal A, Bjornstad K, et al. Strain rate imaging by ultrasonography in the diagnosis of coronary artery disease. J Am Soc Echocardiogr 2000;13:1053–1064.

Sutherland GR, Kukulski T, Voight JU, D'hooge J. Tissue Doppler echocardiography. Future developments. Echocardiography 1999; 16:509–520.

Taniguchi DK, Martin RW, Trowers EA, et al. Changes in esophageal wall layers during motility: Measurements with a new miniature ultrasound suction device. Gastrointest Endosc 1993;39:146–152.

Taniguchi DK, Martin RW, Trowers EA, Silverstein FE. Simultaneous M-mode echoesophagram and manometry in the sheep esophagus. Gastrointest Endosc 1995;41:582–586.

Uematsu M, Nakatani S, Yamagishi M, Matsuda H, Miyatake K. Usefulness of myocardial velocity gradient derived from two-dimensional tissue Doppler imaging as an indicator of regional myocardial contraction independent of translational motion assessed in atrial septal defect. Am J Cardiol 1997;79:237–241.

Urheim S, Edvardsen T, Torp H, Angelsen B, Smiseth OA. Myocardial strain by Doppler echocardiography. Validation of a new method to quantify regional myocardial function. Circulation 2000;102:1158–1164.

Published with permission



Voigt JU, Arnold MF, Karlsson M, et al. Assessment of regional longitudinal myocardial strain rate derived from doppler myocardial imaging indexes in normal and infarcted myocardium. J Am Soc Echocardiogr 2000;13:588–598.

## APPENDIX

This appendix describes the concept of strain and strain rate, and how these entities can be estimated from the Doppler velocities. In general terms, strain means relative deformation, and strain rate means rate of deformation. If an object has an initial length $L_0$ that, after a certain time, changes to $L$, strain is defined as:

$$e = \frac{L - L_0}{L_0}. \tag{1A}$$

The instantaneous change in length (d$L$) in a small time increment (d$t$) is related to the velocities ($\nu_1$ and $\nu_2$) of the end points of the object:

$$dL = (\nu_2 - \nu_1)dt \tag{2A}$$

By dividing eqn (2A) with $L$, we see that the instantaneous change in length per unit length equals the velocity gradient times the time increment:

$$\frac{dL}{L} = \frac{\nu_2 - \nu_1}{L} dt. \tag{3A}$$

Because it is not feasible to track the end points of the object, the velocity gradient is estimated from two points with a fixed distance:

$$\frac{dL}{L} \approx \frac{\nu(r + \Delta r) - \nu(r)}{\Delta r} dt = \text{SR } dt. \tag{4A}$$

The velocity gradient estimate is termed strain rate (SR). Finally, by integrating this equation, we arrive at:

$$\log \frac{L}{L_0} = \int_{t_0}^{t} \text{SR } dt, \tag{5A}$$

where "log" denotes the natural logarithm. This gives the following relation between strain rate estimated by velocity gradient and strain:

$$e = \exp\left(\int_{t_0}^{t} \text{SR } dt\right) - 1. \tag{6A}$$

CHAPTER 9

# THREE-DIMENSIONAL ULTRASONOGRAPHY IN GASTROENTEROLOGY

ODD HELGE GILJA AND ROY MARTIN

Ultrasonography is widely used in the diagnosis and follow-up of patients with gastrointestinal diseases, and is incorporated into the daily routine in many clinics worldwide. Dedicated methods, such as endoscopic ultrasonography, has further expanded the options for diagnostic ultrasound in the field of gastroenterology and hepatology. The digital revolution has made 3D ultrasonography a natural extension of 2D ultrasound scanning. Most frequently, this is made by stacking serial 2D ultrasonograms together and utilizing computerized algorithms and equipment to process and display the data. However, in recent years, 2D array matrix probes has been developed to enable real-time 3D scanning.

## 1. Formation of 3D Ultrasonographic Images

If the relative position in space of a series of 2D sonograms is recorded along with the image data, three-dimensional (3D) ultrasonographic images can be constructed. For most applications, the process of making 3D images based on ultrasonography is divided into 5 major steps: Data acquisition, digitization, storage, processing, and display.

### 1.1. *Data acquisition*

Principally, data acquisition by 3D ultrasonography can be performed in 3 different ways (1). Sampling of data may be carried out either by using a 2D probe attached to a motor which moves the probe in a computer-defined way, or by a spatial localizing system connected to a 2D probe, or by electronic 3D probes with the possibility of direct volume acquisition in real time.

First, and most frequently used, are ordinary 2D probes which are inserted into motorized holders and either rotated (2, 3), translated (4–8), or tilted (9–15) to acquire a data volume. The rotation scanning is often applied to cardiac imaging while acquisition by tilting or translating is frequently used for transcutaneous abdominal and obstetric scanning. Pullback devices have also been constructed to aid intravascular and intraductal scanning where the transducer is positioned at a distant site in relation to the mechanical holder (16–18).

Second, acquisition of ultrasonographic data can be assisted by devices that record the exact position and movements of the transducer in space. This has been obtained by utilizing mechanical arms (19) (20–24), acoustic sensors (25–29), or magnetic sensors (30–34). A magnetic sensor and a transducer is depicted in Fig. 1. Furthermore, gyroscopic and optical devices can be applied to follow the position of the scanhead.

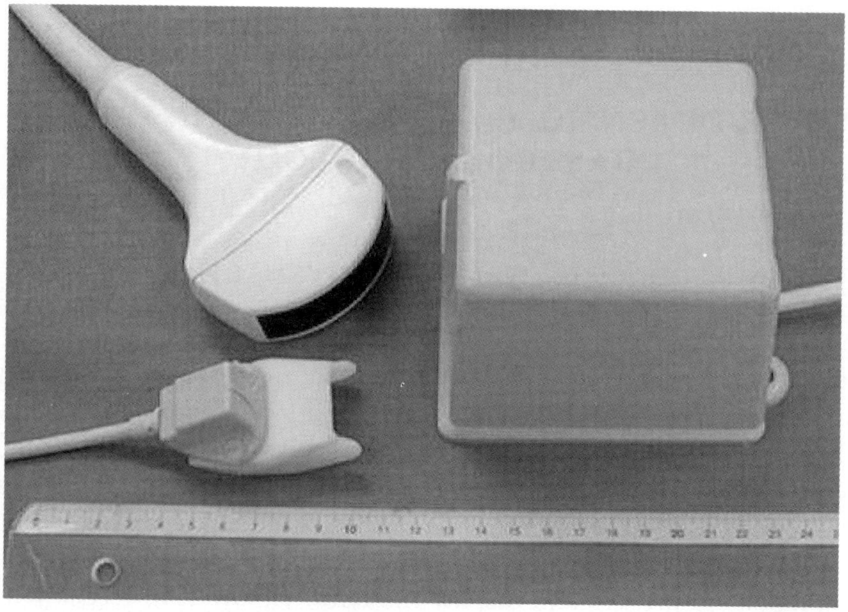

Fig. 1. Photo showing an electromagnetic sensor, a field generator and a 3.5 MHz curved array scanhead. This system enables handheld, flexible scanning of large volumes of interest and position, orientation, and image data can be combined to facilitate 3D reconstruction of organs.

Third, true volumetric 2D array transducers have been developed (35). Such complex transducers will generate a pyramidal volume of ultrasound data, enabling dynamic real-time 3D ultrasonography.

### 1.2. *Data digitization*

Ultrasound raw data are available in a digital format within most scanners. However, many of the commercially available ultrasound scanners generate analogue output signals. Therefore, in order to be processed by a computer, conversion of ultrasonographic data into a digital format is necessary. Frequently, this is done by video frame grabbing using designated hardware cards in the computer or in the scanner. However, frame grabbing of video signals impairs image resolution. Preferably, the raw data of the ultrasound images is digitized directly maintaining the original resolution.

### 1.3. *Data storage*

Following data capture and digitization, the image data is normally stored temporarily until computer processing can take place. Analogue videotape is still sometimes used as a storage medium for ultrasonographic images because of its availability and low cost. However, its inherent deficiencies include signal degradation, noise, and the need to digitize images before 3D processing. High resolution 3D ultrasound data give rise to large image files necessitating high capacity storage media's like magneto-optical disks, digital tapes, or hard disks. The ultimate goal in 3D ultrasonography is to obviate the data storage operation and perform direct data processing and volume estimation in real time, and subsequently store only the clinically relevant images and measurements.

### 1.4. *Data processing*

Depending on the mode of acquisition, the image data can be prepared in different ways (36). Only the mainstream flowchart of processing will be outlined here.

First, the image data must be converted to a rectangular (Cartesian) co-ordinate system. Image points are assigned to new positions within a cuberille (regular data volume) on the basis of their pyramidal (if tilting acquisition) co-ordinates. This scan-conversion is usually relatively time consuming and is performed by computer algorithms.

Second, mathematical interpolation is performed to generate values that "fill in the gaps" between 2D slices that are stacked together in the cuberille. After scan-conversion and interpolation, the pixels can be treated as spatially correct 3D image elements known as voxels.

Third, methods for image enhancement are usually applied to improve the contrast of the image and remove artifacts. These techniques include filtering, histogram stretching and sliding, and morphologic operations. This step may be important to the overall quality of the final 3D ultrasound image but may not be of great importance in volume measurements. Image enhancement represents an uncertainty because significant clinical information can be lost in the operation.

Fourth, the cube of image data is now ready for segmentation; that is the procedure where the object of interest is separated from the surrounding structures in order to be displayed meaningfully (37). Three fundamental approaches to segmentation have been utilized in 3D ultrasonography: extraction by visual inspection and manual outlining of contours; semi-automatic separation using visualization algorithms (38) aided by operator interaction; and fully automatic computer segmentation. The latter method is capable of detecting edges with high contrast, but is subject to inaccuracies and artifact production. Therefore, automatic segmentation must be used with great care if applied to patient data. Manual segmentation of structures in the 3D data set makes accurate volume estimation and reconstruction of organs or pathologic tissue achievable. This method, which primarily supplies quantitative information, is applicable to all areas of sonographic imaging where volume calculation is indicated.

### 1.5. *Data display*

The final step in the formation of 3D ultrasound images is to display the data so that the inherent voxel information is communicated accurately. Commonly, simple rotation of the object on the computer monitor can provide some 3D effects. Tomographic display of orthogonal sections or even arbitrary sections are widely used to depict the results of 3D ultrasonography. In particular, arbitrarily slicing in the 3D image allows the user to define unique planes to demonstrate structures that may not be oriented along a rectangular 3D grid. To further enhance the 3D outcome of the images, stereoglasses have been applied (39, 40). Projection of images by optical holography enables the observer to move around the

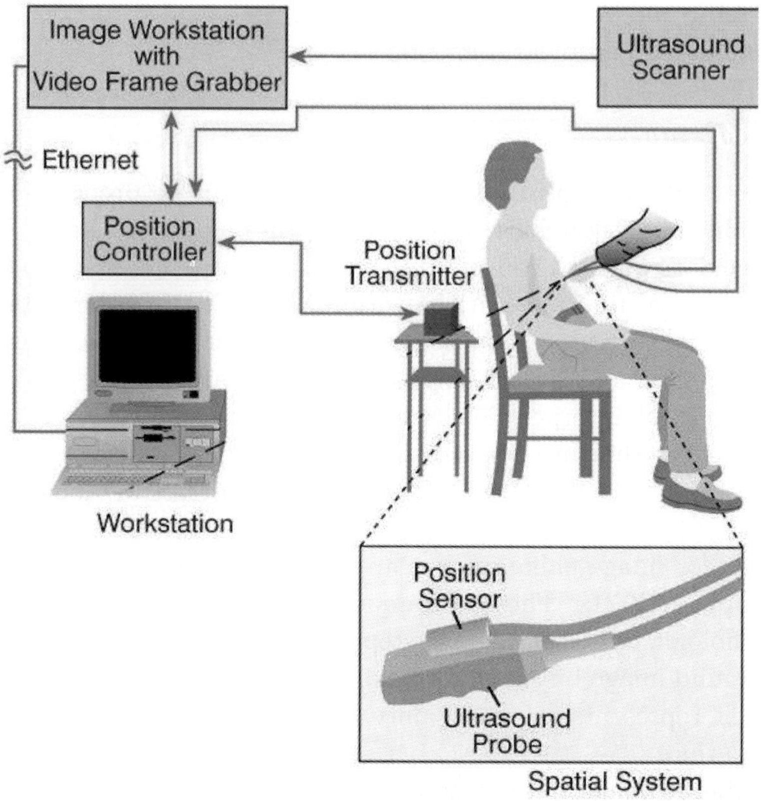


Fig. 2. Block diagram of a 3D ultrasound system based on magnetic position and orientation measurement (POM). Image and POM data are acquired simultaneously and the ultrasonograms are digitized from the video output of the scanner by use of a frame grabber board or directly from raw data from scanner. The data is ultimately analyzed on a PC workstation.

object and examine the spatial relationships from different viewpoints (41–43). A typical setup of a 3D ultrasound system is shown in Fig. 2.

Data processing and display requires specialized computer software to handle the ultrasound images. We have, in collaboration with Christian Michelsen Research (Bergen, Norway) and Vingmed Sound (Horten, Norway) developed a software package; EchoPac3D® (44). EchoPac3D enable import of image data that are acquired both with mechanical devices and magnetic position sensors, as well as endosonographic acquisitions. Manual segmentation or semiautomatic rendering of structures in the 3D data set makes accurate volume estimation and reconstruction of organs or pathologic tissue achievable. The accuracy of volume estimation in this software package has been evaluated in several studies (45–47). A display of the EchoPac3D software is shown in Fig. 3. The 3D ultrasound system used in our lab is outlined more in depth in a previous review (48).

Ultrasound data contains a significant amount of noise and speckle and may exhibit boundary regions several pixels wide. It is important to keep in mind that the quality of the final 3D data display strongly depends on the resolution of the raw data. Transducer frequency and lateral resolution, frame rate of the scanner, accuracy of 3D probe, speed of scanning, methods of filtering and segmentation, are all factors that influences the final

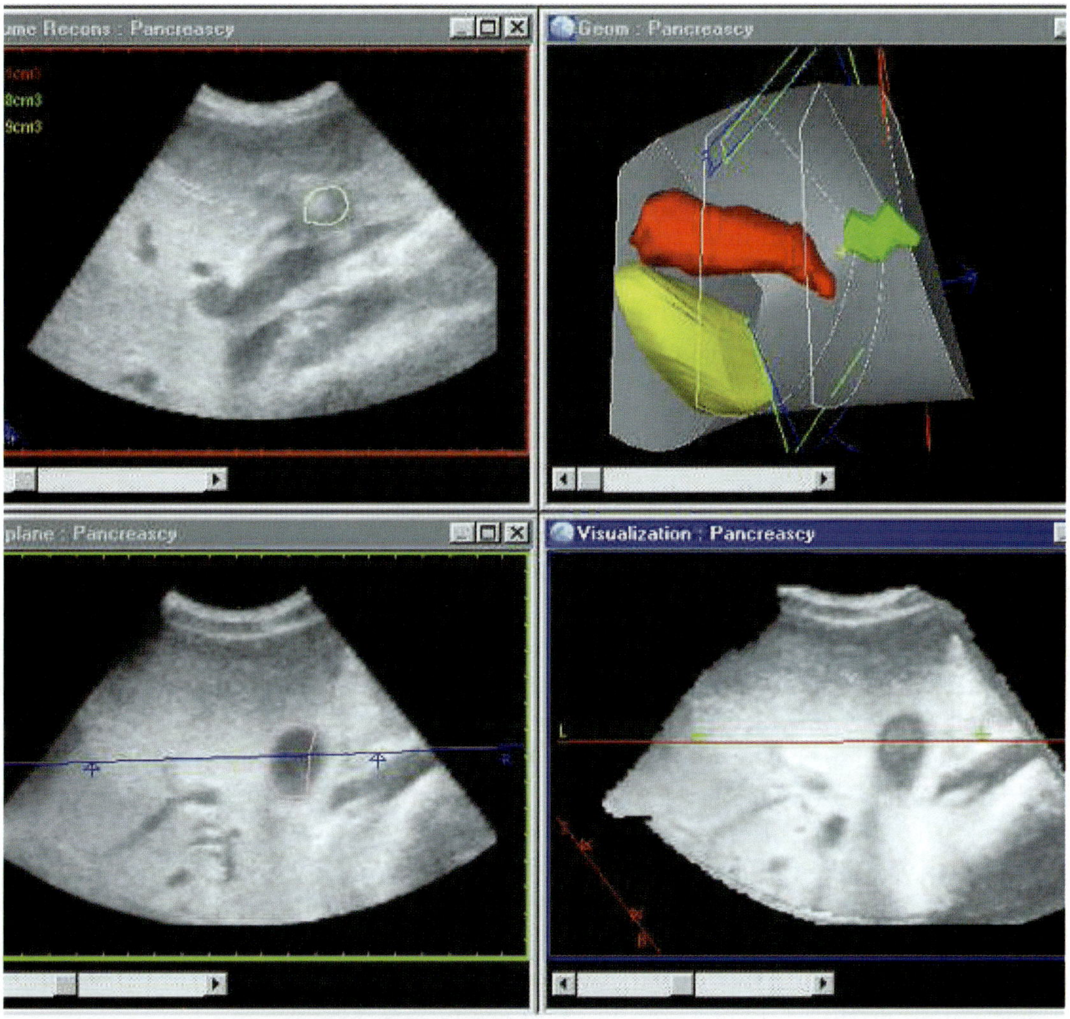


Fig. 3. A display of EchoPac3D® software manufactured by GE-Vingmed Sound (Horten, Norway). In the upper right panel, the green volume is a pancreatic cyst, the red volume is the gallbladder, and the yellow volume depicts part of the liver. In the upper left panel, the measurement and analysis window is shown. The visualization window, enabling application of numerous algorithms, is shown in the lower right panel. In the lower left panel, a slicer window is shown. The EchoPac3D® software enables quick and intuitive post-processing of 3D ultrasonographic images.

image and subsequently volume measurements. Furthermore, there is no advantage in sampling over a spatial scale that is much smaller than the resolution cell of the display system. The ultrasound sampling conditions using a specific transducer is closely related to the display parameters.

## 2. 3D Ultrasonography of the Stomach

Two-dimensional (2D) ultrasonography has been utilized to assess gastric emptying in patients with functional dyspepsia (49–51), diabetes mellitus (52), and in infants with gastroesophageal reflux (53). In several studies, repeated single 2D ultrasonic sections of the antrum have been applied to measure gastric emptying rates (50–52, 54, 55). To estimate volumes of the gastric antrum by means of 2D ultrasound, a sum-of-cylinders method (56) and simple formulas (49) have been used. Early attempts were also made to calculate total stomach volumes, but were never properly validated (19, 57). Volume estimation based on 2D sonograms is subject to significant error because assumptions regarding geometrical shape of the antrum need to be made before reliable volume measurements can be performed.

To overcome these limitations, a method for volume estimation of organs and tissue based on three-dimensional (3D) ultrasonography was developed (45). Using a motor device, the transducer was tilted through an angle of 90, capturing sequential 2D-frames before the data set was transferred to a graphic workstation for final 3D processing. This 3D ultrasound system demonstrated excellent accuracy *in vitro* both on phantoms (46) and on animal organs (45), and intra- and interobserver variation was low. When validated *in vivo* against Magnetic Resonance Imaging, this 3D ultrasound system was in good agreement and presented high precision (47). This system has also been used to study diseases of the liver (58), and to evaluate patients with functional dyspepsia (59–61). Despite the significant achievements with respect to accuracy in volume estimation and 3D reconstruction of tissue and organs, this 3D system could only acquire a 90° fan-like data set from a pre-determined, single position of the transducer. Accordingly, a mechanical system like this poses a great limitation to acquisition, because only relatively small volumes can be captured.

Random acquisition of 3D ultrasound data has been achieved by utilizing different devices to locate the exact position and orientation of the transducer in space. To enable scanning of a large organ like the fluid-filled stomach, a commercially available magnetometer-based position and orientation measurement (POM) device was interfaced. This system for magnetic scanhead tracking was validated both with respect to its precision in locating specific points in space (30) and to its accuracy in volume estimation (31, 62). In these studies, the sensor system worked satisfactorily in scanning human organs, and high precision and accuracy were revealed in volume estimation. For the first time, total gastric volumes and intragastric distribution of meals could be studied by ultrasonography (63). In this study, the depth of scanning was adjusted to fit each individual's habitus, averaging 17.6 cm. Sagittal sections of the stomach were recorded throughout its entire length, starting in the proximal part where the transducer was positioned by the left subcostal margin and tilted cranially to image the most superior part of the stomach. After stepwise scanning of the proximal stomach angling from left to right, the transducer was moved and held to insonicate normally to the skin surface. Then the distal stomach was scanned stepwise moving distally to the gastroduodenal junction. The image data and the position and orientation data were transferred to a workstation for final processing. A 3D reconstruction of the total stomach volume based on magnetic scanhead tracking is depicted in Fig. 4. The most difficult part of this scanning technique is to ensure that the complete proximal part of the stomach volume is captured.

However, the stomach is a large and geometrically complex organ to study by ultrasonography. Therefore , we have made some efforts trying to validate this 3D ultrasonographic method *in vivo* in healthy controls. A barostat bag were positioned in the proximal stomach

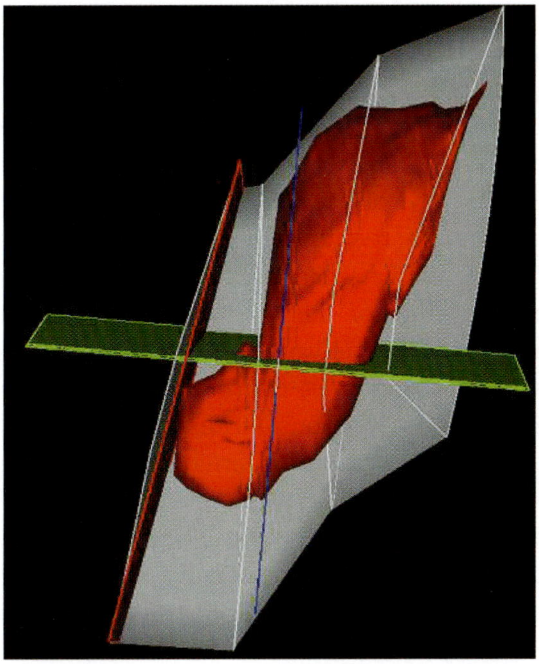

Fig. 4. An outline of the total stomach volume after ingestion of a soup meal that serves as a contrast medium. The images used for 3D reconstruction are acquired by ordinary ultrasonography assisted by magnetic scanhead tracking. The light gray area denotes the total volume that is acquired, and vertical and horizontal sections are displayed.

of six healthy subjects who underwent scanning with the Bird® magnetic system. In steps of 100 ml, up to 700 ml of meat soup was instilled into and subsequently aspirated from the barostat bag while simultaneous 3D scanning was performed. This 3D ultrasound system correlated very good to infused volumes and showed very good agreement with true volumes, as well as low interobserver variation (64).

Hausken and co-workers developed a non-invasive method for evaluating transpyloric flow and duodenogastric reflux stroke volumes using a three-dimensional guided digital color Doppler imaging model (65). They studied healthy subjects during ingestion of a soup meal and 10 minutes postprandially. Cross-sectional color Doppler digital images of duodenogastric reflux episodes were acquired with a 5–3 MHz phased array transducer. The 3D position and orientation data were acquired using a magnetic sensing system. They found high intra- and inter individual variations of the stroke volumes of transpyloric flow episodes during the initial gastric emptying. The duodenogastric reflux episodes lasted on average 2.4 seconds with a volume of an average of 8.3 ml. This novel method minimized geometric assumptions and angular ambiguity.

## 3. 3D Ultrasonography of the Liver

Liver size assessment is an essential part of the clinical examination and is usually deduced by palpation and percussion. Despite training and experience, such evaluation can only be crude, and is at times inaccurate and misleading (66, 67). Using two-dimensional (2D) ultrasonography, liver volume can be estimated by ultrasonic planimetry i.e. calculation of liver volume from sagittal or transverse liver slices of 1 cm thickness (68–70). The techniques have been validated using CT with good correlation between methods. Thiel *et al.* found that the sonographic technique was more accurate than the computed tomography scan method as it allowed the use of sagittal scanning of the liver, which is superior to the transverse scanning technique required by the computed tomography scanner (70). Therefore, Hausken *et al.* utilized the same 3D system for the stomach based on magnetic scanhead tracking to study volumes of the liver (71). They positioned the transducer at the epigastrium and intercostally. Scans were obtained in three separate 8-second periods of suspended mid-inspiration. Images were captured continuously while freely moving the ultrasound probe in standardized directions (translation and tilting) to cover the entire liver. The three image sets (120 images each) were obtained in a total of 60 seconds, which included the time between breath holds. In this study, Duplex Doppler ultrasonography was also used to measure portal and hepatic vein blood flow fasting and postprandially. In Fig. 5, a reconstruction of the total liver volume is displayed.

Liver volume is an indirect measure of hepatic reserve and can be used to assess the ability of the liver to tolerate injury and resection. Patients with cirrhosis and a small liver may have less hepatic reserve than cirrhotics with normal size livers and the ability to identify these patients might influence therapeutic decisions. Accurate pre-operative assessment of liver volume is important prior to liver resection in patients with liver tumors. Patients with predicted inadequate residual liver volume following liver resection are at substantial risk for post-operative liver failure and death. Ultrasonic volume estimates could also be

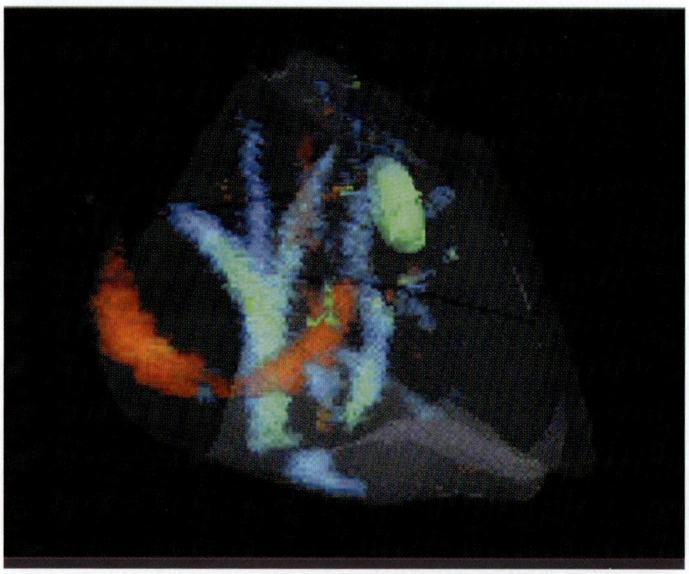

Fig. 5. A 3D reconstruction of the liver (gray) in a patient with a malignant tumor (green) undergoing pre-operative evaluation. Liver veins in blue and the portal vein in red are visualized using a color flow Doppler rendering technique. The image demonstrates tumor-vessel relationship and enables careful image analysis for the surgeon.

used to accurately measure the volume of tumors within the liver over time. The effective treatment of encapsulated hepatocellular carcinomas by ethanol injection requires injecting volumes of ethanol approximating the total tumor volume, which is most commonly estimated using the formula for a sphere. A 3D ultrasound method of following tumor volume has the potential to become the preferred method for monitoring response to therapy for many cancers involving the liver.

Liess and co-workers estimated the size of hepatic tumors by three-dimensional ultrasonography and performed volume measurement by computer-linked planimetry. Initial tests with water filled balloons revealed good accuracy and high reproducibility of the method applied by one investigator as well as by four different investigators. Circumscribed hepatic lesions of 63 patients were investigated by using conventional sonography (ellipsoid formula), computed tomography (ellipsoid formula) and three-dimensional-sonography (ellipsoid formula, orthogonal triplet, planimetry). As a volume of reference, a mathematical approximation for infinite sonographic slices (planimetry) of a very well circumscribed haemangioma of the liver was defined. Based on these results a mean error of −6% (SD +/−39%) was determined for conventional sonography. For computed tomography, a mean error of 2% (SD +/−35%) was found, for three-dimensional-sonography that figure was −6% (SD +/−5%). Follow up investigations can only demonstrate significant alterations of volume when the SD-interval is exceeded. Therefore, three-dimensional-sonography provides a more sensitive and reliable recognition of volumetric changes of liver tumors than conventional sonography or computed tomography does. Other authors compared the accuracy of *in vivo*, three-dimensional ultrasonography to 3D CT scanning (72). They found that planimetric 3D ultrasonography was independent of the investigator and substantially more accurate than measurements with conventional sonography and comparable with those measurements made using CT investigations. 3D sonography seemed as compared with CT examination, an economical procedure for the follow-up of tumor disease. In Osler-Weber-Rendu disease, three-dimensional ultrasonography has been utilized to visualize porto-venous shunting (73).

Intra-operative hepatic ultrasonography provides significant information about tumor location and vascular anatomy in the liver, and is an indispensable procedure during hepatic resection. Motohide *et al.* developed a new three-dimensional ultrasonography image processing method by applying of the intensity projection method (74). The minimum and maximum intensity projection displayed the arrangement of blood vessels (hepatic veins and portal veins) and hyperechoic regions, respectively. Moving the probe manually, images were taken and processed on a real-time basis (in about 10 seconds). 3D-US was used in 24 patients undergoing hepatic resection, and allowed easy visualization of the tumors and vascular anatomy. The authors considered 3D ultrasonography to be an efficient and safe navigation system in liver surgery.

## 4. 3D Ultrasonography of the Gallbladder

The volume of the gallbladder is significant to measure in order to enable the calculation of gallbladder emptying. Usually, the volume of the gallbladder is estimated by 2D ultrasonography using different formulas that assume a certain shape of the organ. The size of the

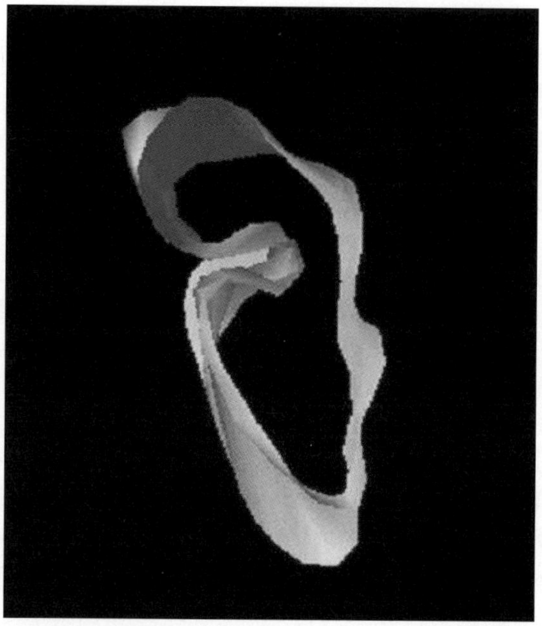

Fig. 6. This image shows a 3D reconstruction of a human gallbladder with a polyp inside. The data was acquired by a stepping motor that was triggered on the frame rate of the scanner, and during 3 seconds a total of 81 2D-frames were recorded. Computer based volume estimation started with interactive contour indication on scan-converted data. Planar contours were selected and drawn with a mouse before the object was reconstructed in 3 dimensions.

fasting gallbladder was similar in patients with non-ulcer-dyspepsia and healthy controls as measured by 3D ultrasonography (59). The volume estimations of the gallbladder in this study were consistent with those obtained by 2D ultrasonography in more than 2000 patients analyzed by Palasciano *et al.* (75). The meal reduced the volume of the gallbladder both in the patients and in the healthy persons. The reduction in gallbladder volume, i.e. gallbladder emptying, was less pronounced in patients with non-ulcer-dyspepsia, consistent with a report by Marzio *et al.* (76). They found that the rate of gastric emptying of liquids did not influence the emptying of the gallbladder. Assessment of gallbladder emptying was also evaluated in another study by 3D ultrasonography (7, 77). A gallbladder polyp is visualized in Fig. 6. 3D ultrasonography has also been used to visualize bile ducts (78) and to locate gallstones in therapy as lithotripsy (79).

## 5. 3D Endoscopic Ultrasonography

Endoscopic ultrasonography has gained acceptance as a valuable tool to obtain diagnostic information in patients with digestive diseases, as it enables detailed visualization of small structures along the gastrointestinal tract. However, its use has been limited to a few centers, partly due to the high demands for skills in both endoscopy and ultrasound scanning. Interpretation of 2D endosonographic images can be challenging, even for experienced operators. Therefore, we have investigated the applicability of new acquisition units allowing endosonographic recordings to be imported into the general 3D reconstruction systems.

(80–83). So far, 3D endosonography has been based on sequential sampling of 2D images, mainly during the pull-back of radial scanning probes. The 3D data are usually displayed in a orthogonal window or by anyplane slicing (Fig. 7).

In a recent study, endoluminal ultrasound examinations were performed with 360° radial scanning 7.5 & 12 MHz echoendoscope and miniature probes, 8 F., 12 and 20 MHz (Olympus CO LTD, Tokyo, Japan). Acquisition of 2D ultrasound images was achieved by

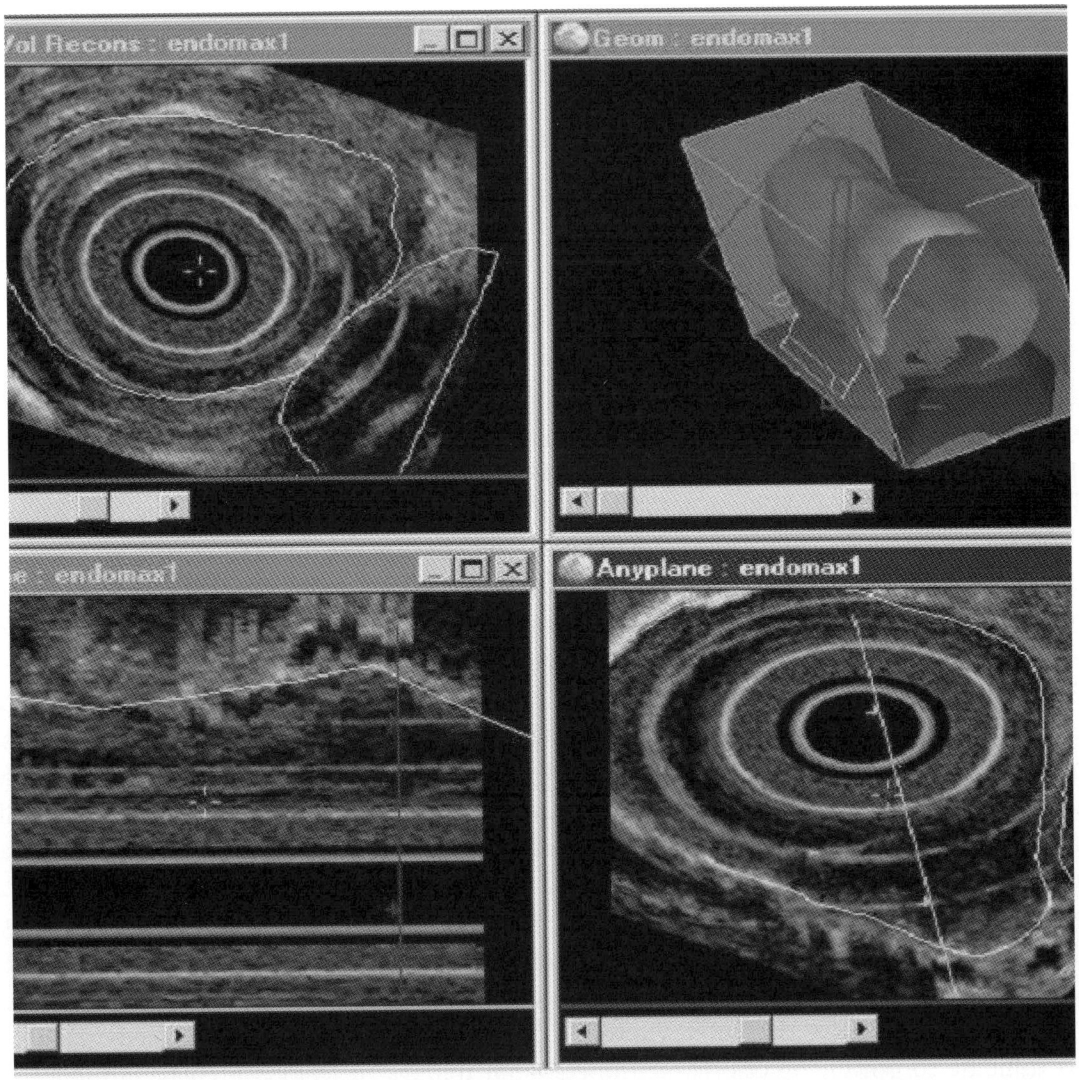


Fig. 7. Three-dimensional display of a mediastinal tumor with lymph node metastases, as imaged by endoscopic ultrasonography during constant-rate pull-back of the endoscope. *Upper left*: Original radial ultrasound scan showing the transducer-containing esophagus in cross-section and the adjacent mediastinal echo-poor tumor. Green and blue lines indicate the positions of the two reconstructed longitudinal planes displayed below. *Upper right*: Geometric window indicating the relative position of the displayed image planes. Lower left: Reconstructed longitudinal image comprising the ultrasound probe and the mediastinal tumor. *Lower right*: Longitudinal image showing part of the main tumor and two enlarged lymph nodes located cranially to it.

connecting the probes to a computer controlled linear stepping motor device (Prototype, MKAB, Gothenburg, Sweden) with an acquisition length of 0.5–15 cm and an operating speed at 10 $mmsec^{-1}$, resulting in a distance between serial images of 0.1–0.2 mm. Further post-processing was performed using EchoPac3D®. These studies demonstrated that 3D-endosonography enabled accurate volume estimation of a wide range of tumors, and improved global display of tumor extensions and topographic relations, thus enabling better preoperative planning (84, 85).

In order to improve image quality of the 3D data set by avoiding artifacts from pulsatile organs, ECG triggered 3D EUS reconstructions was attempted (86). The authors found that ECG triggered 3D EUS images could easily be obtained using a stepping motor device during routine examinations, resulting in a clear demonstration of the different wall layers in the longitudinal image axis. The 3D volumes acquired were approx. $12 \times 8 \times 5$ cm in size and the optimal frame distances in ECG trigged acquisitions were 1.0–1.25 mm. The lateral dislocation was 2.40 mm (SD 0.56) in non-ECG trigged examinations resulting in a fuzzy image in the axial display, compared to 0,19 mm (SD 0.23) in the ECG trigged scans ($p < 0.0027$). This resulted in higher accuracy in the evaluation of small and superficial lesions of the esophageal wall and fundic region of the stomach.

Other researchers have also assessed the clinical usefulness and problems of three-dimensional images obtained by endosonography (87). Nishimura and co-workers studied 18 resected specimens of gastrointestinal lesions and 21 patients. In the resected specimens, the surface images were quite consistent with the macroscopic findings in 17 cases. In 2 esophageal cancers, 7 of 10 gastric cancers, and 2 colonic cancers the depth of tumor invasion was assessed accurately from the reconstructed images. In the *in vivo* study, although 3D displays had some limitations, it was particularly useful for esophageal and rectal lesions. They concluded that this new diagnostic method enabled visualization of the total extent of gastrointestinal lesions and appeared to have useful clinical applications.

Another Japanese group used a system of three-dimensional endoscopic ultrasonography to analyze the surface, the echo-density, and the echo-patterns of cross-sectional images of submucosal lesions. They evaluated the quality of the three-dimensional image and cross-sectional images of lipomas, leiomyomas, and cysts. They stated that analysis of 3D-EUS images was useful in making a diagnosis of submucosal lesions (88). Tsutsui and co-workers evaluated the usefulness of three-dimensional sonography using Olympus ultrasound 3D imaging system to spatially clarify digestive lesions (89). They converted the sequential 2D data into volume data by an image processing software (Medical Design Composer 1.0) developed by the authors. They found that determination of the depth and the extent of tumor invasion was more correctly viewed when arbitrary slicing was applied. However, it was difficult to obtain precise three-dimensional images in lesions greatly influenced by heart beats. In another study, volume measurement using tissue characterization of 3D endoscopic ultrasonographic images was performed (90), showing good correlation between the volume measured with 3D-EUS and the volume obtained using tissue characterization. The tissue characterization volumes were only relatively slightly larger than the volumes measured using 3D-EUS, and the authors suggested that there is some promise for tissue characterization in 3D-EUS.

Hunerbein *et al.* aimed at developing a technique for three-dimensional endoscopic ultrasound of the esophagus based on standard endosonographic images (91). They attached a high-resolution miniprobe (360 degrees, 12.5 MHz) to a stepping motor that enabled ECG-triggered withdrawal of the transducer for imaging of esophageal cancer patients. The system enabled the acquisition of accurate three-dimensional ultrasound data within 30–50 s. Computed image processing allowed display of the data in transverse, longitudinal, and oblique sections, or as a 3D reconstruction. Three-dimensional imaging provided accurate visualization of the tumor and surrounding structures in all cases. Longitudinal scan planes and 3D views improved the assessment of longitudinal tumor infiltration and the spatial relation of the tumor to relevant mediastinal structures. They concluded that three-dimensional endoscopic ultrasound of the esophagus was technically feasible and it allowed the assessment of local tumor spread in previously unattainable scan planes.

### 5.1. *3D ultrasonography of the rectum*

Transrectal ultrasound is the most sensitive technique for per-operative staging and follow-up of rectal cancer. Major limitations of this technique include the complexity of image interpretation and the inability to examine stenotic tumors or to identify recurrent rectal cancer. Therefore, Hunerbein and co-workers conducted a prospective study to investigate the value of three-dimensional endosonography for staging rectal cancer (92). Three-dimensional endosonography was performed in 100 patients with rectal tumors. Transrectal volume scans were obtained using a 3D multiplane transducer (7.5/10.0 MHz). Stenotic tumors were examined with a 3D front-fire transducer (5.0/7.5 MHz). The volume scans were processed and analyzed on a Combison 530 workstation (Kretztechnik, Zipf, Austria). Display of volume data in three perpendicular planes or as 3D view facilitated the interpretation of ultrasound images and enhanced the diagnostic information of the data. The accuracy of 3D endosonography in the assessment of infiltration depth was 88% compared to 82% with the conventional technique. In the determination of lymph node involvement, 3D and two-dimensional endosonography provided accuracy rates of 79% and 74%, respectively. The 3D scanning allowed the visualization of obstructing tumors using reconstructed planes in front of the transducer. Correct assessment of the infiltration depth was possible in 15 of 21 patients with obstructing tumors (accuracy, 76%). Three-dimensional endosonography displayed suspicious pararectal lesions in 30 patients. Transrectal ultrasound-guided biopsy was extremely precise (accuracy, 98%) and showed malignancy in 10 of 30 patients. They concluded that the 3D imaging and ultrasound-guided biopsy seemed capable to improve staging of rectal cancer and should be evaluated in further studies. The same authors also investigated the value of three-dimensional endorectal ultrasonography for staging of obstructing rectal cancer (93). In this study, they concluded that this technique may improve therapy planning in advanced rectal cancer by selecting patients who require preoperative adjuvant therapy.

Williams and co-workers used three-dimensional endosonography to determine the incidence and functional consequences of external sphincter trauma (94). They examined 55 women after delivery and found ultrasound evidence of postpartum trauma in 13 of 45 women who had a vaginal delivery, involving the external sphincter in five, the pubo-analis in nine, and the transverse perineii in three. They concluded that coronal imaging enabled by 3D ultrasonography of the external anal sphincter was a useful adjunct to the assessment of trauma.

Hydrosonography of the colon (hydrocolonic sonography) has made possible nearly complete visualization of the colon by transabdominal scanning. By retrograde instillation of water or another echo-poor liquid into the colon, tumors and inflammation of the colon can be detected at a higher rate than by conventional ultrasonography. A 3D ultrasonogram of the ileocoecal valve based on transabdominal hydrosonography is depicted in Fig. 8.

## 6. Conclusion

The introduction of 3D ultrasonographic imaging in the field of gastroenterology seem to improve standardization of data acquisition and analysis, particularly relevant for endosonographic imaging. Moreover, acquisition time during an unpleasant procedure for the patient, can be reduced. 3D imaging also make ultrasonography less operator dependant and facilitates easier interpretation of ultrasonographic images. For volume estimation, there are several studies that demonstrate high accuracy of 3D ultrasonography. Furthermore, when conventional 2D scanning is compared with 3D ultrasonography, studies conclude that 3D ultrasonography perform better than 2D ultrasonography with respect to accuracy and precision in volume calculation (95–97).

For mapping of complex anatomy, e.g. to aid surgical planning, 3D ultrasonography appear to be a promising tool (98–101). Vascular imaging was improved with three-

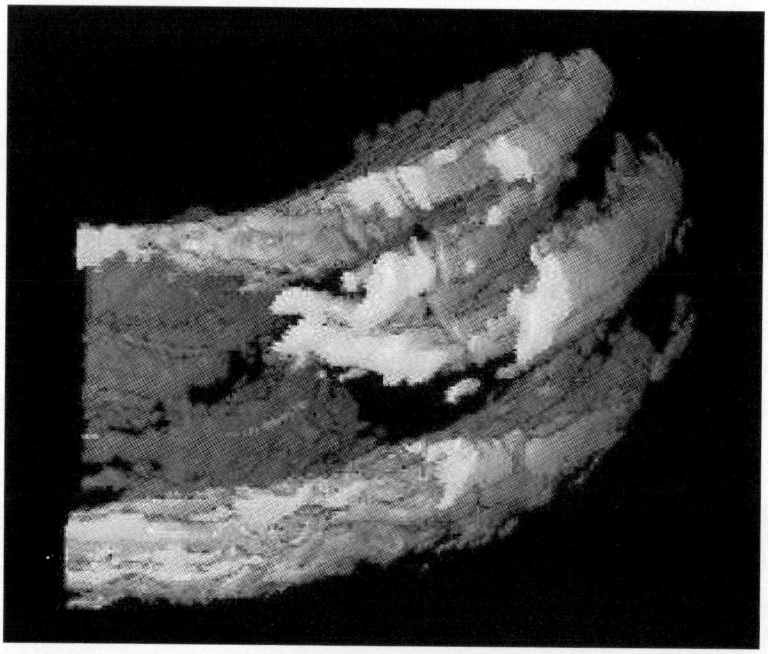

Fig. 8. 3D ultrasonogram of the ileocoecal valve (Valvula Bauhini) based on transabdominal acquisition using a 3.5 MHz mechanical transducer and a tilting motor. The colon was prepared by retrograde installation of water, so-called hydrosonography. The distal ileum is seen to the right and coecum to the left.

dimensional ultrasonography, and this imaging method may provide additional assistance in decision making when evaluating abdominal vessels (102).

However, there are limitations of 3D ultrasonography that needs to be acknowledged. The whole process from acquisition to display of 3D images is time consuming and requires dedicated, well-trained operators. The importance of high quality raw data enabled by careful acquisition cannot be overestimated, as there is principally no new image data in the 3D file compared to the original 2D image.

There is an exiting future for 3D ultrasonography as development in acquisition devices, transducer technology, and computer software and hardware will permit real-time data acquisition and image rendering. On-line display and volume calculation will enhance diagnostic value and allow smooth patient examination and work-up. Further development of contrast agents may aid 3D automatic rendering and speed up volume estimation. 3D ultrasonography may become, not only an excellent diagnostic tool, but also an important imaging modality in interventional medicine.

## References

1. Salustri, A. and Roelandt, J. R., Ultrasonic three-dimensional reconstruction of the heart. Ultrasound Med Biol 1995; 21: 281–293.
2. Ghosh, A., Nanda, N. C. and Maurer, G., Three-dimensional reconstruction of echocardiographic images using the rotation method. Ultrasound Med Biol 1982; 8: 655–661.
3. Roelandt, J. R., ten Cate, F. J., Vletter, W. B. and Taams, M. A., Ultrasonic dynamic three-dimensional visualization of the heart with a multiplane transesophageal imaging transducer. J Am Soc Echocardiogr 1994; 7: 217–229.
4. Picot, P. A., Rickey, D. W., Mitchell, R., Rankin, R. N. and Fenster, A., Three-dimensional colour Doppler imaging. Ultrasound in Medicine and Biology 1993; 19: 95–104.
5. Ross, J. J., Jr., D'Adamo, A. J., Karalis, D. G. and Chandrasekaran, K., Three-dimensional transesophageal echo imaging of the descending thoracic aorta. Am J Cardiol 1993; 71: 1000–1002.
6. Sohn, C. and Grotepass, J., [3-dimensional organ image using ultrasound]. Ultraschall Med 1990; 11: 295–301.
7. Sackmann, M., Pauletzki, J., Zwiebel, F. M. and Holl, J., Three-dimensional ultrasonography in hepatobiliary and pancreatic diseases. Bildgebung 1994; 61: 100–103.
8. Sehgal, C. M., Broderick, G. A., Whittington, R., Gorniak, R. J. and Arger, P. H., Three-dimensional US and volumetric assessment of the prostate. Radiology 1994; 192: 274–278.
9. Martin, R. W., Bashein, G., Zimmer, R. and Sutherland, J., An endoscopic micromanipulator for multiplanar transesophageal imaging. Ultrasound Med Biol 1986; 12: 965–975.
10. Martin, R. W. and Bashein, G., Measurement of stroke volume with three-dimensional transesophageal ultrasonic scanning: Comparison with thermodilution measurement. Anesthesiology 1989; 70: 470–476.
11. Belohlavek, M., Foley, D. A., Gerber, T. C., Greenleaf, J. F. and Seward, J. B., Three-dimensional ultrasound imaging of the atrial septum: Normal and pathologic anatomy. J Am Coll Cardiol 1993; 22: 1673–1678.
12. Pretorius, D. H. and Nelson, T. R., Fetal face visualization using three-dimensional ultrasonography. J Ultrasound Med 1995; 14: 349–356.

13. Hamper, U. M., Trapanotto, V., Sheth, S., DeJong, M. R. and Caskey, C. I., Three-dimensional US: Preliminary clinical experience. Radiology 1994; 191: 397–401.
14. Wagner, S., Gebel, M., Bleck, J. S. and Manns, M. P., Clinical application of three-dimensional sonography in hepatobiliary disease. Bildgebung 1994; 61: 104–109.
15. Zoller, W. G. and Liess, H., [3-D ultrasound in gastroenterology]. Bildgebung 1994; 61: 95–99.
16. Rosenfield, K., Losordo, D. W., Ramaswamy, K., Pastore, J. O., Langevin, R. E., Razvi, S. *et al.*, Three-dimensional reconstruction of human coronary and peripheral arteries from images recorded during two-dimensional intravascular ultrasound examination. Circulation 1991; 84: 1938–1956.
17. Mintz, G. S., Pichard, A. D., Satler, L. F., Popma, J. J., Kent, K. M. and Leon, M. B., Three-dimensional intravascular ultrasonography: Reconstruction of endovascular stents *in vitro* and *in vivo*. J Clin Ultrasound 1993; 21: 609–615.
18. Chandrasekaran, K., Sehgal, C. M., Hsu, T. L., Young, N. A., D'Adamo, A. J., Robb, R. A. *et al.*, Three-dimensional volumetric ultrasound imaging of arterial pathology from two-dimensional intravascular ultrasound: An *in vitro* study. Angiology 1994; 45: 253–264.
19. Whittingham, T. A. and Bateman, D. N., Measurement of stomach volume by real-time ultrasound. Ultrasound Med Biol 1983; Suppl 2: 459–463.
20. Dekker, D. L., Piziali, R. L. and Dong, E. Jr., A system for ultrasonically imaging the human heart in three dimensions. Comput Biomed Res 1974; 7: 544–553.
21. Nikravesh, P. E., Skorton, D. J., Chandran, K. B., Attarwala, Y. M., Pandian, N. and Kerber, R. E., Computerized three-dimensional finite element reconstruction of the left ventricle from cross-sectional echocardiograms. Ultrason Imaging 1984; 6: 48–59.
22. Raichlen, J. S., Trivedi, S. S., Herman, G. T., St. John Sutton M. G. and Reichek, N., Dynamic three-dimensional reconstruction of the left ventricle from two-dimensional echocardiograms. J Am Coll Cardiol 1986; 8: 364–370.
23. Sawada, H., Fujii, J., Aizawa, T., Kato, K., Onoe, M., Kuno, Y. *et al.*, Three dimensional reconstruction of the human left ventricle from multiple cross-sectional echocardiograms: Comparison with biplane cineventriculography using Simpson's rule. J Cardiogr 1985; 15: 439–447.
24. Geiser, E. A., Christie, L. G. J., Conetta, D. A., Conti, C. R. and Gossman, G. S., A mechanical arm for spatial registration of two-dimensional echocardiographic sections. Cathet Cardiovasc Diagn 1982; 8: 89–101.
25. Moritz, W. E., Shreve, P. L. and Mace, L. E., Analysis of an ultrasonic spatial locating system. IEEE Trans Instrum Meas 1976; 25: 43–50.
26. Levine, R. A., Handschumacher, M. D., Sanfilippo, A. J., Hagege, A. A., Harrigan, P., Marshall, J. E. *et al.*, Three-dimensional echocardiographic reconstruction of the mitral valve, with implications for the diagnosis of mitral valve prolapse. Circulation 1989; 80: 589–598.
27. King, D. L., King, D. L., Jr. and Shao, M. Y., Three-dimensional spatial registration and interactive display of position and orientation of real-time ultrasound images. J Ultrasound Med 1990; 9: 525–532.
28. Handschumacher, M. D., Lethor, J. P., Siu, S. C., Mele, D., Rivera, J. M., Picard, M. H. *et al.*, A new integrated system for three-dimensional echocardiographic reconstruction: Development and validation for ventricular volume with application in human subjects. J Am Coll Cardiol 1993; 21: 743–753.
29. King, D. L., King, D. L., Jr. and Shao, M. Y., Evaluation of *in vitro* measurement accuracy of a three-dimensional ultrasound scanner. J Ultrasound Med 1991; 10: 77–82.
30. Detmer, P. R., Bashein, G., Hodges, T. C., Beach, K. W., Filer, E. P., Burns, D. H. *et al.*, 3D ultrasonic image feature localization based on magnetic scanhead tracking: *In vitro* calibration and validation. Ultrasound Med Biol 1994; 20: 923–936.

31. Hodges, T. C., Detmer, P. R., Burns, D. H., Beach, K. W. and Strandness, Jr. D. E., Ultrasonic three-dimensional reconstruction: *In vitro* and *in vivo* volume and area measurement. Ultrasound Med Biol 1994; 20: 719–729.
32. Kelly, I. M., Gardener, J. E., Brett, A. D., Richards, R. and Lees, W. R., Three-dimensional US of the fetus. Work in progress. Radiology 1994; 192: 253–259.
33. Pretorius, D. H. and Nelson, T. R., Prenatal visualization of cranial sutures and fontanelles with three-dimensional ultrasonography. J Ultrasound Med 1994; 13: 871–876.
34. Leotta, D. F., Detmer, P. R., Gilja, O. H., Jong, J. M., Martin, R. W., Primozich, J. F. *et al.*, Three-dimensional ultrasound imaging using multiple magnetic tracking systems and miniature magnetic sensors. Proc IEEE Int Ultrasonics Symp 1995; Seattle, WA, USA: pp. 1415–1418.
35. Snyder, J. E., Kisslo, S., von Ramm, O. Real-time orthogonal mode scanning of the heart. I. System design. J. Am. Coic. Caudiol. 1986; 7: 1279–1285.
36. Belohlavek, M., Foley, D. A., Gerber, T. C., Kinter, T. M., Greenleaf, J. F. and Seward, J. B., Three- and four-dimensional cardiovascular ultrasound imaging: A new era for echocardiography. Mayo Clin Proc 1993; 68: 221–240.
37. Greenleaf, J. F., Belohlavek, M., Gerber, T. C., Foley, D. A. and Seward, J. B., Multidimensional visualization in echocardiography: An introduction. Mayo Clin Proc 1993; 68: 213–220.
38. Visualization in scientific computing. 1st ed. IEEE Computer Society Press, Los Alamitos. 1989.
39. Nelson, T. R. and Pretorius, D. H., Visualization of the fetal thoracic skeleton with three-dimensional sonography: A preliminary report. AJR Am J Roentgenol 1995; 164: 1485–1488.
40. Martin, R. W., Legget, M., McDonald, J., Li, X.-N., Leotta, D. F., Bolson, E. *et al.*, Stereographic viewing of 3D ultrasound images: A novelty or a tool? Proc IEEE Int Ultrasonics Symp 1995; 2: 1431–1434.
41. Baum, G. and Stroke, G. W., Optical holographic three-dimensional ultrasonography. Science 1975; 89: 994–995.
42. Koivukangas, J., Ylitalo, J., Alasaarela, E. and Tauriainen, A., Three-dimensional ultrasound imaging of brain for neurosurgery. Ann Clin Res 1986; 18 Suppl 47: 65–72.
43. Redman, J. D., Walton, W. P., Fleming, J. E. and Hall, A. M., Holographic display of data from ultrasonic scanning. Ultrasonics 1969; 7: 26–29.
44. Martens, D., Hausken, T., Gilja, O. H., Steen, E. N. and Alker, H. J., 3D processing of ultrasound images using a novel echopac-3D software. Ultrasound Med Biol 1997; 23(S1): 136.
45. Gilja, O. H., Thune, N., Matre, K., Hausken, T., Odegaard, S. and Berstad, A., *In vitro* evaluation of three-dimensional ultrasonography in volume estimation of abdominal organs. Ultrasound Med Biol 1994; 20: 157–165.
46. Thune, N., Hausken, T., Gilja, O. H. and Matre, K., A practical method for estimating enclosed volumes using 3D ultrasound. Eur J Ultrasound 1996; 3: 83–92.
47. Gilja, O. H., Smievoll, A. I., Thune, N., Matre, K., Hausken, T., Odegaard, S. *et al.*, *In vivo* comparison of 3D ultrasonography and magnetic resonance imaging in volume estimation of human kidneys. Ultrasound Med Biol 1995; 21: 25–32.
48. Gilja, O. H., Hausken, T., Berstad, A. and Odegaard, S., Measurements of organ volume by ultrasonography. Proc Inst Mech Eng [H] 1999; 213: 247–259.
49. Bolondi, L., Bortolotti, M., Santi, V., Calletti, T., Gaiani, S. and Labo, G., Measurement of gastric emptying time by real-time ultrasonography. Gastroenterology 1985; 89: 752–759.
50. Duan, L. P., Zheng, Z. T. and Li, Y. N., A study of gastric emptying in non-ulcer dyspepsia using a new ultrasonographic method. Scand J Gastroenterol 1993; 28: 355–360.
51. Hou, X. H., Deng, Y. B. and Zhang, J. K., [Measurement of gastric emptying in non-ulcer dyspepsia]. Chung Hua Nei Ko Tsa Chih 1992; 31: 623–5, 658.

52. Dorlars, D., Schilling, D. and Riemann, J. F., [The feasibility of ultrasonography for the evaluation of stomach motility disorders]. Dtsch Med Wochenschr 1994; 119: 575–580.
53. LiVoti, G., Tulone, V., Bruno, R., Cataliotti, F., Iacono, G., Cavataio, F. *et al.*, Ultrasonography and gastric emptying: Evaluation in infants with gastroesophageal reflux. J Pediatr Gastroenterol Nutr 1992; 14: 397–399.
54. Desaga, J. F. and Hixt, U., [Sonographic determination of gastric emptying]. Ultraschall Med 1987; 8: 138–141.
55. Newell, S. J., Chapman, S. and Booth, I. W., Ultrasonic assessment of gastric emptying in the preterm infant. Arch Dis Child 1993; 69: 32–36.
56. Radberg, G., Asztely, M., Cantor, P., Rehfeld, J. F., Jarnfeldt Samsioe A. and Svanvik, J., Gastric and gallbladder emptying in relation to the secretion of cholecystokinin after a meal in late pregnancy. Digestion 1989; 42: 174–180.
57. Stein, W. W., Brettel, H. F. and Garten, T., [Stomach volume determination using the ultrasonic B picture method]. Munch Med Wochenschr 1972; 114: 1871–1873.
58. Hokland, J. and Hausken, T., An interactive volume rendering method applied to ultrasonography of abdominal structures. IEEE Ultrason Symp Proc 1994; 3: 1567–1571.
59. Hausken, T., Thune, N., Matre, K., Gilja, O. H., Odegaard, S. and Berstad, A., Volume estimation of the gastric antrum and the gallbladder in patients with non-ulcer dyspepsia and erosive prepyloric changes, using three-dimensional ultrasonography. Neurogastroenterol Mot 1994; 6: 263–270.
60. Gilja, O. H., Hausken, T., Odegaard, S. and Berstad, A., Three-dimensional ultrasonography of the gastric antrum in patients with functional dyspepsia. Scand J Gastroenterol 1996; 31: 847–855.
61. Berstad, A., Hausken, T., Gilja, O. H., Thune, N., Matre, K. and Odegaard, S., Volume measurement of gastric antrum by 3-D ultrasonography and flow measurements through the pylorus by duplex technique. Dig Dis Sci 1994; 39: 97–100.
62. Matre, K., Stokke, E. M., Martens, D. and Gilja, O. H., *In vitro* volume estimation of kidneys using three-dimensional ultrasonography and a position sensor. Eur J Ultrasound 1999; 10: 65–73.
63. Gilja, O. H., Detmer, P. R., Jong, J. M., Leotta, D. F., Li, X.-N., Beach, K. W. *et al.*, Intragastric distribution and gastric emptying assessed by 3D-ultrasonography. Gastroenterology 1997; 113: 38–49.
64. Tefera, S., Gilja, O. H., Olavsdottir, E., Hausken, T., Hatlebakk, J. G. and Berstad, A., Intragastric maldistribution of a liquid meal in patients with reflux oesophagitis assessed by three dimensional ultrasonography. Gut 2002; 50: 153–158.
65. Hausken, T., Li, X.-N., Goldman, B., Leotta, D. F., Odegaard, S. and Martin, R. W., Quantification of gastric emptying and duodenogastric reflux stroke volumes using three-dimensional guided digital color Doppler Imaging. Eur J Ultrasound 2001; 13: 205–213.
66. Meyhoff, H. H., Roder, O. and Andersen, B., Palpatory estimation of liver size. Within- and between-observer variation. Acta Chir Scand 1979; 145: 479–481.
67. Sullivan, S., Krasner, N. and Williams, R., The clinical estimation of liver size: A comparison of techniques and an analysis of the source of error. Br Med J 1976; 2: 1042–1043.
68. Raeth, U., Johnson, P. J. and Williams, R., Ultrasound determination of liver size and assessment of patients with malignant liver disease. Liver 1984; 4: 287–293.
69. Wynne, H. A., Cope, L. H., Mutch, E., Rawlins, M. D., Woodhouse, K. W. and James, O. F., The effect of age upon liver volume and apparent liver blood flow in healthy man. Hepatology 1989; 9: 297–301.

70. Van Thiel D. H., Hagler, N. G., Schade, R. R., Skolnick, M. L., Heyl, A. P., Rosenblum, E. *et al.*, *In vivo* hepatic volume determination using sonography and computed tomography. Validation and a comparison of the two techniques. Gastroenterology 1985; 88: 1812–1817.
71. Hausken, T., Leotta, D. F., Helton, S., Kowdley, K. V., Goldman, B., Vaezy, S. *et al.*, Estimation of the human liver volume and configuration using three-dimensional ultrasonography: Effect of a high-caloric liquid meal. Ultrasound Med Biol 1998; 24: 1357–1367.
72. Wolf, G. K., Lang, H., Prokop, M., Schreiber, M. and Zoller, W., Volume measurements of localized hepatic lesions using three-dimensional sonography in comparison with three-dimensional computed tomography. Eur J Med Res 1998; 3: 157–164.
73. Matsuo, M., Kanematsu, M., Kato, H., Kondo, H., Sugisaki, K. and Hoshi, H., Osler-Weber-Rendu disease: Visualizing portovenous shunting with three-dimensional sonography. AJR Am J Roentgenol 2001; 176: 919–920.
74. Motohide, S., Go, W., Masahirö, O., Hiroshi, H. and Masaki, K., [Clinical application of three-dimensional ultrasound imaging as intraoperative navigation for liver surgery]. Nippon Geka Gakkai Zasshi 1998; 99: 203–207.
75. Rovetta, G., Galactosaminoglycuronoglycan sulfate (matrix) in therapy of tibiofibular osteoarthritis of the knee. Drugs Exp Clin Res 1991; 17: 53–57.
76. Marzio, L., DiFelice, F., Laico, M. G., Imbimbo, B., Lapenna, D. and Cuccurullo, F., Gallbladder hypokinesia and normal gastric emptying of liquids in patients with dyspeptic symptoms. A double-blind placebo-controlled clinical trial with cisapride. Dig Dis Sci 1992; 37: 262–267.
77. Pauletzki, J., Sackmann, M., Holl, J. and Paumgartner, G., Evaluation of gallbladder volume and emptying with a novel three-dimensional ultrasound system: Comparison with the sum-of-cylinders and the ellipsoid methods. J Clin Ultrasound 1996; 24: 277–285.
78. Fine, D., Perring, S., Herbetko, J., Hacking, C. N., Fleming, J. S. and Dewbury, K. C., Three-dimensional (3D) ultrasound imaging of the gallbladder and dilated biliary tree: Reconstruction from real-time B-scans. Br J Radiol 1991; 64: 1056–1057.
79. Sohn, C. and Bastert, G., [Three-dimensional ultrasonic imaging. Its clinical use]. Dtsch Med Wochenschr 1992; 117: 467–472.
80. Molin, S. O., Nesje, L. B., Gilja, O. H., Hausken, T. and Odegaard, S., Modalities for Three-Dimensional Endoscopic and Laparoscopic Ultrasonography: *In vitro* and *in vivo* Evaluation. Endoscopy 1996; 28: S38.
81. Molin, S., Nesje, L. B., Gilja, O. H., Hausken, T., Martens, D. and Odegaard, S., 3D-endosonography in gastroenterology: Methodology and clinical applications. Eur J Ultrasound 1999; 10: 171–177.
82. Molin, S. O., Nesje, L. B., Gilja, O. H., Hausken, T. and Odegaard, S., Adoption of conventional endosonography for 3D visualization of GI tract. Scand J Gastroenterol 1996; 31: 33.
83. Molin, S. O., Jirås, A., Hall-Angerås, M., Falk, A., Martens, D., Gilja, O. H. *et al.*, Virtual Reality in Surgical Practice. *In vitro* and *in vivo* evaluations. In: Eds. Sieburg, H., Weghorst, S., Morgan, K., Studies in Health Technology and Informatics. IOS Press and Ohmsha, 1997; 246–253.
84. Bismuth, H., Galmiche, J. P., Huguier, M. and Jaeck, D., Eds. Diseases of the gastrointestinal tract examined with 3D endoscopic ultrasonography. 98 A.D. Apr 15; Monduzzi Editore, 1998.
85. Odegaard, S., Nesje, L. B., Molin, S. O., Gilja, O. H. and Hausken, T., Three-dimensional intraluminal sonography in the evaluation of gastrointestinal diseases. Abdom Imaging 1999; 24: 449–451.
86. Molin, S. O., Engstrøm, A., Nesje, L. B., Gilja, O. H. and Odegaard, S., Improvement of 3D EUS using ECG- and respiratory triggered acquisition. Eur J Ultrasound 1998; 7: 54.

87. Nishimura, K., Niwa, Y., Goto, H., Hase, S., Arisawa, T. and Hayakawa, T., Three-dimensional endoscopic ultrasonography of gastrointestinal lesions using an ultrasound probe. Scand J Gastroenterol 1997; 32: 862–868.
88. Miyamoto, M., Aoyama, N., Sakashita, M., Shirasaka, D., Sakai, S., Ikemura, T. *et al.*, Three-dimensional endoscopic ultrasonography for SMT. Digestion 1998; 59(S3): 194.
89. Tsutsuii, A., Okamura, S., Okita, Y., Fukuda, T., Hayashi, S., Muguruma, N. *et al.*, Usefulness of three-dimensional display of digestive lesions by endoscopic ultrasonography. Digestion 1998; 59(S3): 194 (Abstract).
90. Yoshino, J., Nakazawa, S., Inui, K., Wakabayashi, T., Okushima, K., Kobayashi, T. *et al.*, Volume measurement using tissue characterization of three-dimensional endoscopic ultrasonographic images. Endoscopy 2000; 32: 624–629.
91. Hunerbein, M., Gretschel, S., Ghadimi, B. M. and Schlag, P. M., Three-dimensional endoscopic ultrasound of the esophagus. Preliminary experience. Surg Endosc 1997; 11: 991–994.
92. Hunerbein, M. and Schlag, P. M., Three-dimensional endosonography for staging of rectal cancer. Ann Surg 1997; 225: 432–438.
93. Hunerbein, M., Below, C. and Schlag, P. M., Three-dimensional endorectal ultrasonography for staging of obstructing rectal cancer. Dis Colon Rectum 1996; 39: 636–642.
94. Williams, A. B., Bartram, C. I., Halligan, S., Spencer, J. A., Nicholls, R. J. and Kmiot, W. A., Anal sphincter damage after vaginal delivery using three-dimensional endosonography. Obstet Gynecol 2001; 97: 770–775.
95. Riccabona, M., Nelson, T. R., Pretorius, D. H. and Davidson, T. E., Distance and volume measurement using three-dimensional ultrasonography. J Ultrasound Med 1995; 14: 881–886.
96. Sapin, P. M., Schroeder, K. D., Smith, M. D., DeMaria, A. N. and King, D. L., Three-dimensional echocardiographic measurement of left ventricular volume *in vitro*: Comparison with two-dimensional echocardiography and cineventriculography. J Am Coll Cardiol 1993; 22: 1530–1537.
97. Kyei Mensah, A., Zaidi, J., Pittrof, R., Shaker, A., Campbell, S. and Tan, S. L., Transvaginal three-dimensional ultrasound: Accuracy of follicular volume measurements. Fertil Steril 1996; 65: 371–376.
98. Borges, A. C., Witt, C., Bartel, T., Muller, S., Konertz, W. and Baumann, G., Preoperative two- and three-dimensional transesophageal echocardiographic assessment of heart tumors. Ann Thorac Surg 1996; 61: 1163–1167.
99. Trocino, G., Salustri, A., Roelandt, J. R., Ansink, T. and van Herwerden, L., Three-dimensional echocardiography of a flail tricuspid valve. J Am Soc Echocardiogr 1996; 9: 91–93.
100. Vannier, M. W. and Marsh, J. L., Three-dimensional imaging, surgical planning, and image-guided therapy. Radiol Clin North Am 1996; 34: 545–563.
101. Vogel, M., Ho, S. Y., Lincoln, C., Yacoub, M. H. and Anderson, R. H., Three-dimensional echocardiography can simulate intraoperative visualization of congenitally malformed hearts. Ann Thorac Surg 1995; 60: 1282–1288.
102. Spaulding, K. A., Kissner, M. E., Kim, E. K., Pretorius, D. H., Rose, S. C., Garroosi, K. *et al.*, Three-dimensional gray scale ultrasonographic imaging of the celiac axis: Preliminary report. J Ultrasound Med 1998; 17: 239–248.

Published with permission

GASTROENTEROLOGY 1997;113:38–49

# Intragastric Distribution and Gastric Emptying Assessed by Three-Dimensional Ultrasonography

ODD HELGE GILJA,* PAUL R. DETMER,† JING MING JONG,† DANIEL F. LEOTTA,§ XIANG–NING LI,§ KIRK W. BEACH,† ROY MARTIN,§ and D. EUGENE STRANDNESS, Jr.†

*Medical Department A, Haukeland Hospital, University of Bergen, Bergen, Norway; and Departments of †Surgery and §Anesthesiology and Center for Bioengineering, University of Washington, Seattle, Washington

*Background & Aims:* **Three-dimensional (3D) ultrasound imaging of the total stomach volume has not yet been achieved. The aim of this study was to investigate whether a magnetic position sensor system for acquisition of 3D ultrasonograms could be used to determine gastric emptying rates and intragastric distribution.** *Methods:* **A system for position and orientation measurement was interfaced to an ultrasound scanner. In vitro accuracy was evaluated by scanning a porcine stomach. Fourteen volunteers, with a median age of 35 years, were scanned fasting and postcibally by two-dimensional (2D) and 3D ultrasound after ingesting a 500-mL soup meal.** *Results:* **This 3D system yielded a strong correlation ($r = 0.997$) between true and estimated volumes in vitro. The limits of agreement were −9.1:70.1 mL in the volume range 1200–1900 mL. The intersubject variability of the total gastric volumes ranged from 12.5% to 46.0%, less than for antral area variability. The average half-emptying time was 22.1 ± 3.8 minutes. Intragastric distribution of the meal, expressed as proximal distal volume, varied on average from 3.6 ± 2.1 (5 minutes postpradially) to 2.7 ± 1.9 (30 minutes postprandially).** *Conclusions:* **This 3D ultrasound system using magnetic scanhead tracking showed excellent in vitro accuracy, calculated gastric emptying rates more precisely than by 2D ultrasound, and enabled estimation of intragastric distribution of a soup meal.**

Assessment of gastric emptying rates is frequently performed to evaluate patients with motility disorders of the upper gastrointestinal tract. Recently, estimation of intragastric distribution of meals has been added to provide further information on gastric pathophysiology, particularly in patients with functional dyspepsia[1–3] and diabetic visceral neuropathy.[4] The gold standard method to measure these gastric parameters is scintigraphy. However, radionuclide methods expose the subject to radiation and have relatively poor image resolution. Thus, we investigated whether ultrasonography, a radiation-free method, may improve gastric imaging and enhance our understanding of gastric motor function.

Transabdominal two-dimensional (2D) ultrasonography of the stomach has mainly been applied to study antral contractions,[5–7] to calculate standardized areas of the distal stomach,[8–11] to monitor antroduodenal fluid movements,[12–14] and to estimate volumes of the antrum attempting to predict gastric emptying rates.[15–18] The proximal stomach has long been considered inappropriate for ultrasonic imaging because of its position behind the costal margins and the frequent presence of air pockets.[19] In an effort to overcome these limitations, a novel method was recently developed that enabled postprandial scanning of the corpus-fundus while the patients were seated.[20] By using a low-fat soup meal, which served as an excellent contrast agent for the gastrointestinal tract, this method was not restricted to slender individuals and was not dependant on high fat content of the meal. By combining real-time images of the different parts of the stomach, the total stomach volume is now available from transabdominal ultrasonographic examinations.

An early system for acquisition and processing of three-dimensional (3D) ultrasound data was developed in an attempt to enhance the accuracy of volume computation of the distal stomach.[21] Using a motor device, the transducer was tilted through an angle of 90°, capturing sequential 2D frames before the data set was transferred to a graphic workstation for final 3D processing. This 3D ultrasound system was validated both in vitro and in vivo and yielded high accuracy and precision in volume estimation of abdominal organs.[22,23] The system has been used to measure gallbladder volume,[24] to study diseases of the liver,[25] and to evaluate patients with functional dyspepsia.[24,26,27] Despite the significant achievements with respect to accuracy in volume estimation and 3D reconstruction of tissue and organs, this 3D system could

*Abbreviations used in this paper:* 2D, two-dimensional; 3D, three-dimensional; P/D, ratio between the proximal and distal volumes; POM, position and orientation measurement; RMS, root mean square; $V_c$, coefficient of variation.


0016-5085/97/$3.00

only acquire a 90° fan-like data set from a predetermined, single position of the transducer.

Random or free-hand acquisition of 3D ultrasound data has been achieved using mechanical,[28,29] acoustic,[30–33] or electromagnetic[34,35] devices to locate the exact position and orientation of the transducer in space. Magnetic systems maintain the flexibility and smoothness of free-hand scanning, in contrast to mechanical devices. The acoustic systems are limited by the fact that they do not tolerate physical interruptions of the acoustic wave, e.g., a hand coming in its way, before accuracy is compromised substantially. Accordingly, to enable scanning of a large organ like the fluid-filled stomach, we chose to interface a commercially available magnetometer-based position and orientation measurement (POM) device, which is relatively immune to metallic influence and electronic noise from the scanner. This system for magnetic scanhead tracking has been validated both with respect to its precision in locating specific points in space[35] and to its accuracy in volume estimation.[36,37] In these studies, the sensor system worked well in scanning human organs, and high precision and accuracy were revealed in point location and volume estimation.

The objectives of this study were threefold. First, we aimed to determine the in vitro accuracy of the magnetic POM system in volume estimation of a porcine stomach. Second, we wanted to assess whether this system for 3D imaging was applicable for scanning of both the proximal and the distal stomach in humans. Third, if the system worked appropriately for gastric scanning, our purpose was to estimate the intragastric distribution of a meal and the gastric emptying rates.

## Materials and Methods

### Study Design

Healthy volunteers on the staff at the University of Washington were recruited to participate in the trial. Before inclusion into the study, a medical history was obtained and ultrasound examination of the liver, pancreas, and biliary tract was performed to rule out diseases of the upper gastrointestinal system.

Criteria of exclusion from the study were previous surgery in the upper gastrointestinal tract, previous peptic ulcer disease, alcoholism, or use of any medication.

### Subjects

Sixteen healthy individuals, by design all men, entered the trial. The data of 2 subjects could not be analyzed because of derangement of the POM data. The included 14 individuals had a median age of 35 years (range, 26–54 years), weighed 74 ± 8 kg (mean ± SD), and their heights were 178 ± 6 cm. Thirteen of the subjects were nonsmokers. To study intraindividual variability, 1 healthy man (age, 34 years; weight, 72 kg; height, 178 cm) was examined on 6 consecutive weekdays.

Scanning humans with the POM ultrasound system received human subject approval. The study was conducted in accordance with the revised Declaration of Helsinki. All volunteers gave written, informed consent to participate in the trial.

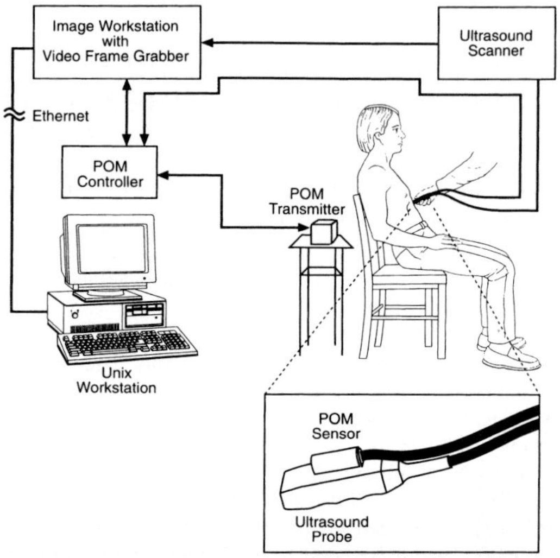


**Figure 1.** Block diagram of the 3D ultrasound system based on magnetic POM. Image and POM data were acquired simultaneously, and the ultrasonograms were digitized from the video output of the scanner by use of a frame grabber board. The POM transmitter was positioned just behind the back of the examined subject and within the performance range of the miniature sensor (60 cm). The data were ultimately transferred via ethernet to a Unix workstation for outlining and volume computation.

### Experimental Setup

The 3D imaging system uses a commercial ultrasound scanner (HDI 3000; Advanced Technology Laboratories, Bothell, WA) and a pulsed magnetic field POM system (Miniature Flock of Birds Model 6D FOB; Ascension Technology Corp., Burlington, VT) attached to the ultrasound scanhead. A custom-designed adapter was glued onto the scanhead at a distance of 2 cm from the transducer face, and the miniature sensor was securely mounted into the adapter. The scanner and the Bird system were interfaced to an image acquisition workstation (Image Vue, Nova Microsonics, Mahwah, NJ). The particular scanhead used in this study was a broadband 5–3 MHz hand-held phased array HDI scanhead. Full-frame ultrasound images from the video output of the ultrasound scanner were digitized by a frame grabber board and saved with the POM data to a hard disk. The setup of the system is shown in Figure 1.

The POM system is based on a quasi-DC pulse-flux magnetometer. It consists of an electronic system control unit, a transmitter module, and a receiving sensor. In-depth description of the POM system and the calibration procedure has been reported previously.[35,38] To calibrate the system, we first determined the precision of the miniature POM system by itself at nine different distances from the transmitter's origin. The miniature sensor alone demonstrated a root mean square (RMS) uncertainty of 2.1 mm over its normal operating range of 500 mm. Second, we measured the precision of the combined POM/ultrasound 3D imaging system, and the RMS uncertainty in point target location was 2.4 mm.

## Test Meal

A liquid meal (500 mL) of commercial meat soup (Toro clear meat soup; Rieber & Søn A/S, Bergen, Norway) containing 1.8 g protein, 0.9 g bovine fat, and 1.1 g carbohydrate (20 kcal) was ingested during a period of 4 minutes. The soup was preheated and then cooled to 37°C, thus improving image quality by reducing the number of air bubbles after ingestion. The pH of the soup varied between 5.4 and 5.7, and the osmolarity was 350 mOsm/kg $H_2O$. Fat, protein, and carbohydrate were all soluble in water. In addition, the soup contained nonsoluble seasoning (0.4 g/L). In previous studies, this soup meal has induced antral contractions at a frequency of 3/min (fed state) in >85% of both patients with functional dyspepsia and healthy controls.[8,13]

## Experimental Protocol

All participants in the trial ingested the soup meal between 8:25 and 9:52 AM after an overnight fast. The 1 smoker in the study was not allowed to smoke in the morning of the examination. The subjects were scanned while sitting in a chair made of plastic material, leaning slightly backwards at an angle of 120° between the thighs and the spine. The electromagnetic transmitter was positioned close to the back of the volunteer to minimize the distance to the receiver on the scanhead (Figure 2). On average, this distance was approximately 30 cm. Time zero was defined at the start of soup ingestion, and scanning was performed while fasting, and after 5, 10, 15, 20, 25, and 35 minutes. Just before ingestion of the soup, the occurrence of antral contractions was observed for at least 2 minutes to evaluate whether the subject's interdigestive migrating motor complex was in phase III (regular contractions with a frequency of 3/min). If phase III was observed, ingestion of soup was postponed until phase I (quiescence) was observed. All the ultrasound examinations were performed by the same physician (O.H.G.). The test meal may induce dyspepsia in a small proportion of healthy subjects.[9,39] Accordingly, the participants were asked to evaluate their total symptoms after the soup meal on a Likert scale from 0 to 9. Zero denotes no symptoms at all, and 9 denotes excruciating symptoms.

## Data Acquisition

Using the current prototype system, 2 investigators were needed to perform the procedure, 1 to run the image workstation and 1 to scan the volunteer. The ultrasound scanner was programmed to the same settings before each examination. The depth of scanning was adjusted to fit each individual's habitus, averaging 17.6 cm. The sector angle of the ultrasound image was 80° in all examinations. The sonographer needed approximately 30 seconds per examination just after the meal to determine the optimal starting position for the 3D image scan. Sagittal sections of the stomach were recorded throughout its entire length, starting in the proximal part where the transducer was positioned by the left subcostal margin and tilted cranially to image the most superior part of the stomach. After stepwise scanning of the proximal stomach angling from left to right, the transducer was moved and held to insonify normally to the skin surface. Then the distal stomach was scanned stepwise moving distally to the gastroduodenal junction (Figure 2). The distance between slices of the stomach during acquisition was approximately 0.5 cm. This interslice distance was not kept constant at various degrees of filling because we had no feedback of its magnitude during scanning. That information could only be obtained after computerized postprocessing of the image and position/orientation data.

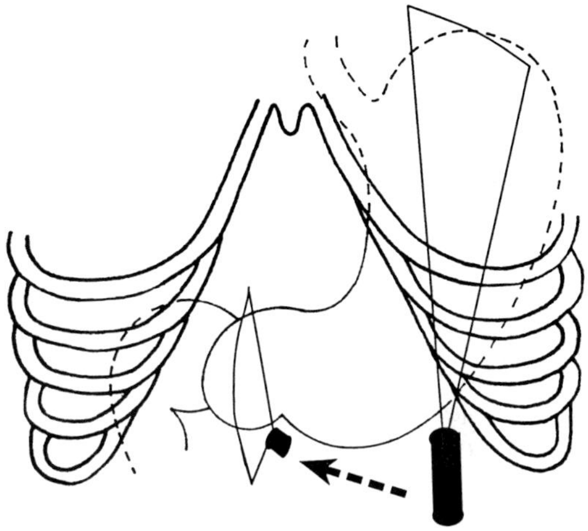

**Figure 2.** Ultrasound scanning of the proximal and distal stomach using magnetic scanhead tracking. Sagittal sections of the stomach were recorded throughout its entire length, starting in the proximal part where the transducer was positioned by the left subcostal margin and tilted cranially to image the most superior part of the stomach. After stepwise scanning of the proximal stomach, the transducer was moved and held to insonify normally to the skin surface. Then the distal stomach was scanned stepwise moving distally to the gastroduodenal junction. Computerized postprocessing of the image, position, and orientation data enabled reconstruction of the total stomach and calculation of volumes, gastric emptying, and intragastric distribution of the meal.

Gastric contractions can be seen on ultrasonography as pulsatile reductions in antral circumference that occur regularly at a frequency of 3/min postcibally and propagate distally. The delay in time between acquisition of sequential 2D sections

Published with permission



enabled the operators to bypass contractions by receiving visual feedback from the monitor. When gastric contractions were observed, the acquisition was paused until the contraction wave passed the position of the image sector, and then scanning continued "surfing" on the postcontraction wave. In some subjects, particularly in slim individuals, a minor influence of the diaphragm's movement during respiration on the gastric configuration could be observed. If this respiration effect was seen, we aimed to record the largest size of the gastric section, which usually was in passive end expirium. Because each image had to be saved to disk after digitization, the workstation required 5 seconds before the next sonogram could be acquired. On average, the time spent to scan the total gastric volume was 2 minutes, which included the short pauses during contractions. One stepwise scan of the whole stomach usually consisted of 4–5 Mb of data depending on the number of 2D sonograms captured in the 3D scan. The image data and the position and orientation data were transferred to a Unix workstation (DEC Alpha, Digital Equipment Corp., San Jose, CA) for final processing.

In conventional ultrasonography of the distal stomach, a 2D sagittal section is often used, in which the aorta, the superior mesenteric vein, and the gastric antrum are visualized simultaneously,[8,10] permitting repeatable measurements to be taken at the same site. To correlate the volumes of the total and distal stomach obtained by 3D ultrasound to the area of this standardized section, we also acquired 2D images of this section at every time point. The built-in caliper system of the scanner was used to estimate the antral areas by tracing the outer profile of the muscularis propria of the gastric wall.

## Volume Estimation

Computerized volume estimation was performed by using custom software developed within the Application Visualization System software package V5.01 (Advanced Visual Systems Inc., Waltham, MA). This began with interactive manual contour indication on the computer display. The inner echo interface of the gastric mucosa was chosen for manual outlining in all samples. In this study, the two compartments of the stomach were scanned in two separate transducer movements, resulting in overlapping volumes between the proximal and distal stomach often being captured. This problem was overcome by providing the user with a 3D display of the outlines on the workstation, which was updated in real time as the operator traced the sonographic sections. The distal stomach was outlined first, and then the outlines of the proximal stomach were "sewed" onto the distal reconstruction. Overlapping volume regions in the acquisition could thus be separated on the workstation, making volume calculations more straightforward. For the volume estimation of the distal and the proximal stomach, we assume that the gastric compartments do not change volumes significantly during the scanning period of 2 minutes. However, it is likely that small volumes of the soup meal flow from the proximal to the distal compartment in this time span, and also that redistribution may occur. This may lead to inaccuracies in volume estimation. To address this issue, we calculated an emptying rate of this meal and we determined how often and how much the volume of the proximal stomach increased compared with the previous measurement in the same individual. Thus, an assessment of the antegrade and retrograde flow between the proximal and the distal stomach could be obtained.

Random acquisition of data implies that adjacent sections and contours may intersect, particularly in organs like the stomach where curvatures deep in the abdominal cavity are seen. Thus, a volume computation method for the total stomach volume should take this into account and not simply calculate the volume by summing the volumes between consecutive contours. Surface tiling of the initial 3D point set is very difficult and time consuming and may introduce errors because of the haphazard spacing between the surface points. A volume computation algorithm by Moritz et al.[40] and Martin et al.[41] was reported to provide accurate volume estimation of the cardiac left ventricle after image acquisition by free-hand nonparallel scanning. In this method, the major axis of the ventricle was first derived by linear least square moment analysis among all the outlined points. With the major axis as the center, all the outlined contours were resampled at fixed angles. Then, the resampled points at the same angle from all the contours were sorted to form a link. Subsequently, the total volume was computed by integrating all of the link sections. In the original cardiac algorithm, the main axis needed to be inside all the contours. Applying this algorithm was not a problem for the calculation of the proximal stomach volume if the main axis was derived from the centroids of the contours at both ends. However, because of the curvature of the distal stomach, it was often impossible to find one axis for this part of the gastric cavity. Accordingly, we divided the distal stomach into three parts and assigned one axis for each part. The default ratio for these three parts was 1:2:1 in terms of the number of outlined contours, but the operator could interactively change the joint location of the axis groupings, if necessary. The decision of where to divide the distal stomach into three parts was made during data analysis and did not bear any relationship to anatomic landmarks. The volume of the total stomach was calculated as the sum of the proximal part and three distal parts of the gastric outlines.

The two acquired compartments of the gastric cavity did not necessarily correspond to the actual division between the proximal and the distal stomach. Accordingly, an algorithm was added to the computer program that enabled the line of intersection between the proximal and the distal stomach to be interactively determined. For this study, the intersection line was defined as the 2D section that was located nearest to the angular incisure at the lesser gastric curvature and directed sagittally toward the greater curvature. After this operation, the volumes of the proximal and distal parts of the stomach were computed automatically. A ratio between the proximal (P) volume and the distal (D) volume was calculated at each time point, and this figure (P/D) was used as a measure of intragastric distribution of the meal. The time needed for manual tracing and volume estimation of a scan of the whole stomach was approximately 7 minutes.

### In Vitro Validation

A pig stomach was obtained from a slaughterhouse, thoroughly washed to remove food remnants and debris, and fixed in 20% formalin. The length of the empty stomach measured 26 cm, and the maximum width was 16 cm. A 2.0-mm catheter with Luer lock was surgically attached to the gastroesophageal junction, enabling known volumes of fluid to be infused. Adjacent to the pylorus, a plastic clamp was mounted firmly to seal the gastric cavity, and a syringe (50 mL) was used to infuse tap water. This gastric preparation was positioned between 6 and 19 cm below the surface in a rubber tank of tap water (23°C). Tap water (1200 mL; 23°C) was infused into the gastric lumen, and air pockets trapped in the cavity were carefully removed using the syringe. A 3D scan of the stomach was obtained by stepwise acquisition of 2D images starting at the surface of the water by the proximal end of the stomach. Subsequently, 100 mL of water was added incrementally before the next 3D scan took place. After the last scan at 1900 mL, blue ink was infused to the gastric lumen to confirm that no leakage was occurring.

### Statistical Analysis

The measurements are given as mean values ± SD of each parameter, if not stated otherwise. As an initial measure of association between true and estimated volumes, Pearson's correlation coefficient was determined. Furthermore, limits of agreement were estimated as suggested by Bland and Altman.[42] The percent error of the measurements was defined as Mean ([Estimated Volume − True Volume]/True Volume) × 100%. Linear regression analysis was applied to estimate the gastric emptying rates and half emptying times; $y$ denotes volume (milliliter) and $x$ denotes time (minutes). The distribution of data was evaluated by inspecting a probability plot and by using Kolmogorov–Smirnov test with Lilliefors subanalysis. If the data appeared normally distributed, Student's $t$ test with two-sided probabilities was used to compare differences between the groups. If not normally distributed, a nonparametric test was applied. A $P$ value <0.05 was chosen as the level of statistical significance. All calculations and graphic designs were performed using commercially available computer software: Microsoft Excel V5.0 for Windows (Microsoft, Redmond, WA) and Systat V5.0 for Windows (Systat Inc., Evanston, IL).

## Results

The magnetometer-based 3D ultrasound system for acquisition and processing of 3D data proved to be applicable both for in vitro and in vivo imaging of the stomach. The conventional free-hand scanning technique was useful for locating the best suitable acoustic windows for 3D imaging. Neither the scanhead sensor mount plus wiring nor the transmitter mount interfered with the normal scanning procedure.

### In Vitro Validation

To scan a pig stomach with this 3D ultrasound system, 15–19 (median, 17) sonograms were recorded depending on the volume of the organ. The 3D system yielded an excellent correlation ($r$ = 0.997) between true volumes and estimated volumes in a range of 1200–1900 mL. There was no significant correlation between the true and difference between true and estimated volumes ($r$ = 0.21; $P$ = 0.62). The 3D ultrasound system overestimated the stomach volumes by an average of 30.5 mL over a range of 1200–1900 mL, and the limits of agreement were from −9.1–70.1 mL (Figure 3). The mean error over the volume range was 2.1% ± 1.1%.

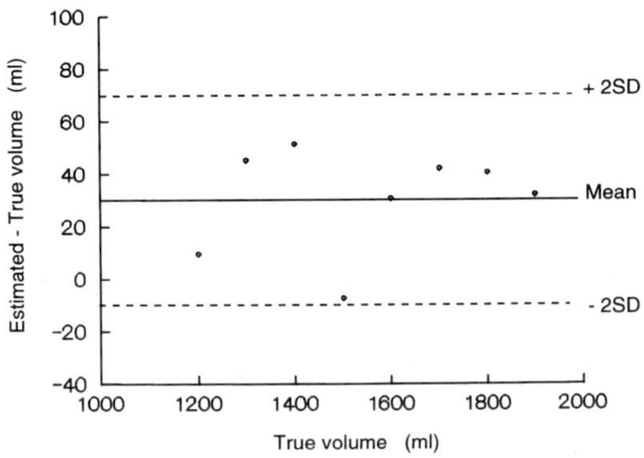


**Figure 3.** Plot displaying the limits of agreement in volume estimation in vitro of the scanning of a porcine stomach by magnetic scanhead tracking. The difference between true volumes (TV), obtained by syringe infusion through a catheter attached to the gastroesophageal junction, and estimated volumes (EV) are depicted on the $y$-axis. The true volumes are plotted along the $x$-axis. The 3D ultrasound system overestimated the volume by an average of 30.5 mL over the range of volumes, displaying no proportional error effect.

### In Vivo Scanning

We acquired a number of 2D scans in the range of 9 ± 2 (fasting) to 19 ± 1 (5 minutes) images to estimate the total stomach volume. The number of sections scanned at 10, 15, 20, 25, and 35 minutes was 18 ± 2, 17 ± 2, 16 ± 2, 15 ± 2, and 14 ± 2, respectively. The depths of scanning used to image the stomach were 12.0 ± 1.6 cm for fasting and 17.9 ± 0.8 cm for postprandial acquisitions.

Ultrasonic imaging of 1 healthy volunteer on 6 consecutive days revealed antral area measurement variability postcibally from 3.8% (5 minutes) to 18.2% (35 minutes), given as coefficient of variation ($V_c$). The intraindividual variability of the total gastric volumes ranged from 5.6% (5 minutes) to 34.3% (35 minutes). Full descriptive statistics are listed in Tables 1 and 2. The regression equation describing the total gastric emptying was y = 451 − 8.0 × (SE of estimate, 16; SE of slope, 0.7; SE of intercept, 14), and the corresponding emptying

Published with permission



**Table 1.** Intraindividual Variability in Healthy Subjects of Sagittal Antral Area Measurements in the Aorto-Mesenteric Section Made by 2D Ultrasonography

| Antral area | Intraindividual variability (n = 6) | | | | Interindividual variability (n = 14) | | | |
|---|---|---|---|---|---|---|---|---|
| | Mean | SEM | SD | Range | Mean | SEM | SD | Range |
| Antecibally | 5.3 | 0.5 | 1.1 | 3.2 | 4.3 | 0.5 | 1.8 | 6.0 |
| 5 min pc | 23.4 | 0.4 | 0.9 | 2.6 | 20.7 | 1.4 | 5.1 | 17.0 |
| 10 min pc | 21.1 | 1.2 | 3.0 | 8.1 | 18.3 | 1.7 | 6.3 | 24.3 |
| 15 min pc | 19.0 | 1.3 | 3.2 | 8.2 | 14.0 | 1.3 | 4.7 | 16.5 |
| 20 min pc | 15.6 | 1.0 | 2.5 | 7.1 | 11.9 | 1.1 | 4.1 | 15.7 |
| 25 min pc | 14.4 | 0.5 | 1.3 | 3.4 | 10.4 | 1.0 | 3.8 | 14.4 |
| 35 min pc | 11.7 | 0.9 | 2.1 | 5.7 | 8.3 | 1.2 | 4.3 | 16.0 |

NOTE. All values are given as centimeters squared. Range is given as the difference between upper and lower limits.
pc, postcibally.

rate was 1.8%/min. In the 2-minute scan time period, 3.6% of the soup meal was emptied from the stomach. The proximal, distal, and the total emptying curves are displayed in Figure 4.

The 14 healthy controls demonstrated postprandial antral area measurement variability in the range of 25% (5 minutes) to 52% (35 minutes). Using the antral 2D measurement as a basis for calculation, we found a half emptying time of 31 ± 22 minutes, and $V_c$ was 70%. The corresponding variability in total gastric volumes was in the range of 13% (5 minutes) to 46% (35 minutes), showing increasing variability with time. The average total gastric emptying was expressed by y = 479 − 11.2 × (SEE, 24; SE of slope, 1.0; SE of intercept, 21). The corresponding values were y = 361 − 8.8 × (SEE, 21; SE of slope, 0.9; SE of intercept, 18) for the proximal stomach, and y = 115 − 2.2 × (SEE, 6; SE of slope, 0.2; SE of intercept, 5) for the distal stomach. The average half

**Table 2.** Intraindividual and Interindividual Variability of Volume Measurements of the Stomach Based on Image Acquisition by 3D Ultrasonography in Healthy Subjects After Ingestion of a 500-mL Soup Meal

| | Intraindividual variability (n = 6) | | | | Interindividual variability (n = 14) | | | |
|---|---|---|---|---|---|---|---|---|
| | Mean | SEM | SD | Range | Mean | SEM | SD | Range |
| Antecibally | | | | | | | | |
| Total volume | 32.9 | 3.2 | 8.0 | 20.0 | 27.8 | 5.6 | 20.9 | 78.9 |
| 5 min pc | | | | | | | | |
| Proximal volume | 318.0 | 8.9 | 21.8 | 55.0 | 327.7 | 15.6 | 58.3 | 257.3 |
| Distal volume | 113.7 | 8.0 | 19.6 | 53.4 | 108.7 | 10.2 | 38.1 | 118.7 |
| Total volume | 431.7 | 9.9 | 24.2 | 74.6 | 436.4 | 14.6 | 54.7 | 171.4 |
| 10 min pc | | | | | | | | |
| Proximal volume | 252.1 | 10.9 | 26.6 | 76.8 | 285.0 | 16.0 | 60.0 | 196.1 |
| Distal volume | 100.7 | 6.4 | 15.6 | 39.7 | 86.2 | 9.0 | 33.5 | 109.1 |
| Total volume | 352.7 | 12.8 | 31.3 | 94.5 | 371.2 | 17.3 | 64.9 | 235.4 |
| 15 min pc | | | | | | | | |
| Proximal volume | 228.5 | 14.6 | 35.7 | 94.4 | 220.7 | 20.0 | 74.7 | 291.5 |
| Distal volume | 90.2 | 7.5 | 18.3 | 44.1 | 84.6 | 6.8 | 25.4 | 78.4 |
| Total volume | 318.7 | 13.3 | 32.6 | 94.1 | 305.4 | 17.7 | 66.4 | 232.2 |
| 20 min pc | | | | | | | | |
| Proximal volume | 224.5 | 19.7 | 48.2 | 102.3 | 172.5 | 16.1 | 60.2 | 188.9 |
| Distal volume | 73.4 | 3.8 | 9.3 | 26.2 | 72.2 | 6.0 | 22.5 | 88.1 |
| Total volume | 297.9 | 20.0 | 49.0 | 102.2 | 244.7 | 16.2 | 60.4 | 164.6 |
| 25 min pc | | | | | | | | |
| Proximal volume | 183.0 | 13.7 | 33.5 | 95.8 | 114.6 | 14.7 | 55.0 | 167.3 |
| Distal volume | 63.5 | 4.8 | 11.7 | 32.1 | 52.5 | 5.4 | 20.1 | 69.5 |
| Total volume | 246.4 | 12.4 | 30.3 | 80.9 | 167.1 | 16.4 | 61.4 | 205.3 |
| 35 min pc | | | | | | | | |
| Proximal volume | 117.4 | 17.1 | 42.0 | 126.8 | 76.1 | 12.1 | 45.1 | 132.6 |
| Distal volume | 59.8 | 8.3 | 20.2 | 55.0 | 40.9 | 6.2 | 23.1 | 80.5 |
| Total volume | 177.2 | 24.8 | 60.7 | 181.8 | 117.0 | 14.4 | 53.9 | 153.6 |

NOTE. All volumes are given as milliliters. Range is given as the difference between upper and lower limits.
pc, postcibally.

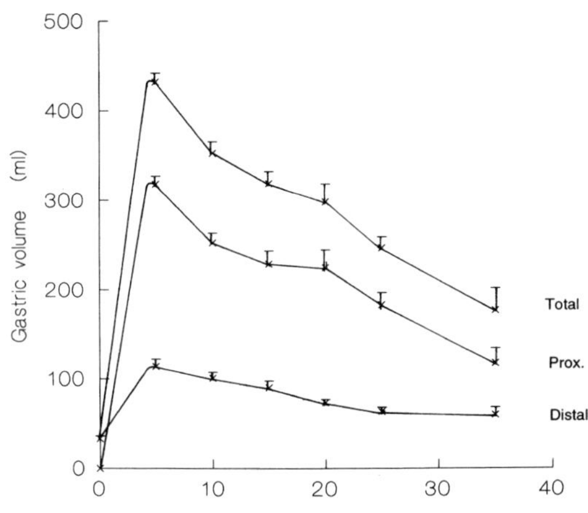


**Figure 4.** Proximal, distal, and total gastric volumes plotted against time to show the day-to-day variability of 1 healthy subject who was scanned on 6 consecutive days. Mean values and SEM are depicted, originating from data acquired by 3D ultrasonography by means of magnetic scanhead tracking.

emptying time of this meal was 22.1 ± 3.8 minutes, based on 3D data, significantly different from half emptying time estimates based on conventional scanning ($P$ = 0.026). The proximal, distal, and the total emptying curves are displayed in Figure 5, and the gastric emptying parameters are listed in Table 3.

Intragastric distribution of the meal, expressed as P/D, varied on average from 3.6 ± 2.1 (5 minutes postcibally) to 2.7 ± 1.9 (30 minutes postcibally) (Table 4). Taking all the scans together, the occurrence of retrograde flow was 11/100 (11%) and it was observed in 10 of 20 examinations. The mean volume of retrograde flow was 28.2 mL when measured in intervals of 5 minutes. The only period in which retrograde flow was not observed was the last observation period (30–35 minutes). Wireframe 3D reconstructions of fasting and postprandial stomach volumes are depicted in Figure 6.

None of the healthy subjects experienced any symptoms during or after the meal. No significant correlation was found between age, weight, or height and gastric areas or volumes. When correlating the standard 2D area measurement of the distal stomach with the corresponding 3D distal volume, only the 35-minute estimates were significantly associated ($r$ = 0.77; $P$ = 0.035, Bonferroni). There was no significant correlation between distal area and total gastric volume or between distal volume and total volume at any time point. However, we found an overall correlation between distal area measurements and distal stomach volumes ($r$ = 0.67; n = 98; $P$ < 0.0005), and between antral area measurements and total stomach volumes ($r$ = 0.53; n = 84; $P$ < 0.005).

## Discussion

The present study shows that a noninvasive and radiation-free method enabled calculation of gastric emptying rates and intragastric distribution of a soup meal in healthy subjects. The use of 3D ultrasonography based on magnetic scanhead tracking permitted images of both the proximal and the distal stomach to be acquired in a translational, stepwise scan. An easy-to-use computer program facilitated outlining of gastric contours and computation of volumes of the gastric compartments. When validated in vitro on a porcine stomach, high accuracy was yielded in volume estimation.

In previous in vitro studies, other investigators reported accuracy of 3D ultrasound systems using mechanical acquisition that was in the same range or lower than in our present study.[40,43,44] Although the present 3D ultrasound system displayed high accuracy in vitro, we cannot immediately extrapolate these results to in vivo conditions. Nevertheless, we have reason to believe that the results obtained in vivo are of acceptable accuracy. First, the mean intercept of the emptying curves of 14 healthy controls was 479.1 mL. Taking into account a mean fasting volume of 27.8 mL, a meal size of 500 mL, and some emptying of the meal during the consumption period,[13] the intercept seems to be at a plausible level.

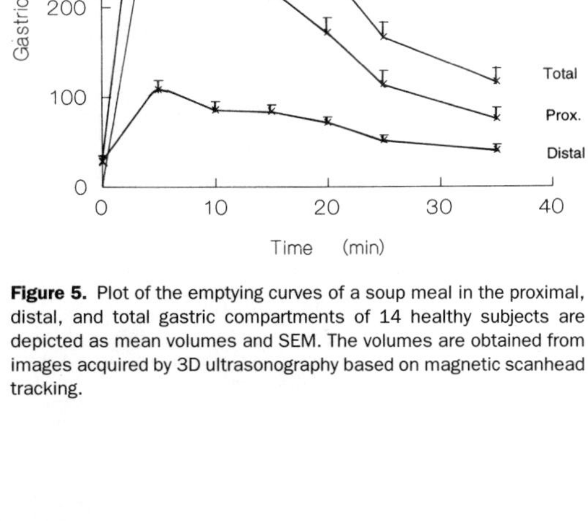


**Figure 5.** Plot of the emptying curves of a soup meal in the proximal, distal, and total gastric compartments of 14 healthy subjects are depicted as mean volumes and SEM. The volumes are obtained from images acquired by 3D ultrasonography based on magnetic scanhead tracking.

Published with permission



**Table 3.** Parameters for Gastric Emptying and Intragastric Distribution of a Soup Meal in 1 Healthy Subject Who Was Scanned on 6 Different Days With a 3D Ultrasonographic System

| Case | Slope | Intercept | $T_{1/2}$ | $P/D_5$ | $P/D_{10}$ | $P/D_{15}$ | $P/D_{20}$ | $P/D_{25}$ | $P/D_{35}$ |
|---|---|---|---|---|---|---|---|---|---|
| 1 | −10.8 | 468.7 | 21.7 | 2.2 | 2.1 | 2.5 | 3.4 | 2.4 | 1.4 |
| 2 | −4.5 | 414.0 | 46.0 | 2.8 | 2.8 | 3.6 | 3.8 | 3.0 | 2.0 |
| 3 | −8.7 | 462.4 | 26.6 | 2.9 | 2.5 | 1.7 | 2.3 | 2.5 | 1.8 |
| 4 | −7.5 | 454.9 | 30.3 | 2.9 | 3.5 | 2.4 | 3.2 | 5.5 | 2.6 |
| 5 | −7.9 | 439.6 | 27.8 | 4.1 | 2.2 | 3.6 | 3.7 | 2.5 | 2.2 |
| 6 | −8.8 | 464.7 | 26.4 | 2.4 | 2.3 | 2.0 | 2.1 | 2.4 | 1.8 |
| Mean | −8.0 | 450.7 | 29.8 | 2.9 | 2.6 | 2.7 | 3.1 | 3.0 | 2.0 |
| SD | 2.1 | 20.7 | 8.4 | 0.6 | 0.5 | 0.8 | 0.7 | 1.2 | 0.4 |
| SEM | 0.8 | 8.5 | 3.4 | 0.3 | 0.2 | 0.3 | 0.3 | 0.5 | 0.2 |
| CV | 0.26 | 0.05 | 0.28 | 0.22 | 0.21 | 0.31 | 0.24 | 0.41 | 0.21 |

NOTE. Slope and intercept (milliliters) denotes the time coefficient (α) and the constant (β) derived from linear regression analysis. $P/D_{5-35}$ denotes the ratio between proximal and distal gastric volumes at different time points after start of soup ingestion (minutes). $T_{1/2}$ denotes half emptying time.

Second, the soup in use was also used in a study where gastric emptying was monitored in healthy controls by radionuclide methods.[45] In this study, a mean half emptying time of 22.9 ± 12.1 minutes was found using scintigraphy, which is close to our finding of 22.1 ± 3.8 minutes. Accordingly, the in vivo data presented in this article appear to be valid and relevant for interpretation of human gastric physiology.

It is well known from scintigraphic studies that gastric emptying data display substantial variability, both intraindividually and interindividually. The variability of the ultrasonic measurements found in our study is comparable to previous radionuclide methodological studies.[46,47] The interindividual variation of antral area measurements using a single 2D sagittal section was greater than the corresponding variation in gastric volumes (Tables 1 and 2). Interestingly, the variability in ultrasound measurements, both within subject and between subjects, increased as emptying proceeded. This observation may be explained by increasing activation of duodeno- and intestino-gastric reflexes throughout the meal-emptying period, inducing relaxation of the proximal stomach to various degrees in different subjects, thus facilitating a wider spectrum of intragastric distribution of the meal.[48,49]

The gastric half emptying rates demonstrated that estimates based on 3D data acquisition were significantly smaller and less variable compared with those based on conventional 2D scanning of the antrum. Actually, the variability ($V_c$) of the 2D data was four times higher than the variability of the 3D data, concerning gastric

**Table 4.** Parameters for Gastric Emptying and Intragastric Distribution of a Soup Meal in 14 Healthy Subjects Who Were Scanned With a 3D Ultrasonographic System Based on Magnetic Scanhead Tracking

| Case | Slope | Intercept | $T_{1/2}$ | $P/D_5$ | $P/D_{10}$ | $P/D_{15}$ | $P/D_{20}$ | $P/D_{25}$ | $P/D_{35}$ |
|---|---|---|---|---|---|---|---|---|---|
| 1 | −9.7 | 481.5 | 24.8 | 2.4 | 2.7 | 2.6 | 1.5 | 1.8 | 1.2 |
| 2 | −8.8 | 480.4 | 27.3 | 4.7 | 3.8 | 3.7 | 3.6 | 3.5 | 3.0 |
| 3 | −11.9 | 440.9 | 18.5 | 1.5 | 2.1 | 1.1 | 0.8 | 0.4 | 0.2 |
| 4 | −8.8 | 466.2 | 26.5 | 3.0 | 2.5 | 1.7 | 2.3 | 2.5 | 1.8 |
| 5 | −11.5 | 487.0 | 21.2 | 2.2 | 2.8 | 2.0 | 1.4 | 1.5 | 2.2 |
| 6 | −12.7 | 445.2 | 17.5 | 6.1 | 2.5 | 6.9 | 8.6 | 7.3 | 5.9 |
| 7 | −13.1 | 441.9 | 16.9 | 2.7 | 4.1 | 2.6 | 1.9 | 0.7 | 0.0 |
| 8 | −7.0 | 376.8 | 26.9 | 3.7 | 1.8 | 2.1 | 1.8 | 1.7 | 1.5 |
| 9 | −12.8 | 453.7 | 17.7 | 1.9 | 1.7 | 0.8 | 1.9 | 1.2 | 0.4 |
| 10 | −8.7 | 440.9 | 25.3 | 3.4 | 3.4 | 2.2 | 2.3 | 1.6 | 1.1 |
| 11 | −14.6 | 601.3 | 20.6 | 2.2 | 2.7 | 2.6 | 3.4 | 5.7 | 3.9 |
| 12 | −14.0 | 595.4 | 21.3 | 9.7 | 9.3 | 7.4 | 4.2 | 2.9 | 8.9 |
| 13 | −9.8 | 492.4 | 25.1 | 3.3 | 7.8 | 4.3 | 3.9 | 4.2 | 5.3 |
| 14 | −12.9 | 504.3 | 19.5 | 3.4 | 2.8 | 2.9 | 2.3 | 2.1 | 3.7 |
| Mean | −11.2 | 479.1 | 22.1 | 3.6 | 3.6 | 3.1 | 2.8 | 2.7 | 2.8 |
| SD | 2.3 | 59.5 | 3.8 | 2.1 | 2.2 | 2.0 | 1.9 | 1.9 | 2.5 |
| SEM | 0.6 | 15.9 | 1.0 | 0.6 | 0.6 | 0.5 | 0.5 | 0.5 | 0.7 |
| CV | 0.21 | 0.12 | 0.17 | 0.59 | 0.63 | 0.64 | 0.68 | 0.73 | 0.91 |

NOTE. Slope and intercept denotes the time coefficient (α) and the constant (β) derived from linear regression analysis. $P/D_{5-35}$ denotes the ratio between proximal and distal gastric volumes at different time points.

half emptying time. Most previous ultrasonic methods to study gastric emptying have used different measures of the antrum to predict total gastric volumes and emptying rates. In this study, there was no significant correlation between antral area and distal or total gastric volume at any time point. In addition, most of the meal was stored in the proximal rather than the distal stomach (Figures 4 and 5); subsequently, the total gastric emptying curve more closely parallels that of the proximal than the distal stomach. Furthermore, phasic contractions change the geometry of the distal stomach to a larger degree than that of the proximal stomach and therefore are more likely to influence the area over the curve in the distal stomach. One of the advantages of 3D ultrasonography is that no assumptions regarding shape of the stomach have to be made before volume estimation. Accordingly, this 3D ultrasound system may represent a significant step forward with respect to measuring gastric emptying by ultrasound.

Using radionuclide methods, different approaches have been used to divide the stomach into a proximal and a distal region of interest.[50,51] Collins et al.[52,53] reported that the proximal stomach region was defined as the "reservoir" area seen in all subjects for at least the first

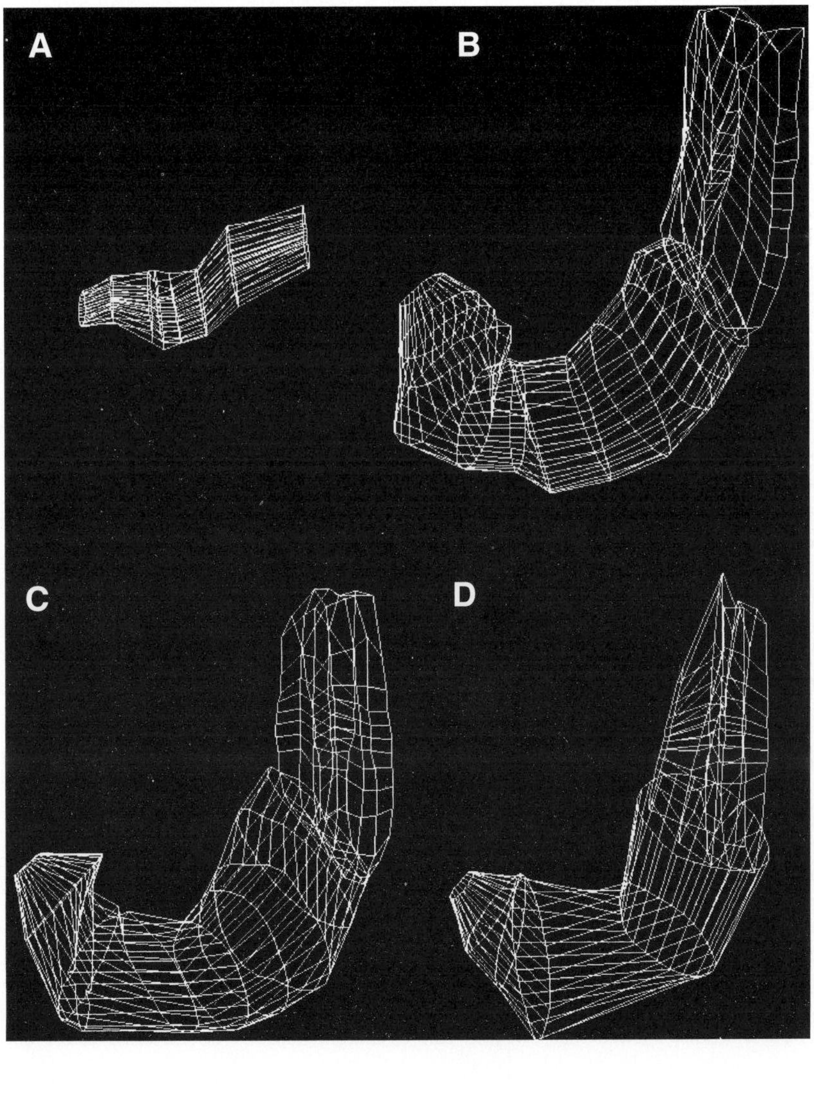


**Figure 6.** 3D wireframes of the stomach of a healthy subject reconstructed from ultrasound images obtained by magnetic scanhead tracking. Panel *A* is made of antecibal scans, and *B, C,* and *D* are outlined from scans 5, 10, and 15 minutes after the soup meal, respectively. Computerized volume reconstruction was performed by using custom software developed within the Application Visualization System software package V5.01 (Advanced Visual Systems Inc., Waltham, MA).

Published with permission



few postcibal frames, and a proximal/distal dividing line was drawn immediately below this region. Another investigator divided the gastric outline at its midpoint by a computer program, with the two regions produced defined as fundus and antrum.[1] In one study, the gastric region of interest was divided into two equal areas, designated the proximal and the distal stomach, by using the cursor facility of the machine to place a line across the stomach so that 50% of the isotope containing pixels was present in each area.[2] Apparently, there seems to be no consensus on how to exactly divide the stomach into a proximal and distal region after scintigraphic scanning. Using ultrasonography, access to anatomic landmarks is provided by the images, giving the operator the choice to base the decision on either anatomic or functional considerations. Contrary to radionuclide methods, ultrasonography offers high image resolution and frame rates that enable exact delineation of the stomach wall without inducing repositioning errors during the examination. In our study, we chose the angular incisure located at the minor curvature as guidance for the division between the distal and the proximal stomach. This anatomic landmark is easily visualized by ultrasonography. In our opinion, the use of ultrasonography to determine the division line is more precise than the radionuclide methods outlined above.

Intragastric distribution is a parameter that has mainly been adopted for studies of patients with functional dyspepsia. Several investigators have indicated that these patients show abnormal intragastric distribution of the meal, as evaluated by scintigraphy.[1–3] In our study on healthy subjects, we observed a relatively high P/D initially, declining as the meal emptied. Interestingly, we found that retrograde flow from the distal to the proximal stomach occurred in 11% of measurement periods, and it was observed in half of the examinations. It is worth noting that the high intersubject variability in the P/D data makes it questionable if intragastric distribution is a useful parameter in diagnosis and work-up of patients. Nevertheless, further development of hardware and software for 3D ultrasonic image acquisition are in progress and may improve spatial and temporal resolution of this technique significantly, thus enabling a more precise and consistent division of the gastric compartments.

This study was subject to the same limitations of ultrasound scanning that are generally observed in other studies. The method is fairly operator-dependent and may be influenced by the presence of air pockets within the fundus, which dramatically reduces image quality. This problem was addressed in previous studies using the same soup meal, both in healthy controls[20] and in patients with functional dyspepsia.[39] These studies showed that air in the gastric fundus was not a critical factor for ultrasonic imaging using this meal, and no subjects had to be excluded for this reason. Similarly, in the present study, gas pockets in the fundus did not impair visualization of the proximal stomach to such an extent that data could not be analyzed. We believe that the method of heating the meal to the boiling point and then cooling it to body temperature generates less air bubbles in the stomach than a meal at room temperature that is ingested. Furthermore, the seated position with the individuals leaning slightly backward was probably optimal with respect to distribution of air within the stomach. If any of the volunteers experienced an urge to burp during or just after the ingestion of the soup, they were encouraged to do so.

Compared with ordinary ultrasound equipment, this 3D system based on magnetic scanhead tracking, although less than for comparable magnetic systems, is susceptible to metallic influence and to interference from external magnetic fields. Therefore, it is of major importance that the laboratory environment is evaluated carefully to avoid spatial distortion of data. The distance from the scanner itself to the sensor on the scanhead should preferably be at least 60 cm, and the bed or chair must be made of material that does not influence magnetic fields. Despite our efforts to remove watches, belts, coins, etc. from both the operators and the participants, two of the data sets were distorted, probably because of magnetic interference from nearby experiments in the laboratory.

An acquisition time of 2 minutes was used in this study because the image workstation design required that it store each captured image to hard disk before the next acquisition. By using image acquisition systems that enable storing of data in random access memory, the acquisition of a total gastric volume could easily be reduced to less than 30 seconds. The long scanning time experienced in this study may have caused a small intragastric volume to empty through the pylorus or possibly to change compartments during the scanning procedure. Conversely, the slow pace of data capture gave the operator time to carefully select images of high quality and to avoid capturing gastric contractions in the data set, thus minimizing potential errors in volume calculation.

This novel ultrasonographic method to scan the human stomach may be used to evaluate patients with functional dyspepsia, diabetes mellitus, and other conditions in which gastroparesis and maldistribution is a prominent feature. However, before further application of this method in clinical settings, validation against the gold standard at present, scintigraphy, would be reasonable. Furthermore, caution needs to be exercised before our

Published with permission



results can be extrapolated to gastric emptying of solids. In conclusion, we found that the present 3D ultrasonographic method based on magnetic scanhead tracking demonstrated high accuracy in vitro. The 3D system computed gastric emptying parameters more precisely than conventional 2D ultrasonography in healthy individuals. Furthermore, intragastric distribution of a meal could be determined based on detailed segmentation of gastric compartments.

## References

1. Scott AM, Kellow JE, Shuter B, Cowan H, Corbett AM, Riley JW, Lunzer MR, Eckstein RP, Hoschl R, Lam SK, Jones MP. Intragastric distribution and gastric emptying of solids and liquids in functional dyspepsia. Lack of influence of symptom subgroups and *H. pylori*-associated gastritis. Dig Dis Sci 1993;38:2247–2254.
2. Troncon LEA, Bennett RJ, Ahluwalia NK, Thompson DG. Abnormal intragastric distribution of food during gastric emptying in functional dyspepsia patients. Gut 1994;35:327–332.
3. Mangnall YF, Houghton LA, Johnson AG, Read NW. Abnormal distribution of a fatty liquid test meal within the stomach of patients with non-ulcer dyspepsia. Eur J Gastroenterol Hepatol 1994;6:323–327.
4. Jones KL, Horowitz M, Wishart MJ, Maddox AF, Harding PE, Chatterton BE. Relationships between gastric emptying, intragastric meal distribution and blood glucose concentrations in diabetes mellitus. J Nucl Med 1995;36:2220–2228.
5. Holt S, McDicken WN, Anderson T, Stewart IC, Heading RC. Dynamic imaging of the stomach by real-time ultrasound—a method for the study of gastric motility. Gut 1980;21:597–601.
6. Hausken T, Odegaard S, Berstad A. Antroduodenal motility studied by real-time ultrasonography. Effect of enprostil. Gastroenterology 1991;100:59–63.
7. Vogelberg KH, Rathmann W, Helbig G. Sonographic examination of gastric motility in diabetics with autonomic neuropathy. Diabetes Res 1987;5:175–179.
8. Hausken T, Berstad A. Wide gastric antrum in patients with non-ulcer dyspepsia. Effect of cisapride. Scand J Gastroenterol 1992; 27:427–432.
9. Hausken T, Svebak S, Wilhelmsen I, Tangen Haug T, Olafsen K, Pettersson E, Hveem K, Berstad A. Low vagal tone and antral dysmotility in patients with functional dyspepsia. Psychosom Med 1993;55:12–22.
10. Dorlars D, Schilling D, Riemann JF. The feasibility of ultrasonography for the evaluation of stomach motility disorders. Dtsch Med Wochenschr 1994;119:575–580.
11. Duan LP, Zheng ZT, Li YN. A study of gastric emptying in non-ulcer dyspepsia using a new ultrasonographic method. Scand J Gastroenterol 1993;28:355–360.
12. King PM, Adam RD, Pryde A, McDicken WN, Heading RC. Relationships of human antroduodenal motility and transpyloric fluid movement: non-invasive observations with real-time ultrasound. Gut 1984;25:1384–1391.
13. Hausken T, Odegaard S, Matre K, Berstad A. Antroduodenal motility and movements of luminal contents studied by duplex sonography. Gastroenterology 1992;102:1583–1590.
14. Brown BP, Schulze Delrieu K, Schrier JE, Abu Yousef MM. The configuration of the human gastroduodenal junction in the separate emptying of liquids and solids. Gastroenterology 1993;105: 433–440.
15. Bateman DN, Whittingham TA. Measurement of gastric emptying by real-time ultrasound. Gut 1982;23:524–527.
16. Bolondi L, Bortolotti M, Santi V, Calletti T, Gaiani S, Labo G. Measurement of gastric emptying time by real-time ultrasonography. Gastroenterology 1985;89:752–759.
17. Ricci R, Bontempo I, Corazziari E, La Bella A, Torsoli A. Real time ultrasonography of the gastric antrum. Gut 1993;34:173–176.
18. Holt S, Cervantes J, Wilkinson AA, Wallace JH. Measurement of gastric emptying rate in humans by real-time ultrasound. Gastroenterology 1986;90:918–923.
19. Tomooka Y, Onitsuka H, Goya T, Koga T, Uchida S, Russell WJ, Torisu M. Ultrasonography of benign gastric ulcers. Characteristic features and sequential follow-ups. J Ultrasound Med 1989;8: 513–517.
20. Gilja OH, Hausken T, Odegaard S, Berstad A. Monitoring postprandial size of the proximal stomach by ultrasonography. J Ultrasound Med 1995;14:81–89.
21. Thune N, Hausken T, Gilja OH, Matre K. A practical method for estimating enclosed volumes using 3D ultrasound. Eur J Ultrasound 1996;3:83–92.
22. Gilja OH, Thune N, Matre K, Hausken T, Odegaard S, Berstad A. In vitro evaluation of three-dimensional ultrasonography in volume estimation of abdominal organs. Ultrasound Med Biol 1994;20: 157–165.
23. Gilja OH, Smievoll AI, Thune N, Matre K, Hausken T, Odegaard S, Berstad A. In vivo comparison of 3D ultrasonography and magnetic resonance imaging in volume estimation of human kidneys. Ultrasound Med Biol 1995;21:25–32.
24. Hausken T, Thune N, Matre K, Gilja OH, Odegaard S, Berstad A. Volume estimation of the gastric antrum and the gallbladder in patients with non-ulcer dyspepsia and erosive prepyloric changes, using three-dimensional ultrasonography. Neurogastroenterol Motil 1994;6:263–270.
25. Hokland J, Hausken T. An interactive volume rendering method applied to ultrasonography of abdominal structures. IEEE Ultrason Symp Proc 1994;3:1567–1571.
26. Gilja OH, Hausken T, Berstad A. Three-dimensional ultrasonography of the gastric antrum in patients with functional dyspepsia (abstr). Gastroenterology 1995;108:A605.
27. Berstad A, Hausken T, Gilja OH, Thune N, Matre K, Odegaard S. Volume measurement of gastric antrum by 3-D ultrasonography and flow measurements through the pylorus by duplex technique. Dig Dis Sci 1994;39:97–100.
28. Dekker DL, Piziali RL, Dong EJ. A system for ultrasonically imaging the human heart in three dimensions. Comput Biomed Res 1974; 7:544–553.
29. Nikravesh PE, Skorton DJ, Chandran KB, Attarwala YM, Pandian N, Kerber RE. Computerized three-dimensional finite element reconstruction of the left ventricle from cross-sectional echocardiograms. Ultrason Imaging 1984;6:48–59.
30. Moritz WE, Shreve PL, Mace LE. Analysis of an ultrasonic spatial locating system. IEEE Trans Instrum Meas 1976;25:43–50.
31. Brinkley JF, Muramatsu SK, McCallum WD, Popp RL. In vitro evaluation of an ultrasonic three-dimensional imaging and volume system. Ultrason Imaging 1982;4:126–139.
32. Handschumacher MD, Lethor JP, Siu SC, Mele D, Rivera JM, Picard MH, Weyman AE, Levine RA. A new integrated system for three-dimensional echocardiographic reconstruction: development and validation for ventricular volume with application in human subjects. J Am Coll Cardiol 1993;21:743–753.
33. Levine RA, Handschumacher MD, Sanfilippo AJ, Hagege AA, Harrigan P, Marshall JE, Weyman AE. Three-dimensional echocardiographic reconstruction of the mitral valve, with implications for the diagnosis of mitral valve prolapse. Circulation 1989;80:589–598.
34. Kelly IM, Gardener JE, Brett AD, Richards R, Lees WR. Three-dimensional US of the fetus. Work in progress. Radiology 1994; 192:253–259.
35. Detmer PR, Bashein G, Hodges TC, Beach KW, Filer EP, Burns

Published with permission



DH, Strandness DE, Jr. 3D ultrasonic image feature localization based on magnetic scanhead tracking: in vitro calibration and validation. Ultrasound Med Biol 1995;20:923–936.

36. Hodges TC, Detmer PR, Burns DH, Beach KW, Strandness DE, Jr. Ultrasonic three-dimensional reconstruction: in vitro and in vivo volume and area measurement. Ultrasound Med Biol 1994; 20:719–729.
37. Gilja OH, Hausken T, Olafsson S, Matre K, Odegaard S. In vitro evaluation of three-dimensional ultrasonography based on magnetic scanhead tracking (abstr). Ultraschall Med 1995;16:24.
38. Leotta DF, Detmer PR, Gilja OH, Jong JM, Martin RW, Primozich JF, Beach KW, Strandness DE, Jr. Three-dimensional ultrasound imaging using multiple magnetic tracking systems and miniature magnetic sensors. Proc IEEE Int Ultrasonics Symp 1995, Seattle, WA: 1415–1418.
39. Gilja OH, Hausken T, Wilhelmsen I, Berstad A. Impaired accommodation of the proximal stomach to a soup meal in functional dyspepsia. Dig Dis Sci 1996;41:689–696.
40. Moritz WE, Pearlman AS, McCabe DH, Medema DK, Ainsworth ME, Boles MS. An ultrasonic technique for imaging the ventricle in three dimensions and calculating its volume. IEEE Trans Biomed Eng 1983;30:482–491.
41. Martin RW, Bashein G, Detmer PR, Moritz WE. Ventricular volume measurement from a multiplanar transesophageal ultrasonic imaging system: an in vitro study. IEEE Trans Biomed Eng 1990; 37:442–449.
42. Bland JM, Altman DG. Statistical methods for assessing agreement between two methods of clinical measurements. Lancet 1986;1:307–310.
43. Ariet M, Geiser EA, Lupkiewicz SM, Conetta DA, Conti CR. Evaluation of a three-dimensional reconstruction to compute left ventricular volume and mass. Am J Cardiol 1984;54:415–420.
44. Basset O, Gimenez G, Mestas JL, Cathignol D, Devonec M. Volume measurement by ultrasonic transverse or sagittal cross-sectional scanning. Ultrasound Med Biol 1991;17:291–296.
45. Hveem K, Jones K, Chatterton BE, Horowitz M. Scintigraphic and ultrasonographic measurement of the antral area—relationship to appetite. Gut 1996;38:816–821.
46. Lawaetz O, Dige Petersen H. Gastric emptying of liquid meals. A study in 88 normal persons. Ann Chir Gynaecol 1989;78:267–276.
47. Brophy CM, Moore JG, Christian PE, Egger MJ, Taylor AT. Variability of gastric emptying measurements in man employing standardized radiolabeled meals. Dig Dis Sci 1986;31:799–806.
48. Azpiroz F, Malagelada JR. Isobaric intestinal distension in humans: sensorial relay and reflex gastric relaxation. Am J Physiol 1990;258:G202–G207.
49. De Ponti F, Azpiroz F, Malagelada JR. Reflex gastric relaxation in response to distention of the duodenum. Am J Physiol 1987; 252:G595–G601.
50. Barker MC, Cobden I, Axon AT. Proximal stomach and antrum in stomach emptying. Gut 1979;20:309–311.
51. Lawaetz O, Aritas Y, Brown NJ, Ralphs DN, Sjontoft E. Distribution of a liquid meal within the stomach and gastric emptying after vagotomy and drainage operations. Gut 1982;23:683–691.
52. Collins PJ, Horowitz M, Chatterton BE. Proximal, distal and total stomach emptying of a digestible solid meal in normal subjects. Br J Radiol 1988;61:12–18.
53. Collins PJ, Houghton LA, Read NW, Horowitz M, Chatterton BE, Heddle R, Dent J. Role of the proximal and distal stomach in mixed solid and liquid meal emptying. Gut 1991;32:615–619.

**Received September 4, 1996. Accepted March 13, 1997.**

**Address requests for reprints to: Odd Helge Gilja, M.D., Ph.D., Medical Department A, Haukeland Hospital, University of Bergen, N-5021 Bergen, Norway. e-mail: Odd.Gilja@meda.uib.no; fax: (47) 55-972950.**

**Supported by The Norwegian Research Council, Odd Fellow Medical Research Foundation (Norway), Astri and Edvard Riisøen's Legacy, and Nycomed Pharma (Norway) and a grant from the University of Washington Royalty Research Fund. The 3D acquisition system was provided by National Institutes of Health grants HL41464 and R43RR07741 and the processing and display equipment by National Institutes of Health HL42270.**

**The authors thank Prof. Svein Ødegaard, who facilitated the collaboration between the University of Washington and the University of Bergen, and Advanced Technology Laboratory (Bothell, WA) for providing the ultrasound system.**

## CHAPTER 10

# THE EchoPAC-3D SOFTWARE FOR 3D IMAGE ANALYSIS

DITLEF MARTENS AND ODD HELGE GILJA

## 1. Introduction

EchoPAC-3D is the GE Vingmed Ultrasound 3D port-processing system. Prototype development started at Christian Michelsen Research (CMR, Bergen Norway) in 1992, working in close collaboration with Haukeland University Hospital with funding from the Norwegian Research Council. A mechanical motorized adapter tilting an annular array probe was developed at SINTEF in Trondheim, Norway. CMR developed software for display of slices from the 3D volume and for volume estimation (1). Methodological and clinical evaluation started at Haukeland UH showing good accuracy of the methods (2). GE Vingmed Ultrasound developed algorithms for interactive volume rendering (3). Support for 3D acquisition using a position-sensing device (Flock of Birds, Ascension Technologies, Burlington, USA) was added to the GE Vingmed System Five scanner. EchoPAC-3D development was in two directions: product development for the first release of EchoPAC-3D and research features to support clinical research at Haukeland UH and other sites. The first product release of EchoPAC-3D ran on a built-in Apple Macintosh on the System-FiVe scanner with position sensor acquisition. A second release for trigged 3D cardiac scanning using multi-plane transesophageal (TEE) probe and transthoracic scanning with rotation adapter was released for the new Vivid-5 scanner in 2000 (4).

EchoPAC-3D supports analysis, measurements and visualization of 3D and triggered data. This paper gives an overview of the features available in the research version of EchoPAC-3D. 3D data acquisition is not an integrated part of EchoPAC-3D, but the system interfaces to raw data format from the scanner (providing 3D acquisition). Being able to view any cutplane (sometimes called C-Mode) through the 3D volume is a natural extension of the B-Mode (2D view) used for 2D scanning. EchoPAC-3D provides this functionality in the AnyPlane window. User-friendly tools to navigate through the 3D volume to select clinically interesting cutplanes and visualizations of the data are important and EchoPAC-3D has a set of tools for navigation. These are used in combination with the Geometry window giving an overview of the 3D volume together with the position and orientation of the cut-planes and visualization. 2D measurements, volume measurements and flow velocity traces provide quantitative analysis of the data. Data can be exported to spreadsheets for further analysis and tools are available to make presentations with bitmaps and video.

Techniques for 3D ultrasound acquisition, analysis and display for medical applications now cover a large field (5). This chapter will focus on the main features developed in EchoPAC-3D.

## 2. Data Acquisition

Three-Dimensional ultrasound data acquisition is a challenging field. Extending from 2D to cover a 3D volume implies that a lot more beams have to be sent into the body. To obtain a resolution comparable to a 2D image the number of beams to be acquired may be 50–200 times larger. Given a typical 2D frame rate of 10 to 50 frames per second a comparable 3D scan will give very low volume rate. Scanning using a low volume rate will give imaging artefacts if the operator holding the probe, the patient or bodily parts moves during the acquisition. For cardiac imaging acquiring only a few frames/volumes per second is not acceptable as the heart contains rapid moving walls and valves. Motion artefacts from respiration and heart movement can also be seen in vascular and radiology applications. A probe for 2D ultrasound sweeps its field of view using either a mechanical motor as used for annular array probes or having an array of elements and using electronically focused beams as available in most modern systems. This idea is extended to 3D ultrasound. A 2D sweep can be either mechanically moved to cover a 3D volume or electronically acquired in 3D.

For mechanical acquisition, the common approaches are:

### 2.1. *3D scanning using mechanical probe movement*

#### 2.1.1. *Tilted scan*

The 2D scanplane is rotated about and axis parallel to the probe surface and in the plane defined by the 2D scan. First 3D ultrasound using EchoPAC-3D at Haukeland University Hospital were acquired using an annular phased array (APAT) probe with an externally attached stepper motor that could tilt the probe 90 degrees. A simple push-button would start the 3D sweep. No changes were required in the scanner. The operator would manually select the correct images to be saved. Some newer systems have the stepper motor built into the probe to avoid the extra attachment and making the system easier to use. Using this system, the beam density in 3D will be similar to the beam density of a 2D sector probe. If the tilt-axis is close to the probe surface the near-field of the probe will cover only a small volume. The advantage is, however, that the probe surface can be kept still avoiding any artefacts from a probe moving along the skin.

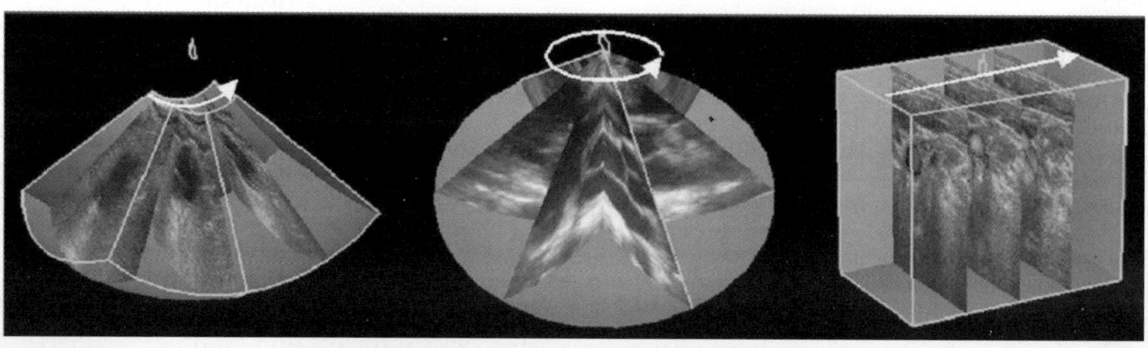

Fig. 1. Different methods for mechanical 3D scanning each shown with three acquired 2D frames. Arrow indicates probe movement. Left: Tilted scan. Centre: rotated scan. Right: translated scan.

### 2.1.2. *Rotated scan*

The probe is rotated about its main axis to cover a cylindrical volume for linear scan and conical volume for sector scan. This acquisition method is quite common for cardiac 3D imaging. Many TEE probes have a built-in motor to rotate the scanplane and for transthoracic imaging, the probe surface must be small to fit in the acoustical window between the ribs.

When using rotational 3D scanning it is very easy to get imaging artefacts along the rotation axis, as all acquired 2D images will cover this area. Any movement during acquisition will cause imaging artefacts in this centre area. The advantage is that all segments of the heart chamber can be covered, also with a short scan with low 3D resolution.

### 2.1.3. *Translated scan*

In a translated scan all 2D scanplanes are parallel. Translated scan is suitable for vascular imaging where imaging with high frequency probes at shallow depth is used. A translated scan gives uniform sampling density in the third dimension, but the mechanical adapter is larger as the probe is moved over a larger distance compared to a rotational and tilted scan.

Translated scan can also be used for endoscopic ultrasound. The probe or endoscope is pulled inside the patient at a constant speed. At Haukeland UH a simple fixture driven by a electric screwdriver has been successfully applied to pull back the endoscope. The pullback speed was measured and 2D images were imported to EchoPAC-3D via a video tape (6).

## 2.2. *Freehand position sensor scan*

A device to sense the position and orientation is attached to the ultrasound probe. Several different systems are available on the market. EchoPAC-3D has been adapted to use a system where a transmitter generates a magnetic field and a small receiver is mounted on the ultrasound probe (Flock of Birds, Ascension Technologies, Vermont, USA). This system operates at a limited range (<60–80 cm) and can be influenced by metal or other magnetic fields.

A freehand system allows the operator to perform a 3D scan quite similar to a 2D scan. Subsequently, the best acoustical windows can be selected. This enables large organs like the liver and stomach to be covered (7). Motion of the probe or operator during scanning may be a problem with the mechanical systems. This motion is detected by the freehand system and adjusted for during reconstruction. The operator needs training to adjust the motion of the probe to the frame rate of the scanner and the desired resolution of the 3D scan. Fast movements of the probe induce gaps in the 3D data. Feedback during acquisition and fast reconstruction time after completing the 3D scan is desirable to make the method practical and clinically useful.

Freehand systems have also been applied to cardiac scanning. A slow tilt during 20–40 cardiac cycles has been found to be accurate and give ventricular volumes rendering with high frame rate (8).

### 2.3. *3D scanning using 2–Dimensional transducer arrays*

A 2D array of elements makes it possible to electronically focus the beams in both azimuth and elevation direction. A large number of elements are required. For 2D scanning 64–128 elements is typical, for 3D scanning a probe containing $64 \times 64$ elements gives a total of 4096 elements. Attaching each element to a separate channel in the scanner is not practically possible because the cable and scanner beam processing modules would be 30 times bigger that of a 2D scanner.

Various techniques have been attempted to reduce the complexity.

(1) Thinned arrays send and receive on fewer elements (10–20% of total).

(2) Doing partial beam forming in the probe makes it possible to attach a 3D probe to a conventional scanner.

(3) A 2D array can be connected so that only one row at a time is active with separate electronic signalling to select active row. The matrix can be flat or curved. This type of probe works like 2D probe with tilted or translated 3D mechanical scan.

Two dimensional transducer array probes are well suited for real-time cardiac scanning where time to acquire a 3D volume needs to be very short (<30 ms) due to the cardiac motion.

## 3. Data Representation and Scan Conversion

When used in radiology applications, EchoPAC-3D will combine the 2D images into one 3D volume. For cardiac data, the ECG trace is used to sort the data into a cineloop of 3D volumes where each volume will contain the 2D frames from the same time offset from the systole. The scanner can detect respiration and limits can be set to reduce respiration artefacts.

To utilize the advantages of the raw data format, EchoPAC-3D will, if possible, extract cut planes directly from the raw data. When using the magnetic sensor for freehand scanning the algorithm to extract cut planes is too slow for interactive use. Therefore, EchoPAC-3D first convert the image data into a regular Cartesian coordinate system and assign each image value to new positions (voxel) within a regular data volume (cuberille).

The visualization algorithms process data in a sub-volume of the raw data. First, data for visualization is always scanconverted to a cuberille to improve the rendering speed. Supporting fast raw data scanconversion for tilted, rotated, translated and freehand 3D formats for both sector and linear 2D probes adds a lot of complexity to the system but avoids an extra transformation. This enables the user to zoom into the data with maximal resolution and allows the calculation of velocity from flow data.

Flow and tissue is time filtered and mixed using the same algorithms used on the scanner. Utilizing raw data also enables parameters like Gain, Compress and Tissue Priority to be modified the same way as in the Freeze mode on the scanner. It is also possible to remove the flow signal to view only the pure tissue image.

### 3.1. *Position sensor data scan conversion*

There are two main methods utilized for scan conversion from 2D planes at arbitrary positions to a regular cuberille where each element (voxel) is stored in Cartesian coordinates.

(a) Scanconvert each 2D frame as a thin 3D slice into the cuberille. If output of other 2D frames overlaps, output is mixed.

(b) For each voxel in the cuberille, find 2D frames close to the voxel and mix based on distance from voxel.

The ultrasound beam has an elevation beam width. This width determines the thickness of the 2D scanplane. If two neighbouring scanplanes have a distance greater than the elevation beam width, the part of the body between the scanplanes has not been scanned. When showing the results from a 3D scan there could be black stripes in the image marking areas that have not been scanned. Using a freehand scan with a position sensor this will occur if the probe is moved too fast (Fig. 2).

For position sensor scan conversion, EchoPAC-3D will estimate the slice thickness based on the position sensor data and show black stripes only if the plane distance is greater than 5 millimetres (configurable) to avoid too many black stripes (Fig. 2). It is common also for motorized 3D scanning to increase inter-plane distance beyond the elevation beam width to save scanning time.

EchoPAC-3D uses the first method. We estimated the performance of both algorithms and the first algorithm was found to be superior in terms of processing speed and comparable in quality to the second algorithm. Areas scanned by several 2D scanplanes can be processed similarly to 2D compound imaging where the scan contains beams sent from different directions to improve image quality. Different algorithms are in use: maximal, median or mean value (9) designed to remove imaging artefacts like shadowing and speckle. EchoPAC-3D uses a weighted mean based on the distance to each 2D scanplane to determine the intensity of each voxel in the cuberille (Fig. 3).

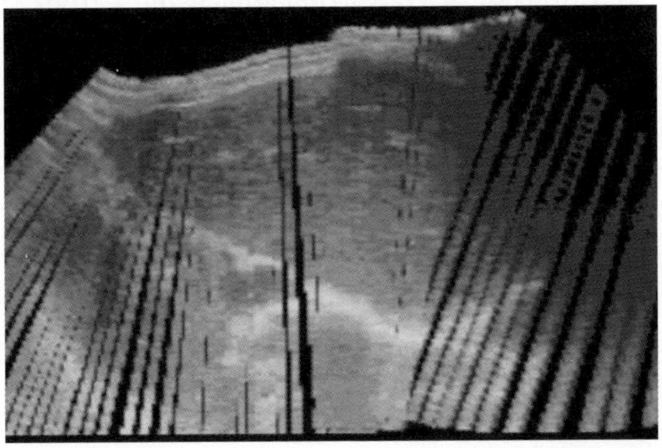

Fig. 2. Moving the probe too fast when scanning a liver using freehand scanning with the Bird system. Each ultrasound slice and gaps can be seen.

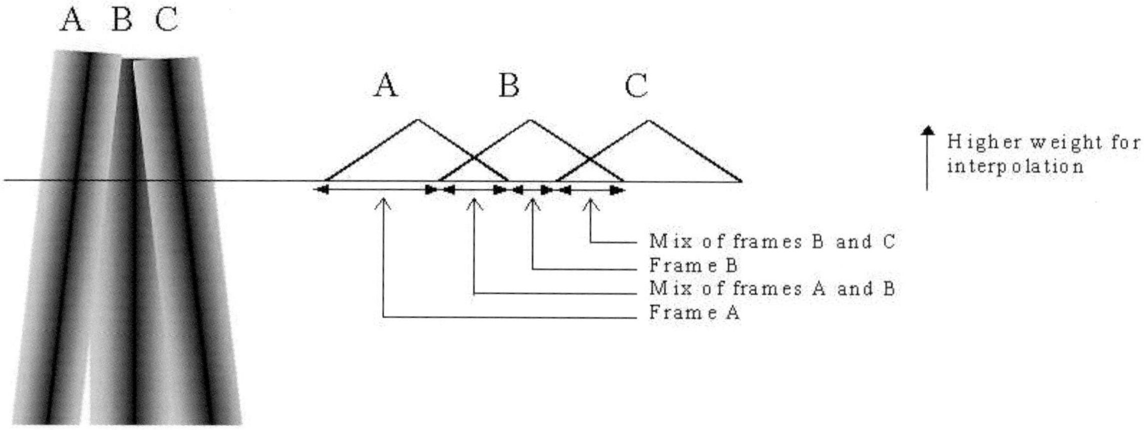


Fig. 3. Position sensor scan conversion of 3 frames showing inter-frame interpolation. Frames will be mixed where they overlap. Black stripes will be shown where they don't.

## 4. Main Features of EchoPAC-3D

The main features of EchoPAC-3D are:

(1) Data Acquisition and Data Import

Several other 3D processing packages does 3D acquisition by grabbing the video signal from the ultrasound scanner and simultaneously controlling the 3D adapter. This allows a very loose coupling to the scanner and is easy to adapt to different probes and scanners. EchoPAC-3D has been connected to scanners supporting 3D acquisition with raw data export for maximal data quality and post processing capabilities. All main modes of 3D and triggered 3D acquisition is supported by EchoPAC-3D. The research version also supports import of video grabbed data for endoscopic ultrasound and Magnetic Resonance (MR) or Computed Tomography (CT) for multi-modality research.

(2) Scan Scanconversion

Scanconversion is the process of converting image data from the geometry from the scanning to a regular geometry (bitmap) that can be displayed on the screen. To fill in gaps between each ultrasound beam for flow imaging the tissue and flow signals must be mixed. 3D scan conversion is similar to 2D, but must handle larger data volumes and more scan formats. Scan conversion is also needed for 3D flow velocity calculations.

(3) Anyplane Slicing

An important basic functionality in a 3D system is to show slices of the 3D volume. A software system should be able to show both original 2D planes and arbitrarily oriented planes.

(4) Quantitative Analysis

EchoPAC-3D support simple 2D measurements in any 2D plane, volume measurements and flow velocity profiles. Ejection fraction can be calculated based on volume measurements on triggered data.

(5) Geometry Visualization

Geometric 3D representation is a fundamental way of presenting 3D data. Points, lines and planes and surfaces can be coloured and presented in an effective way on PC graphics adapters. EchoPAC-3D converts the volumetric ultrasound data into geometric representations to aid orientation in 3D, show orientation of anyplane slice planes, and guide which part of the volume is shown in the visualization window. Reconstructed volumes are shown to aid the interpretation of the shape of the volumes. It is also possible in EchoPAC-3D to mix volume visualization with geometric data to obtain more information in one image.

(6) Volume Visualization

Volume visualization is used to extract the object of interest from the image data. EchoPAC-3D supports both surface and volume rendering. Surface rendering is suitable for images with high contrast between the object and its surroundings often found in cardiac, vascular and fetal imaging where the heart or fetus is adjacent to low contrast liquids. Volume rendering has the capacity to visualize more data in depth by applying various degrees of transparency.

(7) Data Export

Several methods are available to export raw data and measurements for further analysis. It is also possible to export images and video for presentations.

## 5. EchoPAC-3D User Interface

The centre area contains the working area with windows of different types showing ultrasound data (Fig. 4). Usually four windows are shown simultaneously, but it is possible to maximize a window or to have more windows, for example, if more than one examination is open.

Menus, toolbars and command panels surround the working area. One of the windows is always active. Colormap, control, and zoom commands affect all windows of the examination. Toolbars and command panel contents depend on the active window and controls only this window.

Features and user interface is defined in more detail in the following sections.

### 5.1. *Data import*

EchoPAC-3D can operate stand-alone or connected to a GE Vingmed Ultrasound scanner. Data can be transferred directly from the image store button on the scanner into a simple data archive on the EchoPAC-3D host computer. It is also possible to fetch data from a GE Vingmed data archive or read directly from the file system on the PC. EchoPAC-3D works with GE Vingmed TruScan ultrasound data. A TruScan data file is a file that contains tissue and flow images in beam-space format with ECG and Respiration traces for cardiac triggering and position sensor data for freehand scanning.

In the research version, additionally import of data from videotapes is possible. This feature is used for data import of endoscopic ultrasound where 3D data is acquired using a pullback mechanism attached to the endoscopic probe. This type of import requires manual

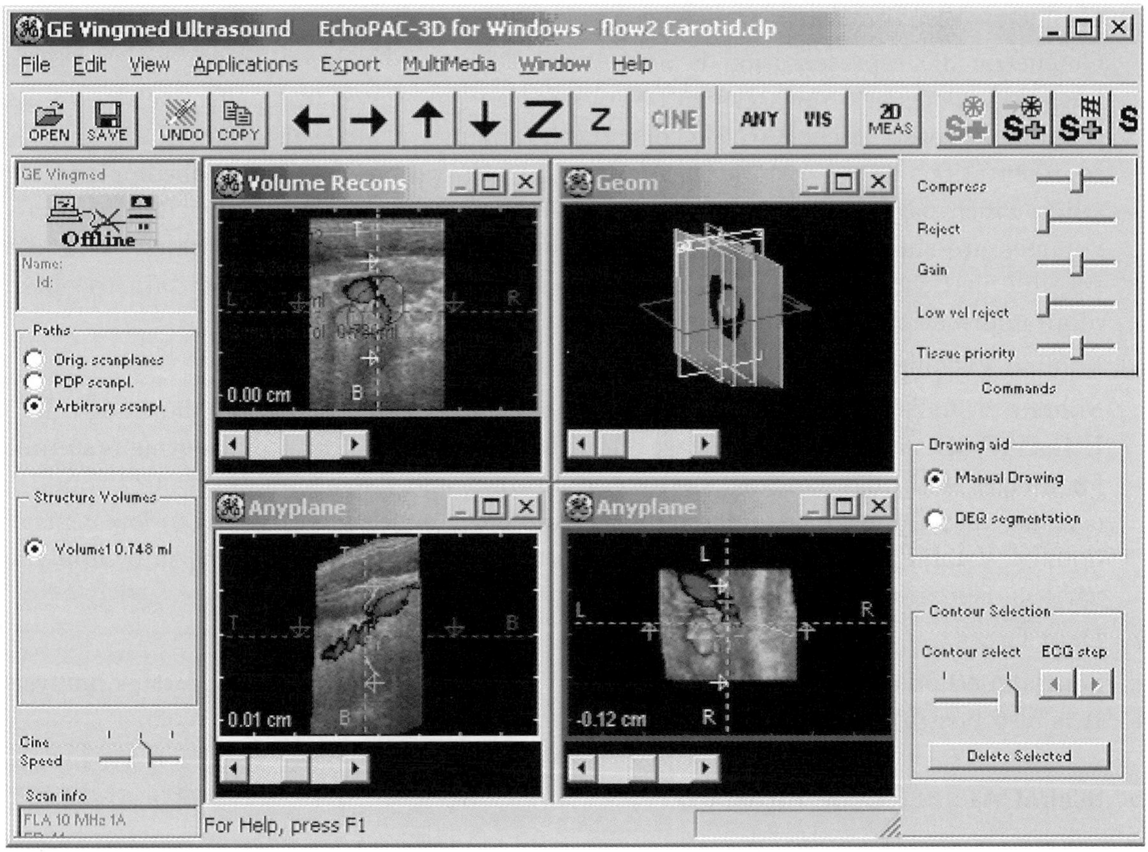


Fig. 4. EchoPAC-3D User Interface. Menus and toolbars are shown above the images. The left side shows selection of path for navigation through the volume and calculated volume of reconstructed objects. The right side contains dialogs for command input.

calibration on the 2D image of the videotape and calibration of the motor speed to calculate the pullback length.

Import of MR and CT volumes has been used in pilot studies to investigate the benefits of combining endoscopic ultrasound with MR and CT. Simple co-registration of two data volumes of different imaging modalities is possible. Viewing the same anatomy in two EchoPAC-3D windows of different imaging modality enables new research possibilities.

### 5.2. *AnyPlane window*

Determining a direction of view by positioning a slice in the 3D data set is often the first step when doing volume estimation and volume visualization. The examiner will quickly scan through the data set, choose one slice as a basis, rotate this slice to get a good direction for volume estimation and reconstruct the volume based on rotation or non-intersecting slices. An overview of the AnyPlane navigation is shown in Fig. 5. When opening an unknown examination, it is possible to view how the volume was scanned by selecting a path containing all original 2D scan planes. The depth slider allows shifting through each scan plane. The geometry window will show the position of the scan plane in relation to

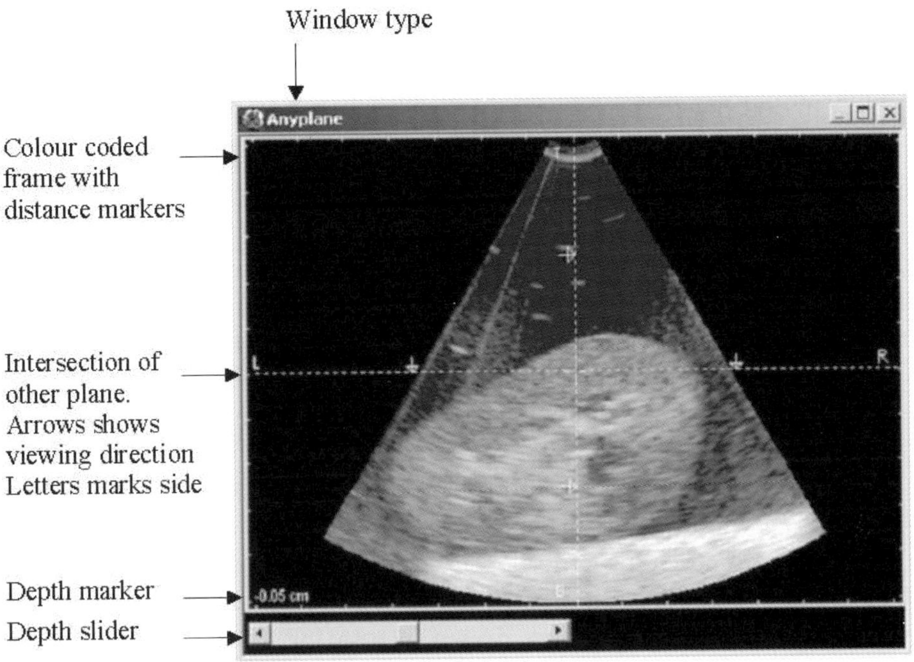


Fig. 5. Overview of contents and controls in the AnyPlane window of EchoPAC-3D.

the full 3D scan. In this mode, EchoPAC-3D scanconverts the data in full resolution based only on the 2D scanplane data the same way as reviewing on a scanner, while the geometry window shows the position of the probe.

The next step is to navigate freely through the 3D data.On a 2D scanner, the examiner has several tools to change the view of a 2D scanplane. Left/Right and Up/Down mirrors the image in horizontal and vertical direction, Rotated view allows rotation in steps of 90 degrees and read-zoom is used to magnify an interesting part of the image.

In 3D imaging there is an additional degree of freedom giving improved viewing possibilities. However, it is also easier to get lost in 3D space. EchoPAC-3D builds its viewing capabilities on the following principles:

(1) Flexibility. The examiner is allowed to select any view of the data. There is no limitation, as seen in some other software programs where views must be orthogonal.

(2) Efficiency. There is a set of orientation tools to aid the examiner quickly to get the desired view. Context menus and toolbars are used for some operations, but keyboard shortcuts are available for the experienced user.

(3) Direct manipulation of the views. Some 3D systems use three sliders to change orientation in $X$, $Y$ and $Z$ plus one slider for depth. We have found higher user acceptance for an alternative approach where the mouse is changing the orientation view by pointing and dragging in the ultrasound data.

(4) Feedback. We use the shape of the mouse cursor extensively to indicate the effect of the mouse in its current location. Interactive response and immediate feedback of a change is also a goal in all working situations.

(5) Help for orientation. The position and orientation of other views are indicated. The Geometry window gives an overall view of the volume and the available views.

(6) It is possible to quickly reset orientation of all views.

In addition to the ultrasound image, each window contains several markers and annotations (Fig. 5). The border with distance markers is colour-coded and this colour is used when information about this window is shown in other windows. Depth and ECG (Frame sliders) are used for navigation in space and time. The header contains window type and icons to maximize and close the window.

Navigation in the 3D volume is a basic feature of a 3D processing and viewing system. If the mouse is dragged near the centre of the window the volume is rotated in the same direction as the mouse is moved. The centre of rotation is in the centre of the window (Fig. 6).

To rotate the ultrasound image around the $z$-axis (2D rotation) the mouse is positioned along the edge of the window and dragged in a clockwise or counter-clockwise direction. The depth slider is used to change the depth of the cut-plane. If original scanplanes are shown in the window the depth slider is used to select which scanplane to show. When doing surface reconstruction based on contours drawn in rotating scanplane the depth slider will change the rotation angle of the plane.

When triggered 3D data is imported, an ECG curve is shown to the right of the depth slider. This curve has a current time marker that can be dragged to change current time.

In some applications it is easiest to see where a cut-plane should be positioned in another window. This also applies for visualizations. For fetal imaging, it is obvious that the visualization should start just in front of the face (Fig. 7). EchoPAC-3D allows positioning of another view by pointing to the intersection line of another view and moving or rotating it to the requested location. Dragging the intersection line at its centre moves the other view plane and dragging near the end of the line rotates the other view.

Toolbar buttons activates zoom and pan. Function keyboard shortcuts enables zoom and pan by dragging the mouse. Important factors for user friendliness are that these

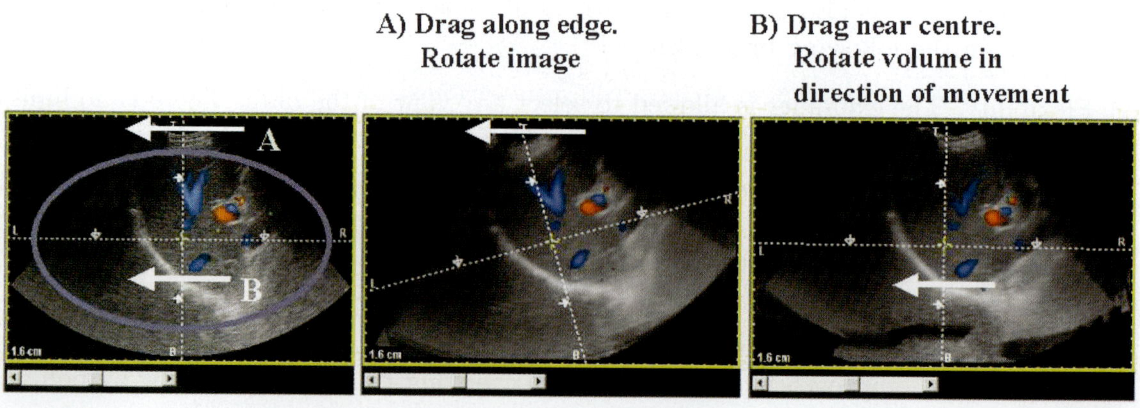


Fig. 6. Areas sensitive for slice rotation in 2D and 3D. Click and drag outside ellipse means rotate image (A). Click and drag inside ellipse is for 3D rotation.

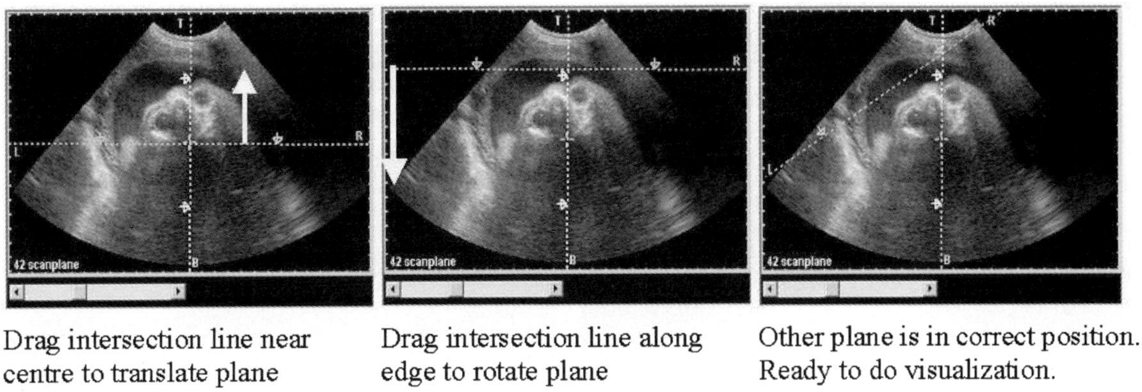


Fig. 7. Commands for translation and rotation of another cut-plane. The ultrasonogram depicts a fetal face.

commands are available in all views and that cursor feedback will always show which tool is about to be applied.

## 5.3. *Geometry window*

The EchoPAC-3D geometry window (Fig. 8) is used to give an overview of the 3D volume and shows how the anyplane windows are oriented. It will also show reconstructed volumes and it is possible to combine this with several ultrasound slices and anatomical B-mode images where the ultrasound sections are shown to mapce to the reconstructed geometry.

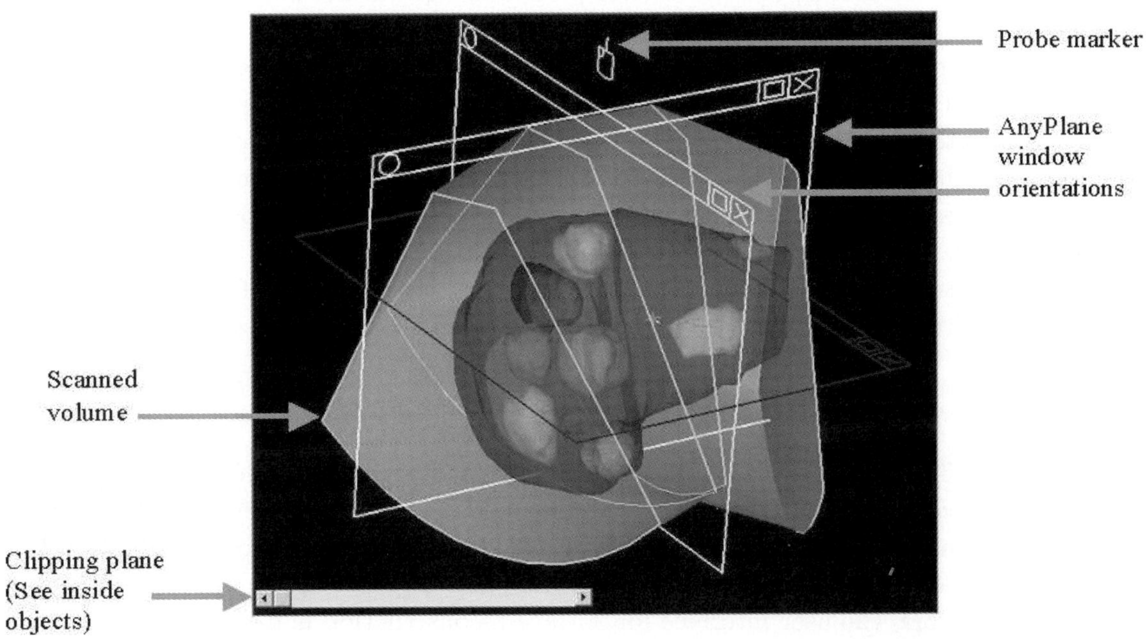


Fig. 8. Geometry window showing reconstruction of a liver with several metastases.

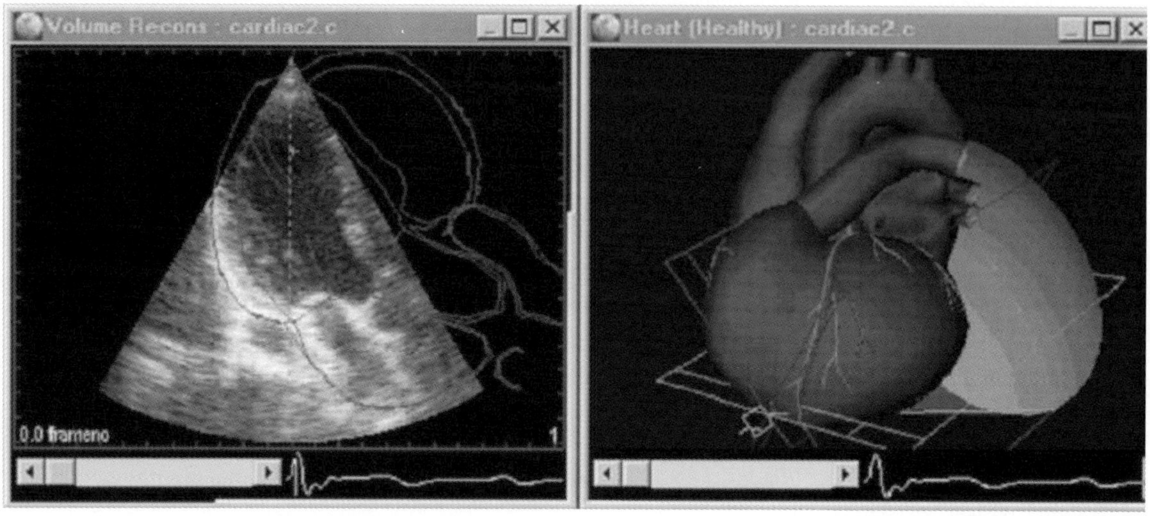


Fig. 9. Ultrasound and geometric model of the heart. Left image shows ultrasound anyplane slice with indication of how the slice intersects the heart model. Right image shows full heart model in geometry window. Ultrasound volume is outlined.

The orientation of the Geometry window is changed by using the same direct manipulation commands as used in the anyplane window. The orientation of each anyplane window is shown by drawing an outline using the window's own colour for identification. It is possible to show the ultrasound image of each slice plane in the Geometry window. This feature aids the interpretation of complex anatomical structures. The surface of reconstructed objects can be displayed as either an opaque or transparent shaded surface or as ultrasound mapped to the curved surface, in effect anatomical curved B-mode.

The Geometry window can support a display of imported geometric models (Fig. 9). A version has been developed in a project funded by the European Union where a model of the heart is calibrated to the ultrasound data (10). Similar functionality can be implemented for models of abdominal organs. This can be used as a familiarization aid for ultrasound where the ultrasound image is shown together with the approximate position in the organ scanned.

The Geometry window is continuously updated as the contents of the other windows changes. The probe marker and the extents of the 3D scan are shown to aid orientation.

## 6. Surface Reconstruction and Volume Measurements

The EchoPAC-3D reconstruction window is the main tool to provide quantitative measurements in EchoPAC-3D. The systems handle surface reconstruction of both static and dynamic structures (Fig. 10) and the algorithms (11) has through clinical evaluation been shown to calculate the volumes with high accuracy (12–14).

In EchoPAC-3D, the user interface for surface reconstruction is based on the principles of flexibility, user feedback and ease of use. To do a reconstruction, the user creates a structure and draws a number of contours in different planes to outline the structure. The system allows the user to select the number of contours to be drawn and which planes to

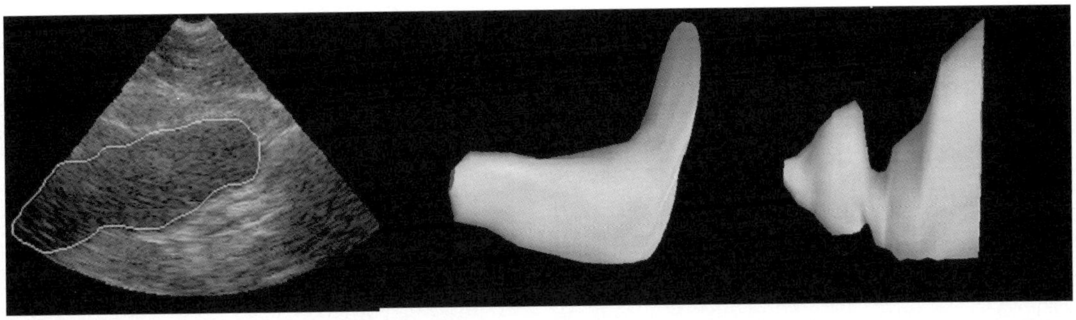

Fig. 10. Volume reconstruction of the gastric antrum. Left: One slice of the 3D volume with manually drawn contour. Centre: Reconstructed volume. Right: Reconstruction of another volume acquired during an antral contraction.

draw them. Feedback is provided by showing the shape of the reconstructed surface in the Geometry window and how the surface intersects the ultrasound image in other windows. This enables the user to quickly verify if the surface matches the underlying data and to modify the volume if the mismatch is too large (Fig. 11).

Reconstruction serves several purposes:

(1) Accurate volume estimation of static and dynamic structures.

(2) Help for orientation in 3D and in communication with a surgeon. Even a very rough reconstruction of a volume will help, for example, outlining of blood vessels.

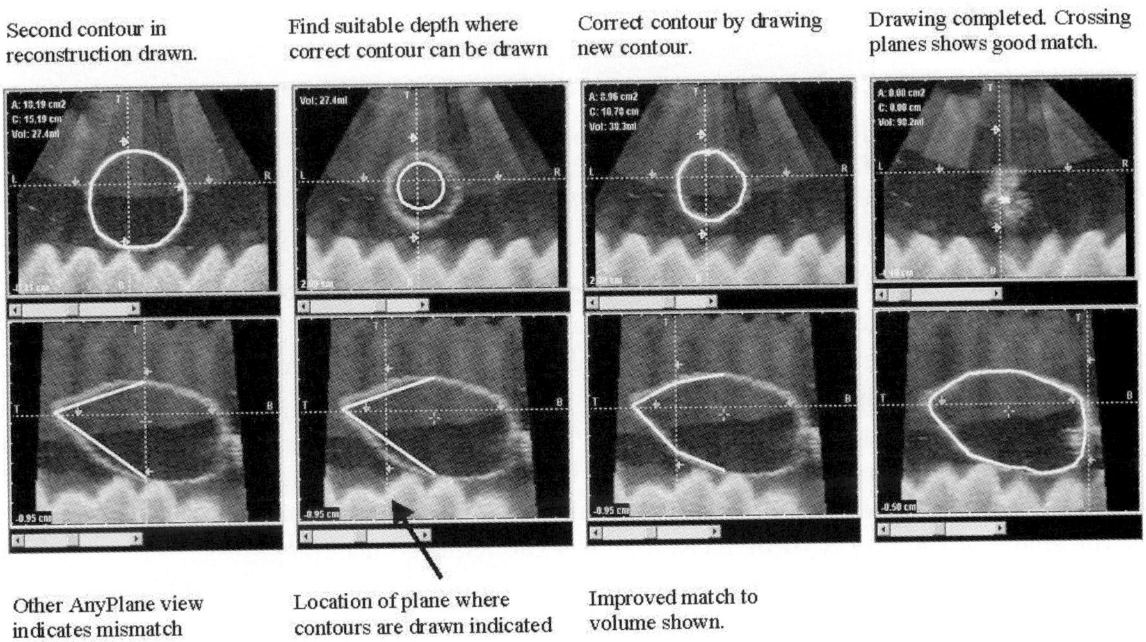


Fig. 11. Volume reconstruction. The windows shown in top row are used for reconstruction of data. The windows shown in bottom row are also shown on the screen and are used to verify the accuracy of the reconstruction.

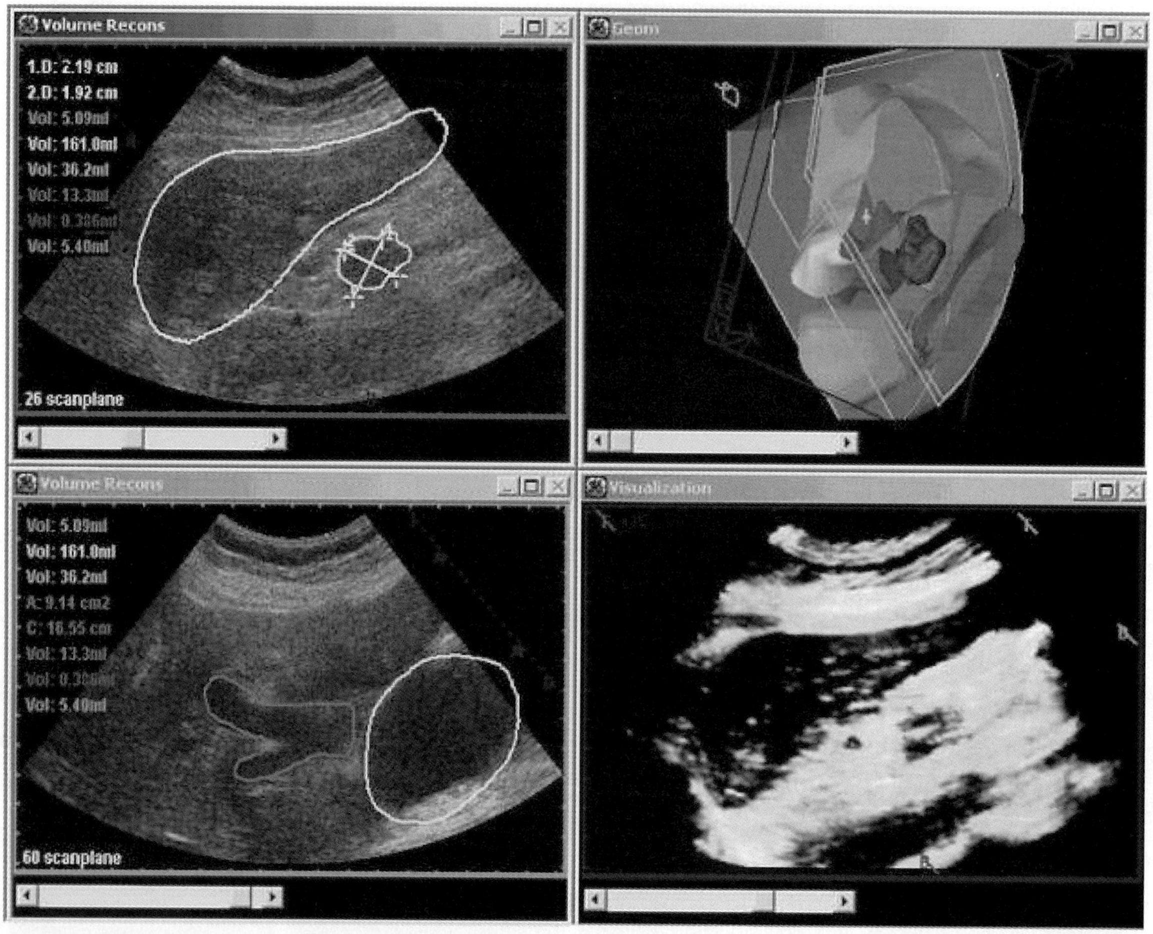


Fig. 12. This 3D ultrasound reconstruction shows a pancreatic tumour and its surrounding structures. The tumour is depicted in grey, the liver in yellow, the gallbladder in light blue, the hepatic duct in pink, the aorta in green, and the superior mesenteric vein in red.

This window supports 3D measurements and surface reconstruction of static and dynamically varying structures, based on manual contour tracing (Fig. 12). Contours must be drawn in either non-crossing slices or slices that cross each other in a common axis. More details of algorithms used are given below.

Contours can be drawn using the mouse to outline the border. The system will automatically interpolate contours between existing contours. Parts of these can be modified where the surface does not match the contours. The number of contours required depends on the shape of the object to be measured and the required accuracy.

The current algorithms support geometries without branches only. This has so far not been a serious limitation. An object with a branch, for example the carotid bifurcation, can be measured by creating two objects, one for the main object, and another for the branch. This technique has been used to create complex reconstructions for research purposes (15).

## 6.1. *Algorithms for volume reconstruction*

Combining contours into volumes is a field with a lot of research interest. The following requirements were defined for a practical implementation in EchoPAC-3D:

(1) Ease of use.

(2) Possibility for the user to visually verify the results of the algorithm. There is a trade-off between how much work is required and the accuracy of volume estimation.

(3) Algorithms should be available for static 3D and dynamic reconstruction. Static reconstruction is applicable for radiology applications and dynamic reconstruction is used for cardiac measurements like ejection fraction.

(4) Stability. Local changes to a contour should not give global changes to volume.

Handling structures with complex geometry involve complex computations and the user interface may be complex. In EchoPAC-3D, we have opted to limit our support to simpler structures without branches. Two algorithms are available:

(1) A set of non-intersecting planar contours. This algorithm is used for all our radiology applications.

(2) From planar contours rotated around a common rotation axis. This algorithm is especially suited for cardiac reconstruction of the left ventricle. When using a rotational 3D scan an advantage is that the contours may be drawn in original 2D scanplanes with maximal image quality.

## 6.2. *Algorithm for reconstruction from non-intersecting planar contours*

This algorithm converts a set of non-intersecting planar contours into a closed polyhedron described by triangles. A triangular representation is easy to handle and triangles can be shaded to draw smooth surfaces in the Geometry window. The algorithm to calculate the volume of any closed polyhedron is described below.

In general, there is no way to join contours together correctly since all the connectivity information is limited to the contour plane and there exists no information about the relationship between adjacent contours.

Several authors have addressed the problem of reconstructing a surface from serial cross-sections. Fuchs *et a1.* (16) reconstructed the surface between contiguous serial contours by minimizing the surface area. Such an optimal surface cannot be found using only local decision-making and therefore efficient methods of global graph searching were needed.

We based our work on the heuristic method described by Ganapathy and Dennehy (17) based on inter-contour coherence. The reconstruction of the polyhedron from the set of contour data is accomplished in three separate steps:

(1) Resampling of the contours.

(2) Sort the contours to place them in correct depth order and check for intersections.

(3) Choosing the starting point for each contour and contour triangulation (Fig. 13).

Step (1). The first step is to resemble each contour such that it consists of a fixed number of vertices, which are evenly spaced. This resembling step is necessary because the number of vertices and their individual spacing along the contour depends on the speed by which the user moves the mouse. We also ensure that all contours are internally stored in counter-clockwise order.

Step (2). The second step is to sort the contours because the user is free to draw and edit the contours in any order. We sort the contours by finding the plane the contours is drawn in and calculating which side of this plane the points in the other contours are at. A requirement for the algorithm is that contours do not intersect.

Step (3). The third step is to match two consecutive contours. For contours $A[0\dots N]$ and $B[0\dots N]$ we do triangulation by connecting $A[m]$ with $B[m]$ and calculate the sub-volume described by the two contours (see Fig. 14). We try all alternative start points of contour B. The start point giving the maximal volume is selected. The best match is given by:

$$\text{Max volume (for } i \text{ in } [0\dots N] \text{ trianglulate } A[m] \text{ with } B[m+i])$$

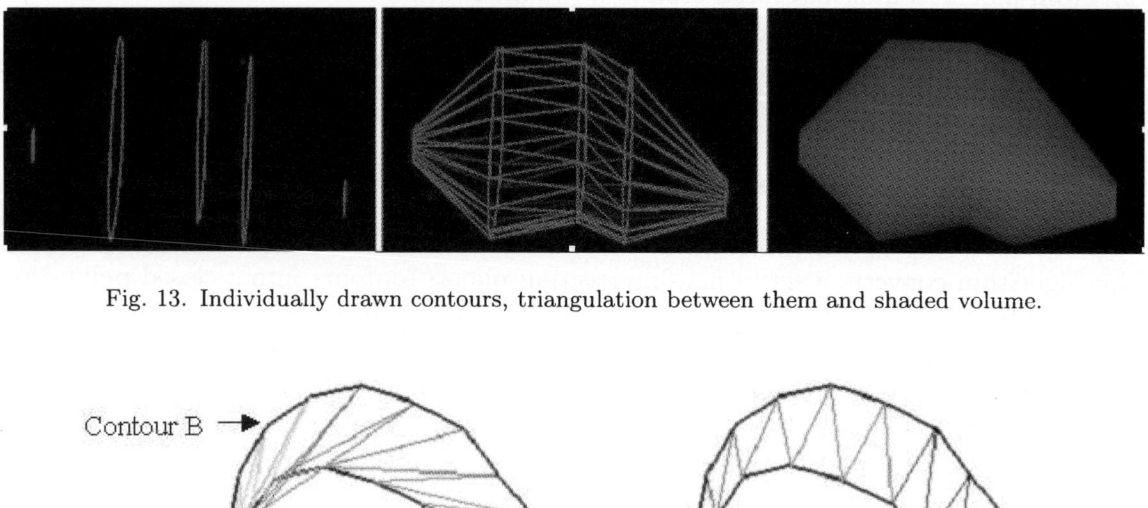

Fig. 13. Individually drawn contours, triangulation between them and shaded volume.

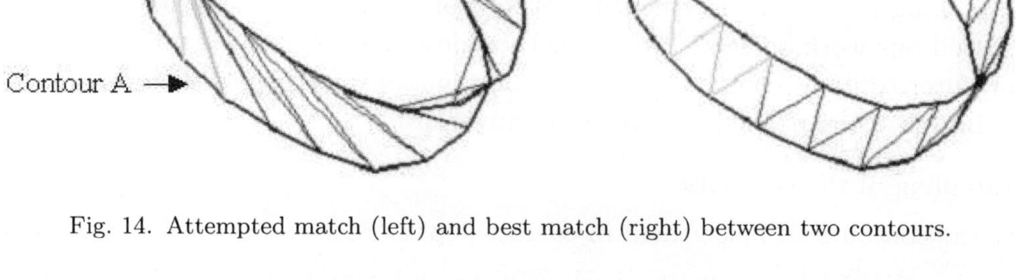


Fig. 14. Attempted match (left) and best match (right) between two contours.

### 6.2.1. *Algorithm for reconstruction from planar contours rotated around a common rotation axis*

This algorithm converts a set of contours drawn in planes rotated round a common rotation axis to a closed polyhedron. All contours must intersect the rotation axis. The output representation is the same as the algorithm for non-intersecting contours.

The algorithm works in three steps.

(1) Split contours along rotation axis.

(2) Resampling of the left and right halves of each contour.

(3) 3D Interpolation to add new contours if difference in angle is too large.

(4) Contour triangulation.

Step (1). Split contours along rotation axis. In this step, clipping the contours along the rotation axis splits the contours in a left and right part. Each contour part is stored in a two-dimensional coordinate system with an attached rotation angle. The left part of the contour is mirrored around the rotation axis and given rotation angle equal to its right part plus 180 degrees. This step also includes verification that the contours are consistently drawn. All contours must intersect the rotation axis.

Step (2). Resampling. The points on the left and right side of the contour are first reordered to make all contour parts start at the "bottom" part of the intersection. Then the contours are resampled to make each contour contain the same number of points.

Step (3). 3D Interpolation. If the rotation angle between two successive contours is larger than a given angle (10 to 20 degrees) new contours are inserted by doing a linear interpolation between the two successive contours. This step will give the resulting polyhedron a smoother appearance that (usually) closer matches the structure to be reconstructed.

Step (4) Contour triangulation. This step just creates triangles between each pair of part contours and transforms the point from the two dimensional coordinate system to 3D probe coordinates (Fig. 15).

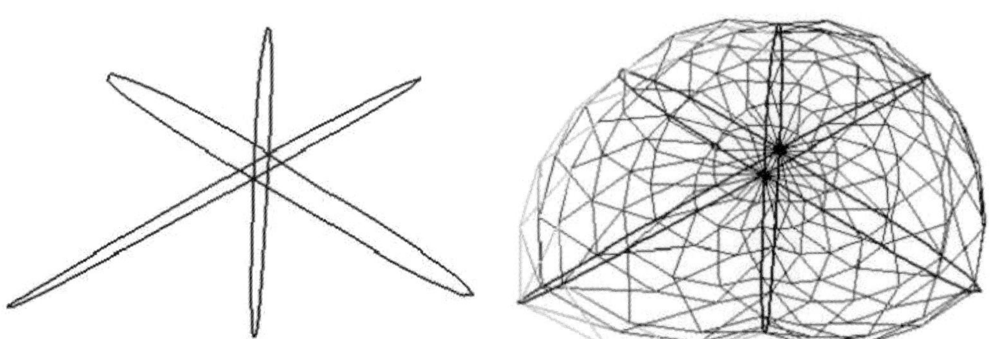

Fig. 15. Result of algor'thm for surface reconstruction from three rotated contours.

### 6.3. *Algorithm for reconstruction of a dynamic volume from planar contours rotated around a common rotation axis*

For reconstruction of a surface with a shape that varies over time (for example the left ventricle) the algorithm above can be expanded to cover dynamic volumes. A minimal requirement is that the contours are defined for the systolic and diastolic phase of the heart cycle. To calculate in-between volumes the contours for that volume are first interpolated in time using linear interpolation based on adjacent contours in time of the defined volume. Then the basic algorithm is applied to do the surface reconstruction and volume calculation.

#### 6.3.1. *Volume of a polyhedron defined by triangles*

The volume of a closed polyhedron (18) formed from triangles can be expressed as:

$$v = \frac{1}{3}\left|\sum_j A_j(Q_j \cdot N_j)\right|$$

where $A_j$ is the surface area of the triangle $j$ in the polyhedron; $Q_j$ is a point in the triangle and $N_j$ is an outward pointing unit vector normal to triangle $j$.

### 6.4. *Discussion and applications of the reconstruction algorithms*

We have chosen very conservative algorithms for volume reconstruction. No complex structures and only linear interpolation between contours. In our experience, the results in volume estimation are accurate and robust.

Visual feedback is very important. The intersection between the reconstructed structure and the ultrasound image is shown in the reconstruction window and the geometry window shows the geometric model of the structure. A manual check allows the user to verify the results and existing contours can be modified or new contours inserted if the mismatch is too large.

A benefit of using this formula is that it applies to any polyhedron. EchoPAC-3D applies it to both volume estimation algorithms and also for calculating the volume of part of a structure. The polyhedron can be clipped through a plane and new triangles added to close the new polyhedrons created. The above algorithm is then used to calculate the sum of sub-volumes.

#### 6.4.1. *Algorithms for automatic object detection*

Ultrasound images often have low contrast between different structures making automatic detection difficult. Most successful approaches have been detecting liquid filled structures like cardiac chambers and the uterus. We have also done work in automatic and semi-automatic detection in EchoPAC-3D, but the results have not been good enough for general release. If extensive manual correction is needed, it is faster to perform manual border detection.

### 6.4.2. *Alternative interpolation methods*

A spline interpolation between contours might give reconstructions that closer match organs that are regular and smooth in appearance and may thus give accurate volume estimation from fewer contours (19). Splines with local properties are recommended to avoid a change to one contour, giving oscillating changes through the whole structure thus making verification harder. We have not yet implemented this feature in EchoPAC-3D, but it may be a topic for further research.

### 6.4.3. *Reconstruction accuracy*

A future research issue may be to find how many contours are needed to obtain a given accuracy for different structures. EchoPAC-3D has a feature to step forward or backward a given distance used for manual reconstruction, but we have not tuned this distance specifically to different organs. The availability of accurate 3D volume measurements could be used to do *in vivo* qualification of standard 2D methods and perhaps select improved measurement methods for 2D ultrasound.

## 7. Volume Rendering

The Volume rendering function in EchoPAC-3D allows volume visualization of both flow and tissue images. Volume rendering can improve the 3D understanding of acquired data (20). EchoPAC-3D supports two types of volume visualization (Fig. 16) (21, 22):

(1) *Gradient shading* use a light model to shade the surface of the object of interest. When light is reflected, the part of the surface facing the light will reflect more light than surfaces facing away from the light (Fig. 17).

    A vital criterion for this rendering mode is that it is possible to detect the surface of the object. Gradient shading is therefore appropriate for the visualization of well-defined tissue/blood (or liquid) transitions found in cardiac, vascular and ob-gyn applications.

(2) *Transparent rendering* is used to view simultaneously different levels and depths of an object. Each tissue value is assigned opacity. The system simulates a ray of light sent into the data volume.

The rendering algorithms tries to separate interesting structures from the neighbouring tissue based on the amount of echo received of the structures. For 3D data acquisition for volume rendering it is therefore important to adjust the scan settings on the scanner to maximize the contrast between the structures.

The result of the visualization is very much dependent on the settings of the visualization controls. When doing surface rendering, the separation between tissue and blood is determined by setting a threshold. If the threshold is set too high, part of the tissue may be falsely classified as blood and removed from the rendering. When evaluating a rendering, the result should be verified by also analysing the 2D anyplane image in interesting locations. EchoPAC-3D supports verification by allowing an anyplane image to intersect the rendering and remove the rendering on one side of the anyplane image. Where the rendering intersects the plane the part of the plane being in front of the rendering is kept

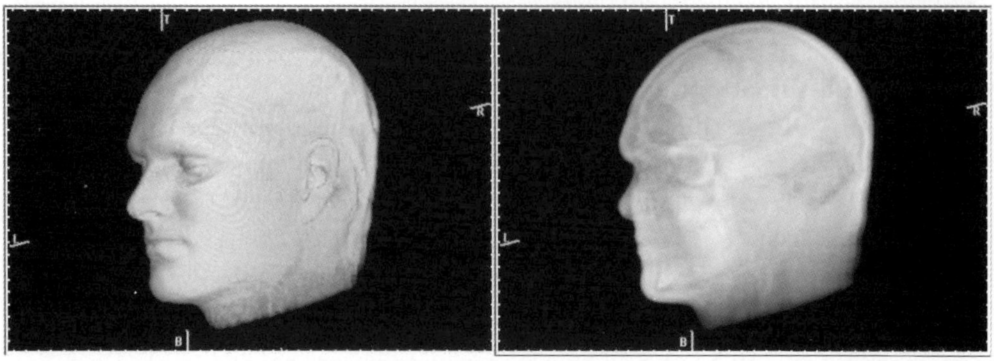

Fig. 16. Visualization of a head scanned by a Magnetic Resonance (MR) scanner. The left image show gradient shading of the surface. The image is lightest on the parts facing the light and darker on the forehead facing away. The right image shows a highly transparent rendering where part of the brain is visible. It is possible to apply a mixture of surface and transparent rendering.

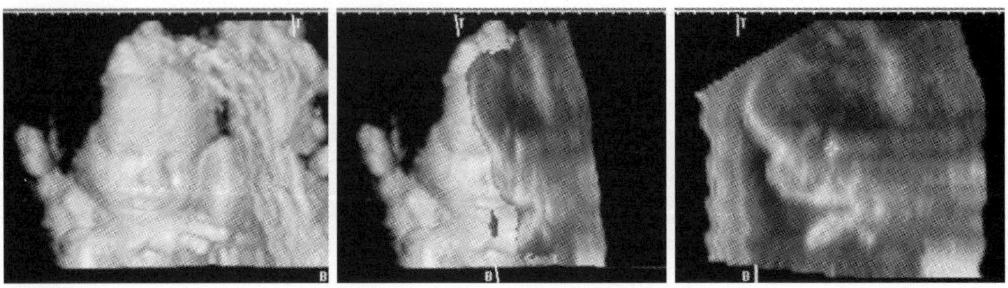

Fig. 17. Verification of fetal gradient shading rendering. Left image shows normal rendering. In the middle image an anyplane image is used to cut the rendering. Internal structures are shown using normal ultrasound image. Right image shows anyplane image used for cutting.

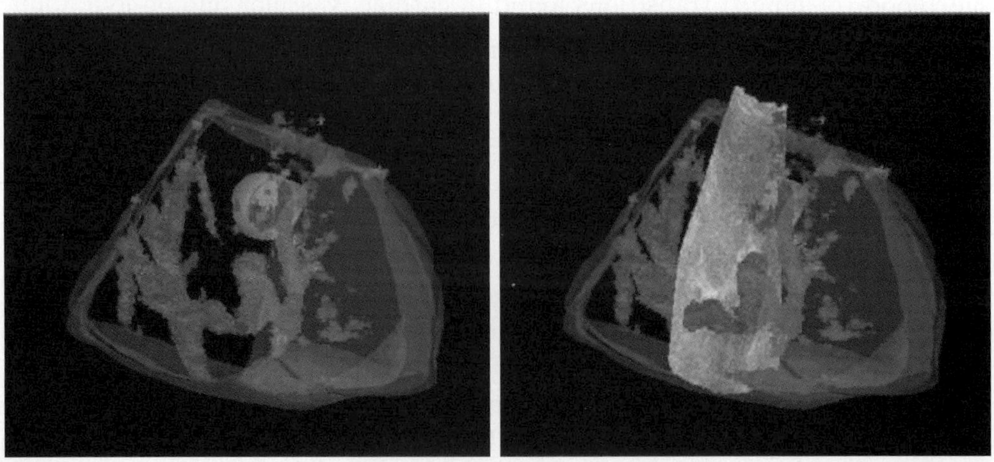

Fig. 18. Tools to verify visualization of liver blood vessel. Left image shows visualization combined with reconstructed liver and tumor. In the right image an anyplane tissue image is added to aid location of tumor relative to important blood vessels.

invisible and the part inside the structure is shown using data from the anyplane image. In this way, it is easy to verify that the rendering matches the surface seen in the anyplane and gives an accurate representation of the data.

The volume visualization is interactive; the examiner can change the orientation and depth of the front plane using the same tools as used in the anyplane window. Volume rendering is done in the Visualization window.

Flow rendering use the same methods as tissue rendering (Figs. 18 and 19). The raw ultrasound data stores separate tissue and flow data. The arbitration information is used to find the visible part of the flow signal.

The quality of ultrasound volume visualization may be impaired by obscuring structures in front of the area of interest. Using the 3D scalpel the examiner can remove such structures. For obscuring structures that are parallel to the visualization sectionss, the examiner should rotate the visualization section about 90 degrees to ensure not to discard parts of the structure of interest. The examiner outlines the area to be removed and the system cuts away everything inside the area. Figure 20 show interactive sequence of steps needed to improve fetal rendering.

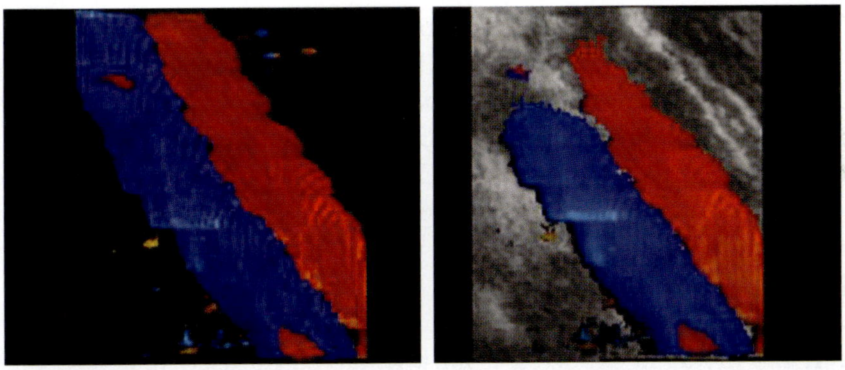

Fig. 19. Flow visualization of the carotid artery. Colour indicates direction of flow. Variation along the vessel is caused by the data acquired at different times in the cardiac cycle, i.e. not triggered. On the right side the same visualization is shown with tissue signal for verification.

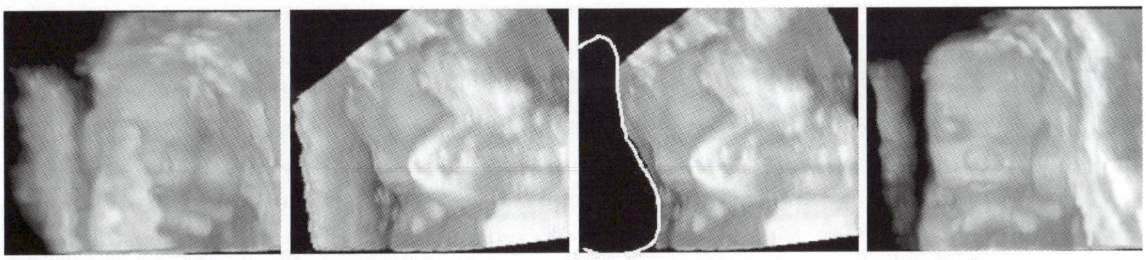


Fig. 20. Fetal rendering showing the application of of a 3D scalpel. Three steps are required to remove undesirable pixels to improve the rendering.

## 8. Data Export

The structure of the GE Vingmed Ultrasound scan file format is proprietary. For very basic 3D research it may be desirabe to provide own algorithms for reconstruction from 2D images into 3D volumes. As this will require disclosure information, EchoPAC-3D provides the possibility to import the data as one long 2D cineloop and export all images as a sequence of scan converted 2D bitmaps in an open format.

The same format can be applied to export 3D volume data. A single or a sequence of 3D cubes can be exported. Such cubes can easily be read or converted into a suitable format for import into other research tools. Tissue data is always exported as 8bit grey level data. Flow data can be exported separately, but this will require access to proprietary algorithms used to mix tissue and flow. It is possible to export mixed tissue and flow data as RGB volumes. The colour information can then be used to deduce flow direction and velocity.

## 9. Measurements and Reconstructed Volume Export

For further analysis, it is possible to export 2D distance and area measurements, 3D volume measurements and flow velocity profiles to a text file in a format suitable for analysis in a spreadsheet.

The shape of the surface of a reconstructed organ has been used to analyse the strain forces that applies to each segment of the surface using special strain analysis software and to analyse cardiac ventricular wall movement. In EchoPAC-3D we have chosen to use the VRML97 format (23) for this purpose. A VRML file describes the 3D graphic primitives in a text format that can easily be interpreted. EchoPAC-3D adds comments to aid parsing the VRML data of a reconstructed volume and of time dependent data for dynamic structure export. By installing a VRML plugin in an internet browser the file can be viewed in an internet environment.

The VRML file contains a full 3D model and commands to view the model from different perspectives. If the model is exported from a triggered dataset, it is also possible to view its dynamic behaviour in the VRML plugin.

## 10. Making Multimedia Presentations

An important feature in a research tool like EchoPAC-3D is the possibility to make illustrations for publications and presentations at conferences. EchoPAC-3D offers several tools to ease these tasks. EchoPAC-3D does not contain built-in reporting tool, but works in combination with slide presentation tools and video-editing systems. Most presentation tools support import of bitmaps graphics and video files. A video-editing system can be used to add video clips to make a complete video presentation. The functionality to make presentations in EchoPAC-3D also works for 2D data.

Presentations are made by starting the presentation software and then use EchoPAC-3D copy commands to transfer the contents of the current window, all windows or the whole EchoPAC-3D user interface bitmap to the software. The Windows clipboard is used for intermediate storage. (It is also possible to store the bitmaps to file and later include them in presentations.)

Video generation does not require special hardware. The requirements are both to be able to document results and to demonstrate how to work using EchoPAC-3D. Video generation supports generation of video files showing use of either of the active window, the whole working area or the complete user interface. For extensive work in video generation it may be an advantage to buy a graphics card with video output capabilities or third party tool to capture screen contents to digital video while working.

For triggered data, it is common to run a cineloop to show how the data varies across a cardiac cycle. EchoPAC-3D has commands to capture a cineloop of the current window to video file.

Graphics image overlays like volume contours and slice markers can often be hard to see on video and in presentations. EchoPAC-3D will enhance the contrast of this graphics by drawing thicker lines.

## 11. Summary

EchoPAC-3D has been developed over a period of nearly 10 years. A close working relationship between physicians and the development team has been an important factor for the development of the software program. Being able to keep EchoPAC-3D as a combination of a product where a rigorous release process is required and a research tool with more frequent updates and extra features for special research has been a fruitful combination. The modular structure of the program has allowed building new windows for research purposes without interfering with the functionality and stability of the basic product.

Systems using probes with built-in 3D support are emerging on the market. These probes use either mechanical or electronic steering to provide 3D volumes. For several abdominal applications we have seen that a probe with a position sensor is required to cover the necessary scan volume. The position sensor device has so far been clipped on externally. Future will tell whether systems with a built-in miniature position sensor will be available on the market, or whether mechanical and electronic probes will be the main focal point. Our experience has shown us that both types are required to cover all applications, but problems making an easy to use and portable position sensor system may favor mechanical and electronic probes.

EchoPAC-3D is a post-processing package. Meeting the goal of facilitating regular clinical 3D examinations is never reached until the scanner provides tools for online 3D analysis. There is also a need to define standard protocols for 3D ultrasound imaging. Image quality will always be an issue. Having full volume data scanned by real-time 3D ultrasound provides new possibilities for display and analysis. A lot of work has been done in research environments. As scanners with real-time 3D capabilities penetrate the markets, we can expect to see more research work being moved to specific clinical applications.

## References

1. Martens, D., Hausken, T., Gilja, O. H. *et al.*, 3D processing of ultrasound data using a novel EchoPAC-3D software. Ultrasound Med Biol, 1997; 23: 136.

2. Gilja, O. H., Thune, N., Matre, K., Hausken, T., Ødegaard, S., Berstad, A., *In vitro* evaluation of three dimensional ultrasonography in volume estimation of organs. Ultrasound Med Biol 1994; 20: 157–165.
3. Steen, E. and Olstad., B., Volume rendering of 3D medical ultrasound data using direct feature mapping. IEEE Trans on medical Imaging, 1994; 13: 517–525.
4. EchoPAC-3D for Windows User's Manual, GEVU part number FB292261 Rev A, May 2000.
5. Nelson, T. R., Downey, D. B. and Pretorius. D. H., Three-Dimensional Ultrasound, Lippincott Williams & Wilkins, 1999.
6. Molin, S. O., Nesje, L. B., Gilja, O. H., Hausken, T., Martens, D. and Ødegaard, S., 3D-endosonography in gastroenterology: Methodology and clinical applications. Eur J Ultrasound 1999; 10: 171–177.
7. Hausken, T., Thune, N., Matre, K., Gilja, O. H., Ødegaard, S. and Berstad, A., Volume estimation of the gastric antrum and the gallbladder in patients with non-ulcer dyspepsia and erosive prepyloric changes, using three-dimensional ultrasonography. Neurogastroenterol. Mot. 1994; 6: 263–270.
8. Berg, S., Torp, H., Martens, D. *et al.*, Dynamic three-dimensional freehand echocardiography using raw ditical ultrasound data. Ultrasound Med Biol 1999; 25: 745–753.
9. Rohling, R., Gee, A. and Berman, L., Three-dimensional spatial compounding of ultrasound images. Med Image Anal. 1997; 1: 177–93.
10. Berlage, T., Augmented-reality communication for diagnostic tasks in cardiology. IEEE Trans Inf Technol Biomed. 1998; 2: 169–73.
11. Thune, N., Gilja, O. H., Hausken, T. and Matre, K., A practical methods for estimating enclosed volumes using 3D ultrasound. European Journal of Ultrasound. 1996; 3: 83–92.
12. Gilja, O. H., Hausken, T., Olafsson, S., Matre, K. and Ødegaard, S., *In vitro* evaluation of three-dimensional ultrasonography based on magnetic scanhead tracking. Ultrasound Med Biol 1998; 24: 1161–1167.
13. Matre, K., Stokke, E. M., Martens, D. and Gilja, O. H., *In vitro* volume estimation of kidneys using three-dimensional ultrasonography and a position sensor. Eur J Ultrasound. 1999; 10: 65–73.
14. Gilja, O. H., Smievoll, A. I., Thune, N., Matre, K., Hausken, T., Ødegaard, S. and A. Berstad., *In vivo* comparison of 3D ultrasonography and Magnetic Resonance Imaging in volume estimation of human kidneys. Ultrasound Med Biol 1995; 21: 25–32.
15. Blaas, H. G., Eik-Nes, S. H., Berg, S. and Torp, H., *In vivo* three-dimensional ultrasound reconstructions of embryos and early fetuses. Lancet. 1998; 352: 1182–6.
16. Fuchs, H., Kedem, Z. M. and Uselton, S. P., Optimal surface reconstruction from planar contours. Communications of the ACM 1977; 20: 693.
17. Ganapathy, S. and Dennehy, T. G., A new general triangulation methods for planar contours. Computer Graphics 1982; 16: 69.
18. Goldman, R. N., Areas of planar polygons and volume of polyhedra. Graphic Gems II, Academic press Inc, 1991: 170.
19. Maehle, J., Bjoernstad, K., Aakhus, S., Torp, H. G. and Angelsen, B. A., Three-dimensional echocardiography for quantitative left ventricular wall motion analysis: A method for reconstruction of endocardial surface and evaluation of regional dysfunction. Echocardiography. 1994; 11: 397–40.
20. Drebin, R. A., Carpenter, L. and Hanrahana, P., Volume Rendering. Computer Graphics. 1988; 22: 65–74.

21. Steen, E. and Olstad, B., Volume rendering of 3D medical images using direct feature mapping. IEEE Trans on Medical Imaging, 1994; 13: 517–525.
22. Steen, E. N., Analysis and visualization of multi-dimensional medical images. PhD thesis, Dept. of Computer Systems and Telematics, Norwegian Institute of Technology, 1996
23. VRML97. International Standard. ISO/IEC 14772-1:1997, ISO/IEC 14772-2:2002, http://www.vrml.org/

Published with permission

ELSEVIER

European Journal of Ultrasound 10 (1999) 171–177

EUROPEAN JOURNAL OF ULTRASOUND

www.elsevier.com/locate/ejultrasou

Review

# 3D-endosonography in gastroenterology: methodology and clinical applications

S.-O. Molin [a,*], L.B. Nesje [a], O.H. Gilja [a], T. Hausken [a], D. Martens [b], S. Ødegaard [c]

[a] *Department of Surgery, Sahlgrenska University Hospital, S-431 80 Mölndal, Sweden*
[b] *Christian Michelsen Research, Bergen, Norway*
[c] *Department of Medicine, Haukeland University Hospital, Bergen, Norway*

Received 17 April 1999; received in revised form 11 August 1999; accepted 13 August 1999

**Abstract**

Endoluminal ultrasonography allows detailed imaging of the gastrointestinal wall and adjacent structures. Three-dimensional (3D) imaging may improve visualisation of topographic relations and the nature of pathologic lesions. The objective of this report is to summarise current status of 3D-endosonography and to discuss the possible clinical impact of this new modality. 3D ultrasonographic images are usually generated from a series of digitised two-dimensional ultrasound pictures acquired in a manner that enables registration of their relative spatial position. Such acquisition can be accomplished with different ultrasound probes, but in most cases of endosonography, a controlled pullback of radial-scanning probes has been applied. Digital ultrasound images are obtained by frame grabbing of analogue video recordings or by direct transmission from digital scanners. Dedicated software programs have been developed for 3D reconstruction and visualisation, allowing interactive display and measurements. 3D endosonography provides new possibilities for clinical imaging, but the impact on therapeutic strategies and clinical outcome has yet to be established. © 1999 Elsevier Science Ireland Ltd. All rights reserved.

*Keywords:* Ultrasound; Imaging; Endosonography; Three-dimensional; Gastroenterology

## 1. Introduction

Advances in ultrasonography (US), together with improved computer technology, offer a great potential for progress in the field of medical imaging. Probes or US catheters can be inserted into hollow organs, such as the gastrointestinal (GI) tract (Rösch, 1993) or vessels (Lee et al., 1995) in

* Corresponding author. Tel.: +46-31-3431000; fax: +46-31-861811.
*E-mail address:* sven-olov.molin@sahlgrenska.se (S.-O. Molin)


PII: S0929-8266(99)00061-0

Published with permission



order to monitor the organ wall and its close vicinity. Endoscopic ultrasonography (EUS) has become a well-established tool in the diagnoses of GI diseases (Rösch and Classen, 1992; Ødegaard et al., 1999; Van Dam and Sivak, 1999) and the method is highly accurate in staging oesophageal, gastric, pancreatic and rectal cancers (Tio et al., 1990, 1992; Lightdale, 1992).

The concept of three-dimensional (3D-) US was first described by Baum and Greenwood (Baum and Greenwood, 1961). The method has been applied mainly for cardiac (Roelandt et al., 1994), vascular (Coatrieux et al., 1994), and obstetric imaging (Riccabona et al., 1997), but recently also in the diagnosis of GI disorders (Zoller and Liess, 1994; Gilja et al., 1997). The objectives of 3D-imaging comprise improved understanding of topographic anatomy and the ability to perform exact distance and volume measurements (Riccabona et al., 1995). By two-dimensional (2D-) US, spatial information may be gained by a combination of different image frames with the operator's hand–eye co-ordination as well as knowledge of depth and surface anatomy. Computerised 3D-US, however, allows concomitant display in several planes and various options for spatial imaging (Belohlavek et al., 1993). 3D-imaging and measurements, as compared with 2D-applications, have certain technical and practical advantages in visualising anatomic and pathologic structures, but its impact on clinical decision-making and outcome has to be established.

Since Hashimoto first reported the use of 3D-EUS (Hashimoto et al., 1989) several investigators have applied 3D-EUS methods for in vitro studies and in vivo examinations of the GI-tract (Kalimanis et al., 1995; Huenerbein et al., 1997; Kanemaki et al., 1997; Molin et al., 1997b; Nishimura et al., 1997; Kaneko and Nakao, 1998). The aim of this report is to summarise the present experience with 3D-EUS and to discuss advantages and limitations of the method as compared with conventional 2D-EUS. Current technologies for image acquisition and digitisation, 3D-reconstruction, and display are shortly described and illustrated with clinical examples.

## 2. Methodological aspects

The main steps of current 3D-EUS technology are: acquisition and digitalisation, 3D-reconstruction, and image display.

### *2.1. Image acquisition*

The 3D-image is usually generated from ultrasound data acquired in a series of US scan planes that are either parallel to each other or separated by regular angular increments. For trans-esophageal examination of the heart, the transducer can be pivoted or rotated, either manually or with a mechanical device (Belohlavek et al., 1993), using linear array or multiplane probes, and similar probes can be applied for gastrointestinal use (Fig. 3(A–B)). The easiest way to acquire parallel 2D-images by radial-scanning EUS is a controlled withdrawal using a motor device (Ødegaard et al., 1998), preferably a stepping motor unit (Fig. 1) (Molin et al., 1997b). Ideally, then, the only probe motion occurring during the acquisition period is due to the transducer being moved axially (Fig. 1).

For cardiac examination several systems have been used with external US to obtain position and orientation information, including articulated arms (Dekker et al., 1974), spark gap microphone (Moritz and Shreve, 1976), laser or infrared sensors, and electromagnetic positioning systems (Detmer et al., 1994).

### *2.2. Image digitisation*

Digitisation of analogue video signals can be performed on conventional multimedia PC workstations. Most 3D-EUS studies have been performed using analogue video tape recordings, but US scanners with integrated computer systems for immediate signal digitisation are currently available. When analogue video recordings are applied, it is necessary to calibrate the image scaling and relative position of individual image frames in order to convert the original recordings into a 3D-data set. At present, digitised image files may require extensive data storage capacity, but new compression algorithms may reduce the size of

Published with permission



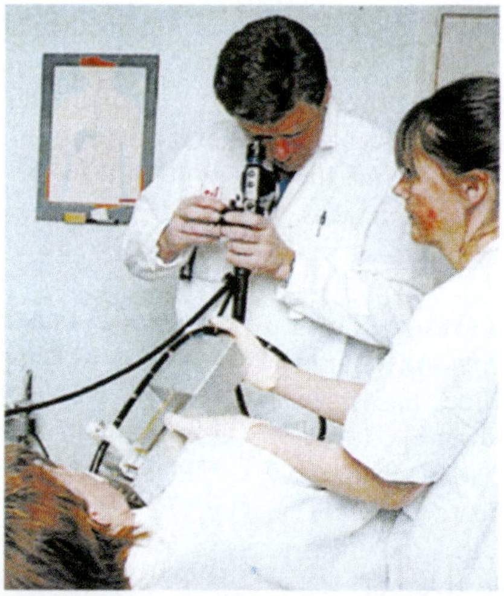

Fig. 1

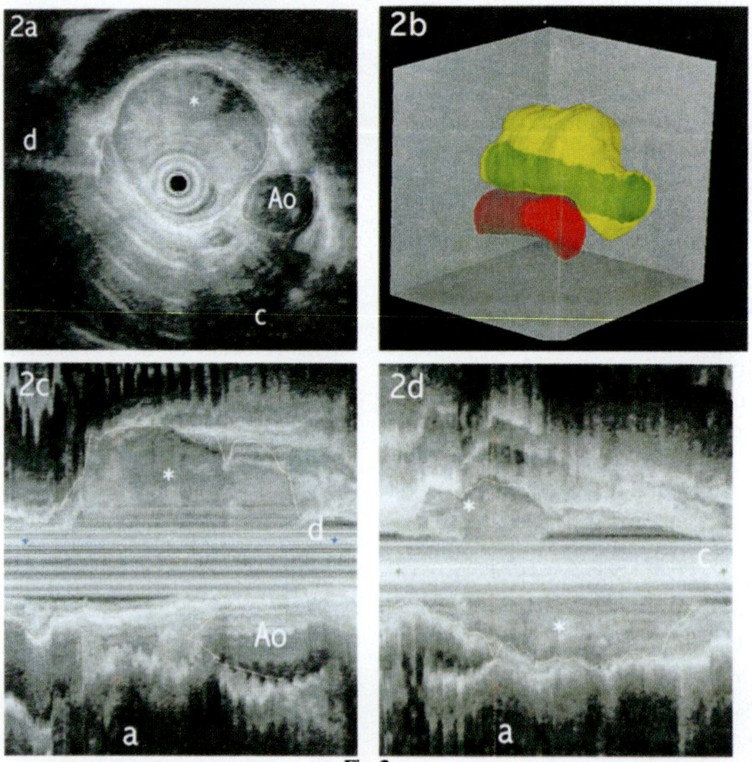


Fig. 2

Fig. 1. A mechanical withdrawal device as in this case a stepping motor, attached to the ultrasound probe can easily be positioned in front of the patient and used on demand for routine examinations.

Fig. 2. Planar slicing with manual contour outlining. Original scanning plane (a) and two orthogonal reconstructed image planes (c, d) in a patient with oesophageal cancer. The reconstructed images can be interactively moved to depict any plane. Manual outlining of tumour (*) borders (b) allows volume estimation and 2D-measurement. Note that outlining is recorded in all planes (a, c, d), and spatial relationships are visualised (B: green = echoendoscope, yellow = tumour, red = descending aorta (Ao)).

Published with permission



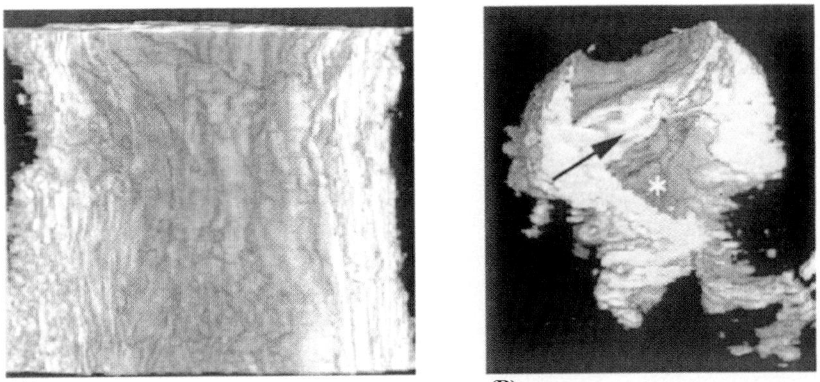

(A) (B)

Fig. 3. Surface rendering. (A) Surface reconstruction of a normal gastric body with visualisation of mucosal folds. (B) Similar data displayed as an 'endoscopic view' from the body of the stomach into the distal part with the prepyloric antrum (*) and angular fold (arrow). Acquisition obtained during mechanical withdrawal of a 4.5 MHz biplane transesophageal probe (A) and mechanically rotating multiplane probe (B).

data files, allowing US acquisitions to be stored directly on digital media. Future EUS systems will probably contain integrated functions for image storage, digital image processing and 3D-display functions.

### 2.3. 3D-reconstruction and display

Reconstruction is the process of transforming pre-processed data into a 3D format. Four different techniques are applied for 3D-visualisation (Belohlavek et al., 1993): planar slicing, surface reconstruction, volume rendering, and slicer-view.

With *planar slicing* (Fig. 2(a–d)), the 3D data can be manipulated interactively to obtain two-dimensional gray-scale images in any plane. *Surface reconstruction* delineates surface features of selected objects and can be accomplished by manual outlining of structures (Fig. 2(b)) or automated rendering techniques (Fig. 3). The rendering technique is mainly used in structures with a fluid–tissue interface, (i.e. in cardiac, vascular and obstetric imaging), and variable shadowing and lighting effects can be applied to enhance surface features. *Volume rendering* (Fig. 4(A)) is a method for imaging internal structures of a recorded volume. Graded transparency permits visualisation of elements beyond a surface, and various filtering algorithms can be applied to enhance object features. Volume rendering can also be combined with planar gray-scale images, in order to obtain a topographic overview together with the details of a 2D-image (Fig. 4(A–B)). In most cases, and especially when imaging solid structures, *slicer-view* (Fig. 5) and planar slicing have appeared to be the preferable visualisation methods for 3D-EUS data from the GI tract.

*Segmentation* is a method for selective display of regions or volumes of interest and can be accomplished either by manual outlining (Fig.

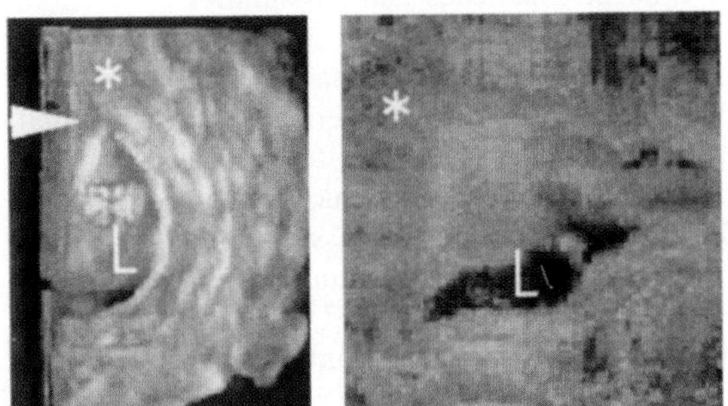


(A) (B)

Fig. 4. Volume rendering. (A) 3D-reconstruction of an intraductal US obtained by a 12 MHz miniprobe in conjunction with ERCP in a patient with cholangiocarcinoma. (B) Reconstructed longitudinal image displayed when the rendered volume is 'sliced' from left to right (arrow). Lumen (L), tumour (*).

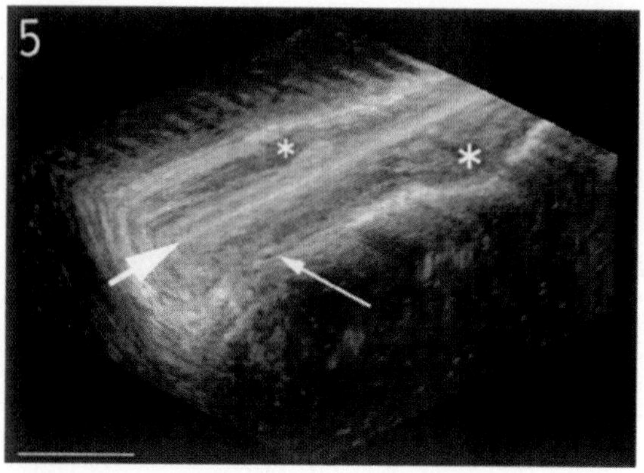


Fig. 5. Slicer-view. 3D-imaging of oesophageal cancer (stage T2), illustrating the projection of 2D-images on a reconstructed ultrasound data volume. Acquisition obtained with pullback of a 20 MHz miniprobe. Tumour infiltrate (*), US probe (thick arrow), outer muscle layer (thin arrow). Bar = 2 cm.

2(b)) or by automated algorithms (Figs. 3 and 4). By manual tracing, a structure (i.e. lesion) is outlined in consecutive 2D-images, constituting a 3D-element by interpolation of traced contours (Fig. 2(b)). Several reconstructed objects can be displayed simultaneously in order to visualise the spatial relationship between adjacent structures.

## 3. Clinical experience and possibilities

The role of 3D-US in clinical practice has yet to be defined. Preliminary experience with 3D-visualisation allows us, however, to speculate on situations in which the technique may be useful. 3D-EUS examinations are well tolerated in patients undergoing routine endoscopy. Our experience with the present 3D-EUS systems comprises approximately 260 examinations, included in a prospective protocol since 1996 (Molin et al., 1997a).

Computer reconstruction is currently not a method for real-time imaging. Production and interpretation of 3D-images are time-consuming, dependent on the complexity of the imaged structures. However, the ability for re-evaluation of details in the recorded volume may in some instances contribute to reduced time of endoscopic procedures. Since 3D-imaging requires new knowledge on image interpretation, there is also a learning curve, which should be accounted for before the full advantage of this new modality can be realised. A certain advantage of 3D-EUS is the possibility for delayed studies and demonstration of data exactly as they were acquired.

### 3.1. Tumour staging

A few clinical studies have been performed on tumour staging using 3D-EUS in the upper GI tract. Huenerbein (Huenerbein et al., 1997) examined five patients with oesophageal cancer using vascular miniprobes and determined tumour stage correctly in 4/5 patients. In our own experience, we have found that valuable clinical information can be obtained using 3D-EUS. In many instances, no further diagnostic work-up was necessary when 63 patients with GI tumours were evaluated (Molin et al., 1997a). Significant interobserver correlation exists for the assessment of tumour extent as well as for visualisation of the normal GI wall (Molin et al., 1998b).

Intraductal 3D-EUS application gained certain advantages when portal vein infiltration was evaluated in patients with pancreatic cancer (Kalimanis et al., 1995). Kaneko and co-workers (Kaneko et al., 1998) demonstrated subtle cancer invasion into the portal vein and found that intravascular surface rendering provided a valuable display for this evaluation.

In the colorectal area, several studies have been performed using 3D-US (Mueller et al., 1992). Ivanov (Ivanov and Diavoc, 1997) reported 15 patients in whom a complete 3D-reconstruction of rectal cancers was accomplished. In a study of recurrent rectal cancers (Huenerbein et al., 1996), the accuracy of 3D-EUS for assessing infiltration depth was 88% as compared with 82% for 2D-EUS. In the evaluation of lymph node involvement, the accuracy rates for 3D- and 2D-EUS were 79 and 74%, respectively.

In tumour staging, a major benefit of 3D- versus 2D-US appears to be the possibility for visualisation of otherwise unattainable planes, with improvement of the ability to explore and find

Published with permission

176 S.-O. Molin et al. / European Journal of Ultrasound 10 (1999) 171–177

representative image planes. This may lead to an increased understanding of the interrelation between normal and pathologic structures and help to obtain an exact preoperative staging and a subsequent appropriate treatment.

## 4. General considerations

Several factors may cause problems in 3D-EUS. A major critical factor is the acquired image quality. Organ motion and catheter displacement may impair a correct 3D-reconstruction. By 2D-EUS, an oblique probe tip position or a curved lumen may cause overestimation of the cross-sectional area. This problem may to a large degree be overcome by 3D-imaging. Several authors have also noticed that pulsative movements from the heart and large arteries may cause image distortion (Hashimoto et al., 1989; Kalimanis et al., 1995). The solution of this obstacle is ECG-gated 3D-EUS, which in our experience improves the image resolution in longitudinal 3D-reconstructions and allows higher accuracy in the evaluation of superficial and early lesions of the oesophagus (Molin et al., 1998a).

Posterior abdominal wall structures including the pancreas are less suitable for 3D-EUS with linear pullback systems, since the curved shapes of the stomach and the duodenum may lead to lateral probe displacement and subsequent erroneous 3D-reconstruction. Other technical solutions for 3D-image acqisition, i.e. electromagnetic positioning systems (Detmer et al., 1994) or multiplane probes, may correct for such errors.

Automated algorithms for image display, such as surface and volume rendering, may be particularly vulnerable to artefacts and insufficient image contrast in the ultrasound image (Belohlavek et al., 1993). This may lead to difficulties in extracting the right objects during the segmentation process, and the reliability of the displayed images can thus be challenged. Consequently, the automated methods, especially surface rendering, have gained limited use in 3D-imaging of GI structures, particularly in the evaluation of tumour infiltration.

Different studies on 3D-EUS may be difficult to compare due to variations in US systems and computer technology, as well as differences in software programs and display methods. Standardisation of the 3D-procedure as well as careful consideration of indications and methodological limitations should therefore be a prerequisite in future evaluations.

In conclusion, 3D-visualisation may become a valuable supplement to conventional endosonography, providing practical and intuitive visual interfaces and new possibilities for measurements and spatial imaging. Further studies are wanted to confirm the clinical impact of 3D-EUS in the diagnosis of gastrointestinal diseases.

## References

Baum G, Greenwood I. Orbital lesion localization by three-dimensional ultrasonography. NY State J Med 1961;61: 4149–57.

Belohlavek M, Foley D, Gerber T, Kinter T, Greenleaf J, Seward J. Three- and four-dimensional cardiovascular ultrasound imaging: a new era for echocardiography. Mayo Clin Proc 1993;68(3):221–40.

Coatrieux JL, Garreau M, Collorec R, Roux C. Computer vision approaches for the three-dimensional reconstruction of coronary arteries: review and prospects. Crit Rev Biomed Eng 1994;22(1):1–38.

Dekker D, Pizali R, Dong EJ. A system for ultrasonically imaging the human hearth in three dimensions. Comput Biomed Res 1974;7:544–53.

Detmer P, Bashein G, Hodges T, et al. 3D ultrasonic image feature localization based on magnetic scanhead tracking: in vitro calibration and validation. Ultrasound Med Biol 1994;20(9):923–36.

Gilja OH, Detmer P, Jong J, et al. Intragastric distribution and gastric emptying assessed by three-dimensional ultrasonography. Gastroenterology 1997;113(1):38–49.

Hashimoto H, Mitsunaga A, Suzuki S, Kurokawa K, Obata H. Evaluation of endoscopic ultrasonography for gastric tumor and presentation of three-dimensional display of endoscopic ultrasonography. Surg Endosc 1989;3:173–81.

Huenerbein M, Dohmoto M, Haensch W, Schlag PM. Evaluation and biopsy of recurrent rectal cancer using three-dimensional endosonography. Dis Colon Rectum 1996; 39(12):1373–8.

Huenerbein M, Gretschel S, Ghadimi BM, Schlag PM. Three-dimensional endoscopic ultrasound of the esophagus. Preliminary experience. Surg Endosc 1997;11(10):991–4.

Ivanov K, Diavoc C. Three-dimensional endoluminal ultrasound: new staging technique in patients with rectal cancer. Dis Colon Rectum 1997;40(1):47–50.

Published with permission



Kalimanis G, Garra SB, Tio T, et al. The feasability of three-dimensional endsoscopic ultrasonography: a preliminary report. Gastrointest Endosc 1995;41(3):235–9.

Kaneko T, Nakao A, Nomoto S, Endo T, Ito S, Takagi H. Intraportal endovascular ultrasonography for assessment of vascular invasion by biliary tract cancer. Gastrointest Endosc 1998;47(1):33–41.

Kaneko T, Nakao A. Three-dimensional imaging of intraportal endovascular ultrasonography for pancreatic cancer. Gastrointest Endosc 1998;48(2):217–8.

Kanemaki N, Nakazawa K, Inui K, Yoshina K, Okushima K. Three-dimensional intraductal ultrasonography: preliminary results of a new technique for the diagnosis of diseases of the pancreatobiliary system. Endoscopy 1997; 29:726–31.

Lee DY, Eigler N, Luo H, et al. Effect of intracoronary ultrasound imaging on clinical decision making. Am Heart J 1995;129(6):1084–93.

Lightdale C. Endoscopic ultrasonography in the diagnosis, staging, and follow-up of esophageal and gastric cancer. Endoscopy 1992;24:297–303.

Molin S-O, Engström A, Nesje LB, et al. Improvement of three-dimensional EUS using ECG-triggered acquisition. Endoscopy 1998a;30(Suppl. 1):A147.

Molin S-O, Falk A, Gilja OH, Nesje LB, Ødegaard S. 3D-endosonography improves the assessment of tumors in the upper gastrointestinal tract. [Abstract]. Gastroenterology 1997a;112(4)(Suppl.):A30.

Molin S-O, Falk A, Hall-Angerås M, Gilja O, Hausken T, Nesje LB, Ødegaard S. Virtual reality in surgical practice in vitro and in vivo evaluations. In: Morgan KS, Hoffman HM, Stredney D, Weghorst SJ, editors. Medicine Meets Virtual Reality: Global Healthcare Grid, in Studies in Health Technology and Informatics. Amsterdam, ISSN: 0926-9630: IOS Press, Ohmsha, 1997b:246–53.

Molin S-O, Nesje LB, Ødegaard S. Critical acquisition of ultrasound data in 3D-EUS. [Abstract]. Eur J Ultrasound 1998b;7(Suppl.1):S43.

Moritz W, Shreve P. A microprocessor-based spatial locating system for use with diagnostic ultrasound. Proc IEEE 1976;64:966–74.

Mueller M, Stamos M, Cavaye D, Kopchok G, Laas T, White R. Three-dimensional transrectal ultrasound: preliminary patient evaluation. J Laparoendosc Surg 1992;2(5):223–7.

Nishimura K, Niwa Y, Goto H, Hase S, Arisawa T, Hayakawa T. Three-dimensional endoscopic ultrasonography of gastrointestinal lesions using an ultrasound probe. Scand J Gastroenterol 1997;32(9):862–8.

Riccabona M, Nelson T, Pretorius D, Davidson T. Distance and volume measurement using three-dimensional ultrasonography. J Ultrasound Med 1995;14(12):881–6.

Riccabona M, Pretorius D, Nelson T, Johnson D, Budorick N. Three-dimensional ultrasound: display modalities in obstetrics. J Clin Ultrasound 1997;25(4):157–67.

Roelandt JR, di Mario C, Pandian NG, et al. Three-dimensional reconstruction of intracoronary ultrasound images. Rationale, approaches, problems, and directions. Circulation ISSN: 0009-7322 1994;90(2):1044–55.

Rösch T, Classen M. Gastroenterologic Endosonography. Stuttgart: Tieme Verlag, 1992.

Rösch T. Endosonography of the gastrointestinal tract—an assessment of current status. Bildgebung ISSN: 1012-5655 1993;60(3):169–75.

Tio TL, Coene PP, Luiken GJ, Tytgat GN. Endosonography in the clinical staging of esophagogastric carcinoma. Gastrointest-Endosc ISSN: 0016-5107 1990;36(2):S2–S10.

Tio TL, Weijers O, Hulsman F, et al. Endosonography of colorectal diseases. Endoscopy 1992;1:309–14.

Van Dam J, Sivak M, editors. Gastrointestinal endosonography. ISBN 0-7216-7989-7, WB Saunders Company 1999.

Zoller WG, Liess H. 3D ultrasound in gastroenterology. Bildgebung ISSN: 1012-5655 1994;61(2):95–9.

Ødegaard S, Nesje LB, Gilja O, Hausken T, Molin S-O, Martens D. Diseases of the gastrointestinal tract axamined with 3D endoscopic ultrasonography. In: Bismuth H, Galmiche JP, Hughuier M, Jaeck D, editors. 8th World Congress of the International Gastro-Surgical Club. Bologna: Monduzzi Edittore, International proceedings division, 1998:827–31.

Ødegaard S, Nesje LB, Ohm M, Kimmey MB. Endoscopy in gastrointestinal diseases. Acta Radiologica 1999;40:119–34.

CHAPTER 11

# GASTRIC EMPTYING AND DUODENO-GASTRIC REFLUX ASSESSED BY DUPLEX SONOGRAPHY

TRYGVE HAUSKEN AND SVEIN ØDEGAARD

Information concerning movement of luminal contents in humans can be obtained by fluoroscopy, scintigraphy, magnetic resonance imaging (MRI) and duplex sonography. The disadvantages of fluoroscopy and scintigraphy are the radiation exposure, the non-physiological stimulus of barium (1), and the relatively low time resolution that can be obtained using these techniques. Studies based on scintigraphy and standard ultrasound of the stomach and duodenum will indirectly measure overall rates of gastric emptying, but these methods do not have the temporal resolution to assess at a second to second basis. Promising new MRI methods are developed. Echo planar imaging, an ultrafast variant of MRI, can provide excellent images of both gastric wall movements and movements of solid and liquid meals (2–4).

Ultrasonographic studies by King, *et al.* (5) using test meals containing bran particles showed that gastric emptying occurred in episodes lasting a few seconds in healthy subjects. The emptying period usually started immediately after relaxation of the antropyloroduodenal segment and was finished before the next peristaltic contraction approached the distal antrum. A brief episode of duodenogastric reflux occurred in about 60% of the peristaltic cycles shortly before the terminal antral contraction. A similar type of reflux was shown in dogs by Malbert, *et al.* (6), who used operatively implanted electromagnetic flowmeter probes. Hausken *et al.* (7–9) showed that by using pulsed Doppler combined with real-time ultrasonography (Duplex sonography), it is possible to visualize antroduodenal motility and transpyloric flow simultaneously. Antegrade and retrograde transpyloric flow is visualized using bidirectional velocity curves. Most contractions of the proximal duodenal bulb preceed closure of the pylorus (and the terminal antrum), and duodenal bulb contraction is often accompanied by a short burst of duodenogastric reflux occurring immediately before closure of the pylorus.

## 1. Ultrasound Methods

### 1.1. *The meal*

A liquid meal of meat soup has been used in our motility studies. The test meal consists of a liquid meal of commercial meat soup. Five hundred ml was pre-warmed to 37°C, and the soup was gradually ingested during 3 minutes. The meal contained 0.9 g protein, 0.9 g fat, and 0.9 g carbohydrate (15 kcal). The soup is hypoechoic, gives a clear image of the intestinal wall, and makes transpyloric movements of the luminal contents visible. The meal induces antroduodenal motility typical of the fed state.

The emptying curve for this meal follows an exponential curve with more emptying initially and 50% of the meal is emptied after 22 minutes.

### 1.2. *In vitro validation*

*In vitro* measurements of back-scattered ultrasound from selected fluids were carried out using a flow rig designed for blood flow calibration. Back-scattered ultrasound from orange juice, vegetable juice, meat soup, and blood was measured using an ultrasound pulsed Doppler meter (SD 100; Vingmed sound A/S, Horten, Norway). A 3-MHz ultrasound beam was directed toward a silicone rubber tube that received the fluid under study from a roller pump.

The nutrient liquids examined all gave good reflection of Doppler-shifted ultrasound and are thus useful for ultrasound Doppler studies. The velocity curves registered with the ultrasound Doppler meter were similar for blood and meat soup. The maximum velocity was within ±10%, suggesting the speed of ultrasound in the two media to be comparable at room temperature. Assuming the relationship between speed and temperature to be similar for blood and meat soup, the measured velocities for movement of the meat soup would be within ±10% of the recorded velocities.

### 1.3. *Procedure*

The subjects were studied in the morning after an overnight fast, immediately after ingesting 500 mL of meat soup. Subjects sat upright during the procedure. The ultrasound probe was positioned at the level of the transpyloric plane with the antrum, the pylorus, and the proximal duodenum visualized simultaneously. The sample volume of the pulsed Doppler was positioned across the pylorus and the angle between the Doppler beams and the transpyloric plane was always $< 60°$. With this view, it was possible to simultaneously record real-time images of the antroduodenal contractions, movements of the luminal contents across the pylorus, and bidirectional velocity curves. To estimate antral retropulsion, the sample volume of the pulsed Doppler was positioned in the distal antrum.

### 1.4. *Problems with duplex sonography*

Several problems are associated with duplex sonography of transpyloric flow and peristalsis. Individual anatomic variations sometimes make it impossible to visualize the pyloric channel and the proximal duodenum in one single plane. In addition, the sample volume of the pulsed Doppler must be positioned precisely across the pylorus, a position that is easily lost by respiration and movements. In addition, subcutaneous fat and abdominal gas may impair the image. Slim and calm persons are most suitable for this investigation.

## 2. Definitions of Transpyloric Flow and Antral Contractions

An **antral contraction** was defined as an indentation of the gastric wall greater than one antral wall thickness, which was not due to respiration, pulsation transmitted from the aorta or heart, or to movements of adjacent intestine, and which was observed to propagate in space and time. **First gastric emptying** was defined as the first occurrence of gastric emptying after the start of drinking the soup. An **episode of gastric emptying** was defined as the flow across the pylorus with a mean velocity of more than 10 cm/sec lasting more than 1 sec.

**Occluding peristaltic-related transpyloric emptying** was defined as gastric emptying associated with contractile activity in which the ultrasound image showed an occlusion of the stomach wall.

**Non-occluding peristaltic-related emptying** was defined as transpyloric emptying of gastric contents associated with contractile activity of the gastric wall which not occluded the lumen. During maximal contractions transpyloric flow could still be seen passing back and forth through the open pylorus.

**Non-peristaltic-related transpyloric emptying** was defined as transpyloric emptying of gastric contents, without contractions detected on ultrasound or manometry.

## 3. Relationship Between Antroduodenal Motility and Transpyloric Flow

Although several studies have suggested that the incidence of gastrointestinal contractions and their amplitude are important determinants of luminal flow, the motor mechanisms responsible for gastric emptying are still poorly understood (1–5, 10–17).

In order to study the relation between motility and flow in detail, techniques with a high temporal and spatial resolution are required for the assessment of antropyloroduodenal pressure waves and transpyloric flow. Subjects were intubated after an overnight fast with a 21-lumen manometric assembly, which was introduced trans-nasally and positioned in the antropyloroduodenal region using fluoroscopy.

## 4. Synchronization of Doppler/Ultrasound and Manometric Recordings

The UD-2000 Video-Mix and imaging digitizing, version 5.10 (MMS, Medical Measurements Systems, Enschede, The Netherlands) was used to synchronize the recorded data. The image digitizing allowed simultaneous display of Doppler/ultrasound data and manometry signals on one PC monitor (Fig. 1). The Doppler/ultrasound data were digitized during the investigation, and the digitized images were saved on disk together with the digitized manometry signals. The computer controlled video recorder recorded all the Doppler/ultrasound images. The computer kept a database with tape information. During recording, the tapes were formatted with coded information. This allowed the system to verify that the correct tape was used. The tape also contained timing information, to allow synchronized playback during analysis. Also, images could be digitized from tape during analysis.

## 5. Relationship Between Transpyloric Flow and Motor Activity

Transpyloric emptying occurred as emptying-reflux-emptying sequences. $45.3 \pm 28\%$ (mean $\pm$ SD) of the sequences were associated with occluding antral peristalsis, $21.5 \pm 18\%$ were

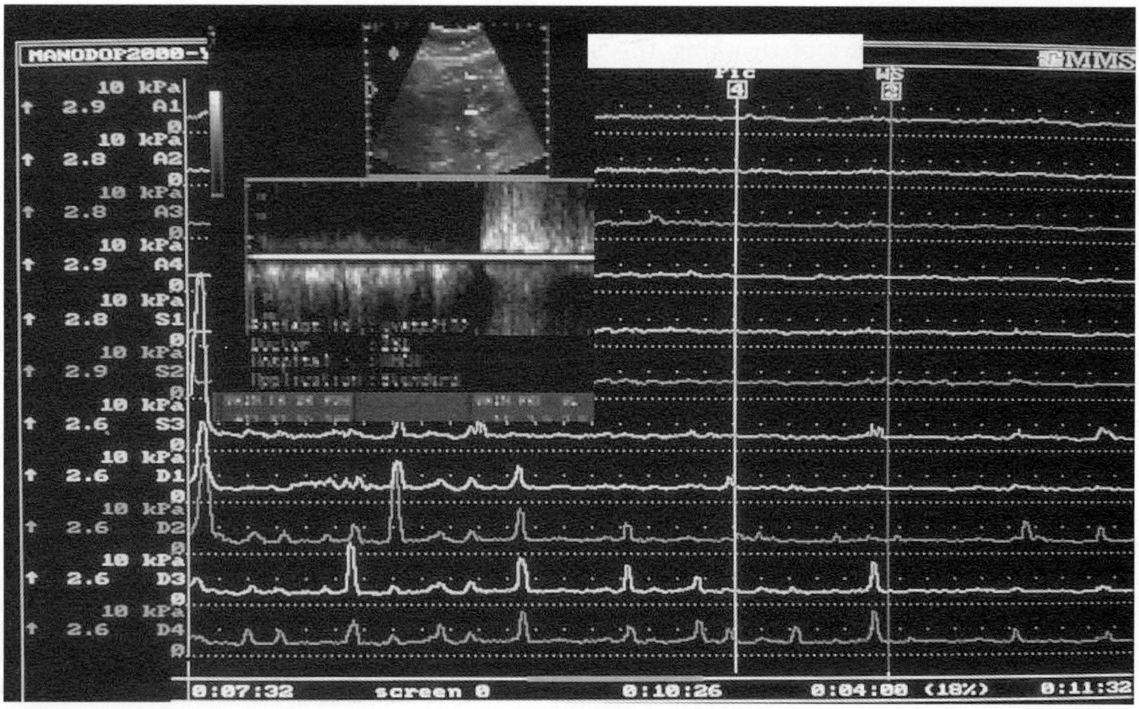


Fig. 1. Simultaneous display of Doppler/ultrasound data and manometry signals on one PC monitor.

associated with non-occluding peristaltic related antral contractions, and $35.7 \pm 36\%$ of the sequences were not associated with peristalsis. Peristaltic related flow occurred as emptying alone, emptying followed by reflux, or as sequences of emptying-reflux-emptying pulses. The flow events occurred always in front of the peristaltic wave. The non-peristaltic related flow was often seen as longer periods of alternating emptying-reflux sequences.

## 6. Relationship Between Transpyloric Emptying and Occluding Peristaltic Contractions

When peristaltic related flow was observed, propagated pressure waves were recorded manometrically over three or more side holes.

Seventy-four percent of the emptying periods showed a sequence of emptying-reflux-emptying. All emptying periods were followed by a reflux period, which was caused by duodenal contraction in 93% of the periods. The proximal duodenal pressure change was in 50% of the periods recorded in only one channel. The reflux periods in association with 2 duodenal contractions or more were caused by propagated (42%) and retroperistaltic (58%) duodenal contractions with a mean amplitude of $4.8 \pm 3.2$ kPa.

## 7. Relationship Between Transpyloric Emptying and Non-Occluding Peristaltic Contractions

When non-occluding peristaltic related flow was seen this corresponded with pressure waves recorded only in the most distal antral sidehole. The gradients at onset of emptying periods were low. The reflux periods were caused by duodenal contractions with a mean amplitude of $2.4 \pm 0.1$ kPa.

## 8. Non-Peristaltic Related Emptying

Non-peristaltic related flow sequences could be seen with more alternating emptying-reflux episodes than those associated with peristalsis. The pressure gradients during non-peristaltic related emptying were significantly lower than during peristaltic related emptying (non-peristaltic: $0.15 \pm 0.6$ kPa, occluding peristaltic $1.7 \pm 2.3$ kPa, $p < 0.005$) (Fig. 2). The reflux periods were in 75% related to a duodenal contraction with a mean amplitude of $4.4 \pm 5.5$ kPa. 25% of the emptying-reflux-emptying periods were followed by a second reflux period, which was related to a duodenal contraction with a mean amplitude of 2.8 kPa.

## 9. Duration of Flow Episodes

In total, the duration of non-peristaltic related emptying pulses were longer than those seen during peristaltic related emptying (non-peristaltic: $6.5 \pm 4.7$ sec, occluding peristaltic $4.4 \pm 2.2$ sec ($p = 0.05$)). The reflux episodes were significantly longer during non-peristaltic related emptying than during peristaltic related (non-peristaltic: $2.6 \pm 0.7$ sec, peristaltic $2.0 \pm 0.8$ sec, $p < 0.03$).

## 10. Interpretation

Gastric emptying of a low caloric liquid meal follows sequences of emptying-reflux-emptying pulses. About half of the sequences are peristaltic related, but both non-occluding, peristaltic related and non-peristaltic related emptying sequences occur. Non-peristaltic related flow sequences have often more alternating emptying-reflux episodes than those associated with peristalsis, and the duration of non-peristaltic related emptying and reflux pulses are

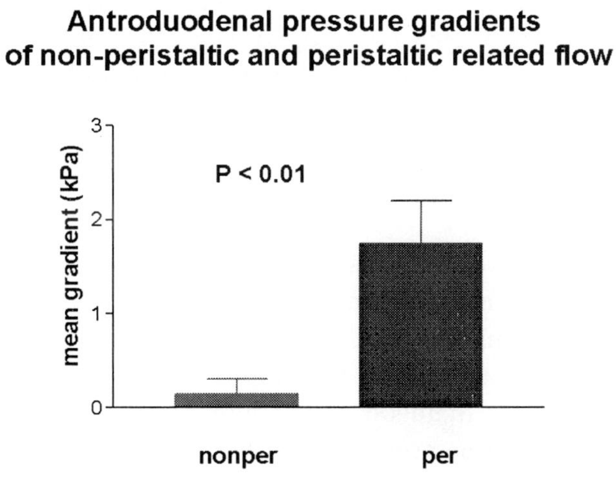


Fig. 2. Histogram of antroduodenal pressures.

longer. The pressure gradients for all types of emptying are low and the pressure gradients during non-peristaltic related emptying are significantly lower than during peristaltic related emptying.

Transpyloric flow can be classified into flow associated with a local increase in the pressure gradient between antrum and duodenum (Pa–Pd) due to antral propagating pressure waves, and flow associated with a common cavity pressure difference between the distal antrum and the proximal duodenum as was observed during non-peristaltic related flow. The second type of flow is independent of peristalsis and is likely to be caused by changes in gastric tone, or by pressure changes outside the stomach such as aortic pulsation and inspiration (18).

Flow can only occur in the presence of an open pylorus. The rate of transpyloric flow in time is proportional to (Pa–Pd)/$R$, where $R$ is pyloric resistance at that time. $R$ is given by $\mu/D^4$, where $D$ is the average diameter of the pyloric channel and $\mu$ is the gastric fluid viscosity (19). Because $R$ is proportional to $1/D^4$, the rate of transpyloric flow is highly influenced by the pyloric diameter. A large pyloric diameter reflects therefore low pyloric resistance. Consequently, the transpyloric flow can be high in spite of a low pressure gradient between the distal antrum and proximal duodenum (Pa–Pd).

Antroduodenal pressure gradients (Pa–Pd) are very low and they were significantly lower during non-peristaltic than with peristaltic related flow. Despite the lower pressure gradients the duration of emptying episodes were significantly longer during non-peristaltic flow suggesting more emptying during these events. The pyloric channel was therefore probably wide resulting in a low pyloric resistance.

Most of the duodenogastric reflux episodes were associated with duodenal contractions that were both propagated and retroperistaltic. Castedal, *et al.* (20) have recently demonstrated the importance of the duodenum as a retroperistalic pump which can retropel duodenal contents to the stomach. Duodenal pressures were recorded from 4 side holes (1.5 cm apart) in the duodenal bulb and the most proximal part of the duodenum. Pressure rise in the most proximal duodenal side hole close to the open pylorus mediates flow both in antegrade and retrograde direction and may explain why propagated duodenal contractions are associated with duodenogastric reflux. It should be stressed that the results may be specific to gastric emptying of a low-caloric liquid meal. Stimulation of the duodenum with a higher caloric meal increases the antroduodenal resistance and this seems to be consistent with previous findings of a decrease in pyloric diameter after a nutrient meal.

## 11. Transpyloric Flow Volume

Based on electromagnetic flowmeter measurements in dogs or force transducers applied in isolated cat stomachs or determined by continuous collection and weighing of all effluent from the open duodenal cannula in dogs (21–22) the emptying stroke volumes have been found to vary between 0.1–75 ml. Using the Doppler technique, flow volume can be estimated by assuming a constant diameter of the human pylorus and calculating the mean velocity within the sample volume averaged over the reflux period.

$$Q = V_{\text{mean}} \cdot \pi \cdot (d/2)^2 \cdot s$$

where $Q$ is flow volume (mL), $V_{\text{mean}}$ is mean velocity (cm/s) within the sample volume averaged over the reflux period, $d$ is the inner diameter of the pylorus, and $s$ is the duration (seconds) of reflux. $V_{\text{mean}}$ was obtained by freezing the picture and using the built-in calculation program of the apparatus.

The flow volume of a single gush of duodenogastric reflux of a liquid meal has been estimated to be approximately 1.8 ml. However, because the pyloric size and geometric shape, spatial flow profile and Doppler angle vary during the reflux episode, accurate calculation of transpyloric flow is difficult. These limitations of the Doppler technique restrict its clinical applications in calculating transpyloric flow where irregularly shaped flow passage, non-parabolic velocity profiles and ambiguous Doppler angles are expected.

Color Doppler has been used widely as a qualitative and semi-quantitative mean for delineating the existence and the extent of abnormal flow. However, it has not been employed quantitatively for clinical studies due to the difficulties in extracting the velocity information from the image. Digital imaging capability of a few new ultrasound systems suggests the feasibility of using color Doppler as a quantitative tool for assessing a flow field.

Consequently, we have developed an orientation determined digital color Doppler method for volume quantification of irregularly shaped flow passages (23).

## 12. Three-Dimensional Ultrasound System

A commercial magnetic position and orientation measurement system (Flock of Birds model 6DFOB, Ascension Technology Corp., Burlington, VT) was used to track the ultrasound scanhead. The receiver was attached to a 3.5 MHz phased array sector-scan ultrasound scanhead connected to an HDI 3000 ultrasound platform (Advanced Technology Laboratories, Inc., Bothell, WA, USA). The 3D position and orientation data were saved on a PC. The 3D data and the digital color images were transferred to a Silicon Graphics Indigo2 workstation for analysis. The available computer memory established a maximum capture period of 32 seconds (480 images); the capture period was set to 8 seconds for the studies described below.

## 13. 3D Reconstruction

A custom tracing program running on a dedicated Indigo2 workstation (Silicon Graphics, Inc., Mountain View, CA, USA) was used to outline the borders of the flow vessel or organ which appeared in each image. The flow tube was outlined for the *in vitro* experiment and for the *in vivo* study — the terminal antrum, pylorus, and duodenal bulb were outlined. The flow jet and individual color Doppler regions were manually identified. The tracing program was interfaced with the software package AVS (Advanced Visual Systems, Inc., Waltham, MA, USA), providing interactive 3D visualization and editing of outlines. Border registration could be examined with 3D stereo viewing glasses (CrystalEyes, Stereographics Corp., San Rafael, CA, USA).

## 14. Principle of Flow Measurement

The measurement involved several steps.

(1) An imaging plane was selected where the orientation of the plane offered fairly good Doppler angles to the vessel or flow channel.

(2) Using the 3D reconstruction and the outlines, a line was fitted through the centroid of two outlines, which were located distal and proximal to the selected measurement plane. This line was considered the axis of the flow through the vessel or organ ($Ax$) at that point.

(3) Areas in the 2D image were identified which each had a specific color, thus a specific velocity. Such a $m$th area is represented in Fig. 3 as $A_m$. Next, the normal direction of this area in 2D was determined by finding two vectors that lay in the image plane and then taking the cross product of them. The resulting area vector ($An_m$) normal to image plane is illustrated in the figure. The angle between this area vector and the flow axis vector is designated as $\phi$ in the figure. This elemental area Anm is projected onto the flow axis by taking a dot product of it and the axial vector ($An_m \bullet Ax$).

(4) Utilizing a look up table, the color in each region was converted to a velocity value. The fact that these values are already in digital form makes this conversion expeditious and fairly accurate. These velocities represent the Doppler velocity in the direction that the ultrasound propagated from the imaging transducer. An example ($V_m$) is shown in Fig. 3 and the angle ($\theta$) between it and $Ax$. This velocity also is projected onto the flow axis with a dot product vector multiplication ($V_m \bullet Ax$).

(5) The flow in each region then was obtained by multiplying the axial projected area and velocity.

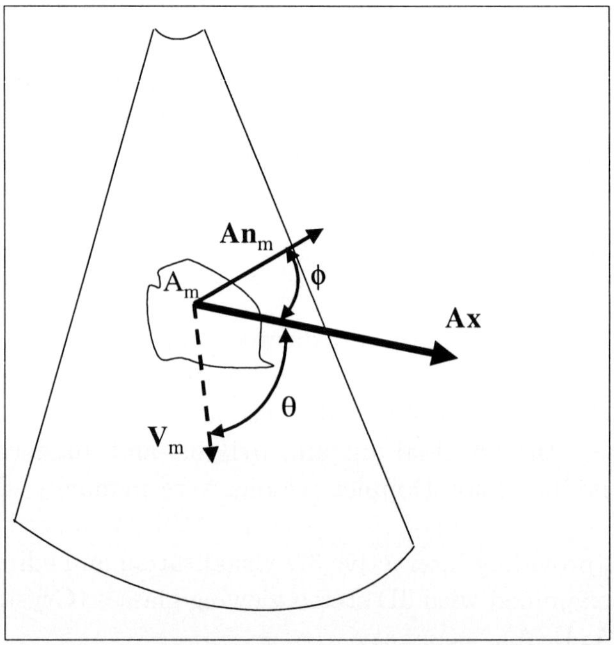


Fig. 3. The various vectors involved in computing flow. $Ax$ is the axis of flow determined for the vessel or organ under study. $A_m$ is a specific area ($m$th area) in the image with a Doppler color and velocity vector, $V_m$. $An_m$ is the area vector with a direction normal to the imaging plane.

(6) The total flow is then a summation of all the regions. The equation for this operation is:

$$\text{Flow} = \sum_{m=1}^{n} (An_m \cdot Ax)(V_m \cdot Ax)$$

The velocity mode (variance off) with no baseline shift and no angle correction was used. Color Gain was set such that the Doppler signal was maximum and restrained within the lumen of the tubular passage and at the highest possible level that no background noise was displayed. The velocity scale was adjusted so that the Nyquist limit was slightly above the maximum velocity, verified by pulse-wave Doppler, in the particular flow field. Other parameters included wall filter low, priority medium, persistence off, and line density medium. These settings were saved and kept consistent for consequential image acquisition.

The velocity extraction was performed by converting the color pixels into a velocity value based on the color component values on the colormap. In color Doppler imaging, velocity is represented by a specified color pixel, with a disparity among its $R$, $G$ and $B$ values. The velocity pixels were identified and segmented by comparing its color components for each pixel. Then, for each color pixel, its velocity value was determined by the inverse of the flow-mapping algorithm. Once the velocity was determined, the flow quantification with velocity-area integration was made using the equation above with the angle correction. The flow quantification was performed for each digital image in the entire transpyloric episode. The duration of the episode was determined by the number of Doppler images that had noticeable Doppler signals. Doppler images acquired at Doppler angles $> 70$ degrees were excluded for the quantification. Integrate the flow rates at each time point yielded the total volume of gastric emptying.

## 15. *In vitro* Flow Study

A custom made flow phantom made of silicon tubing was used to generate static flow rates. The *in vitro* validation was conducted with the consistent and predetermined instrument settings. The flow rate varied from 3–35 ml/sec. Water with fish oil (2%) was used to mimic biological fluid, which scattered ultrasound. The flow settings for the phantom were calibrated by collecting known volumes in a measured time. Images were acquired at angles to the axis of the flow tube over a range of 35° to 65°. Cross-sectional color Doppler digital images were acquired using a HDI-3000 (Advanced Technology Laboratory, Bothel, WA) ultrasound system with a 10 MHz linear transducer. The 3D position and orientation data were acquired with a magnetic sensing system (Ascension Technology) and saved on a PC.

Quantitatively, the ultrasound measured flow rates underestimated the reference flow rates (by average of 8.8%) over the range of 3 to 30 ml/s. The linear regression of the fit had a slope of 0.88 and an intercept of the axis of $-0.59$ ml.

## 16. Transpyloric Flow Volumes in Humans

The investigator moved the transducer in freehand across the pylorus region for 3D reconstruction of the terminal antrum, pylorus, duodenal bulb and the flow jet. This reconstruction was used to determine the orientation of the flow passage. Digital color Doppler images were obtained continuously covering transpyloric flow episode. Images were acquired first with the cineloop memory in the ultrasound scanner and then transferred to workstation for analysis. Duplicated scans were acquired to guarantee the success.

An example of 3D outlines and a reconstruction is shown in Fig. 4. Due to the limitation in computer memory only very small episodes of gastric emptying were captured. In healthy volunteers, high inter-individual variations of the stroke volumes of transpyloric flow episodes were seen during the initial gastric emptying of the present liquid meal. Stroke volume of gastric emptying episodes lasted on average only 0.69 sec (range 0.1–1.5 s ) with a volume of on average of 4.3 ml (range 1.1–7.4 ml). The duodenogastric reflux episodes lasted on average 1.4 seconds (range 0.1–2.7 s) with a volume of on average of 8.3 ml (range 1.3–14.1 ml). The flow volumes varied also in one single person, for emptying periods from 1,1 ml - 7.4 ml (average 4.7 ml), and for reflux episodes from 1.3 ml–2.3 (average 1.7 ml). The angle between flow direction and the ultrasound beam (Doppler angle) was on average 40.3° (range 16.4°–66.9°).

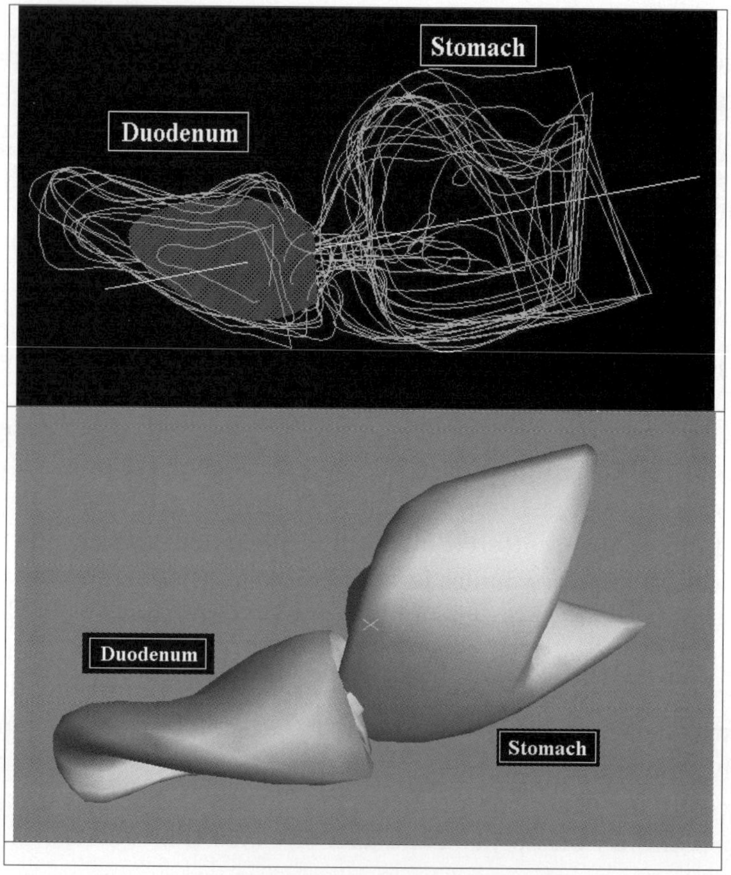


Fig. 4. The upper photograph shows the outlines obtained from one of the *in vivo* studies. The shaded region in the central region of the duodenum illustrates the location of the color Doppler imaging plane. The lower photograph is a shaded reconstruction of the surface of the duodenum and stomach scanned in one subject.

## 17. Interpretation

With appropriate instrument settings, orientation determined color Doppler can be used for dynamic quantification of transpyloric flow pulses in humans. The estimated flow volumes showed high variations, both between subjects and when estimated in one single subject.

Currently available methods for studying gastric emptying do not provide quantitative information about the movement of gastric contents. Studies based on scintigraphy and standard ultrasound at the gastric and duodenal level will indirectly measure overall rates of gastric emptying, but these methods do not have the temporal resolution to distinguish flow through the pylorus at one moment from the flow a few seconds later. The standard ultrasound Doppler technique provides temporal resolution to distinguish flow, but it does not allow accurate quantification of flow volume (ml), due to reasons mentioned above. Stroke volumes of flow have been measured only *in vitro* or on anesthetized animals.

The new orientation determined color Doppler might help the investigator to quantify net gastric emptying and to estimate the amount of duodenogastric reflux. The method can be used to study normal physiology and pathophysiology of the gastro-pyloro-duodenal segment and to monitor the effect of medications on transpyloric flow.

Flow quantification has been a difficulty especially in an irregularly shaped flow vessel and in fluid filled hollow organs such as the gastro-pyloro-duodenal segment. Assumptions of circular cross-sectional shape and uniform velocity profile are insufficient for flow estimation. Color Doppler imaging has been widely used in clinical practice for qualitative and semi-quantitative flow quantification. It is the only non-invasive mean that covers a relative large sampling field that vessels and the gastro-pyloro-duodenal segment can be easily scanned with reasonable Doppler angle. The digital feature of the image, ensuring a faithful velocity extraction, permits an objective and geometry-independent quantification of volume flow. The intersect angle is a major factor that determines the accuracy of flow quantification. In addition, the accuracy of flow rate is also related with the spatial velocity variation that affects the measured velocities and area. The 3D capability provided a quality control for eliminating inappropriate Doppler angles. Thus, the effect of beam thickness and area caused by improper Doppler angle would be minimized.

## 18. Digitized Doppler Patterns of Transpyloric Flow can be Studied by Doppler Ultrasound

We have also developed a software for digitizing the recorded Doppler data (LabVIEW 5.1, National Instruments). Ten healthy volunteers (5F) consumed 500 ml of low caloric soup. Using 3.5 mHz Duplex ultrasound, the transpyloric plane was imaged for 30 min in 10 min intervals to assess the pattern of transpyloric flow, divided into ante- and retrograde flow periods. The bi-directional sound information on the tape was transferred (using audio-out of the video recorder and audio-in on the sound card) to a computer and the digitized Doppler data were saved on disk. The software allowed information of both flow duration and flow velocity. The sum of emptying and reflux periods containing those data over time was used for analysis (Fig. 5). Antral area and proximal stomach volume were assessed for each interval.

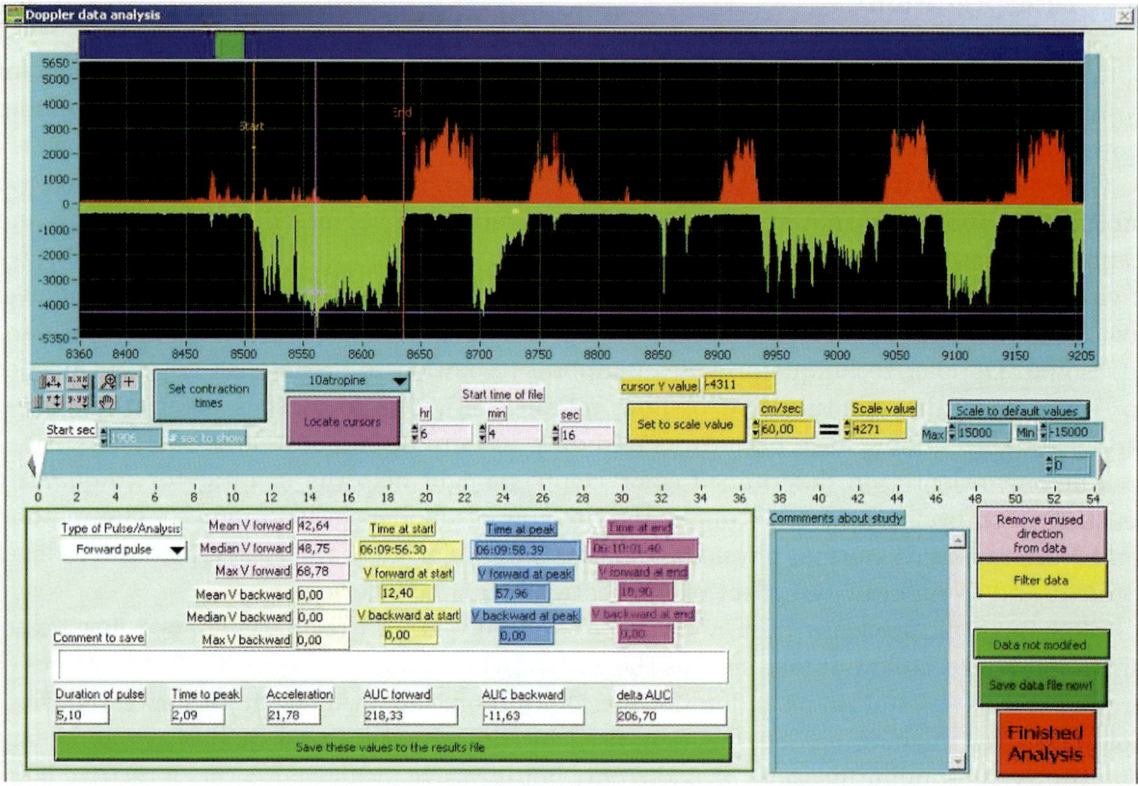


Fig. 5. The analysis screen.

Both proximal stomach volume and antral area over time were significantly reduced ($p < 0.0001$ and $p < 0.001$, respectively). A positive correlation ($r = 0.83$, $p < 0.005$) was found between net forward flow, calculated as Area Under the Curve (AUC) of the difference between AUC of forward flow and AUC of retrograde flow, and reduction of proximal stomach volume over time. No correlation was found between reduction in antral area and net forward flow. The new developed software for digitizing ultrasound Doppler data can be used to study transpyloric flow using the information of both flow duration and flow velocity.

## 19. Duplex Sonography in Patients with Functional Dyspepsia

Patients with functional dyspepsia often experience early satiety and discomfort after a meal. Using duplex sonography it is possible to relate timing of symptoms and early postprandial emptying in patients with functional dyspepsia (9). Twelve patients were investigated during 3 minutes of soup ingestion (500 ml) and in the following 10 minutes postprandial period. Gastric emptying commenced on average 52 seconds after the start of ingestion. In all patients, meal related discomfort was experienced after commencement of transpyloric emptying, on average after 143 seconds. The early occurrence of meal-related symptoms suggests that gastric distension is the main factor in symptom generation. The onset of symptoms after the commencement of gastric emptying suggests that intestinal tasting receptors are involved in symptom generation. An inverse relationship was found between the duration of the tasting period and symptom intensity, suggesting that the time allowed for duodenal tasting might be too short in patients with functional dyspepsia.

## References


1. Rao, S. S., Lu, C. and Schulze Delrieu K., Duodenum as a immediate brake to gastric outflow: A videofluoroscopic and manometric asessment. Gastroenterology 1996; 110: 740–747.
2. Wright, J., Evans, D., Gowland, P. and Mansfield, P., Validation of of antroduodenal motility measurements made by echo-planar magnetic resonance imaging. Neurogastroenterol Mot 1999; 11: 19–25.
3. Boulby, P., Moore, R., Gowland, P. and Spiller, R. C., Fat delays emptying but increases forward and backward antral flow as assessed by flow-sensitive magnetic resonance imaging. Neurogastroenterol Mot 1999; 11: 27–36.
4. Marciani, L., Gowland, P., Fillery-Travis, A., Manoj, P., Wright, J., Smith, P., Moore, R. and Spiller, R. C., Assessment of antral grinding of a model solid meal with echo-planar imaging. Am J Physiol Gastrointestinal Liver Physiol 2001; 280(5): G844–849.
5. King, P. M., Adam, R. D., Pryde, A., Mcdicken, W. N. and Heading, R. C., Relationships of human antroduodenal motility and transpyloric fluid movement: Non-invasive obsevations with real-time ultrasound. Gut 1984; 25: 1384–1391.
6. Malbert, C. H. and Ruckebusch, Y., Relationships between pressure and flow across the gastroduodenal junction in dogs. Am J Physiol 1991; 260: G653–657.
7. Hausken, T., Ødegaard, S., Matre, K. and Berstad, A., Antroduodenal motility and movements of luminal contents studied by duplex sonography. Gastroenterology 1992; 102: 1583–1590.
8. Hausken, T., Gilja, O. H., Odegaard, S. and Berstad, A., Flow across the human pylorus soon after ingestion of food, studies by duplex sonography. Scand J Gastroenterol 1998; 484-490.
9. Hausken, T., Gilja, O. H., Undeland, K. A. and Berstad, A., Timing of postprandial dyspeptic symptoms and transpyloric passage of gastric contents. Scand J Gastroenterol 1998; 33: 822–827.
10. Hveem, K., Jones, K. L., Chatterton, B. E. and Horowitz, M., Scintigraphic measurement of gastric emptying and ultrasonographic assessment of antral area: Relation to appetite. Gut 1996; 38: 816–821.
11. Houghton, L. A., Read, N. W., Heddle, R. *et al.*, The relationship of the motor activity of the antrum, pylorus and duodenum to gastric emptying of a solid-liquid mixed meal. Gastroenterology 1988; 94: 1285–1291.
12. Camilleri, M., Malagelada, J.-R., Brown, M. L., Becker, G. and Zinsmeister, A. R., Relationship between antral motility and gastric emptying of solids and liquids in humans. Am J Physiol 1985; 249: G580–G585.
13. Fraser, R., Horowitz, M., Maddox, A. and Dent, J., Dual effects of cisapride on gastric emptying and antropyloroduodenal motility. Am J Physiol 1993; 264: G195–G201.
14. Verhagen, M. A. M. T., Samsom, M., Kroodsma, J. M., Edmonds, A. and Smout, A. J. P. M., The new motilin agonist ABT-229 strongly stimulates postprandial antral motility in healthy volunteers. Alim Pharm Ther 1997; 11: 1077–1086.
15. Samsom, M., Akkermans, L. M. A., Jebbink, H. J. A., Van Isselt H., vanBerge-Henegouwen, G. P. and Smout, A. J. P. M., Gastrointestinal motor mechanisms in hyperglycemia-induced delayed gastric emptying in type I diabetes mellitus. Gut 1997; 40: 641–646.

16. Hausken, T., Mundt, M. and Samsom, M., Low antroduodenal pressure gradients are responsible for gastric emptying of a low-caloric liquid meal in humans. Neurogastroenterology Mot 2002; 14: 97–105.
17. Hausken, T., Ødegaard, S. and Berstad, A., Effect of respiration on early gastric liquid emptying in healthy subjects. Ultraschall in der Medizin 1999; 20:(suppl): S12.
18. Hausken, T., Ødegaard, S., Gilja, O. H. and Berstad, A., Mixing of gastric contents is evoked by heart contractions and respiration. Neurogastroenterology and Motility 1998; 10: A453.
19. Indireshkumar, K., Brasseur, J. G., Faas, H., Hebbard, G. S., Kunz, P., Dent, J., Feinle, C., Li, M., Boesiger, P., Fried, M. and Schwizer, A., Relative contributions of "pressure pump" and "peristaltic pump" to gastric emptying. Am J Physiol 2000; 278: G604–G616.
20. Castedal, M., Bjornsson, E., Gretarsdottir, J., Fjalling, M. and Abrahamsson, H., Scintigraphic assessment of interdigestive duodenogastric reflux in humans: Distinguishing between duodenal and biliary reflux material. Scand J Gastroenterol 2000; 35: 590–598.
21. Schulze-Delrieu, K., Herman, R. J., Shirazi, S. S. and Brown, B. P., Contractions move contents by changing the configuration of the isolated cat stomach. Am J Physiol 1998; 274: G359–69.
22. Malbert, C. H., Serthelon, J. P. and Dent, J., Changes in antroduodenal resistance induced by cisapride in concious dogs. Am J Physiol 1992; 263: G202–8.
23. Hausken, T., Li, X.-N., Goldman, B., Leotta, D., Ødegaard, S. and Martin, R., Quantification of gastric emptying and duodenogastric reflux stroke volumes using three-dimensional guided digital color Doppler imaging. European Journal of Ultrasound 2001; 13: 205–213.

Published with permission

GASTROENTEROLOGY 1992;102:1583–1590

# Antroduodenal Motility and Movements of Luminal Contents Studied by Duplex Sonography

TRYGVE HAUSKEN, SVEIN ØDEGAARD, KNUT MATRE, and ARNOLD BERSTAD

Section of Gastroenterology, Medical Department A, University of Bergen, Haukeland Hospital, Bergen, Norway

**The motility of the gastroduodenal wall, movement of gastric contents, and velocity curves of transpyloric flow can be synchronously visualized by duplex sonography. In eight healthy individuals, 18 ± 6 (mean ± SD) peristaltic cycles per person in response to the ingestion of 500 mL of meat soup were recorded. Coordinated antroduodenal contractions were seen in 67% of the cycles. Two types of duodenogastric reflux were observed. One type occurred in the middle of the peristaltic cycle (midcycle reflux), whereas the other followed immediately after antegrade flow at the end of the cycle (end-cycle reflux). End-cycle reflux was significantly more frequent in conjunction with coordinated (70%) than with uncoordinated (17%) antroduodenal contractions ($P < 0.005$). Thus, in the fed state, a short gush of duodenogastric reflux normally precedes the peristaltic closure of the pylorus.**

Gastric emptying is a complicated process determined by the coordinated motor activity of the stomach and the proximal small intestine. It is generally assumed that the peristaltic antral wave propels the gastric contents toward the duodenum and that the terminal antrum, pylorus, and proximal duodenum contract in sequence just in time to prevent duodenogastric reflux.[1] This concept is probably an oversimplification. Motility recordings by strain-gauge transducers combined with videofluoroscopy in dogs[2] indicate that in the fed state, contractions of the duodenal bulb often precede pyloric closure and thus do not necessarily represent a continuation of the gastric peristaltic wave. Recent human studies suggest that the duodenum plays an important role in the control of gastric emptying[3] and that reflux across the pylorus is frequent and apparently a normal phenomenon.[4]

In the present study we used duplex sonography to investigate in healthy persons the relationship between antroduodenal motility and transpyloric movements of luminal contents after ingestion of a meat soup. Small particles in the soup reflect the ultrasound beam, and using pulsed Doppler combined with real-time ultrasonography (duplex sonography) it was possible to visualize antroduodenal motility and transpyloric flow simultaneously. Antegrade and retrograde transpyloric flow was visualized using bidirectional velocity curves. Most contractions of the proximal duodenal bulb preceded closure of the pylorus (and the terminal antrum), and duodenal bulb contraction was often accompanied by a short burst of duodenogastric reflux occurring immediately before closure of the pylorus.

## Materials and Methods

### *In Vitro Measurements*

In vitro measurements of backscattered ultrasound from selected fluids were carried out using a flow rig designed for blood flow calibration.[5] Backscattered ultrasound from orange juice, vegetable juice, meat soup, and blood was measured using a standalone ultrasound pulsed Doppler meter (SD 100; Vingmed sound A/S, Horten, Norway). A 3-MHz ultrasound beam was directed toward a silicone rubber tube that received the fluid under study from a roller pump.

### *In Vivo Measurements*

*Subjects.* Fifteen healthy volunteers (10 men, 5 women; age range, 24–62 years, mean, 36 years) without gastrointestinal symptoms participated in the study.

*Apparatus.* A duplex apparatus (ACUSON 128; Mountain View, CA) with a 5-MHz linear probe was used. The scanner was used both in pulsed Doppler and color Doppler mode. For quantitative velocity measurements pulsed Doppler mode was used, and timing of events was read from the spectral curves. Color Doppler, showing antegrade and retrograde transpyloric flows in different colors, was used for rapid orientation, confirmation of posi-


0016-5085/92/$3.00

Published with permission



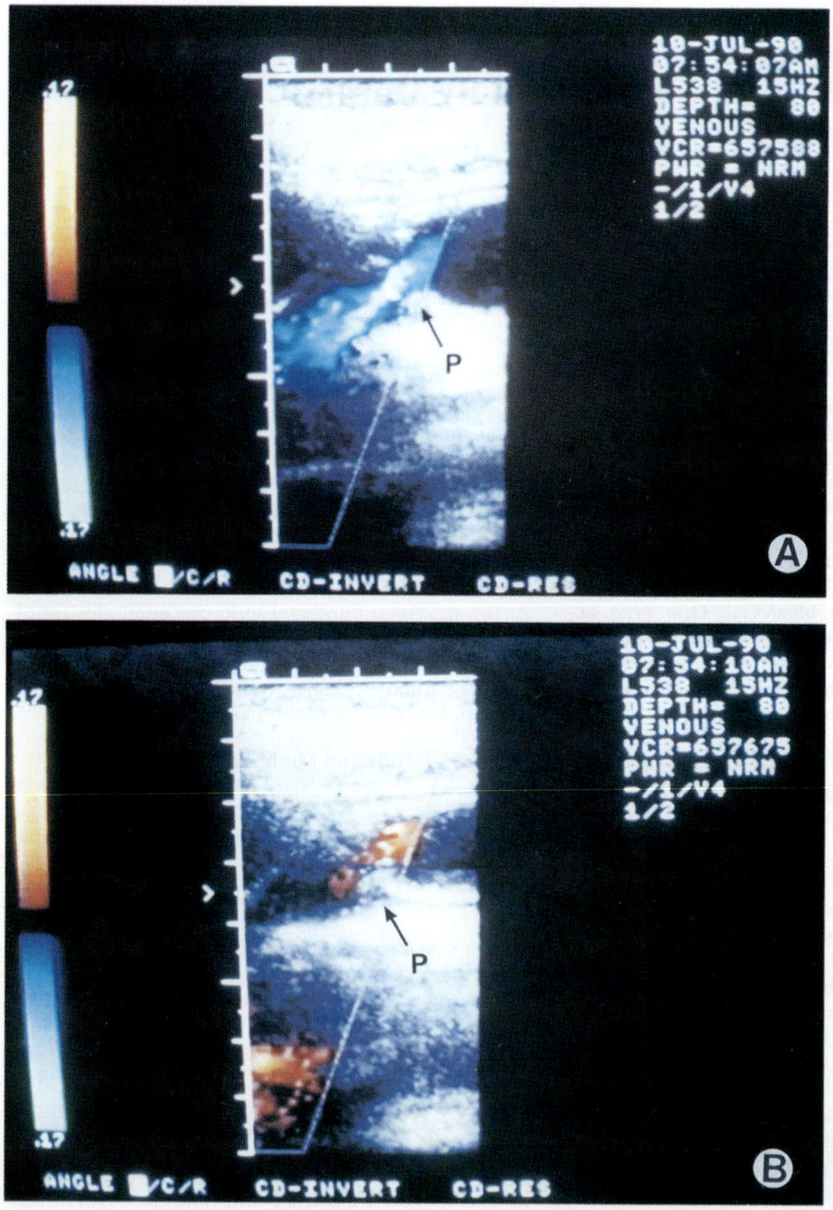


**Figure 1. Color Doppler scan with visualization of transpyloric (P, pylorus) forward flow in blue (*A*) and retrograde flow in red (*B*); *bars* = 0.5 cm.**

tion, and visual support for the pulsed Doppler recordings (Figure 1*A* and *B*).

*Test meal.* A liquid meal of commercial meat soup (Toro clear meat soup; Rieber & Søn A/S, Bergen, Norway; 2 cubes/L) was prewarmed to 37°C, and 500 mL of the soup was ingested during 4 minutes. The meal contained 1.8 g protein, 0.9 g fat, and 1.1 g carbohydrate (20 kcal). The pH varied between 5.4 and 5.7, and the osmolarity was 350 mOsm/kg $H_2O$. Fat, protein, and carbohydrate were all soluble in water. In addition, the soup contained nonsoluble seasoning (0.4 g/L). The seasoning had been ground, and the maximal size of the small nonsoluble particles was

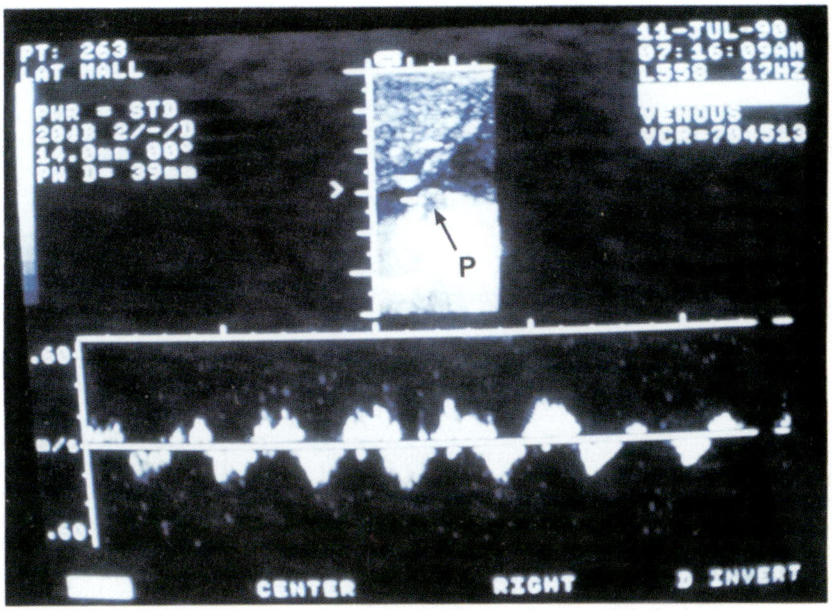


**Figure 2.** Transpyloric scan of the antropyloroduodenal segment (*upper part*) with velocity curve of pendulating pulse (aortic)–mediated movements of gastric content across the pylorus (*lower part*) (P, pylorus); the *calibration bars* on the ultrasound image mark depth in 0.5 cm. On the velocity curves, the *calibration bars* indicate meters per second and 0.2 seconds on the *y*-axis and *x*-axis, respectively.

0.2 mm. In all healthy subjects previously investigated by us (n = 80), ingestion of 500 mL of this soup induced antral contractions at a frequency of 3/min. This motility pattern is typical of the fed state.[6]

*Procedure.* The subjects were studied in the morning after an overnight fast, immediately after ingesting 500 mL of meat soup. Subjects sat upright during the procedure. The ultrasound probe was positioned at the level of the transpyloric plane with the antrum, the pylorus, and the proximal duodenum visualized simultaneously. The sample volume of the pulsed Doppler was positioned across the pylorus, and the angle between the Doppler

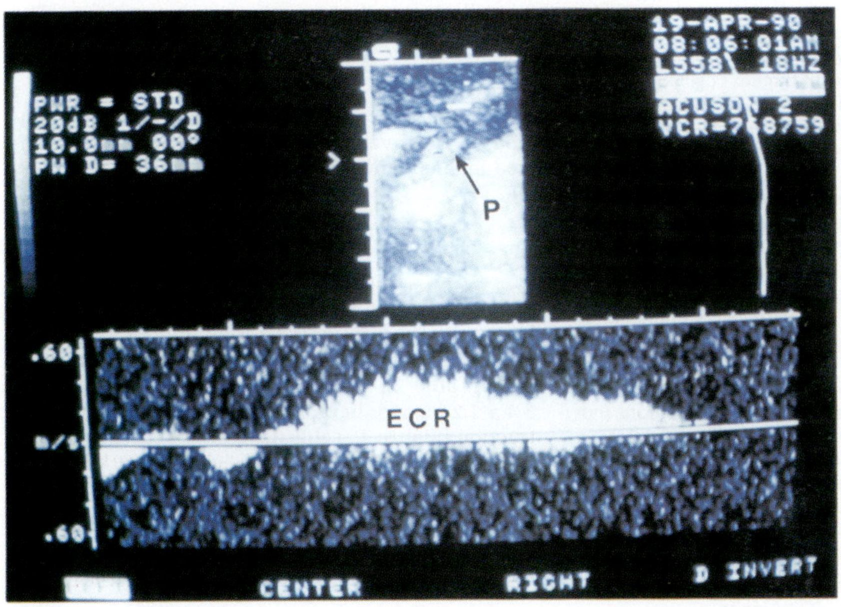


**Figure 3.** Transpyloric scan of the antropyloroduodenal segment (*upper part*) (P, pylorus) with velocity curve of ECR (*lower part*). *Calibration bars* are as in Figure 2.

Published with permission



beam and the transpyloric plane was always <60°. With this view it was possible to simultaneously record real-time images of the antroduodenal contractions, movements of the luminal contents across the pylorus, and bidirectional velocity curves. To estimate antral retropulsion, the sample volume of the pulsed Doppler was positioned in the distal antrum. The motility was recorded on video tape for 15 minutes. Time relationships and velocities were determined by replaying the video tapes several times at varying speeds and with frequent stops.

*Flow volume.* It is possible to calculate flow volume by duplex sonography. Flow volume of duodenogastric reflux was estimated according to the following formula:

$$Q = V_{mean} \cdot \pi \cdot (d/2)^2 \cdot s,$$

where $Q$ is flow volume (mL), $V_{mean}$ is mean velocity (cm/s) within the sample volume averaged over the reflux period, $d$ is the inner diameter of the pylorus, and $s$ is the duration (seconds) of reflux. $V_{mean}$ was obtained by freezing the picture and using the built-in calculation program of the apparatus. Such automatic calculation was not possible when replaying the video. Flow volume estimation was not a primary aim of this study and was therefore attempted only occasionally.

### *Definitions*

A peristaltic cycle is defined as the time between two terminal antral contractions.

Antroduodenal coordination denotes closely time-related contractions of the proximal duodenal bulb and the terminal antrum (i.e., there must be no quiescent interval between the two contractions). Coordinated antroduodenal contractions occurred during the "time window" between the end of forward flow of one peristaltic cycle and the beginning of forward flow of the next cycle.

Duodenogastric reflux is defined as a gush of retrograde flow of duodenal contents across pylorus.

Pendulating flow is defined as to-and-fro movements of luminal contents across the pylorus synchronously with the aortic pulsation. In pulsed Doppler display, this pulse-related flow was superimposed on peristaltic-related flow, unrelated to true gastric emptying and duodenogastric reflux (Figure 2).

End-cycle reflux (ECR) denotes a gush of duodenogastric reflux at the end of the peristaltic cycle immediately before closure of the terminal antrum (and the pylorus) (Figure 3).

Midcycle reflux (MCR) denotes a gush of duodenogastric reflux occurring between two antral contractions (not immediately before closure of the terminal antrum).

Terminal antral contraction (TAC) designates the moment when the pylorus appears to be maximally closed during the period between closure and opening of the terminal antrum.

Retropulsion is defined as retrograde movement of gastric contents within the antrum.

### *Data Treatment and Analysis*

Subjects in whom <10 peristaltic cycles could be accurately observed were excluded. Ten cycles was chosen as a lower limit to be sure that representatives of both coordinated and uncoordinated cycles had been accurately recorded in each person. Statistical analyses were performed using paired Student's $t$ tests (two-tailed), and $P$ values of <0.05 were considered significant. Values for measured variables are given as mean ± SD.

## **Results**

### *In Vitro Results*

The nutrient liquids examined all gave good reflection of Doppler-shifted ultrasound and are thus useful for ultrasound Doppler studies. The velocity curves registered with the ultrasound Doppler meter were similar for blood and meat soup. The maximum velocity was within ±10%, suggesting the speed of ultrasound in the two media to be comparable at room temperature. Assuming the relationship between speed and temperature to be similar for blood and meat soup, the measured velocities for movement of the meat soup would be within ±10% of the recorded velocities.

### *In Vivo Results*

Only 8 (7 men, 1 woman; age 24–62 years; mean, 34 years) of 15 subjects in which investigation was attempted could be evaluated. The reasons for excluding 7 subjects are given in Materials and Methods. The meal was ingested over 4 minutes, and recording started 153 ± 42 seconds thereafter. The mean number of peristaltic cycles recorded per person was 17.6 ± 6.2 (Table 1). The mean duration of the cycles was 19.9 ± 2.6 seconds (Table 2). Figure 4 is a schematic drawing illustrating a typical relationship between velocities of transpyloric flow and antroduodenal contractions during one peristaltic cycle.

### *Timing of Antegrade Flow*

Antegrade transpyloric flow began during the opening phase of the pylorus, 6.1 ± 1.9 seconds (Table 3) after the terminal antral contraction. The duration of the period of forward flow was 8.5 ± 1.2 seconds (Table 2), ending with the pylorus still open 3.4 ± 1.2 seconds before the next terminal antral contraction (Figure 4; Table 3).

### *End-Cycle Reflux*

In 50% of all peristaltic cycles (Table 1), the end of the forward flow period was immediately followed by ECR, the duration of which was 2.1 ± 0.5

*Table 1. Duodenogastric Reflex Related to Motility Variables*

| Subject | No. of cycles | AD/cycles[a] | ECR/cycles[b] | ECR/AD[c] | ECR/A[d] | MCR/cycles[e] |
|---|---|---|---|---|---|---|
| 1 | 10 | 0.70 | 0.40 | 0.43 | 0.33 | 0.20 |
| 2 | 29 | 0.45 | 0.48 | 1.00 | 0.06 | 0.45 |
| 3 | 22 | 0.77 | 0.59 | 0.71 | 0.20 | 0.59 |
| 4 | 15 | 0.40 | 0.27 | 0.67 | 0.00 | 0.33 |
| 5 | 13 | 0.85 | 0.54 | 0.55 | 0.50 | 0.38 |
| 6 | 22 | 0.82 | 0.68 | 0.78 | 0.25 | 0.36 |
| 7 | 15 | 0.60 | 0.53 | 0.89 | 0.00 | 0.53 |
| 8 | 15 | 0.80 | 0.47 | 0.58 | 0.00 | 0.73 |
| Mean | 17.6 | 0.67 | 0.50 | 0.70 | 0.17 | 0.45 |
| SD | 6.2 | 0.17 | 0.12 | 0.19 | 0.19 | 0.17 |

A peristaltic cycle is the period between two antral contractions.
[a]Number of coordinated antroduodenal contractions divided by number of cycles.
[b]Number of ECR episodes divided by number of cycles.
[c]Number of ECR episodes divided by number of coordinated antroduodenal contractions.
[d]Number of ERC episodes divided by number of uncoordinated antral contractions.
[e]Number of MCR episodes divided by number of cycles.

seconds (Table 2). ECR was seen more frequently in conjunction with coordinated (on average 70%) than in conjunction with uncoordinated contractions (average 17%) ($P < 0.005$) (Table 1). The beginning of ECR occurred 1.8 ± 1.1 seconds (Table 3) before the start of the concurrent duodenal bulb contraction. In most instances (84%) this duodenal bulb contraction was seen concomitantly with an M wave in the velocity profile of ECR (Figure 4).

Flow volume of ECR, calculated according to the formula given, ranged between 1.5 mL and 1.8 mL (n = 5).

### *Coordinated Contractions*

Coordinated antroduodenal contractions were seen in 67% of all cycles (Table 1). Duodenal bulb contractions began 2.3 ± 1.3 seconds (Table 3) before the TAC (Figure 4).

Shortly before the duodenal contractions, the cross-sectional area of the duodenal bulb often increased (49% of all coordinated antroduodenal contractions).

### *Uncoordinated Contractions*

In 33% of the peristaltic cycles (Table 1) the antral contractions were uncoordinated (not associated with a duodenal contraction). In these instances the interval between the end of forward flow and the TAC was shorter (1.9 ± 0.6 seconds) than in coordinated contractions accompanied by ECR (4.6 ± 1.3 seconds; $P < 0.001$).

### *Midcycle Reflux*

MCR occurred between and unrelated to the coordinated antroduodenal contractions in 45% of all cycles (Table 1 and 2). In 32% of the MCRs, a duodenal contraction was seen concomitantly.

### *Pendulating Flow*

Pendulating flow was seen during the period of forward flow at times in all persons (Figure 2).

*Table 2. Duration of Peristaltic Cycles, Forward Flow, and Duodenogastric Reflux*

| Subject | Peristaltic cycle (s) | Forward flow (s per cycle) | ECR (s per episode) | MCR (s per episode) |
|---|---|---|---|---|
| 1 | 20.7 ± 1.5 | 6.4 ± 2.9 | 1.5 ± 0.6 | 1.2 ± 0.5 |
| 2 | 17.2 ± 1.8 | 9.2 ± 2.5 | 2.4 ± 0.8 | 2.2 ± 0.6 |
| 3 | 22.9 ± 1.2 | 9.6 ± 2.5 | 3.2 ± 1.5 | 2.0 ± 0.6 |
| 4 | 17.7 ± 1.8 | 7.4 ± 1.8 | 2.1 ± 0.4 | 2.1 ± 0.7 |
| 5 | 18.3 ± 6.2 | 7.5 ± 3.6 | 1.7 ± 0.8 | 1.9 ± 0.6 |
| 6 | 19.0 ± 2.8 | 8.9 ± 2.4 | 1.9 ± 1.2 | 1.8 ± 0.8 |
| 7 | 24.6 ± 3.7 | 9.9 ± 4.3 | 1.9 ± 0.7 | 1.5 ± 0.6 |
| 8 | 18.7 ± 1.6 | 8.8 ± 2.6 | 1.8 ± 0.7 | 1.7 ± 0.5 |
| Mean | 19.9 ± 2.6 | 8.5 ± 1.2 | 2.1 ± 0.5 | 1.8 ± 0.4 |

Results represent individual means ± SD and group means ± SD.

Published with permission



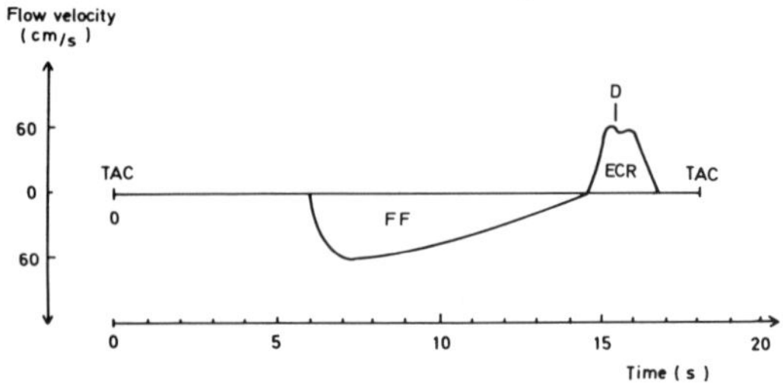


**Figure 4. Schematic drawing of typical Doppler registrations during one peristaltic cycle (the time between two TACs). The curve below the zero line represents the velocity curve of forward flow (FF). The curve above the zero line represents duodenogastric reflux. The ECR follows immediately after the period of forward flow. The duodenal bulb contraction (D) started just after the beginning of ECR, giving an M wave profile of the ECR curve. The timing and velocities are based on the mean values recorded.**

*Retropulsion*

Retropulsion was always associated with an occluding TAC. It was seen in all subjects, but the duration and the maximal velocity of retropulsion were estimated in only two subjects. The results were 2–4 seconds and 20 cm/s, respectively.

*Flow Velocities*

Considering all subjects, peak velocity was 60 cm/s for ECR and MCR, as well as for gastric emptying (forward flow).

## Discussion

By duplex sonography it was possible to relate transpyloric movements of an ingested meat soup to antropyloroduodenal contractions accurately. In most normal peristaltic cycles, the period of transpyloric forward flow was followed by a short gush of duodenogastric reflux. This physiological reflux occurred when the duodenal bulb contraction preceded the pyloric closure. Such ECR was seen in most coordinated antroduodenal contractions and might constitute a hallmark of coordinated antroduodenal peristalsis.

Several problems are associated with duplex sonography of transpyloric flow and peristalsis. Individual anatomic variations sometimes make it impossible to visualize the pyloric channel and the proximal duodenum in one single plane. In addition, the sample volume of the pulsed Doppler must be positioned precisely across the pylorus, a position that is easily lost by respiration and movements. In addition, subcutaneous fat and abdominal gas may impair the image. Slim and calm persons are most suitable for this investigation. Seven of 15 subjects had to be excluded because <10 peristaltic cycles could be investigated accurately during the observation period.

Because of the position of the ultrasound probe, only the first part of the duodenum (the duodenal bulb) was visualized. ECR and MCR were therefore observed as reflux from the duodenal bulb into the antrum. However, it appeared as if ECRs and MCRs were initiated distal to the duodenal bulb. Pendulating transpyloric flow appeared as particles moving <1 cm to and fro across the open pylorus synchronously with the aortic pulsation. This type of flow was superimposed on peristaltic related flow such as forward flow, ECR, and MCR.

A liquid meal of meat soup was used because we have experience with this soup from previous secretion and motility studies.[7–9] The soup is hypoechoic, gives a clear image of the intestinal wall, and makes transpyloric movements of the luminal contents visible. The meal induces antroduodenal motility typical of the fed state.[6,9] In the in vitro model, the soup gave ultrasound Doppler shifts similar to those of blood. The recorded velocities of ECR, MCR, and forward flow should therefore represent accurate values.

One possibility when using the Doppler technique is its ability to measure flow volume. By assuming a constant diameter of the pylorus, the flow volume of a single gush of duodenogastric reflux was estimated as 1.8 mL. However, because the pyloric diameter varies during the reflux period, accurate calculation of the transpyloric flow rate is difficult. Therefore, the estimated flow volume is an approximate value only.

Ultrasonographic studies by King et al.[4,10] using test meals containing bran particles showed that gastric emptying occurred in episodes lasting a few seconds in healthy subjects. The emptying period

*Table 3. Intervals Between TAC and Beginning of Forward Flow, End of Forward Flow and TAC, Start of ECR and Start of Duodenal Bulb Contraction, and Start of Duodenal Bulb Contraction and TAC*

| Subject | TAC–FF | FF–TAC | ECR–D | D–TAC |
|---|---|---|---|---|
| 1 | 9.7 ± 2.3 | 1.3 ± 0.8 | 0.8 ± 0.7 | 0.9 ± 0.4 |
| 2 | 4.4 ± 2.1 | 2.3 ± 1.1 | 1.8 ± 1.7 | 2.3 ± 1.2 |
| 3 | 6.0 ± 1.2 | 4.3 ± 1.5 | 2.4 ± 0.9 | 2.2 ± 1.2 |
| 4 | 6.8 ± 2.5 | 3.2 ± 1.7 | 1.8 ± 0.9 | 1.5 ± 1.8 |
| 5 | 6.0 ± 1.7 | 2.7 ± 1.9 | 0.8 ± 0.7 | 2.8 ± 1.8 |
| 6 | 4.0 ± 1.6 | 5.2 ± 2.2 | 1.2 ± 0.9 | 4.0 ± 1.6 |
| 7 | 7.3 ± 2.4 | 4.2 ± 3.3 | 1.2 ± 0.5 | 4.3 ± 2.3 |
| 8 | 4.3 ± 1.7 | 3.7 ± 2.0 | 4.1 ± 1.1 | 0.9 ± 1.4 |
| Mean | 6.1 ± 1.9 | 3.4 ± 1.2 | 1.8 ± 1.1 | 2.3 ± 1.3 |

Results represent individual means ± SD and group means ± SD. FF, forward flow; D, duodenal bulb contraction (coordinated to an antral contraction).

Published with permission



usually started immediately after relaxation of the antropyloroduodenal segment and was finished before the next peristaltic contraction approached the distal antrum. A brief episode of duodenogastric reflux occurred in about 60% of the peristaltic cycles shortly before the TAC. A similar type of reflux was shown in dogs by Malbert et al.,[11] who used operatively implanted electromagnetic flowmeter probes. Our findings are consistent with these results.

Simultaneous fluoroscopy and pressure recordings in dogs have shown that the timing of contractions of the terminal antrum, pyloric sphincter, and duodenal bulb may vary.[1,2] In the fed state, contractions of the duodenal bulb often occurred before pyloric closure.[2] This early occurrence of a duodenal bulb contraction is consistent with our observations. The duodenal bulb contraction started an average of 1.8 seconds after the beginning of the ECR, apparently increasing the velocity of the ECR (indicated by an M wave of the velocity profile).

Previous studies have suggested that the gastric emptying is regulated by a "brake" in the second part of the duodenum.[3] Our results support this theory. At the end of the period of forward flow, shortly before duodenal bulb contraction, the cross-sectional area of the duodenal bulb often increased. This dilatation of the bulb might be caused by the duodenal brake stopping the antegrade flow and filling the proximal duodenum. We suggest that the resulting duodenogastric pressure gradient causes retrograde flow, beginning as a "passive" reflux (the first part of the M wave of the velocity profile of the ECR) and continuing as an "active" reflux due to the duodenal bulb contraction (the second part of the M wave of velocity profile of the ECR). In cardiology, similar M waves of the flow velocity curves are observed for the flow across the normal mitral valve.[12] Also, it appears that the ECR initiates antral retropulsion and the early duodenal bulb contraction strengthens the pyloric closure. The purpose, if any, of the occasionally occurring MCRs is uncertain.

It is generally assumed that the peristaltic antral waves mix, grind, and retropel the gastric contents to reduce the size of the ingested particles. The period of forward flow lasted longer in peristaltic cycles with uncoordinated than in those with coordinated contractions. This finding indicates an association between lack of coordination and a weak duodenal brake. The latter may reduce the pressure gradient toward the antrum. Antral retropulsion and grinding might then be impaired. It is possible that this is the normal handling of gastric contents that do not require grinding.

Our findings suggest the existence of two phases of the peristaltic cycle: the gastric emptying phase, which begins immediately after relaxation of the antropyloric segment and ceases several seconds before the next pyloric closure, and the retropelling phase, which follows the period of forward flow, begins with an ECR, continues during the pyloric closure, and ends with the pyloric relaxation.

Possibly, both coordinated (with ECR) and uncoordinated (without ECR) antroduodenal contractions are part of the normal peristalsis. Gastric emptying and retropulsion might be regulated by the duodenal brake, the latter being regulated by the quality of the chyme delivered into the duodenum. The degree of retropulsion might thus be regulated from cycle to cycle depending on the quality of the chyme. The various time intervals recorded in the present study might therefore be valid only for the particular meat soup used and not for meals in general.

When the composition of the gastric contents is changed to contain more nutrients and solid particles, antroduodenal contractions are inhibited.[13–15] Similar motility changes are seen after intraduodenal infusion of dextrose,[16] lipids,[17,18] and acid[19] and even in response to exogenous stress.[20,21] The motility pattern after meals, therefore, depends on several factors: among the important factors is the composition of the meal. The meat soup applied in the present study stimulated the motility during the entire observation period and was therefore very suitable for studying normal antroduodenal coordination.

### *Conclusion*

Antroduodenal motility and movements of luminal contents can be visualized by duplex sonography. The peristaltic closure of the pylorus is normally preceded by a short gush of duodenogastric reflux. This physiological reflux might constitute a hallmark of coordinated antroduodenal peristalsis. Duplex sonography is a promising method for studying antroduodenal motility in humans.

## References


1. Carlson HC, Code CF, Nelson RA. Motor action of the canine gastroduodenal junction: a cineradiographic, pressure, and electric study. Am J Dig Dis 1966;11:155–172.
2. Ehrlein HJ, Hiesinger E. Computer analysis of mechanical activity of gastroduodenal junction in unanaesthized dogs. Q J Exp Physiol 1982;67:17–29.
3. Dooley CP, Valenzuela JE. Antropyloroduodenal activity during gastric emptying of liquid meals in humans. Am J Physiol 1988;255:G93–G98.
4. King PM, Adam RD, Pryde A, Mcdicken WN, Heading RC. Relationships of human antroduodenal motility and transpyloric fluid movement: non-invasive observations with real-time ultrasound. Gut 1984;25:1384–1391.
5. Segadal K, Matre K, Engedal H, Resch F, Grip A. Estimation of flow in aortocoronary grafts with a pulsed ultrasound Doppler meter. Thorac Cardiovasc Surg 1982;30:265–268.
6. Malagelada JR. Where do we stand on gastric motility? Scand J Gastroenterol 1990;25:42–51.

Published with permission




7. Frislid K, Berstad A, Guldvog I. Simulated meal test. A new method for estimation of parietal and non-parietal secretion in response to food. Scand J Gastroenterol 1985;20:115–122.
8. Berstad K, Massey H, Berstad A. Effect of enprostil on basal and meal-stimulated gastric acid and pepsin secretion, serum gastrin and gastric emptying in healthy persons. Aliment Pharmacol Ther 1988;2:65–72.
9. Hausken T, Ødegaard S, Berstad A. Antroduodenal motility studied by real-time ultrasonography. Effect of enprostil. Gastroenterology 1991;100:59–63.
10. King PM, Pryde A, Heading RC. Effect of alterations in test meal composition on episodic transpyloric fluid movement in humans. Dig Dis Sci 1988;33:12:1537–1543.
11. Malbert CH, Ruckebusch Y. Duodenal bulb control of the flow rate of digesta in the fasted and fed dog. J Physiol 1989;409:371–384.
12. Nishimura RA, Abel MD, Hatle LK, Tajik AJ. Assessment of diastolic function of the heart: Background and current applications of Doppler echocardiography. Part II. Clinical studies. Mayo Clin Proc 1989;64:181–204.
13. White CM, Poxon V, Williams JA. Effects of nutrient liquids on human gastroduodenal motor activity. Gut 1983;24:1109–1116.
14. Houghten LA, Read NW, Heddle R, Maddern GJ, Downton J, Toouli J, Dent J. Motor activity of the gastric antrum, pylorus, and duodenum under fasted conditions and after a liquid meal. Gastroenterology 1988;94:1276–1284.
15. Houghten LA, Read NW, Heddle R, Horowitz M, Collins PJ, Chatterton B, Dent J. Relationship of the motor activity of the antrum, pylorus, and duodenum to gastric emptying of a solid-liquid mixed meal. Gastroenterology 1988;94:1285–1291.
16. Heddle R, Fone D, Dent D, Horowitz M. Stimulation of pyloric motility by intraduodenal dextrose in normal subjects. Gut 1988;29:1349–1357.
17. Heddle R, Dent J, Read NW, et al. Antropyloroduodenal motor responses to intraduodenal lipid infusions in healthy volunteers. Am J Physiol 1988;254:G671–G679.
18. Heddle R, Collins PJ, Dent J, Horowitz M, Read NW, Chatterton B, Houghten LA. The motor mechanisms associated with slowing of the gastric emptying of a solid meal by an intraduodenal lipid infusion. J Gastroenterol Hepatol 1989;4:437–447.
19. Houghten LA, Kerrigan DD, Read NW. Effect of intraduodenal infusion of acid on the antropyloroduodenal motor unit in human volunteers. J Gastrointest Motil 1990;2:202–208.
20. Fone DR, Horowitz M, Maddox A, Akkermans LM, Read NW, Dent J. Gastroduodenal motility during the delayed gastric emptying induced by cold stress. Gastroenterology 1990; 98:1155–1161.
21. Hausken T, Svebakk S, Wilhelmsen I, Haug TT, Olafsen KS, Petterson E, Murison R, Berstad A. Antral hypomotility—a sensitive response to mental stress. Scand J Gastroenterol 1990;25(Suppl 176):16.


Received January 22, 1991. Accepted October 4, 1991.

Address requests for reprints to: Arnold Berstad, M.D., Section of Gastroenterology, Medical Department A, Haukeland Hospital, N-5021 Bergen, Norway.

Supported by Janssen Pharmaceutica, Belgia and Rhone Poulenc, Norway.

# CHAPTER 12

# HYDROSONOGRAPHY OF THE GASTROINTESTINAL TRACT

GEIR FOLVIK AND TRYGVE HAUSKEN

Transabdominal ultrasound is useful for evaluating parenchymal abdominal organs. It can also be applied for imaging the GI tract (1, 2). However, luminal gas often causes inadequate sonographic imaging of the stomach and intestines. Visualization of the small bowel is also prevented by a collapsed lumen. By filling the GI tract with water or another echo-poor liquid, it is possible to improve the ultrasonographic visualization considerably. In contrast to endoscopy and X-ray, ultrasound allows a detailed evaluation of the wall of the GI tract as well as the subserous fatty tissue (3).

## 1. Hydrocolonic Sonography

By conventional high-resolution transabdominal ultrasound it is possible to disclose pathologically increased wall thickness in the colon. However, it can be difficult and even impossible to obtain a detailed evaluation of the five layer colonic wall. In addition, most often, it is impossible to study the colonic lumen. After retrograde instillation of water into the colon, sonographic visualization is considerably improved. Hydrosonography of the colon (hydrocolonic sonography) has proved useful for imaging the large bowel (4–6). By retrograde instillation of water or another echo-poor liquid into the colon, it is possible to visualize the colon sonographically from the rectosigmoid junction to the caecum in almost all patients (6, 7). However, properly imaging of the colonic flexures and the transverse colon can be very difficult (8). Therefore, small lesions in these areas can be missed. In addition, excessive obesity and bowel gas prevent imaging. Rectum is difficult to evaluate with this technique because of its deep location in the pelvis behind the pubic symphysis.

### 1.1. *Method*

Bowel preparation by laxative intestinal lavage has to be performed the day or night before the examination. Before performing hydrocolonic sonography up to 1,500 ml of water has to be instilled into the colon rectally after an intravenous injection of 20 mg of scopolamine-N-butyl bromide (Buscopan®). The amount of instilled water depends on the distension of the colon. The relaxant injected is necessary for optimal distension of the colon and for suppressing the sense of urgency. Continuous transabdominal ultrasound scanning starts immediately at the time of water instillation. Imaging begins at the rectosigmoid junction and ends at the caecum. High-resolution ultrasound can be applied. Careful analysis of the wall thickness, echogenicity and stratification has to be performed. In addition, the colonic lumen, haustration and the subserous fatty tissue are studied. Total examination time is often 15–20 minutes.

## 1.2. *Sonographic measurement and interpretation*

The normal colon has a wall thickness of less than 3–4 mm. During hydrocolonic sonography, the normal colonic lumen is echo-free and 4–5 cm wide with ribbon-shaped haustra projecting into it. By high-resolution ultrasound, it is possible to identify five layers within the colonic wall. Imaging by hydrocolonic sonography demonstrates an echo-free intestinal lumen, the five individual layers of the colon wall and the connective tissue surrounding the colon (Fig. 1). Layers 1, 3 and 5 are hyperechoic, and layers 2 and 4 an- or hypoechoic. Layers 1 and 2 adjacent to the intestinal lumen represent the mucosa, layer 3 represents the submucosa, layer 4 represents the muscularis propria and layer 5 represents the serosa and the subserous fatty tissue. Wall thickness greater than 4 mm, loss of normal echostratification, intraluminal masses fixed to the colonic wall, luminal narrowing, loss of haustral pattern, or abnormalities of the surrounding connective tissue are considered pathologic. However, the interpretation of the thickness, echogenicity, and the wall layers of the gastrointestinal tract may be influenced by both the intraluminal fluid and the transducer pressure (9). Thus, this has to be taken into consideration when interpreting the ultrasound images.

Polyps and carcinomas in the colon appear sonographically as echogenic structures projecting from the intestinal wall into the lumen (Figs. 2–4). Malignant lesions present with marked thickened colonic walls, predominantly hypoechoic. Most often wall stratification cannot be identified. The intraluminal masses are often heterogeneous. In some cases

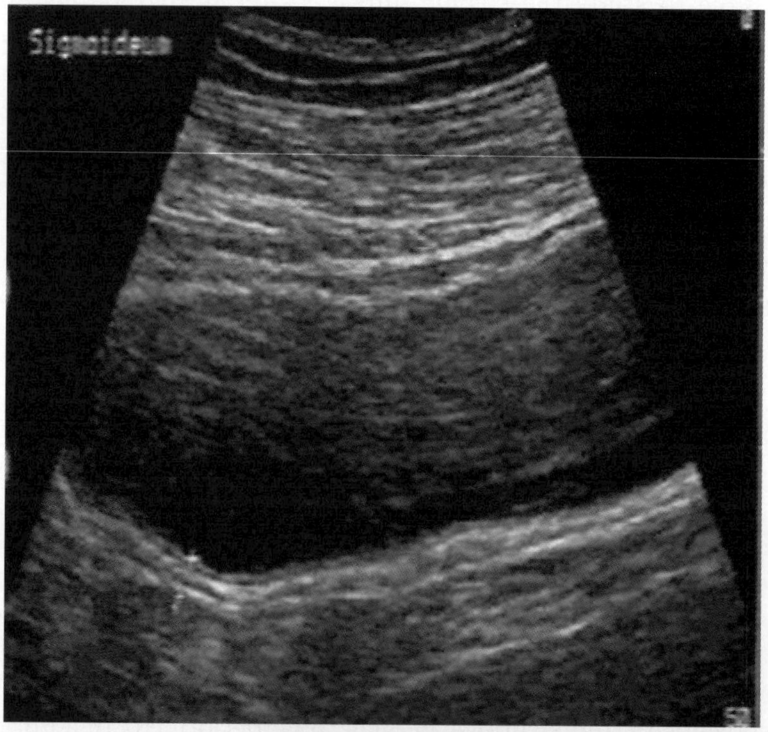


Fig. 1. Normal hydrocolonic sonography (HCS). Note that it is possible to identify the five layers of the colonic wall. Image kindly provided by R. Pedersen, M.D.

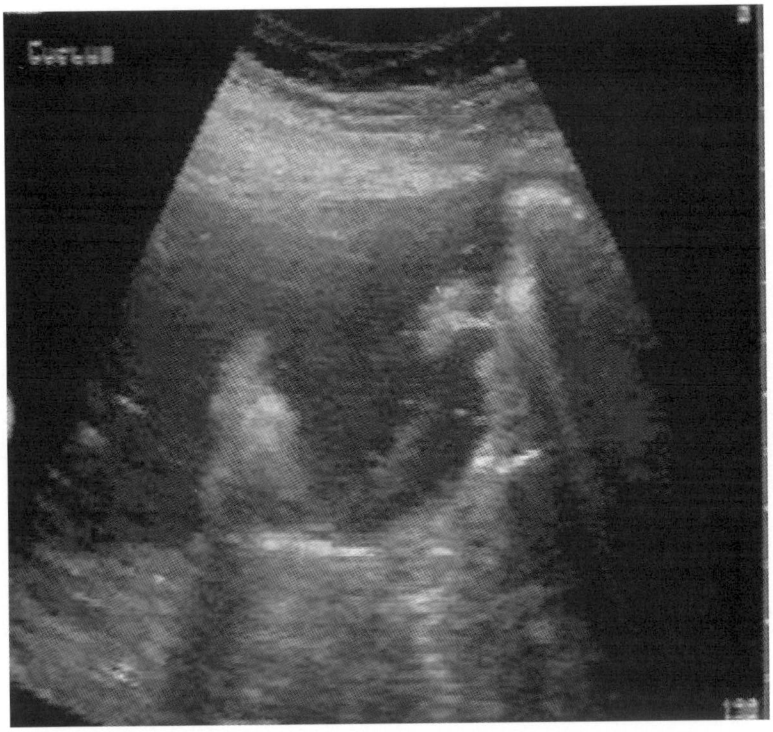

Fig. 2. Sonographic imaging of polyps in the caecum. Image kindly provided by R. Pedersen, M.D.

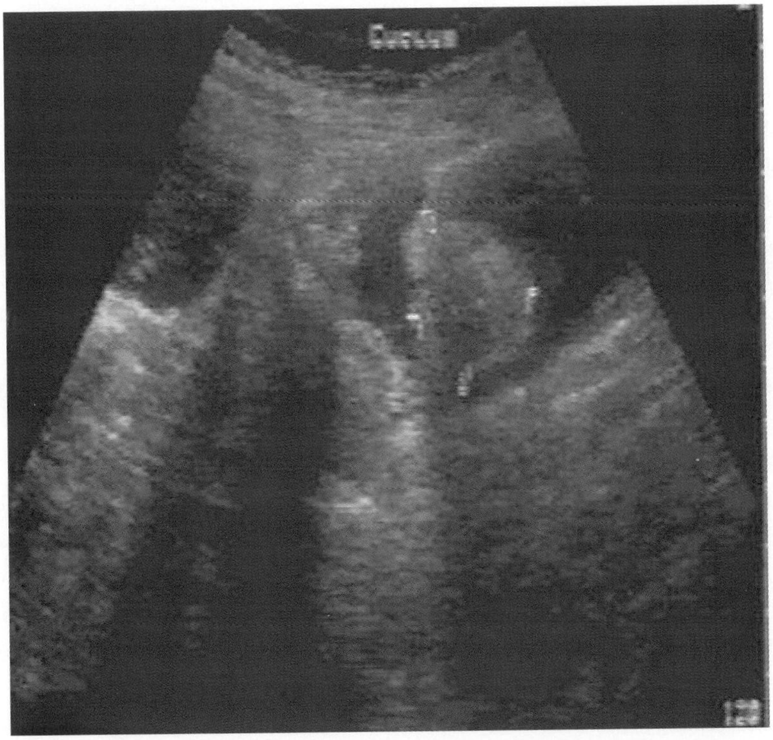

Fig. 3. Large polyp in the caecum. Image kindly provided by R. Pedersen, M.D.

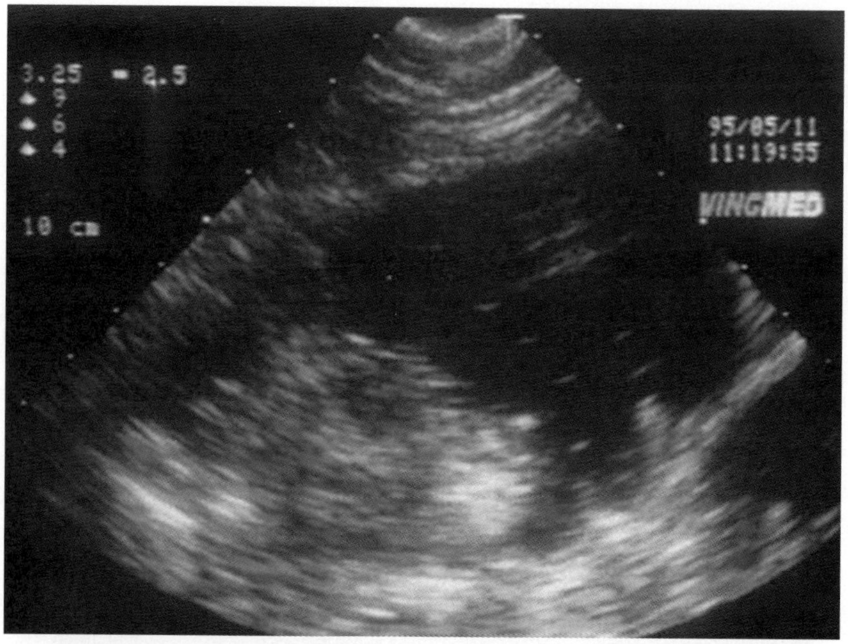


Fig. 4. Cancer coeci. Echogenicity is disturbed at the base of the tumour.

extension of the disease into the pericolonic connective tissue can be seen. However, it is not always possible to distinguish between benign and malignant lesions. Site and length of involvement can be settled. Limberg has demonstrated that polyps larger than 7 mm can be identified in 91% of cases. Smaller polyps are often missed. Sensitivity in detecting colonic carcinomas up to 97% has been demonstrated (6). Hydrocolonic sonography also permits a more precise staging of tumours in the colon. In Crohn's disease the normal stratification of the colonic wall is disturbed, and the wall appears hypoechogenic and thickened. In acute ulcerative colitis, the normal stratification of the wall is most often preserved, and the wall is only slightly thickened. Limberg has also shown that sensitivity in correctly diagnosing colonic Crohn's disease and ulcerative colitis by hydrosonography compared to colonoscopy is 96% and 91%, respectively (10). Specificity was 100 and 98%, respectively. Furthermore, by hydrocolonic sonography it was possible to differentiate Crohn's disease from ulcerative colitis in 93% of the cases.

In contrast to X-ray and endoscopy, sonography discloses both the intra- and extramural lesions of the bowel wall. The examination is easy to perform, well tolerated and safe. In cases of colonic strictures, a common complication in Crohn's disease and carcinomas, colonoscopy can be impossible. In such cases a detailed evaluation of the stenosis and the proximally located segments is made possible by hydrocolonic sonography. Site and length of involvement can be settled. Ultrasound is also applicable in cases where radiation should be avoided.

Because rectum cannot be evaluated with this technique, a large number of colorectal cancers can be missed. In addition, it may be difficult or even impossible to diagnose a small carcinoma ($T1$) and small polyps by hydrosonography. Consequently, hydrocolonic sonography cannot be used for tumour screening. However, it can be very useful for evaluating colonic lesions that already have been diagnosed by endoscopy or X-ray. Extent of the lesion, whether there is a high-grade stenosis, and whether there is infiltration, can be settled.

Hydrocolonic sonography is an accurate method for evaluating and diagnosing inflammatory bowel disease. Limberg has shown that hydrocolonic sonography is superior to conventional transabdominal (10) ultrasound in correctly diagnosing Crohn's disease and ulcerative colitis. Therefore, it can be recommended for follow-up of patients with inflammatory bowel disease. Because minor mucosal abnormalities can be impossible to detect with this technique, the extent of inflammation can be underestimated as compared with colonoscopy. Hydrosonography helps in the judgement whether or not a treatment is successful. Hydrocolonic sonography may reduce the numbers of colonoscopies and barium enema studies in the follow-up of patients with inflammatory bowel disease.

## 2. Hydrosonography of the Small Intestine

High-resolution transabdominal ultrasound can be applied for imaging the small bowel. However, sensitivity in diagnosing pathology in the small intestine is not good enough to allow the use of this technique as a screening method. Marked thickened intestinal wall is often necessary for disclosing pathology in the small bowel by conventional transabdominal ultrasound. Most often, the lumen of the small intestine is collapsed which prevents imaging. Intraluminal changes can be missed. In addition, it is difficult or even impossible to dissociate one loop from another. Often luminal gas results in inadequate ultrasonographic imaging as well. By filling the stomach or the colon with water or another echo-poor liquid, it is possible to improve the visualization of these organs considerably. A similar technique can be applied for studying the small intestine (11). Isotonic non-absorbable polyethylene glycol (PEG) solution is infused through a nasojejunal tube which is placed at the duodenojejunal flexure either by endoscopy or by fluoroscopy. Transabdominal ultrasound is performed during infusion of the PEG solution. In contrast to conventional transabdominal ultrasound, it is possible to study the lumen of the small bowel. In addition, it is possible to obtain a detailed evaluation of the wall of the small intestine.

### 2.1. *Method*

On the day before the examination the patient takes either natrium picosulphate (Pico-Salax®) or bisacodyl (Toilax®) orally for bowel evacuation. The next day a nasojejunal tube is placed at the duodenojejunal fleksure by gastroscopy or fluoroscopy. Ultrasound is performed with the patient in the supine position while 2 l of the PEG solution (Laxabon®) is infused in 40 minutes through the tube. The isotonic polyethylene glycol solution is non-absorbable and non-fermentable. It remains unchanged in the intestinal lumen and thereby distending the intestinal loops. Both curved-array and linear transducers can be applied. It is possible to use high-resolution ultrasound (12 MHz), but for optimal imaging of both the anterior and the posterior wall of the intestine 5–9 MHz-transducers are often recommended. First, the duodenum and the proximal part of the jejunum are examined. As the small intestine is expanded by the PEG solution, the rest of the jejunum and the ileum are studied. Ultrasound is performed to disclose extra-intestinal pathology and for evaluating the subserous fatty tissue. A careful analysis of the wall thickness, echogenicity and stratification is performed. Intraluminal changes are looked for as well. Total examination time is most often 40–45 minutes.

An Italian group (Pallotta *et al.*) has applied a similar technique for imaging the small bowel (small intestine contrast ultrasonography or SICUS) (12–14). Instead of introducing a nasojejunal tube, the PEG solution is given orally in a smaller volume (about 200–800 ml) after an overnight fast, still with excellent imaging of the small intestine. The patient drinks increasing amounts of the PEG solution until the anechoic fluid reaches the jejunum. Pallota et al claim that the entire small bowel can be visualized sequentially by this method, which allows sonographic reconstruction of the entire small intestine. The ultrasound examination starts with the patient in the upright position. When the PEG solution reaches the jejunum, the patient is examined in the supine position. Examination time is about 45 minutes.

## 2.2. *Sonographic measurement and interpretation*

Wall thickness of the normal small bowel should not exceed 3 mm. By high-resolution ultrasound echo stratification is preserved. Peristalsis is present. Normal motor activity of the small intestine can be defined as the presence of intermittent variation of the intestinal luminal diameter, variation in the wall thickness and/or change in the loop axial plane. In addition, no luminal narrowing (stenosis) or distended loops (prestenotic dilatation) can be seen. Luminal diameter more than 30 mm is considered pathologic. Valvulae conniventes are easily identified. By conventional transabdominal ultrasound it can be

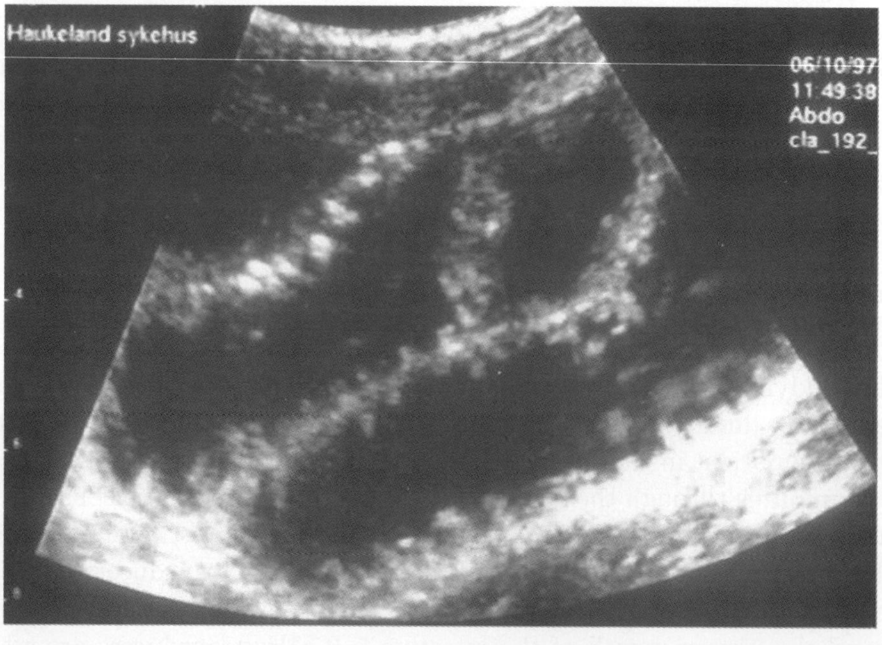


Fig. 5. Normal segments of the small intestine visualized by hydrosonography. Note that it is easy to identify the valvulae conniventes.

difficult to distinguish the small intestine from the colon which is easy with this method. Hydrosonography gives an excellent imaging of the small bowel (Fig. 5), especially the distal part of the ileum and the ileocaecal valve (Fig. 6). Most often the colon is clearly visualized as well. Sensitivity in detecting pathology in the small bowel filled with PEG solution range from 64–100%. Specificity range from 97–100% (11, 14, 15). Pallotta, *et al.* found a diagnostic sensitivity of SICUS to detect small bowel lesions of 100% compared to conventional barium study of the small bowel. However, it is surprising that the diagnostic sensitivity in detecting small intestine pathology is so much higher than found in study by Folvik *et al.* Perhaps this in part could be explained by the fact that the patients in the study by Folvik, *et al.* had low disease activity, and thereby minimal changes in the small bowel. A study by Cittadini, *et al.* could support this explanation (15). They found a diagnostic sensitivity of 72%. False negative findings were mainly due to minimal lesions in the small bowel. In contrast to conventional barium contrast examination of the small bowel a direct measure of the wall thickness of the small bowel is possible (Figs. 7–9). Luminal flow across the ileocoecal valve can be studied by performing Doppler ultrasound examination (Fig. 10). Doppler ultrasound can also be applied for studying the circulation within the wall of the small intestine by measuring the Resistance Index. In addition, extraintestinal complications in inflammatory bowel disease can be seen. As opposed to enteroclysis and CT-studies the method is safe in cases where radiation should be avoided, such as in pregnancy. It is especially useful for evaluating the ascendic part of the colon, the caecum and the distal part of the ileum in cases where endoscopy is unsuccessful. In contrast to CT-studies and MRI (magnetic resonance imaging) it is inexpensive. In addition, ultrasound is harmless and applicable for repeated bedside examinations. It is

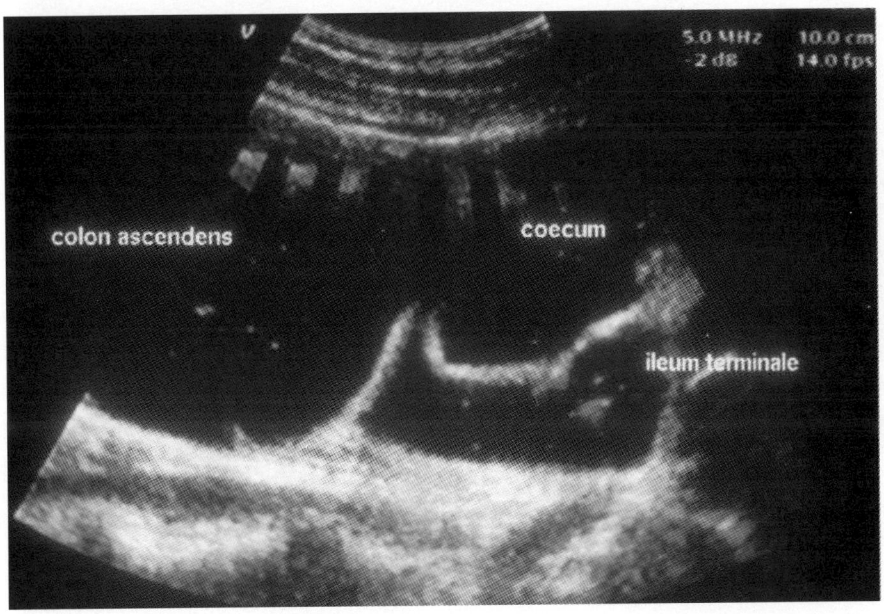


Fig. 6. Normal hydrosonography of the terminal part of the ileum and the ileocaecal valve. The caecum and the ascending part of the colon are clearly visualized, which is necessary for identification of the ileocaecal valve.

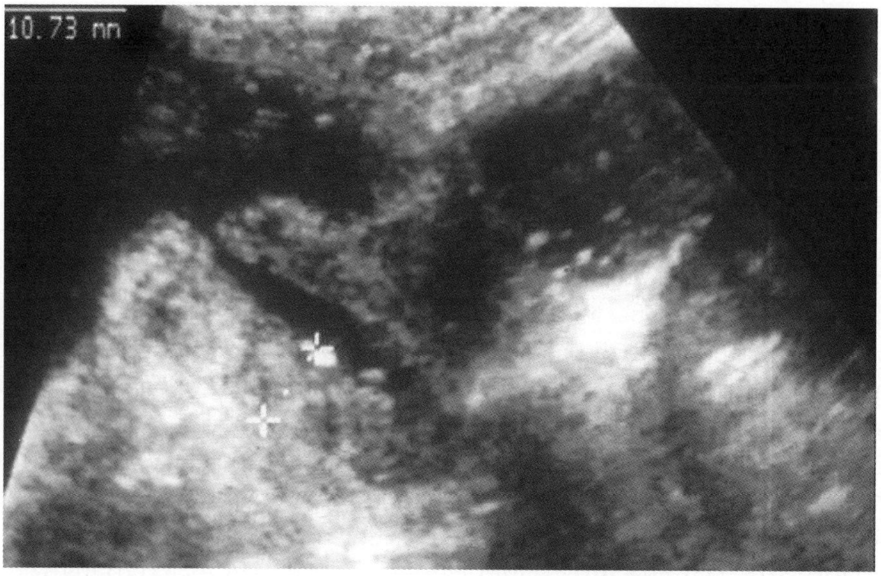


Fig. 7. The hydrosonographic appearance of Crohn disease in the distal part of the ileum. Wall thickness is about 10.7 mm without clear echo-stratification. The wall is slightly hypoechoic as compared with the surrounding tissue.

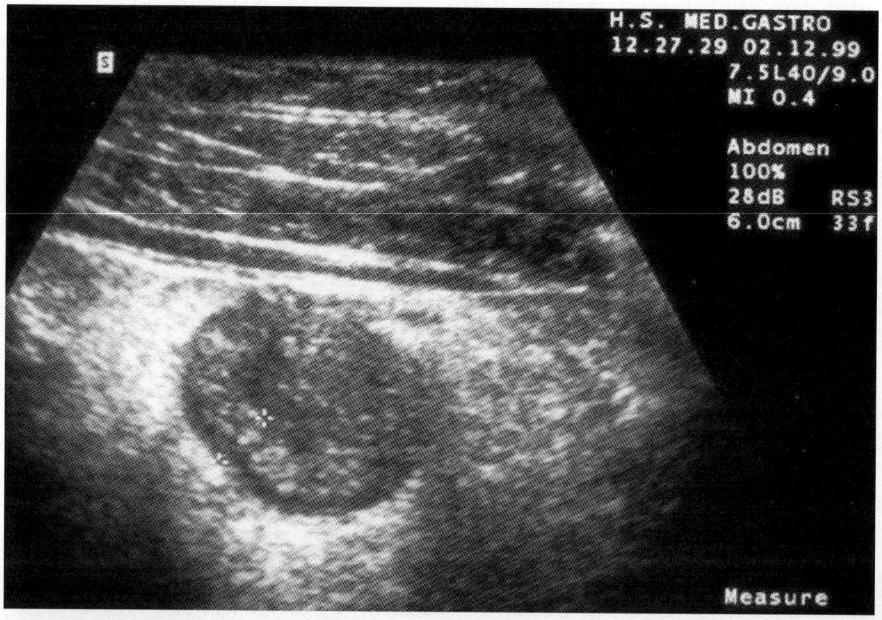


Fig. 8. Cross-sectional image of the small intestine which shows marked thickened wall of the small bowel without clear echo-stratification associated with Crohn's disease.

therefore especially suitable in the follow up of patients with inflammatory bowel disease where repeated examinations often are necessary.

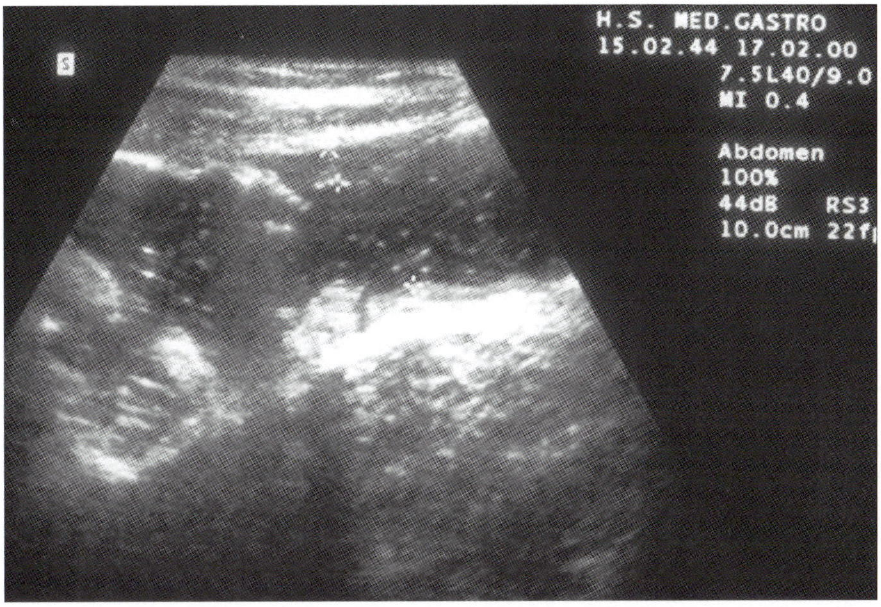


Fig. 9. Hydrosonographic imaging of a thickened ileo-colic anastomosis.

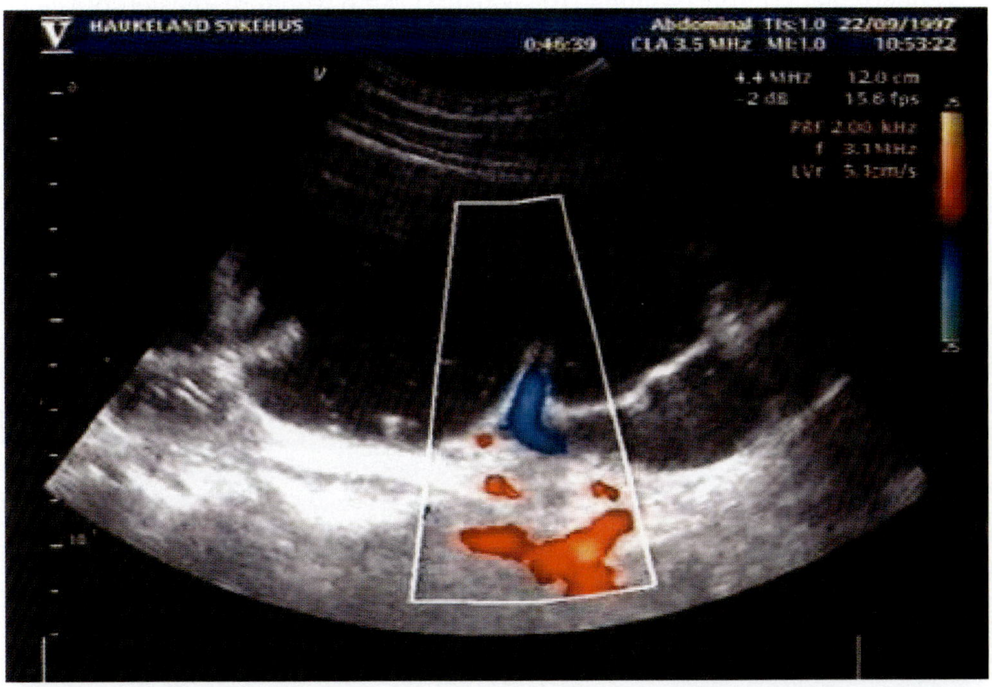


Fig. 10. Color Doppler examination of the ileocaecal valve showing an episode of reflux.

## 3. Hydrosonography of the Upper Gastrointestinal Tract

Oesophagus, stomach and the proximal part of the duodenum are best evaluated by upper endoscopy. X-ray and fluoroscopy are valuable in case of intramural pathology and for studying motility disorders. It can be impossible to disclose linitis plastica by gastroscopy unless for advanced disease. After filling the stomach with water or another echo-poor liquid it is possible to study the wall of the upper GI tract by using transabdominal ultrasound, and thereby raise the suspicion of intramural carcinomas (16). This technique allows evaluation of the pancreas as well, regarding its significance for tumour detection, staging and assessment of tumour resectability. In addition, hydrosonography is useful for studying GI-motility (17).

### 3.1. *Method*

The hydrosonography examination consists of two parts. First, a conventional transabdominal ultrasound to examine the parenchymal organs is performed. Second, the patient is asked to drink 500–1000 ml of regular tap water. Initially, the patient is examined sitting in an upright position. The water collects at the lowest part of the stomach, which allows examination of the pyloric portion and the distal part of the stomach. Subsequently, the patient is examined in supine, left lateral and finally in right lateral position to shift the water within the stomach. This manoeuvre ensures that every part of the gastric wall is distended by fluid. By combining water distension with intravenous administration of 20–40 mg of scopolamine-N-butyl bromide (Buscopan®), an optimal distension of the stomach and the duodenum is achieved. A detailed evaluation of the stomach, the duodenal wall, the pancreas and the peripancreatic vessel relevant for resectability is possible. Destruction

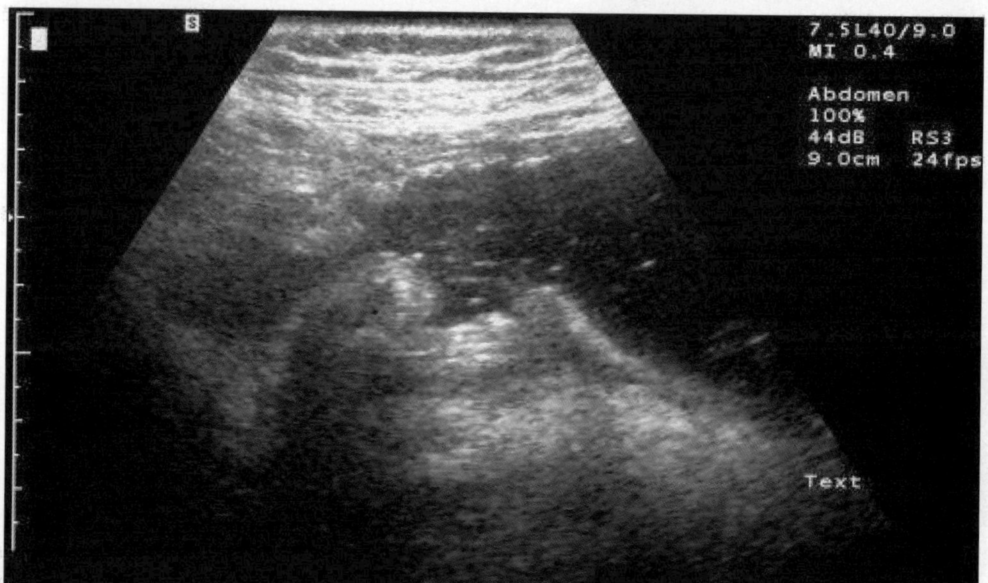


Fig. 11. Hydrosonographic image of a benign prepyloric ulcer on the posterior wall.

and thickening of the bowel wall are well visualized, but not specific for malignant disease (Figs. 11, 12).

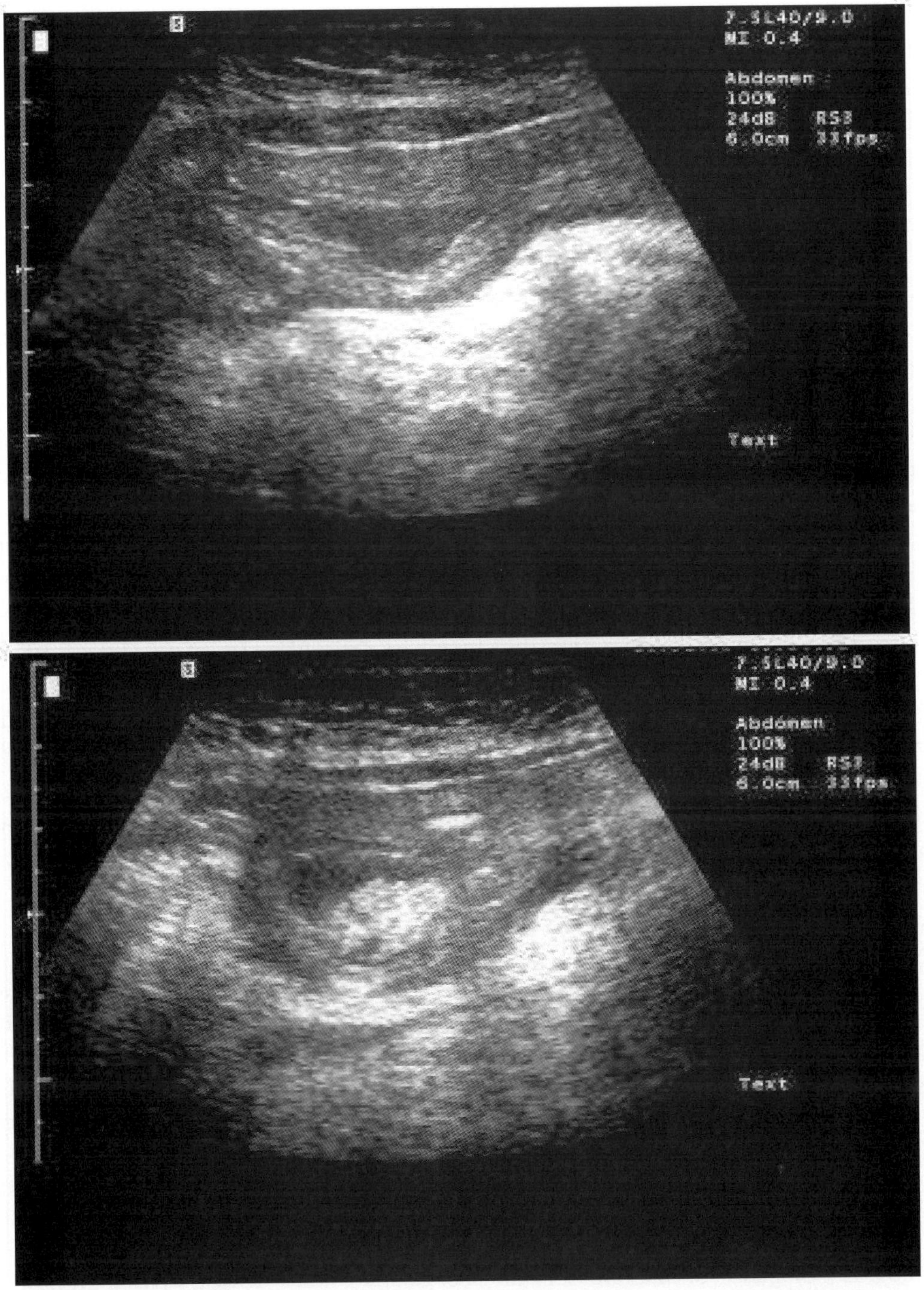


Fig. 12. Hydrosonographic image of gastric cancer (linitis plastica). Upper panel longitudinal section. Lower panel transverse section.

### 3.2. *Clinical interpretation*

Using this technique, Dux, *et al.* examined 25 patients with suspected gastric cancer for TNM staging (18). All patients were operated on, and tumours removed when possible. Hydrosonography was correlated to histopathologic staging. Hydrosonography correctly localised tumours in 75% of patients. T-accuracy was low for gastric cancers (41%). N-staging was accurate in 68% of all cases and highly specific (100%). All patients without cancer were correctly diagnosed by hydrosonography. Gastric ulcer was visualized as homogenous thickening of the gastric wall without destruction of its layers that was correctly classified as inflammation. The major challenge with this method is imaging of tumours located in the cardia region.

Hydrosonography has been compared with endosonography for localization and staging of gastric cancer (19). Fifty-two consecutive patients were examined. The T-staging accuracy of endosonography and hydrosonography were 74% and 46%, respectively. Carcinomas of the cardia were often misclassified by both methods. The N-staging accuracy of endosonography was 86% and 61% for hydrosonography. Based on these results, transabdominal hydrosonography cannot replace endosonography in gastric cancer staging. However, when performed in conjunction with conventional ultrasound, hydrosonography provides useful information about local tumour stage, especially in cases of advanced and stenotic tumours, and can be used in the follow-up after treatment.

In an open prospective study 51 patients with suspected pancreatic cancer were examined using hydrosonography together with scopolamine-N-butyl bromide (Buscopan®) intravenously in order to achieve an optimal distension of the stomach (20). A complete identification of the pancreas was possible in all 51 patients. In 48 of the 51 patients, a positive diagnosis for tumour or other pathology was made. A total of 16 pancreatic cancers and 5 benign tumours were diagnosed. Among other findings, pseudocysts and pancreatitis were diagnosed. For tumour detection, sensitivity was 82% and specificity 100%. For correct assessment of tumour resectability, sensitivity was 86% and specificity 100%.

In conclusion, hydrosonography is a supplement to routine transabdominal ultrasonography and improves imaging accuracy.

## References

1. Solvig, J., Ekberg, O., Lindgren, S., Floren, C.-H. and Nilsson, P., Ultrasound examination of the small bowel: Comparison with enteroclysis in patients with Crohn disease. Abdom Imaging 1995; 20: 323–6.
2. Hollerbach, S., Geissler, A., Schiegl, H., Kullmann, F., Lock, G., Schmidt, J., Schlegel, J., Schoelmerich, J. and Andus, T., The accuracy of abdominal ultrasound in the assessment of bowel disorders. Scand J Gastroenterol 1998; 33: 1201–8.
3. Kimmey, M. B., Martin, R. W., Haggitt, R. C., Wang, K. Y., Franklin, D. W. and Silverstein, F. E., Histologic correlates of gastrointestinal ultrasound images. Gastroenterology 1989; 96: 433–41
4. Limberg, B., Diagnosis of inflammatory and neoplastic colonic disease by sonography. J. Clin. Gastroenterol. 1987; 9: 607–611.
5. Limberg, B., Diagnosis of acute ulcerative colitis and colonic Crohn's disease by colonic sonography. J Clin Ultrasound 1989; 17: 25–31.

6. Limberg, B., Diagnosis of colonic tumours and chronic inflammatory colonic diseases by hydrocolonic sonography. Radiologe 1993 Jul; 33(7): 407–11.
7. Dixit, R., Chowdhury, V. and Kumar, N., Hydrocolonic sonography in the evaluation of colonic lesions. Abdom Imaging 1999; 24: 497–505.
8. Dux, M., Hydrocolonic sonography. Invited commentary. Abdom Imaging 1999; 24: 506–7.
9. Ødegaard, S., Kimmey, M. B., Martin, R. W., Yee, H. C., Cheung, H. S. and Silverstein, F. E., The effects of applied pressure on thickness, layers and echogenicity of gastrointestinal wall ultrasound images. Gastrointest Endosc 1992; 38: 351–6.
10. Limberg, B. and Osswald, B., Diagnosis and differential diagnosis of ulcerative colitis and Crohn's disease by hydrocolonic sonography. Am J Gastroenterol 1994 Jul; 89(7): 1051–7.
11. Folvik, G., Bjerke-Larssen, T., Ødegaard, S., Hausken, T., Gilja, O. H. and Berstad, A., Hydrosonography of the small intestine: Comparison with radiologic barium study. Scan J Gastroenterol 1999; 12: 1247–52.
12. Pallotta, N., Baccini, F. and Corazziari, E., Contrast ultrasonography of the normal small bowel. Ultrasound Med Biol 1999 Nov; 25(9): 1335–40.
13. Pallotta, N., Baccini, F. and Corazziari, E., Small intestine contrast ultrasonography. J Ultrasound Med 2000; 19: 21–6.
14. Pallotta, N., Baccini, F. and Corazziari, E., Small intestine contrast ultrasonography (SICUS) in the diagnosis of small intestine lesions. Ultrasound Med Biol 2001 Mar; 27(3): 335–41.
15. Cittadini, G., Giasotto, V., Garlaschi, G., de Cicco, E., Gallo, A. and Cittadin, G., Transabdominal ultrasonography of the small bowel after oral administration of a non-absorbable anechoic solution: Comparison with barium enteroclysis. Clin Radiol 2001 Mar; 56(3): 225–30.
16. Gilja, O. H., Olafsson, S., Folvik, G., Hausken, T., Ødegaard, S. and Berstad, A., The ultrasound meal accommodation test. A case study. Motility 1999; 46: 14–5.
17. Gilja, O. H., Hausken, T., Wilhelmsen, I. and A. Berstad, Impaired accommodation of the proximal stomach to a meal in functional dyspepsia. Dig Dis Sci 1996; 41(4): 689–96.
18. Dux, M., Roeren, T., Kuntz, C., Richter, G. M. and Kaufmann, G. W., TNM staging of gastrointestinal tumours by hydrosonography: Results of a histopathologically controlled study in 60 patients. Abdom Imaging 1997; 22: 24–34.
19. Kuntz, C., Dux, M., Pollock, A., Buhl, K. and Herfarth, C., Hydrosonographie als Alternative oder Ergaenzung zur Endosonographie beim Magencarcinom. Chirurg 1998; 69: 438–42.
20. Simon, C., Hoffmann, V., Richter, G. M., Seelos, R., Senninger, N. and Kauffmann, G. W., Hydrosonography of the pancreas. Preliminary results of a pilot study. Radiologe 1996; 36: 389–96.

Published with permission

ORIGINAL ARTICLE

# Hydrosonography of the Small Intestine: Comparison with Radiologic Barium Study

**G. Folvik, T. Bjerke-Larssen, S. Ødegaard, T. Hausken, O. H. Gilja & A. Berstad**
Division of Gastroenterology, Depts. of Medicine and Radiology, Haukeland University Hospital, University of Bergen, Bergen, Norway

Folvik G, Bjerke-Larssen T, Ødegaard S, Hausken T, Gilja OH, Berstad A. Hydrosonography of the small intestine: comparison with radiologic barium study. Scand J Gastroenterol 1999;34:1247–1252.

**Background:** Transabdominal ultrasonography of the small intestine is hampered by luminal gas. We have developed a new sonographic method (hydrosonography) that largely eliminates the gas problem and have compared this method with radiologic barium study. **Methods:** Fifty-six patients admitted for X-ray examination of the small bowel because of abdominal pain, diarrhoea, weight loss and/or known inflammatory bowel disease were examined. To remove luminal gas before performing transabdominal ultrasonography, 2 l of polyethylene glycol solution was inserted through a nasojejunal tube by means of a peristaltic pump. Wall thickness, peristalsis, luminal narrowing, prestenotic dilatation, and extraintestinal complications were recorded. **Results:** On ultrasonography we were able to visualize the terminal part of the ileum in 98% of the patients. Perfect agreement between hydrosonography and barium studies was seen in 50 of 55 patients. However, 44 patients had normal findings on both examinations. The sensitivity and specificity of hydrosonography were 64% and 100%, respectively. The positive predictive value was 100%. For X-ray examination sensitivity and specificity were 91% and 100%, respectively. Four patients with minor mucosal abnormalities or pathologic findings in the upper part of the small intestine accounted for the relatively low overall sensitivity found for hydrosonography compared with roentgenography. However, important extraintestinal complications were disclosed by ultrasound. **Conclusions:** Hydrosonography of the small bowel is a new, convenient, and reliable method for examining the lower part of the small intestine. However, it cannot replace barium studies in patients with mucosal abnormalities, especially in the upper part of the small bowel.

**Key words:** Barium studies; extraintestinal complications; hydrosonography; inflammatory bowel disease; small bowel; ultrasonography

*Geir Folvik, M.D., Division of Gastroenterology, Dept. of Medicine, Haukeland University Hospital, NO-5021 Bergen, Norway (fax: +47 55972950)*

Transabdominal ultrasonography has proved very useful for evaluation of parenchymal abdominal organs. It can also be applied for imaging of the gastrointestinal tract (1–6). However, luminal gas often causes inadequate ultrasonographic imaging of the intestines. By filling the stomach (7–11) and the colon (12–18) with water or another echo-poor liquid, it is possible to improve the ultrasonographic visualization of these organs considerably. We have applied a similar technique for studying the wall and the lumen of the small intestine by using a nasojejunal tube for infusion of liquid. The indwelling intestinal tube is also used for infusion of barium contrast for conventional radiologic examination (enteroclysis).

As luminal liquid we have chosen an isotonic non-absorbable polyethylene glycol (PEG) solution, which otherwise is used for bowel cleansing before barium enema, colonoscopy, and colon surgery. The solution can also be used for whole-gut irrigation to quantify gastrointestinal loss of protein (19), blood (20), immunoglobulins, and other inflammatory products (21).

The aim of this study was to examine the applicability, performance, and diagnostic yield of this novel method for ultrasonographic examination (hydrosonography) of the small intestine and to compare the results of this method with those of conventional barium contrast examination.

## Materials and Methods

### *Subjects*

Between January 1997 and November 1998, 56 consecutive patients admitted for barium study of the small intestine were included in the study. There were 31 males and 25 females, and their age ranged between 16 and 69 years (mean, 36.0 years). The indications for examination were abdominal pain, diarrhoea and/or weight loss, or known inflammatory bowel disease. The final diagnosis is based on conventional

Published with permission



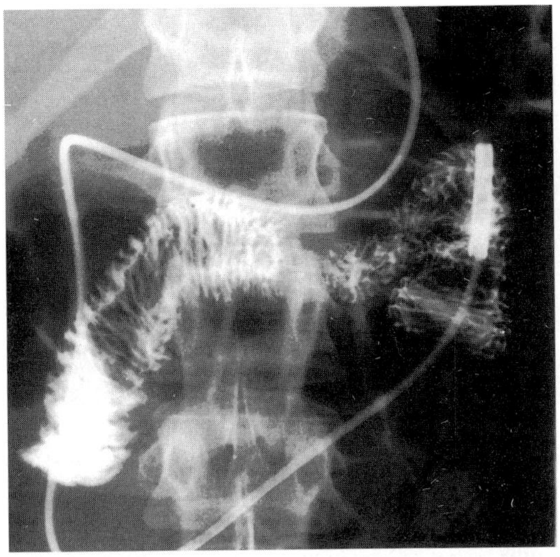

Fig. 1. Nasojejunal tube in correct position with its tip at the duodenojejunal flexure after endoscopic placement.

clinical criteria, including patient history, clinical examination, Crohn simple index, laboratory tests, endoscopy, and biopsy. Five patients had ulcerative colitis and 17 had Crohn disease. Simple index in patients with Crohn disease ranged between 0 and 18 (median, 6). Five patients had been operated on by ileocaecal resection because of Crohn disease.

*Procedure*

On the day before the examinations the patients took either natrium picosulphate (Pico-Salax®) or bisacodyl (Toilax®) orally for bowel evacuation. The next day they were intubated in the following manner: a nasojejunal feeding tube (9 French) for endoscopic placement (Stayput, Compat Biosystems speciality feeding tubes, Sandoz Nutrition Corp., USA) equipped with a guide wire and a black thread at the tip of the tube was passed transnasally into the stomach (22). A gastroscope was introduced into the stomach, and by means of a biopsy forceps the tube was pulled into the descending part of the duodenum. The biopsy forceps and the tube were pushed down as far as possible before the biopsy forceps was opened and withdrawn together with the scope while the tube was hold in position by the guide wire. The tube should be lying with an appropriate bend along the greater curvature of the stomach. Finally, the patient was moved to his/her right side, the guide wire withdrawn, and the tube fastened to the nose at approximately 90 cm. The intubation procedure took about 10 min.

*Ultrasonography*

Ultrasonography was performed with the patient in the supine position while 2 l of the PEG solution (MW 3350, Laxabon®, Tika, Sweden) was infused in 40 min through the tube by means of a peristaltic pump (Watson Marlow, 505S/RL, Falmouth, Cornwall, England). Ultrasonography was performed bedside by an experienced investigator (G. Folvik), using a 3.3- to 5.0-MHz curved-array probe (System Five, VingMed Sound, Horten, Norway). First, ultrasonography of the parenchymal abdominal organs was performed. Second, ultrasonography was performed to disclose extra-intestinal complications such as infiltrates (solid masses/conglomerate tumours), abscesses, fistulas, or hydronephrosis. Third, the duodenum and the upper part of the small bowel were examined, starting with a 3.3-MHz transducer. To visualize the duodenum, an inter-/sub-costal scan at the right side was performed. Then, we examined the proximal part of the jejunum by moving the transducer to the midline, orientating the scanhead transversally. As the small intestine was expanded by the PEG solution, the frequency of the transducer head could be increased to 5.0 MHz, thereby obtaining more detailed imaging. The jejunum and the ileum were examined by moving the 5.0-MHz probe to the left side of the abdomen before successively moving the transducer head on the skin surface to the right side. In case of severe obesity, lower transducer frequency was used. Subsequently, a right longitudinal scan in the medioclavicular line was performed to identify the ascending part of the colon and, in some cases, the caecum and the ileocaecal valve. The terminal part of the ileum and the ileocaecal valve were studied particularly carefully. An oblique scanning plane just cranial to the iliac crest was often used to obtain clear imaging of the caecum, the ileocaecal valve, and the terminal part of the ileum. In a few cases a better access to the ileocaecal valve could be obtained by tilting the transducer head down behind the iliac crest. The caecum and the ascending part of the colon were evaluated in longitudinal and cross sections.

The criteria for a normal ultrasonography of the small bowel were as follows: wall thickness less than 3 mm and

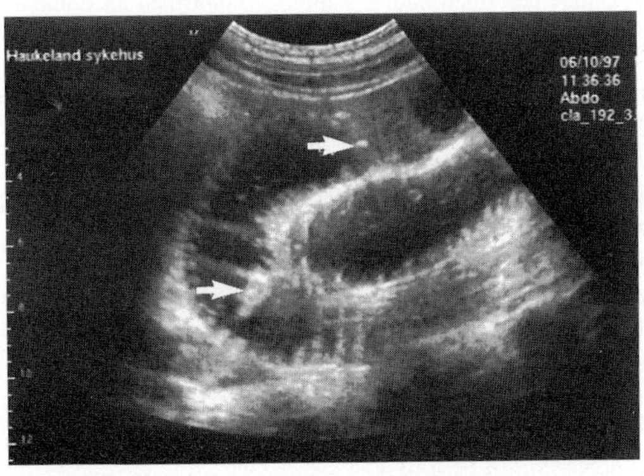


Fig. 2. Normal segments of the small intestine visualized by hydrosonography. Luminal contents are indicated by arrows. Note that it is easy to identify the valvulae conniventes.

Published with permission



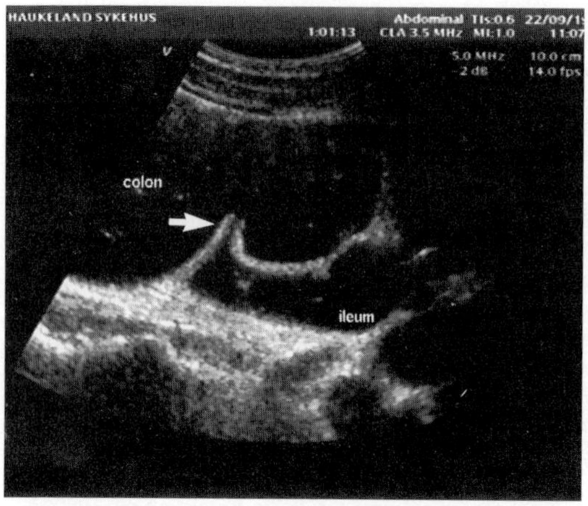


Fig. 3. Normal hydrosonograpy of the terminal part of the ileum and the ileocaecal valve (arrow). The caecum and the ascending part of the colon are clearly visualized, which is necessary for identification of the ileocaecal valve. Wall thickness is less than 3 mm.

preservation of the echo stratification, the presence of peristalsis, and no luminal narrowing (stenosis) or distended loops (prestenotic dilatation). The criteria for pathologic dilatation of the small bowel were defined as a luminal diameter more than 30 mm (23–25). Segments of the small intestine without peristalsis during the examination were assumed to be abnormal. The results of the subsequent small-bowel barium examination were unknown to the investigator.

*Barium study*

With the nasojejunal tube in place, the patient was sent to the Dept. of Radiology, where the correct position of the tube, preferably with the tip in the proximal jejunum, first was checked by fluoroscopy (Fig. 1). By means of the intubation technique described above, radiology confirmed an optimal position of the nasojejunal tube in 52 of 55 consecutive intubations. One patient was not sent to X-ray examination. The barium study followed conventional procedures supervised by an experienced radiologist (T. Bjerke-Larssen).

In an ex vivo study we checked whether the above-mentioned 9 French tube could be perfused with the barium sulphate contrast (Mixobar Colon® suspension, 1 g/ml, Astra, Sweden) in a concentration and at the rate usually used for small-bowel examination. The 640 ml of barium contrast was diluted with 960 ml water and poured into a plastic bag from which the suspension was infused by means of a peristaltic pump delivering 23 ml/min. The tube performed perfectly at this and considerably higher speeds of infusion.

*Ethics*

Informed consent was given by the patients before examination.

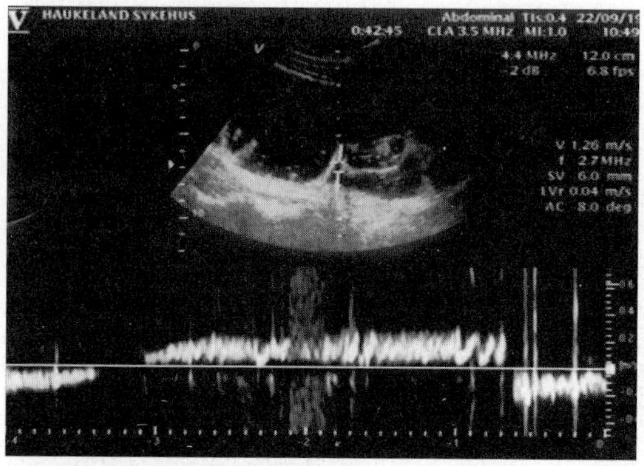


Fig. 4. Doppler examination of the ileocaecal valve, showing both emptying and episodes of reflux. Velocity profiles across the ileocaecal valve are indicated.

## Results

By ultrasonography it was possible to visualize the terminal/neo-terminal (ileocolic anastomosis) part of the ileum in 54 of 55 cases (98%). One patient was not sent to X-ray examination because of symptoms of subileus. It was possible to clearly identify the ileocaecal valve in 43 of 50 cases (86%). Five patients had been operated on with ileocaecal resection. Fig. 2 shows the sonographic appearance of a normal jejunum. The valvulae conniventes were usually clearly visualized within the lumen of the small intestine. Fig. 3 shows the hydrosonographic appearance of the terminal part of the ileum and the ileocaecal valve in a patient without disease. With X-ray examination the terminal/neo-terminal part of ileum was visualized in 51 of 55 cases (93%). In four cases there were problems with either the contrast-filling or the free-projecting of the terminal/neo-terminal part of the ileum. Visualization of the ileocaecal valve was not noted. In most cases the hydrosonographic examination took about 40 min, the time necessary for infusion of 2 l of the PEG solution. However, in some patients we had to prolong the sonographic examination to obtain adequate imaging of the ileocaecal valve and the terminal part of the ileum. In one patient the time needed to reach this goal was almost 90 min. In contrast, in some cases it was possible to visualize the distal part of the ileum and the ileocaecal valve in about 20 min. Moreover, it was possible to study the luminal flow across the ileocaecal valve. The result of a typical Doppler examination of the ileocaecal valve is shown in Fig. 4. Even though the small bowel was filled with PEG solution from above, multiple reflux episodes across the ileocaecal valve were seen, also in patients without disease.

Perfect agreement between the ultrasonographic and the barium contrast examinations was found in 50 of 55 patients. However, as many as 44 patients had normal findings on both examinations. Among these there were four patients with

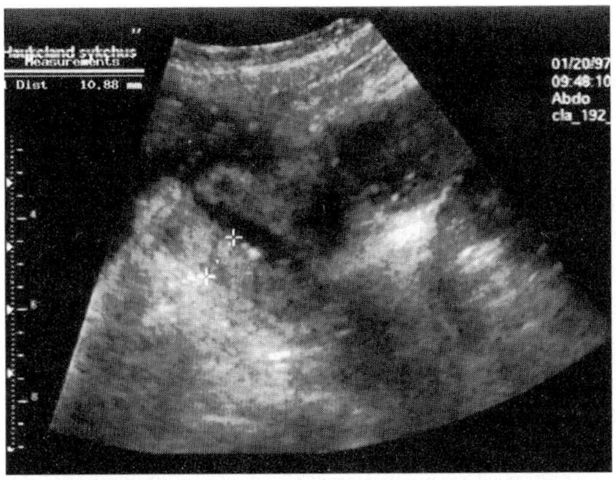


Fig. 5. The hydrosonographic appearance of Crohn disease in the distal part of the ileum. Wall thickness is about 10.9 mm, without clear echo stratification. The wall is slightly hypoechoic as compared with the surrounding tissue. The ileocaecal valve appeared 'stiff', and peristaltic motility was clearly reduced in this area.

Crohn colitis, two patients with Crohn disease in remission, and five patients with ulcerative colitis. One patient (Patient 56) was not sent to barium contrast examination because of symptoms of subileus. In this case the luminal diameter of the small bowel was 35 mm (prestenotic dilatation), and increased motility was seen. This patient started vomiting during the ultrasonographic examination, which disclosed an inflammatory infiltrate in the right lower quadrant in addition to hydronephrosis on the right side. Subsequent surgery confirmed the sonographic findings. Among the 11 patients with Crohn disease in the small intestine, 1 had fistulas, 1 had abnormal findings in the proximal part of the small bowel, 1 had Crohn lesions at several locations, and the other 8 patients had pathologic changes in the terminal/neo-terminal part of the ileum. In four patients radiologic examination showed minor mucosal abnormalities not seen by ultrasound—that is, minor contrast irregularities that could not be classified further. In three of these patients the abnormalities were located in the distal part of the ileum, whereas in the fourth patient they were seen in the duodenum and the proximal part of the jejunum. The radiologic examination also showed widened space between adjacent intestines as an indirect sign of increased wall thickness. In this case transabdominal bowel sonography was disturbed by luminal gas. Agreement between hydrosonography and radiology was seen in the patient with fistulas and in the patient who had Crohn lesions at several locations.

One patient who had undergone surgery had a pathologic ileocaecal valve with luminal narrowing when examined by ultrasound but had a normal barium contrast study. The patient had been operated on with a new method (ileocolic nipple valve anastomosis (26)) for the purpose of reconstructing the ileocaecal valve. Whether the luminal narrowing was caused by the operation or inflammatory changes is not known. However, the valve was not normal as compared with the sonographic findings in patients not being operated on.

Beside loss of stratification, wall thickening appeared to be either hypoechoic or to have mixed echogenicity (luminal liquid was anechoic). Fig. 5 shows the sonographic appearance of Crohn disease in the terminal part of the ileum. However, even in normal subjects it was difficult to distinguish the different wall layers by means of the 3.3- to 5.0-MHz transducers. Moreover, in case of more pronounced wall thickening, motility appeared to be reduced.

When clinical criteria were used for the final diagnosis, the overall sensitivity and specificity of hydrosonography of the small intestine were 64% and 100%, respectively. The positive predictive value was 100%, and the sensitivity and specificity of classical barium studies of the small bowel were 91% and 100%, respectively. The positive predictive value was 100% (Table I).

## Discussion

Hydrosonography of the small intestine gave excellent visualization of the distal part of the ileum and the ileocaecal valve. The caecum, the ascending part of the colon, and, in most cases, the rest of the colon were clearly visualized as well. By conventional transabdominal ultrasonography it is often difficult to distinguish the small intestine from the colon, which turned out to be easy with the present hydrosonographic method. In one case ultrasonography did not detect pathologic changes in the duodenum and the jejunum. This result suggests that it may be difficult to detect abnormalities in the upper part of the small intestine unless there are more pronounced pathologic changes. In a prospective study by Hollerbach et al. (27), similar difficulties in detecting abnormalities in this part of the small bowel were experienced. Probably, inadequate filling of the duodenum and the proximal part of the jejunum is responsible for some of the difficulties experienced in detecting abnormalities in

Table I. Hydrosonography of the small bowel using polyethylene glycol solution and conventional radiologic barium examination of the small bowel

| | Disease status | | |
|---|---|---|---|
| | Disease | Normal | Total |
| Ultrasound* | | | |
| Abnormal | 7 | 0 | 7 |
| Normal | 4 | 44 | 48 |
| Total | 11 | 44 | 55 |
| Radiology† | | | |
| Abnormal | 10 | 0 | 10 |
| Normal | 1 | 44 | 45 |
| Total | 11 | 44 | 55 |

* Sensitivity, 64%; specificity, 100%; and positive predictive value, 100%. Negative predictive value, 92%.

† Sensitivity, 91%; specificity, 100%; and positive predictive value, 100%. Negative predictive value, 98%.

Published with permission



these regions. Given an 'optimal' tube position, inadequate filling of this part of the gastrointestinal tract is not surprising. Luminal gas within the stomach may also contribute to inadequate imaging of the proximal part of the intestine. In some cases it was also difficult to visualize the ileocaecal valve because of a deeply located caecum behind the iliac bone, obesity, or overlying luminal gas. However, such problems were partly eliminated by turning the patient in an upright position when performing ultrasonography. In the case of a deeply located caecum similar difficulties were experienced with barium studies.

Perfect agreement between hydrosonography and barium contrast examination was seen unless the patient had abnormalities in the upper part of the small bowel or mucosal abnormalities solely. These difficulties account for the relatively low sensitivity found on ultrasonography as compared with barium studies. In such cases barium examination seems superior to ultrasonography. Barium studies of the small bowel give an indirect measure of the wall thickness of the small intestine by means of the increased distance between adjacent segments of the small bowel. In contrast, ultrasonography gives a direct measure of the wall thickness, which in some cases may be advantageous. By using high-resolution imaging (5 MHz or higher) it is possible to study the different wall layers of the small intestine more precisely and, possibly, to detect mucosal abnormalities. Even in patients without disease, it was difficult to distinguish the different wall layers by using 3.3- to 5.0-MHz transducers. By using high-frequency ultrasound or high-resolution imaging several studies have shown that it is possible to identify five different wall layers, which correlates well with histology (28–31). However, the interpretation of the thickness, echogenicity, and wall layers of the gastrointestinal tract may be influenced by both the intraluminal fluid and the transducer pressure (32). Thus, this has to be taken into consideration when interpreting the ultrasound images. Moreover, studies have shown that Doppler ultrasound is useful in evaluating patients with active Crohn disease, and by using colour Doppler it is possible to study the circulation within the wall of the intestine (33).

As shown in this and in several other studies (34, 35), ultrasonography is an excellent method for diagnosing extra-intestinal complications of Crohn disease. Hydrosonography may also give a useful evaluation of the patient's response to a volume challenge—that is, if the patient experiences abdominal pain, nausea, and vomiting due to luminal narrowing.

Several authors have reported high sensitivity and specificity for detection of inflammatory bowel disease with transabdominal bowel sonography (2, 4–6). However, in a prospective study by Hollerbach et al. (27) ultrasonography was found to have a rather low sensitivity for detecting abnormalities of the small bowel. Even with an experienced investigator the sensitivity of the present hydrosonographic technique was too low for the method to be used for general screening of inflammatory disorders of the small intestine. Probably, the low sensitivity experienced in our study could partly be explained by the fact that most patients had less severe disease than in studies showing high sensitivity in detecting inflammatory bowel disease.

Ultrasonography of the small bowel has to our knowledge not previously been performed in the manner we present here. We used PEG solution as luminal liquid. Even though we did not use pure water, we have named the present ultrasonographic method hydrosonography. The reason is that the solution is anechoic, like water. Simultaneously, the PEG solution serves as a bowel-cleansing solution. Our intubation procedure is quick and safe and gives an optimal tube position in most cases. For conventional radiologic examination of the small bowel a thicker (14 French) jejunal tube for barium contrast infusion is pushed in position with a guide wire and fluoroscopy. The main drawback of this method is, beside exposure to radiation, the inconvenience of the intubation procedure, which is unpleasant to the patient and takes an unpredictable amont of time.

We conclude that this new ultrasonographic method is convenient and reliable for examining the lower part of the small intestine. It provides additional information as compared with conventional barium studies. However, at the present time it cannot replace the barium contrast examination in patients with disease in the upper part of the small bowel and in patients with minor mucosal abnormalities. The method may be of particular value in patients in whom radiation should be avoided, such as in pregnancy, and when the endoscopic examination of the caecum and the distal part of ileum are unsuccessful. Further studies are indicated to explore the potential of improvement using novel state-of-the-art high-frequency transducers.

## Acknowledgement

This study was supported by Innovest Strategic Research Program (Haukeland University Hospital and University of Bergen), Bergen, Norway.

## References

1. Puylaert JBCM, Groeneveld D, van der Werf SDJ. The role of US in the primary diagnosis of ileocecal Crohn's disease. Eur J Gastroenterol Hepatol 1996;8:A36–7.
2. Solvig J, Ekberg O, Lindgren S, Floren C-H, Nilsson P. Ultrasound examination of the small bowel: comparison with enteroclysis in patients with Crohn disease. Abdom Imaging 1995;20:323–6.
3. Khaw KT, Yeoman LJ, Saverymuttu SH, Cook MG, Joseph AE. Ultrasonic patterns in inflammatory bowel disease. Clin Radiol 1991;43:171–5.
4. Bozkurt T, Richter F, Lux G. Ultrasonography as a primary diagnostic tool in patients with inflammatory disease and tumors of the small intestine and large bowel. J Clin Ultrasound 1994;22:85–91.
5. Hata J, Haruma K, Suenaga K, Yoshihara M, Yamamoto G, Tanaka S, et al. Ultrasonographic assessment of inflammatory bowel disease. Am J Gastroenterol 1992;87:443–7.
6. Hata J, Haruma K, Yamanaka H, Fujimura J, Yoshihara M,

Published with permission



Shimamoto T. Ultrasonographic evaluation of the bowel wall in inflammatory bowel disease: comparison of in vivo and in vitro studies. Abdom Imaging 1994;19:395–9.

7. Hausken T, Ødegaard S, Berstad A. Antroduodenal motility and movements of luminal content studied by Duplex-sonography. Gastroenterology 1992;102:1583–90.
8. Gilja OH, Hausken T, Ødegaard S, Berstad A. Monitoring postprandial size of the proximal stomach by ultrasonography. J Ultrasound Med 1995;14:81–9.
9. Gilja OH, Hausken T, Wilhelmsen I, Berstad A. Impaired accommodation of the proximal stomach to a meal in functional dyspepsia. Dig Dis Sci 1996;41:689–96.
10. Gilja OH, Detmer PR, Jong JM, Leotta DF, Li X-N, Beach KW, et al. Intragastric distribution and gastric emptying assessed by three-dimensional ultrasonography. Gastroenterology 1997;113: 38–49.
11. Hausken T, Gilja OH, Undeland KA, Berstad A. Timing of postprandial dyspeptic symptoms and transpyloric passage of gastric content. Scand J Gastroenterol 1998;33:822–7.
12. Limberg B. Differentialdiagnose akut entzündlicher Dickdarmerkrankungen durch Kolonsonographie. Dtsch Med Wochenschr 1987;112:382–5.
13. Limberg B. Diagnosis of inflammatory and neoplastic colonic disease by sonography. J Clin Gastroenterol 1987;9:607–11.
14. Limberg B. Sonographic features of colonic Crohn's disease: comparison of in vivo and in vitro studies. J Clin Ultrasound 1990;18:161–6.
15. Limberg B. Diagnosis of acute ulcerative colitis and colonic Crohn's disease by colonic sonography. J Clin Ultrasound 1989;17:25–31.
16. Hirooka N, Ohno T, Misonoo M, Kobayashi C, Musha H, Mori H, et al. Sono-enterocolonography by oral water administration. J Clin Ultrasound 1989;17:585–9.
17. Chui DW, Gooding GAW, McQuaid KR, Griswold V, Grendell JH. Hydrocolonic ultrasonography in the detection of colonic polyps and tumors. N Engl J Med 1994;331:1685–8.
18. Limberg B, Osswald B. Diagnosis and differential diagnosis of ulcerative colitis and Crohn's disease by hydrocolonic sonography. Am J Gastroenterol 1994;89:1051–7.
19. Acciuffi S, Ghosh S, Ferguson A. Strengths and limitations of the Crohn's disease acitivity index, revealed by an objective gut lavage test of gastrointestinal protein loss. Aliment Pharmacol Ther 1996;10:321–6.
20. Ferguson A, Brydon WG, Brian H, Williams A, Mackie MJ. Use of whole gut perfusion to investigate gastrointestinal blood loss in patients with iron deficiency anaemia. Gut 1996;38:120–4.
21. Ferguson A, Sallam J, O'Mahony S, Poxton I. Clinical investigation of gut immune responses. Adv Drug Deliv Rev 1995;18:53–71.
22. Brenna E, Kleveland PM, Waldum HL. En enkel metode for endoskopisk plassering av nasojejunal ernæringssonde. Tidsskr Nor Laegeforen 1997;117:2054–5.
23. Ha HK, Kim JS, Lee HJ. Differentiation of simple and strangulated small bowel obstructions. Usefulness of known CT criteria. Radiology 1997;204:507–12.
24. Czechowski J. Conventional radiography and ultrasonography in the diagnosis of small bowel obstruction and strangulation. Acta Radiol 1996;37:186–9.
25. Maglinte DD, Reyes BL, Harmon BH, Kelvin FM, Turner WW Jr, Hage JE, et al. Reliability and role of plain film radiography and CT in the diagnosis of small bowel obstruction. Am J Roentgenol 1996;167:1451–5.
26. Smedh K, Olaison G, Sjødahl R. Ileocolic nipple valve anastomosis for preventing recurrence of surgically treated Crohn's disease: long-term follow-up of six cases. Dis Colon Rectum 1990;33:987–90.
27. Hollerbach S, Geissler A, Schiegl H, Kullmann F, Lock G, Schmidt J, et al. The accuracy of abdominal ultrasound in the assessment of bowel disorders. Scand J Gastroenterol 1998;33: 1201–8.
28. Ødegaard S, Kimmey MB. Location of the muscularis mucosae on high frequency gastrointestinal ultrasound images. Eur J Ultrasound 1994;1:39–50.
29. Kimmey MB, Martin RW, Hagitt RC, Wang KY, Franklin DW, Silverstein FE. Histologic correlates of gastrointestinal endoscopic ultrasound images. Gastroenterology 1989;96:433–41.
30. Cheung AHS, Wang KY, Jiranek KC, Ødegaard S, Kimmey MB, Silverstein FE. Evaluation of a 20 MHz ultrasound system for diagnosis of porcine small bowel ischemia. Invest Radiol 1992;27:217–23.
31. Kimmey MB, Wang KY, Hagitt RC, Mack LA, Silverstein FE. Diagnosis of inflammatory bowel disease with ultrasound. An in vitro study. Invest Radiol 1990;25:1085–90.
32. Ødegaard S, Kimmey MB, Martin RW, Yee HC, Cheung HS, Silverstein FE. The effects of applied pressure on the thickness, layers and echogenicity of gastrointestinal wall ultrasound images. Gastrointest Endosc 1992;38:351–6.
33. Silvan Delgado M, Juanco Pedregal C, Parra Blanco JA, Barreda Gonzalez M. Usefulness of Doppler ultrasound in the evaluation of patients with active Crohn's disease. Rev Esp Enferm Dig 1997;89:677–84.
34. Gasche C, Moser G, Turetschek K, Schober E, Moeschl P, Oberhuber G. Transabdominal bowel sonography for the detection of intestinal complications in Crohn's disease. Gut 1999;44:112–7.
35. Futagami Y, Hata J, Haruma K, Fujimura J, Tani H, Okamoto E, et al. Evaluation of intestinal complications of Crohn's disease by transabdominal ultrasonography. Dig Dis Week Abstract Book; 1997.

Received 23 March 1999
Accepted 9 August 1999

## CHAPTER 13

# APPLICATIONS OF ACOUSTIC MICROSCOPY IN GASTROENTEROLOGY

THOMAS ANDERSEN AND HANS GREGERSEN

## 1. Acoustic Microscopy

The advancement of science follows a trend of wishing to know greater details in physiology, medicine and tissue engineering. The traditionally biomechanical testing models are often based on macroscopically *en bloc* testing i.e. testing of the tissue as one. For this purpose, one has to assume that the tissue consist of a single layer. However, most visceral organs are multi-layered. Obtaining data from several layers is a step towards the next level in the hierarchy of structure of living tissue. Data relating microscale biomechanical properties and gastrointestinal histology are sparse and needed. High frequency acoustics is an obvious candidate for obtaining new knowledge on the distribution of biomechanical properties of gastrointestinal tissue since it is based on mechanical (elastic) waves and has micrometer resolution.

The idea of using sound for studying material structure and properties was first suggested by the Soviet scientist, Sokolov in 1949 (1). The technologies for generating such acoustic waves and processing the signals were not available before the 1970's (2). From then on, the development was carried out at Stanford (USA) and Oxford (UK) universities with the aim of material and component analyses including measurement of elastic properties and inspection for surface and sub-surface flaws (fatigue cracks, dents, voids, delamination and disbonding) as well as establishing in biological analysis (3).

Japan has since then refined the scanning acousic microscopy (SAM) technique by increasing the resolution and implementing methods for quantification of acoustic properties.

Utilization of low-energy high-frequency acoustic waves in SAM makes it an interesting technique in biomedicine. It not only ensures that the object of study remains intact and can be studied repeatedly, but living objects like human cells in culture can be studied microscopically during drug manipulation and movement (4). Also, it allows for examination of even small cell inclusions and tissue constituents since the resolution of SAM normally is in the micrometer range. The best resolution recorded with SAM is 15 nm at 15,300 MHz (5).

The most important property of SAM is its ability to measure acoustic properties with great accuracy. This property resides in the simple fact that acoustic waves are mechanical by nature and thus interacts mechanically with the object under investigation: the object responds to insonification from the microscope lens in accordance with its own mechanical properties (below), and it is that response which is recorded by the microscope.

The remaining of this chapter will show how advanced high-frequency ultrasound and the elementary theory of elasticity can be used to quantify gastrointestinal properties on a micrometer scale. The next sections deals with the reflection mode of SAM microscope. After that, the Scanning Laser Acoustic Microscope (SLAM) is described.

### 1.1. *Microscope design*

Different types of SAM microscopes exist. The most common one is the reflection mode SAM microscope (Figs. 1 and 2). This microscope has a single acoustic lens that is used both for transmitting and receiving reflected acoustic waves. The SAM microscope utilizes ultrasound signal frequencies ($f$) in the GHz-range to image and measure elastic properties in sectioned tissue specimens. In both imaging and measurement mode, operation is by way of a focused acoustic lens with a piezo-electric transducer transmitting and receiving ultrasound to and from the tissue. The microscope may be operated at $f = 500$ MHz using a lens with a numerical aperture (NA) of 0.98 to yield a resolution ($w$) of approximately 1.5 $\mu$m (6):

$$w = \frac{0.51\, C_{\text{couplant}}}{NAf} \tag{1}$$

where $C_{\text{couplant}}$ is the ultrasound propagation speed in the acoustic couplant. $C_{\text{couplant}}$ is 1,482 ms$^{-1}$ at 20°C, according to Kino (7).

Using a 2,000 MHz lens with NA of 0.6 and assuming $v$ is 1520 ms$^{-1}$ (35°C) in the object of study (reasonable for soft biological tissue), the resolution will be approximately 0.65 $\mu$m. It is the combined action of high signal frequency and the focusing sapphire rod that provides the high spatial resolution. A lens is shown in Fig. 3. It has a transducer made

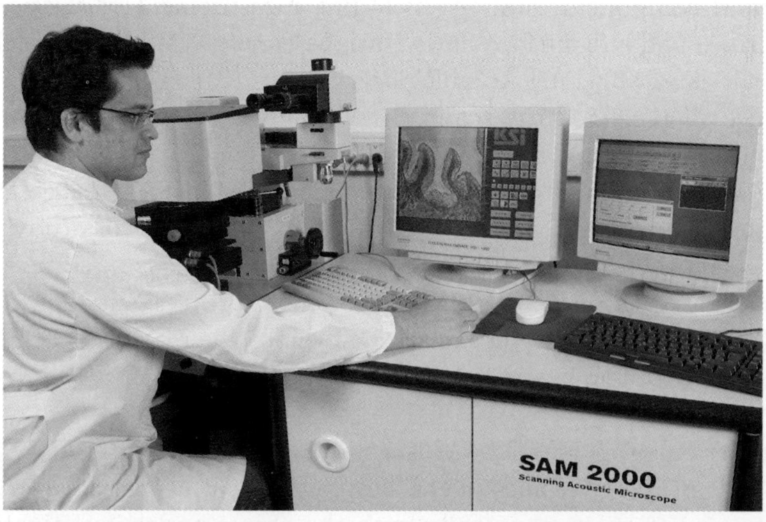


Fig. 1. Photography of the Leica scanning acoustic microscope (SAM2000$^{\text{TM}}$, KSI, Herborn, Germany) in Aarhus, Denmark. The housing in front of the operator is where the lens is located. The screen to the right of the operator shows instant images of the materials investigated under the microscope and the screen to the far right is the control screen with the move-dialogue for the x-y-table.

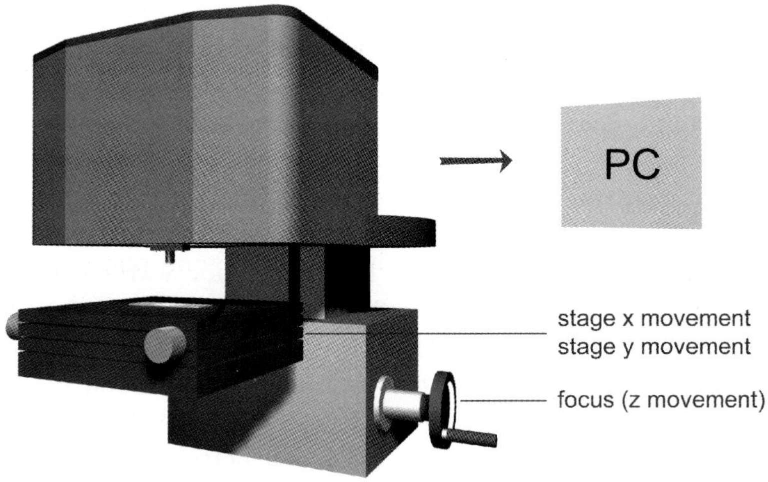


Fig. 2. Schematic diagram of the housing and x-y-table of a *reflection mode scanning acoustic microscope*. The focusing (Z movement) of the lens is done manually. All acoustic signals are transferred through the modulator, and to the PC for imaging. The circled feature in the image is the lens, and is described in detail in Fig. 3. Copyright Skakkebæk Sørensen.

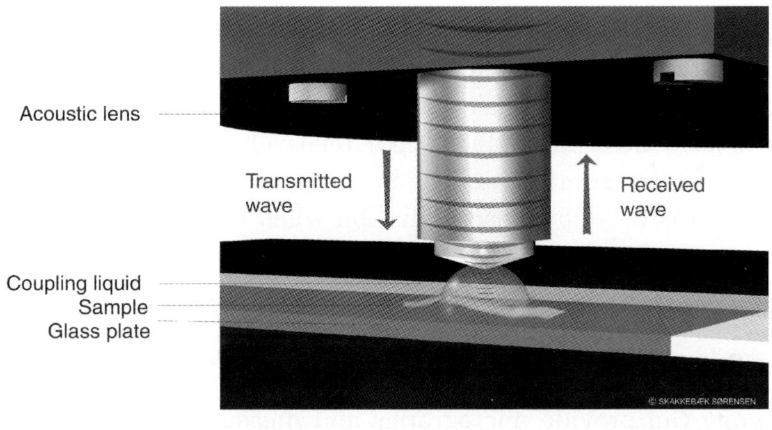


Fig. 3. Drawing of an acoustic lens for a typical *reflection mode scanning acoustic microscope*. The gold-coated zinc oxide ultrasound transducer generates the sound waves that are transmitted to the object and detects the waves reflected from it. Focusing, and thus an increase of resolution is achieved with a small cavity at the tip of the short sapphire rod. The pathway is then: transducer, sapphire rod, couplant, object, sapphire rod, and transducer. The same lens is used for transmission and collection of reflected ultrasound. Note that a liquid (water) is used to couple the ultrasound to the specimen. Copyright Skakkebæk Sørensen.

of a layer of zinc oxide between two gold electrodes at the top. Plane acoustic waves are emitted and travel through a sapphire rod with a hemispherical cavity for focusing at the tip. As the waves pass from the cavity to the couplant and the object of study, they become spherical and travel towards a focus on the axis of the lens. A typical wave path is shown schematically in Fig. 3. Because the acoustic wave velocity is much greater in sapphire than in water, which is usually used as a couplant between the lens and the object of study is almost no spherical aberration even though the lens has only one spherical surface.

Acoustic microscopes may have two oppositely located lenses — one for transmitting and one for receiving. However, in these *transmission mode SAM microscopes*, the lenses are difficult to align and this technique is not commercially available. Another type of acoustic microscope is the *scanning electron acoustic microscope*, where it is the excitation of the acoustic waves that is focused. Yet, another type is the scanning laser acoustic microscope called SLAM, where the waves are transmitted through the object of study and detected by a focused optical probe the measures local surface tilt on the surface of the object. The SLAM has the advantage of live images, but high-frequency waves cannot be used. The following technical descriptions refer to the reflection mode SAM microscope.

A complete description of the electronics in a SAM microscope is beyond the scope of this paper, but detailed description of the pathway can be found in Briggs' book (8). The resolution offered by a SAM microscope is normally comparable to that of the optical counterpart. However, it is possible to achieve a much better resolution with an acoustic microscope than with an optical, but very special techniques must be applied. By using of superfluid liquid helium that has a very low acoustic attenuation due to its low temperature, it is possible to use far higher wave frequencies than those described here. That enables resolution in the nanometer range (9). The magnification offered by conventional acoustic microscopes is of the same magnitude as that of optical microscopes. The resolution sets the limit of the highest usable magnification. In theory, the only factor that limits the magnification of an acoustic microscope is the smallest area of the object that the microscope can scan. The greatest advantages using SAM, is in the field of subsurface imaging. First, many materials are opaque to light but transparent to sound. Second, it is possible to separate subsurface acoustic echoes due to their relatively low travel velocity compared to the velocity of light. Third, an acoustic lens in the reflection mode acoustic microscope is confocal, resulting in greater depth discrimination when compared to a traditional optical microscope.

### 1.2. *Imaging and assessment of acoustic and mechanical properties*

The SAM microscope can provide micrographs and measurements of acoustic and elastic properties of the object. Micrographs of small to large objects, or regions of interest, are made by scanning the lens across the object because of the very limited spatial size of the lens focal zone. The scanning is done in a faster fashion, i.e. a scan in a series of lines. Either the lens or the object is scanned. The latter can be achieved by use of a stage stepper, or DC-motor, and this method usually offers the largest scan field. An acoustic micrograph with a scan field of 1 by 1 mm taken at 500 MHz is shown in Fig. 4, which also shows the velocity (speed of sound), the acoustic impedance and elastic properties of the tissue. In imaging mode, most acoustic microscopes acquire the envelope-detected video signal in each "point" along the lines of scanning for modulation of the micrograph brightness. Thus, in that mode usually no individual and particular acoustic property gives rise to the pixel brightness (10). The brightness is modulated by the interaction of several different properties at various magnitudes. Consequently, a conventional micrograph cannot be used for the quantitative analysis of acoustic properties. However, several SAM techniques exist for such analysis, and that is exactly what gives SAM a leading position in the field of bioacoustics and microelastic analysis.

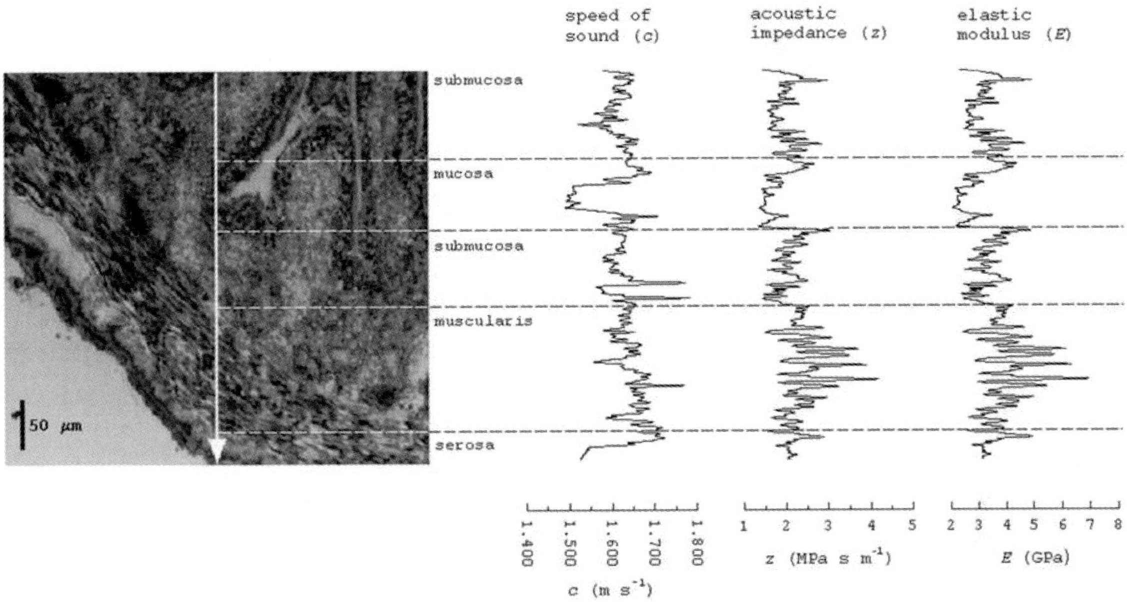


Fig. 4. Micrograph of small intestinal wall acquired at 500 MHz. The field is approximately 1 × 1 mm. The specimen was snab frozen in liquid nitrogen and cryosectioned into 5-$\mu$m-thick transverse sections and mounted on corning glass substrate. The other half of the figure shows the calculated acoustic parameters; the velocity ($C$), the acoustic impedance ($Z$) and the elastic properties ($E$) of the tissue.

In image mode, the lens x-y-scans fields of interest, magnifying between 125× and 600×. In this mode, the reflected ultrasound is converted to 512 by 500 pixels 8-bit greyscale images. Once an image is obtained, the microscope is switched to the time-resolved measurement mode where it scans the lens along a programmed scan-line while digitizing and recording individual reflected ultrasound waves.

## 1.3. *Calculation of elasticity*

Elementary elasticity theory can be applied to SAM measurements for calculation of $c_{11}$, which expresses the elastic stiffness. In acoustics, the speed $C$ and acoustic impedance $Z$, the latter being the ratio of stress or pressure to particle displacement velocity, are the parameters necessary to calculate $c_{11}$. The recorded ultrasound waves contain echoes in the form of voltage amplitude signals originating from the upper tissue surface and the tissue-substrate interface. Briggs and co-workers have described the method of detecting the relevant echoes by way of computer-based signal deconvolution and waveform recognition in detail (8). Determination of $C$ and $Z$ require

- Individual wave amplitudes ($A_1$ and $A_2$) and timings ($t_1$ and $t_2$) (Fig. 5).
- Reference amplitude and timing of an echo in a wave received from a substrate without tissue ($A_0$ and $t_0$).
- Standard $C$ and $Z$ values of the couplant (1,532.9 ms$^{-1}$ and 1.53 MPa sm$^{-1}$, respectively) into:

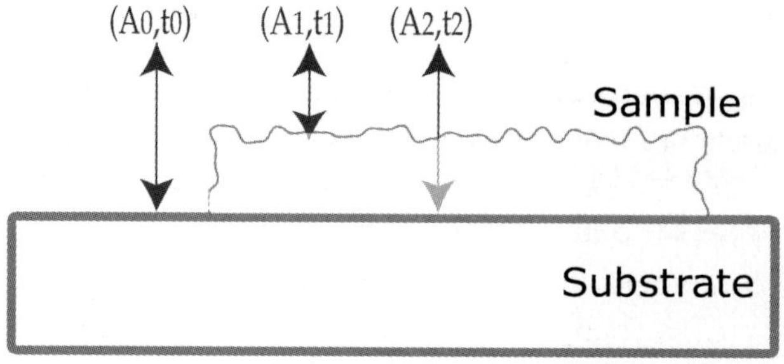


Fig. 5. Specimen on substrate. The arrows indicate where signals are recorded and subsequently analyzed off-line. $A$ is the amplitude and $t$ is the timing.

$$C = C_{\text{couplant}} \frac{t_0 - t_1}{t_2 - t_1} (\text{ms}^{-1}) \tag{2}$$

and

$$Z = Z_{\text{couplant}} \frac{A_0 + A_1}{A_0 - A_1} (\text{Pa sm}^{-1}) \tag{3}$$

In the analysis, absorption in the thickness of the sample is neglected and the variables in Eq. (3) taken to be real-valued. $c_{11}$ is computed from

$$c_{11} = CZ \text{ (Pa)} \tag{4}$$

$c_{11}$ is related to Young's modulus ($E$) by the relationship

$$c_{11} = \frac{(1-\sigma)E}{(1+\sigma)(1-2\sigma)} \tag{5}$$

where $\sigma$ is the Poisson's ratio. Because $\sigma$ is only slightly less than 0.5 for soft tissue, $c_{11}$ may be considerably higher than $E$.

## 1.4. *Tissue preparation for SAM*

High-frequency acoustic waves are highly attenuated resulting in a limited penetration range. At 2,000 MHz, the waves may not penetrate more than a few micrometers into biological tissue. This implicates that most SAM investigations can only be done on tissue sections and analogously to what is done in optical microscopy. There is a need for tissue preparation before micrographs and measurements can be done. Two methods of preparation for soft tissue investigation include formaldehyde fixation and imbedding in paraffin ore cryosection of fresh tissue.

Little scientific proof exists as to what method is the best. The influence of formaldehyde fixation and imbedding in paraffin has showed to change the acoustic properties of tissue in the low-frequency range (11, 12). However, these studies have not been performed at high frequencies used in most SAM studies. Ongoing investigation of the changes due to fixation and imbedding in paraffin, at the SAM laboratory in Aarhus, shows no significant differences on the microscopical level. On the other hand, cryosection has not shown favorable use in investigation above 500 MHz. The investigation has to be done quickly to prevent autolysis. Staining is not needed. The acoustic and elastic heterogeneity among the constituents of most biological tissue ensures that contrast is always present in acoustic micrographs.

### 1.5. *Selected SAM studies*

Several organ systems have been studied with SAM over recent years. Most studies have been done in the cardiovascular system on normal tissue (13–15), atherosclerotic lesions (16), infarcted myocardium (17, 18), and myocardial inflammation and fibrosis (19). Another organ system for which SAM shows great promise is bones (20–22). Because of the good resolution offered by SAM, even single cell acoustic and elastic properties can be measured (23–25). Another study described various distinct motility domains in cells *in vitro* (26). Although mainly qualitative by nature, that study showed a new application for SAM: imaging of movement and how the individual cell *in vitro* prepare and carry out the complex procedure of movement. Even gastric ulcers can be identified and differentiated with SAM *in vitro*. One study examined experimentally induced gastric ulcers in rats and was able to differentiate two distinct types of ulcer healing (27). Recently Jørgensen *et al.*, provided data on the elastic stiffness measured with 500 MHz scanning acoustic microscopy in the guinea pig small intestinal tissue (28). It was found that the speed of sound and the acoustic impedance varied throughout the wall. $C_{11}$ differed between the wall layers with the circular muscle layer being the stiffest and the longitudinal muscle layer, the softest.

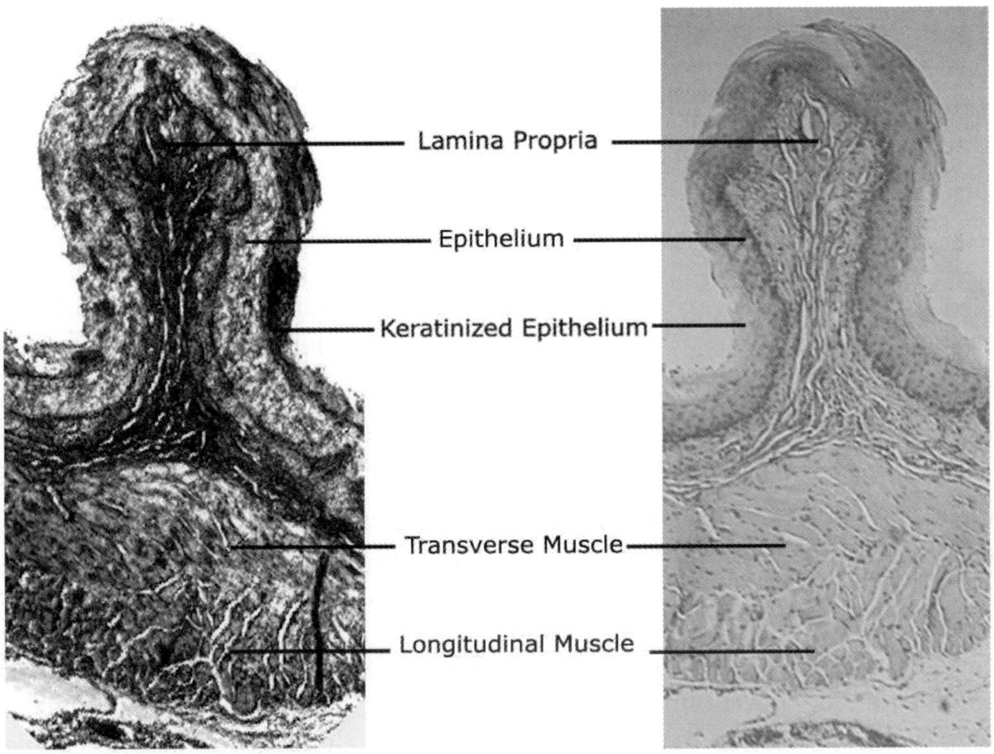


Fig. 6. The esophagus from a Wistar rat. (a) The SAM microscopic image at 1,000 MHz to the left. Variation in tones of grey corresponds to differences in elastic properties. (b) The light microscopic image stained with hematoxylin — eosin to the right. The keratinization of the epithelium is evident. The lamina propria consists of loose connective tissue, smooth muscle cells and vessels. The tunica muscularis consist of muscle arranged in an inner circular and an outer longitudinal layer. Tunica muscularis is surrounded by a tunica adventitia of connective tissue.

Figure 6 shows a section of the esophagus using ultrasound microscopy (SAM) at $f$ = 500 MHz and conventional light microscopy (HE-stained).

### 1.6. *Future SAM investigations*

The times resolve technique is a good method for investigating the elastic properties of tissue at a frequency of 500 MHz. If one wants to investigate tissue at a higher frequency (equals higher resolution), one could benefit from using the $V(f)$ technique (29). This method relies on acquiring amplitude ($V$) at different frequencies ($f$). By obtaining six raw-images at different frequencies, the values of speed and elastic properties can be calculated in the range from 900 MHz to 1,200 MHz. Ongoing pilot studies, reveals that this is a suitable new method for investigating of GI tissue, at a higher frequency. Figure 6 is from the pilot study.

## 2. Scanning Laser Acoustic Microscope

Scanning Laser Acoustic Microscope (SLAM) was introduced by Korpel and coworkers in 1971 (30). SLAM is a transmission mode instrument that creates real-time acoustic images of a sample throughout its entire thickness. A piezoelectric transducer located beneath the sample produces a collimated continuous-wave ultrasound beam at frequencies from 10 to 500 MHz. When the ultrasound wave propagates through the sample, the wave is affected by mechanical inhomogeneities in the material. A scanned laser beam is used as the ultrasound detector. The ability of the SLAM to produce simultaneously optical and acoustic images from which the acoustic properties of the specimen can be calculated facilitates its use in this field of biology. The ultrasonic attenuation and propagation speed can be estimated from the obtained information. Conventional tissue fixation and staining are not required for the SLAM imaging. Living cells and tissues can be studied. The SLAM has been found useful for the *in vitro* assessment of acoustic properties in biological materials such as skin (31), kidney (32) and liver (33).

### 2.1. *Principles of scanning laser acoustic microscopy*

Three SLAM modes produce three different images. For all modes, the sample is located between the SLAM stage and a plastic cover slip. In the *optical mode*, a focused laser beam scans the specimen from above. The beam is transmitted through the cover slip and specimen to a photodiode at the base of the stage. The received photodiode signal is electronically processed and displayed on a TV-monitor; the SLAM's optical image is comparable to that of conventional optical microscopy at a magnification of 100×, but it is not comparable in that the light source is a laser. In the *acoustic mode*, the specimen is insonified with an ultrasonic wave generated by a piezoelectric transducer located below the specimen. The sound wave traverses the specimen and is incident on the lower surface of the cover slip, the surface with the coating. The laser beam that in turn is reflected to a photodiode scans the acoustic generated deflections on this surface of the cover slip. The laser signal is then processed into an acoustic-mode image and displayed in real time on the TV monitor. The ultrasonic attenuation of the specimen can be calculated from this acoustic image according to the method of Tervola (19, 34). In the *interference mode*, the laser beam is detected by the same photodiode as in the acoustic mode and it is then mixed with a reference signal to produce an interference image displayed on the monitor. From the interference image, the acoustic propagation speed is calculated from the lateral shift of the vertical interference lines. The lines shift to the right when the sound waves enter an object having a higher speed relative to the coupling reference medium. Quantitative speed profiles can be obtained from several image regions in different loci. The propagation speed of the specimen is calculated by the method of Goss and O'Brien (35) in relation to that of the reference medium according to the following expression:

$$C_X = \frac{C_0}{\sin\theta_0}\left[\tan^{-1}\left(\frac{1}{\frac{1}{\tan\theta_0} - \frac{\lambda_0 N}{T\sin\theta_0}}\right)\right] \text{ ms}^{-1} \tag{6}$$

where $C_X$ is the propagation speed in the specimen of interest, $C_0$ is the propagation speed in the reference medium, $\lambda_0$ is the wavelength of sound in the reference medium, $T$ is the specimen thickness, $N$ is the measured normalized lateral fringe shift, $\theta_0$ is the angle between the direction of sound propagation in the reference medium and the normal to the stage surface, and is determined from Snell's Law:

$$\theta_0 = \sin^{-1}\left[\frac{C_0}{C_s}\sin\theta_s\right] \tag{7}$$

where $C_s$ is the propagation speed in the fused silica stage (5,968 $\text{ms}^{-1}$), and $\theta_s$ is the angle the sound wave follows through the stage (45°). Measurements of the propagation speed can be done along the vertical line in each layer of the wall to yield a speed profile.

### 2.2. *Gastrointestinal SLAM studies*

Assentoft and coworkers (36) provided preliminary data obtained in the guinea pig esophagus in 1996. To the best of our knowledge, the only thorough gastrointestinal study published with focus on the elastic properties is the paper included in this book following the current review (37). In brief, they aimed to evaluate the propagation speed of sound in the tissue layers of the esophagus at various mechanical loadings. The propagation speed in the esophagus was determined in the no-load state where all external forces are removed, in the distended state and in the zero-stress state (by cutting the esophageal rings radially to release any residual stresses). Differences were found between the layers and between the mechanical states. It was concluded that the esophagus is a composite structure with heterogeneous propagation speed characteristics. Furthermore, the mechanical loading state must be considered in esophageal ultrasound studies.

## Acknowledgement

Dr. Claus Jørgensen, Aarhus University Hospital is kindly thanked for providing input to the manuscript. Medical student Anne Skakkebæk Jensen and architect Rasmus Nørgaard Sørensen are thanked for providing 3D images.

## References


1. Sokolov, S. Y., Ultrasonic microscope. Doklady Akademii Nauk SSR 1949; 63: 333–5.
2. Maugh, T. H., Acoustic Microscopy: A new window to the world of the small. (Editorial). Science 1978; 201: 1110–4.
3. Lemons, R. A. and Quate, C. F., Acoustic microscopy: Biomedical applications. Science 1975; 188: 905–11.
4. Lüers, H., Hillmann, K., Litniewski, J. and Bereiter-Hahn, J., Acoustic Microscopy of cultured cells. Distribution of forces and cytoskeletal elements. Cell Biophysics 1992; 3: 279–93.
5. Muha, M. S, Moulthrop, A. A., Kozlowski, G. C. and Hadimioglu, B., Acoustic microscopy at 15.3 GHz in pressurized superfluid helium. Appl Phys Letter 1990; 56: 1019–21.
6. Kino, G. S., Acoustic Waves: Devices, imaging and analog signal processing. Prentice Hall, New Jersey, N.J., 1987.
7. Kino, G. S., Fundamentals of scanning systems. Scanned image microscopy (ed. E.A. Ash), pp. 1–21. Academic Press, London. 1980.
8. Briggs, G. A., Acoustic Microscopy. Oxford University Press, New York. 1992.
9. Foster, J. S. and Rugar, D., Low-temperature acoustic microscopy. IEEE Trans 1985; SU-32: 139–51.
10. Daft, C. M. W., Briggs, G. A. D. and O'Brien, W. D., Frequency dependence of tissue attenuation measured by acoustic microscopy. J Acoust Soc Am 1989; 85: 416–22.
11. Bamber, J. C., Hill, C. R., King, J. A. and Dunn, F., Ultrasonic propagation through fixed and unfixed tissues. Ultrasound Med Biol 1979; 5: 159–65.
12. van der Steen, A. F., Cuypers, M. H., Thijssen, J. M. and de Wilde, P. C., Influence of histochemical preparation on acoustic parameters of liver tissue: A 5-MHz study. Ultrasound Med Biol 1991; 17: 879–91.
13. Jørgensen, C. S., Knauss, D., Hager, H. and Briggs, G. A. D., Sonography and quantitative measurements. A preliminary study of coronary artery wall topography and mechanical properties. IEEE Med Biol 1996; 15: 35–41.
14. Wickline, S. A., Barzilai, B., Thomas, L. J. I. and Saffitz, J., Quantification of intimal and medial thickness in excised human coronary arteries with 50 MHz acoustic microscopy. Coron Artery Dis 1990; 1: 375–81.
15. Wickline, S. A., Advances in ultrasound methods for high-resolution imaging of the cardiovascular system. Trends in Cardiovascular Medicine 1997; 7: 168–73.
16. Shephard, R. K., Miller, J. G. and Wickline, S. A., Quantification of atherosclerotic plaque composition in cholesterol-fed rabbits with 50 MHz acoustic microscopy. Arterioscler Thromb 1992; 12: 1227–34.
17. O'Brien, W. D., Sagar, K. B., Warltier, D. C. and Rhyne, T. L., Acoustic propagation properties of normal stunned and infarcted myocardium: Morphological and biochemical determinants. Circulation 1995; 91: 154–60.
18. Saijo, Y., Tanaka, M., Okawai, H., Sasaki, H., Nitta, S. I. and Dunn, F., Ultrasonic tissue characterization of infacted myocardium by scanning acoustic microscopy. Ultrasound Med Biol 1997; 23: 77–85.
19. Tervola, K. M. U. and O'Brien, Jr. W. D., Spatial frequency domain technique: An approach for analyzing the scanning laser acoustic microscope interferogram images IEEE Transactions on Sonics and Ultrasonics 1985; 4: 544–54.
20. Katz, J. L. and Meunier, A., Scanning acoustic microscope studies of the elastic properties of osteons and osteon lamellae. J Biomech Eng 1993; 115: 543–48.

21. Meunier, A., Katz, J. L., Christel, P. and Sedel, L., A reflection scanning acoustic microscope for bone and bone biomaterials interface studies. J Orthop Res 1988; 6: 770–75.
22. Hasegawa, K., Turner, C. H., Recker, R. R., Wu, E. and Burr, D. B., Elastic properties of osteoporotic bone measured by scanning acoustic microscopy. Bone 1995; 16: 85–90.
23. Bereiter-Hahn, J., Scanning acoustic microscopy visualizes cytomechanical responses to cytochalasin D. J Microscopy 1987; 146: 29–39.
24. Hildebrand, J. A. and Rugar, E. L., Measurement of cellular elastic properties by acoustic microscopy. J Microscopy 1983; 134: 245–60.
25. Briggs, G. A. D., Wang, J. and Gundle, R., Quantitative acoustic microscopy of individual living human cells. J Microscopy 1993; 172: 3–12.
26. Veslý, P., Lüers, H., Riehle, M. and Bereiter-Hahn, J., Subtraction scanning acoustic microscopy reveals motility domains in cells *in vitro*. Cell Mot Cytoskel 1994; 29: 231–40.
27. Mizutani, K., Tsukamoto, Y., Goto, H., Hase, S., Niwa, Y. and Ohashi, S., Evaluation of acetic acid-induced gastric ulcers in rats by scanning acoustic microscopy. Scand J Gastroenterol 1991; 26: 313–20.
28. Jørgensen, C. S., Assentoft, J. E., Knauss, D., Gregersen, H. and Briggs, G. A. D., Small intestinal wall distribution of elastic stiffness measured with 500 MHz scanning acoustic microscopy. Ann Biomed Eng 2001; 29: 1059–63.
29. Kundo, T., Breiter-Hahn, J. and Karl, I., Cell property determination from the acoustic microscope generated voltage versus frequency curves. Biophys J 2000; 78: 2270–9.
30. Korpel, A., Kessler, L. W. and Palermo, P. R., Acoustic Microscope operating 100 MHz Nature 1971; 232: 110–1.
31. Steiger, D. L., O'Brien, Jr. W. D. and Olerud, J. E., Riederer-Henderson MA, Odland GF. Measurement uncertainty assessment of the scanning laser acoustic microscope and application to canine skin and wound IEEE Trans Ultra Ferroelec Frequency Control 1988; 35: 741–8.
32. Kessler, L. W., Fields, S. I. and Dunn, F., Acoustic microscope of mammalian kidney. J Clin Ultrasound 1974; 2: 317–20.
33. Tervola, K. M. U., Gummer, M. A., Erdman, Jr. J. W., O'Brien and Jr. W. D., Ultrasound attenuation and velocities in rat liver as a function of fat concentration: A study at 100 MHz using a scanning laser acoustic microscope. J Acoust Soc Am 1985; 77: 307–13.
34. Tervola, K. M. U., Foster, S. G. and O'Brien Jr. W. D., Attenuation coefficient measurement technique at 100 MHz with the scanning laser acoustic microscope. IEEE Transactions on Sonics and Ultrasonics 1985; SU-32: 259–65.
35. Goss, S. A. and O'Brien Jr. W. D., Direct ultrasonic velocity measurements of mammalian collagen threads. J Acoust Soc Am 1979; 65: 507–11.
36. Assentoft, J. E., Jørgensen, C. S., Gregersen, H., Christensen, L. L., Djurhuus, J. C. and O'Brien Jr. W. D., Characterizing biological tissue using scanning laser acoustic microscopy IEEE Engineering in Medicine and Biology 1996; 15: 42–5.
37. Assentoft, J. E., Gregersen, H., O'Brien Jr, W. D., Propagation speed of sound assessment in the layers of the guinea-pig esophagus *in vitro* by means of acoustic microscopy. Ultrasonics 2001; 39: 263–8.

Published with permission

ELSEVIER

Ultrasonics 39 (2001) 263–268

Ultrasonics

www.elsevier.nl/locate/ultras

# Propagation speed of sound assessment in the layers of the guinea-pig esophagus in vitro by means of acoustic microscopy

J.E. Assentoft [a], H. Gregersen [a,b], W.D. O'Brien Jr. [c,*]

[a] Institute of Experimental Clinical Research, Skejby Hospital, Section SKS, Denmark

[b] Center for Sensory-Motor Interaction, Aalborg University and Department A, Aalborg Hospital, Denmark

[c] Department of Electrical and Computer Engineering, Bioacoustics Research Laboratory, University of Illinois at Urbana-Champaign, 405 N. Mathews, Urbana, IL 61801, USA

Received 11 August 2000; received in revised form 18 December 2000; accepted 21 December 2000

**Abstract**

The study's purpose was to evaluate the propagation speed of sound in the tissue layers of the esophagus at various mechanical loadings. Scanning laser acoustics microscopy was applied for the estimation of the propagation speed in the mucosa–submucosa and muscle layers of guinea-pig esophagus in vitro ($n = 26$). The propagation speed in the esophagus was determined in the no-load state with all external forces removed, and in the distended and zero-stress states. The zero-stress state was obtained by cutting the esophageal rings radially. The propagation speed in the no-load state differed significantly ($p < 0.001$) between the muscle layer (median 1740, quartiles 1735–1746 m/s) and the mucosa (1607, 1605–1609 m/s). In the distended state the propagation speed in the muscle layer decreased significantly ($p < 0.001$) to 1673 (1666–1681) m/s while it did not change significantly in mucosa (1602, 1600–1607 m/s). When compared to the no-load state, the propagation speed in the zero-stress state in the muscle layers decreased to 1624 (1615–1636) m/s ($p < 0.001$) and in mucosa to 1584 (1566–1603) m/s ($p < 0.001$). In conclusion, the esophagus is a composite structure with heterogeneous propagation speed characteristics. Furthermore, the mechanical loading state must be considered in esophageal ultrasound studies. 

*Keywords:* Ultrasound propagation speed; Mucosa; Muscle; Digestive tract

## 1. Introduction

The advancement of science in recent years follows a trend of needing to know greater details in physiology, medicine and tissue engineering. Obtaining morphometric and biomechanical data from several adjacent layers of tissue is a step towards the next level in the hierarchy of structure of living tissue. Such data are needed in a mechanical analysis of a composite biological structure. Thus far, Yu et al. [1] presented a two-layer model based on bending experiments for determination of stress–strain properties. Gregersen et al. [2] studied the zero-stress state of the layers of guinea-pig esophagus and found significant differences in residual strain between the muscle and mucosa–submucosa layers. Realizing that obtaining mechanical data on individual layers of biological tissues are useful, we need to develop new methods to characterize layered organs to a greater extent. In this study we employed a scanning laser acoustic microscope (SLAM) to obtain a better understanding of the composite properties of the esophagus.

The practical application of ultrasound for imaging was demonstrated by the French physicist Paul Langevin during World War I [3]. In the early 1930s Sokolov explored the usefulness of ultrasound for imaging internal structures in optically opaque objects [3,4] and he was first to suggest ultrasound at 3 GHz for imaging small objects. This technique is now known as *acoustic microscopy*, which is defined as a general term for high resolution, high frequency ultrasonic inspection techniques that produce images of features beneath the surface of the sample. Further developments led to the SLAM which was introduced by Korpel and coworkers [5]. The SLAM is a transmission mode instrument that creates real-time acoustic images of a sample throughout its entire thickness. A collimated continuous-wave ultrasound beam at frequencies from 10 to 500 MHz is

* Corresponding author. Tel.: +1-217-333-2407; fax: +1-217-244-0105.

*E-mail address:* wdo@uiuc.edu (W.D. O'Brien Jr.).

0041-624X/01/$ - see front matter 
PII: S0041-624X(01)00053-1

Published with permission



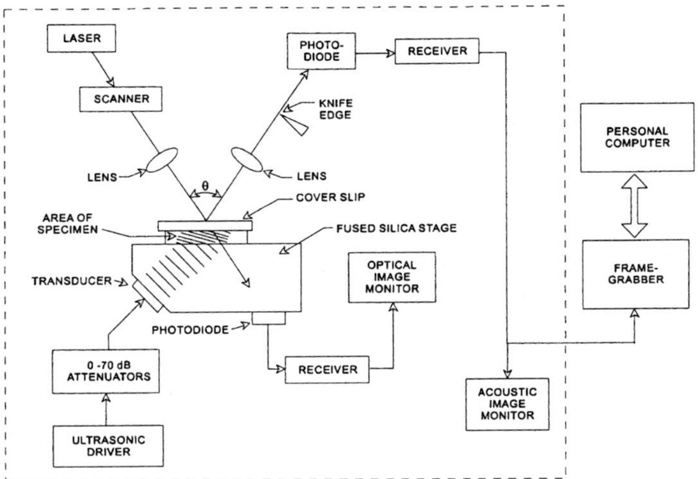


Fig. 1. Block diagram of the SLAM.

produced by a piezoelectric transducer located beneath the sample (for this study, 100 MHz was used). When the ultrasound wave propagates through the sample, the wave is affected by mechanical inhomogeneities in the material. A scanned laser beam is used as the ultrasound detector (Fig. 1). The ability of the SLAM to produce simultaneously optical and acoustic images from which the acoustic properties of the specimen can be calculated make easy its use in this field of biology. The ultrasonic attenuation and propagation speed can be estimated from the obtained information. Conventional tissue fixation and staining are not required for the SLAM imaging; this allows for studies of living cells and tissues [6]. The SLAM has been found useful for the in vitro assessment of acoustic properties in biological materials such as skin [7], kidney [8] and liver [9].

The SLAM technique was thus used as the method for estimating propagation speed in the simple layered structure of the guinea-pig esophagus. The esophagus consists of an innermost mucosa–submucosal layer (hereafter referred to as the mucosal layer) that mainly consists of connective tissue with blood vessels and nerves, and outermost longitudinal and circumferential muscle layers. The esophagus is an important organ to study due to its mechanical function and composite structure. Furthermore, diseases can cause structural and biomechanical remodeling in the esophagus.

The propagation speed in the individual layers of the esophagus has, to the best of our knowledge, not been presented in the literature. The aim of this study was to determine the propagation speed in the individual layers of esophagus in vitro in the no-load state with all external forces removed, in the distended state and in the zero-stress state. The distended state corresponds to the physiological state where a bolus of fluid or food passes through the esophagus. The no-load state is the conditions where no external forces are applied, i.e., zero pressure from outside and inside. The no-load state was for many years considered to be the reference state for mechanical analysis, i.e., the reference length for strain. However, we know now that residual stresses may reside in the no-load state. The cut-open state, also called the zero-stress state, is the condition where also the residual (internal) forces have been released by making a radial cut through the wall. The zero-stress state is important in mechanics because it is the state to where all the stresses and strains refer.

## 2. Material and methods

### 2.1. Specimen preparation

Twenty-six 700–900-g female guinea pigs were euthanized using pentobarbital, and a long midline cut was made in the neck and chest. Calcium-free Krebs solution was poured into the chest cavity. The esophagus was separated from adjacent structures from the tongue to the stomach. A 4-cm-long segment beginning 2 mm from the root of the tongue was excised. The tissue was cleaned and snap-frozen in one of four different states (see below) in liquid nitrogen and stored at −80°C.

At the time of sample evaluation, 100-μm-thick cross-sections were cut in a Lipshaw cryo-microtome. Each specimen was placed on the SLAM stage and allowed 5 min for equilibration to 24.5°C (as measured by an Omega Engineering Inc., Model HH21) before estimates of the propagation speed were performed. A physio-

Published with permission

J.E. Assentoft et al. / Ultrasonics 39 (2001) 263–268 265

logical saline solution was used as coupling medium between the SLAM stage and specimen and served as a reference medium (known acoustic properties) for calculation of the propagation speed. The experimental protocol was approved by the University of Illinois' Laboratory Animal Care Advisory Committee and satisfied all campus and National Institutes of Health (NIH) rules for the humane use of laboratory animals.

The esophagus was studied under four different conditions: distended state ($n = 26$), no-load state ($n = 26$), zero-stress state ($n = 26$) and finally the mucosal layer without the muscle layer attached ($n = 6$). The distended state corresponds to the homeostatic state with a food bolus in the esophagus. The distended state was obtained by infusing Tissue Tek (OCT) in the esophagus to a diameter, $D$, corresponding to an approximate stretch ratio, $D_{\text{distended}}/D_{\text{no-load}}$, at the outer surface of 1.15 before it was snap frozen. The stretch ratio did not change after mounting the specimen on the SLAM stage. The no-load state represents the condition without any external forces applied. The zero-stress state represents the state where residual stresses are not present, and was obtained by a radial cut that caused the esophagus to spring open. About thirty seconds after the radial cut, the sample was snap-frozen. The mucosal layer was studied under no-load conditions by removing the muscle layer surgically under a microscope before it was snap-frozen. Separation was performed without visible damage to the mucosal tissue; optical microscope magnification of 4× was used. The muscle layer was not suitable for investigation after separation.

### 2.2. Scanning laser acoustic microscopy

The technical details and operating principles of the SLAM (Sonomicroscope®, Sonoscan, Inc., Bensenville, Illinois) have previously been described in detail [10]. The three SLAM modes produce three different images. For all modes, the sample is located between the SLAM stage and plastic coverslip (Fig. 1). The coverslip is coated with a partially reflecting optical layer, and that layer is adjacent to the sample. In the *optical mode*, a focused laser beam scans the specimen from above, and is transmitted through the coverslip and specimen to a photodiode at the base of the stage. The received photodiode signal is electronically processed and displayed to a TV-monitor; the SLAM's optical image is comparable to that of conventional optical microscopy at a magnification of 100×, but is not comparable in that the light source is that of a laser. In the *acoustic mode*, the specimen is insonified with a 100-MHz (in this case) ultrasonic wave generated by a piezoelectric transducer located below the specimen. The sound wave traverses the specimen and is incident on the lower surface of the coverslip, the surface with the coating. The acoustic generated deflections on this surface of the coverslip are scanned by the laser beam that in turn is reflected to a photodiode. The laser signal is then processed into an acoustic-mode image and displayed in real time on the TV monitor. The ultrasonic attenuation of the specimen can be calculated from this acoustic image [11]. However, specimen attenuation was not possible for this experiment because the attenuation technique requires different thicknesses of the same sample, and there was insufficient sample material. In the *interference mode*, the laser beam is detected by the same photodiode as in the acoustic mode and it is then mixed with a 100-MHz reference signal to produce an interference image displayed on the TV-monitor (Fig. 2). From the interference image, the acoustic propagation speed is calculated from the lateral (horizontal) shift of the vertical interference lines [12]. The lines shift to the right when the sound waves enter an object having a higher speed relative to the coupling reference medium. Quantitative speed profiles (Figs. 3 and 4) are created from analysis of several image regions in different loci. The propagation speed of the specimen is calculated in relation to that of the 1520-m/s reference medium (calcium-free Krebs–Ringer solution with $10^{-2}$ M $MgCl_2$), hereafter referred to as the Krebs–Ringer solution, according to the following expression [12,13]:

$$C_x = \frac{C_o}{\sin\theta_o}\left[\tan^{-1}\left(\frac{1}{\frac{1}{\tan\theta_o} - \frac{\lambda_o N}{T\sin\theta_o}}\right)\right] \text{ m/s} \quad (1)$$

where $C_x$ is the propagation speed in the specimen of interest, $C_o$ is the propagation speed in the reference

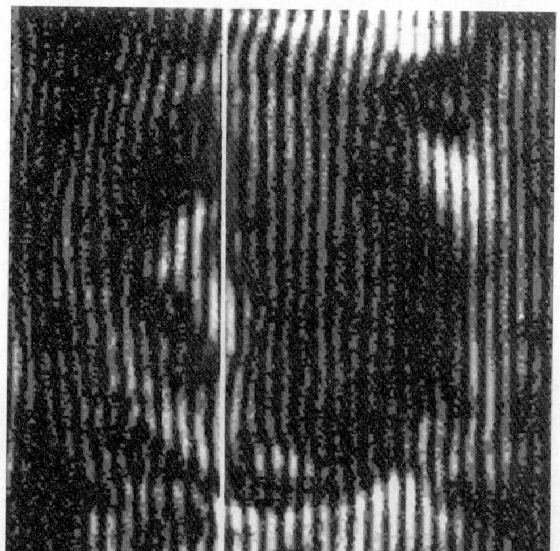

Fig. 2. An interference image of the cross-section of an esophagus. The darker vertical lines are the interference lines. The white vertical line that passes through the center of the esophagus indicates where the propagation speed profile was obtained that is displayed in Fig. 3.

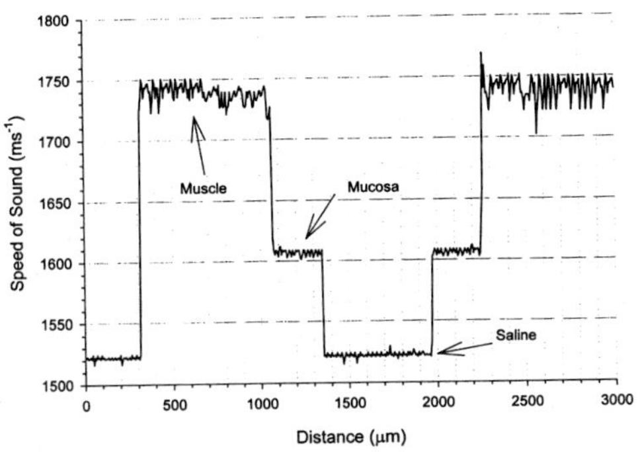


Fig. 3. The propagation speed profile that depicts the speed of muscle and mucosa layers in esophagus at no-load state. The distance axis goes from top to bottom (see vertical white line in Fig. 3) of the interference image. The reference medium is Krebs–Ringer solution.

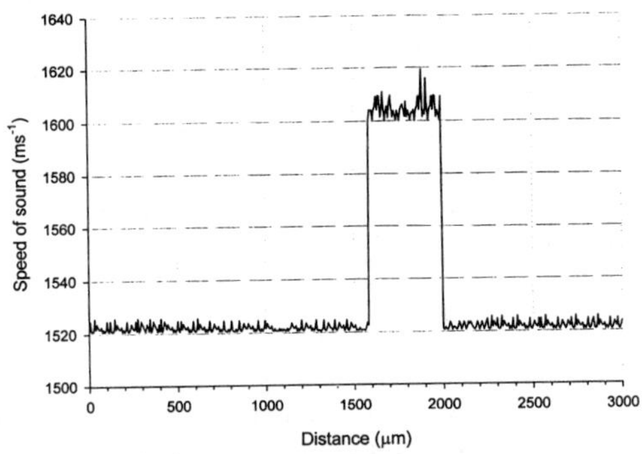


Fig. 4. The propagation speed profile in the mucosa layer of esophagus at the no-load state. The reference medium is Krebs–Ringer solution.

medium (Krebs–Ringer solution, 30°C, 1520 m/s), $\lambda_o$ is the wavelength of sound in the reference medium, $T$ is the specimen thickness, $N$ is the measured normalized lateral fringe shift, $\theta_o$ is the angle between the direction of sound propagation in the reference medium and the normal to the stage surface, and is determined from Snell's law:

$$\theta_o = \sin^{-1}\left[\frac{C_o}{C_s}\sin\theta_s\right] \qquad (2)$$

where $C_s$ is the propagation speed in the fused silica stage (5968 m/s), and $\theta_s$ is the angle the sound wave travels through the stage (45°). Measurements of the propagation speed were done along the vertical line in each layer of the wall (Fig. 2) to yield a speed profile (Fig. 4).

### 2.3. Uncertainty of SLAM measurements

An uncertainty assessment of the SLAM's measurement procedures and results was performed by measuring the propagation speed in a known media (Dow Corning 710, Dow Corning, Midland, MI), a silicone oil for which attenuation coefficient and speed have been characterized acoustically and referenced in the literature [12,14,15]. A droplet of the oil was placed inside a metal spacer surrounded by saline on the scanning stage surface and a coverslip was then placed on top of the metal spacer. The thickness of the metal spacer was measured with a calibrated digital caliper to within ±1 μm. The saline and the oil did not mix. The oil was then allowed to equilibrate to 30°C before the measurement were taken. The propagation speed was determined for varying oil thickness (75 and 120 μm) with all other factors kept constant. Our experiments on Dow Corning 710 gave a propagation speed of 1341 m/s (quartiles 1321–1357 m/s). Hence, the precision was 2.7% $[((1357-1321)/1341)\times 100\%]$ . For accuracy determination the median value of 1341 should be compared to values in the literature of approximately 1350 m/s [14]. Sources of speed error of the Dow Corning 710 included the reference medium speed (Krebs–Ringer solution), the normalized fringe shift, the specimen thickness, noise and other unknown variations in the SLAM system. Krebs–Ringer solution was used as the reference medium, and the temperature was kept stable to reduce the error due to the reference speed. The difference in propagation speed between thicknesses of 75 and 120 μm was less than 10 m/s. An extensive error analysis of SLAM measurements is provided by Steiger et al. [7].

Data are presented as median and quartiles. Statistical test was the Mann–Whitney Rank Sum test using SigmaStat (Jandel Scientific). Results were considered significant when $p < 0.05$.

## 3. Results

The propagation speed from the different layers and preparations are given in Table 1. It was not possible to distinguish the circular and longitudinal muscle layers in any of the preparations, though the sound beam direction was parallel to the longitudinal muscle layer and perpendicular to the circumferential muscle layer. It was a general finding that the propagation speed was higher in the muscle layer than in mucosa ($p < 0.001$ for the distended, no-load and zero-stress states). The most pronounced difference in propagation speed between the layers was found in no-load state (approximately 8% difference, Fig. 3). The propagation speed in the muscle layer differed among the three states ($p < 0.001$) with the highest median value of 1740 m/s in no-load state. The lowest value was found in the zero-stress state (1624, 1615–1636 m/s). In mucosa the propagation speed also varied between the three states ($p < 0.001$) with the lowest values in zero-stress state (1584, 1566–1603 m/s). The propagation speed in the no-load state for mucosa

Table 1
Propagation speed in the different layers of esophagus measured at 100 MHz

| | Esophagus | | | | | | |
|---|---|---|---|---|---|---|---|
| | No-load state | | Distended state | | Zero-stress state | | Separated layer |
| | Muscle | Mucosa | Muscle | Mucosa | Muscle | Mucosa | Mucosa |
| Median speed (m/s) | 1740 | 1607 | 1673 | 1602 | 1624 | 1584 | 1606 |
| Quartiles (m/s) | 1735–1746 | 1605–1609 | 1666–1681 | 1600–1607 | 1615–1636 | 1566–1603 | 1602–1609 |

Muscle differed from mucosa at all three states ($p < 0.001$). The propagation speed for the muscle layer differed between the three states ($p < 0.001$). The propagation speed for the mucosa layer differed between the three state ($p < 0.001$) but the mucosa separated from the muscle layer (last column) did not differ from the mucosa with the muscle layer attached in no-load state.

separated from the muscle layer did not differ from that obtained in mucosa with muscle attached (Figs. 3 and 4, Table 1).

## 4. Discussion

In this paper we show that it is possible with SLAM to image sections of the guinea-pig esophagus and quantitatively distinguish its layered topography. As far as we know there are no other acoustic microscope studies that have investigated the layered structures in esophagus. The wall can be quantitatively characterized and its layers distinguished by use of the SLAM propagation speed profile. We aimed to study the properties at different states of mechanical loading. The distended state corresponds to the in vivo state with bolus passage. In the no-load state, the specimen is not exposed to any external forces but residual stresses may be present in the tissue. Such residual stresses are released by cutting the tissue radially to achieve the zero-stress state. The zero-stress state was first described in biological tissues in 1983 [16,17] and it provides a reference state for morphometric and mechanical analysis. Recently, it was found that the guinea-pig esophagus and duodenum exhibit large residual strains and that the residual strain reduces the stress concentration at the luminal surface during loading [2,18,19]. It is of interest to note from this study that the lowest propagation speed values was indeed found in the zero-stress state. This makes sense considering that the stress-strain properties of biological tissues are exponential-like [18] and that the propagation speed is proportional to the square root of the elastic modulus [13]. Releasing the residual stress causes the elastic moduli to decrease resulting in lowering of the propagation speed. The trend of increasing propagation speed with the loading level was most evident for the muscle tissue. The reason for the lesser response in the mucosa layer is likely that it is compressed in the no-load state and unfolds rather than stretches during low degrees of distension [2,18].

Comparable quantitative ultrasound data to the best of our knowledge have not been reported for the esophagus. However, values of propagation speed obtained from muscle in other organs [7,9,20] are similar to the ones found in the esophageal muscle coat in this study. In addition, the values for mucosa in this study agree with recent measurements in urethra [20,21] where it was also found that the propagation speed was highest in the muscle layer. The similarity with other tissues suggests that the freezing technique used in this study did not change the ultrasonic properties significantly. It was a principal result that the propagation speed was higher in the muscle layer than in mucosa of esophagus. The accuracy and error of SLAM for speed measurements have previously been estimated to be ±2.9% and ±0.4%, respectively [7]. Hence, the difference in propagation speed between the muscle and mucosa layers cannot be explained by measurement uncertainties. It is well known that gastrointestinal mucosa–submucosa contains vessels, nerves, some muscle cells, and loose connective tissue. Only a part of the submucosa contains high amounts of collagen. The muscle tissue contains a high amount of actin–myosin proteins in the muscle cells and collagen fibers between the muscle cells. It is therefore not surprising that the highest propagation speed was found in the muscle layer since connective tissue fibers in other tissues have been shown to have a relatively high propagation speed [22]. Thus, the elastic stiffness will increase with the amount of collagen and the ultrasonic propagation speed will increase with collagen content since the speed is proportional to the square root of the elastic modulus of the material as shown by Fields et al. [23] and Goss and O'Brien [13]. Another contributing factor to the difference in propagation speed between the muscle and mucosa layers may be that the muscle layers are exposed to a higher tensile stress than the mucosa. According to a previous study on residual strains in the layered esophagus [2], it is evident that the mucosa–submucosa layer is compressed by the tension in the muscle layer at the no-load state, at low degrees of distension, and even at the zero-stress state if the muscle layer is not separated surgically from the mucosa–submucosal layer. We were not able to demonstrate differences in propagation speed between the two orthogonal muscle layers. This is in contrast to a previous study on bovine longissimus dorsi, psoas major and lobster extensor, where the speed was significantly higher for ultrasound parallel to the muscle fibers than perpendicular to the muscle fibers [24].

Published with permission



This study focused on the muscle and mucosa layers and showed differences between layers and loading states. Future studies should focus on ultrasonic properties in various directions in order to obtain more detailed data on tissue anisotropy and heterogeneity in the gastrointestinal tract.

## Acknowledgements

This work is partially supported by a grant from The Danish Research Councils (9501709), Karen Elise Jensens Foundation, and the US National Institutes of Health (CA09067). The authors acknowledge the help from James F. Zachary, DVM, Ph.D., Veterinary Pathobiology, and Ann C. Benefiel, Biological Resources, Beckman Institute for Advanced Science and Technology, both at the University of Illinois.

## References

[1] R. Yu, J. Zhon, Y.C. Fung, Neutral axis location in bending and Young's modulus of different layers of arterial wall, Am. J. Physiol. 265 (1993) H52–H60.

[2] H. Gregersen, C. Lee, S. Chien, R. Skalak, Y.C. Fung, Strain distribution in the layered wall of the esophagus, J. Biomech. Engng. 121 (1999) 442–448.

[3] F.V. Hunt, Origins of Acoustics New Haven, Yale University Press, New Haven, CT 1978.

[4] G. Wade, Acoustic Imaging, Plenum Press, New York, 1976.

[5] A. Korpel, L.W. Kessler, P.R. Palermo, Acoustic microscope operating 100 MHz, Nature 232 (1971) 110–111.

[6] J.A. Slobin, D.L. Stocum, W.D. O'Brien Jr., Amphibian limb regeneration curves generated by the scanning laser acoustic microscope, J. Histochem. Cytochem. 34 (1986) 53–56.

[7] D.L. Steiger, W.D. O'Brien Jr., J.E. Olerud, M.A. Riederer-Henderson, G.F. Odland, Measurement uncertainty assessment of the scanning laser acoustic microscope and application to canine skin and wound, IEEE Trans. Ultra Ferroelec. Freq. Contrl. 35 (1988) 741–748.

[8] L.W. Kessler, S.I. Fields, F. Dunn, Acoustic microscope of mammalian kidney, J. Clin. Ultrasound 2 (1974) 317–320.

[9] K.M.U. Tervola, M.A. Gummer, J.W. Erdman Jr., W.D. O'Brien Jr., Ultrasound attenuation and velocities in rat liver as a function of fat concentration: a study at 100 MHz using a scanning laser acoustic microscope, J. Acoust. Soc. Am. 77 (1985) 307–313.

[10] L.W. Kessler, A. Korpel, P.R. Palermo, Simultaneous acoustic and optical microscopy of biological specimens, Nature 239 (1972) 111–112.

[11] K.M.U. Tervola, S.G. Foster, W.D. O'Brien Jr., Attenuation coefficient measurement technique at 100 MHz with the scanning laser acoustic microscope, IEEE Trans. Sonics Ultrason. SU-32 (1985) 259–265.

[12] K.M.U. Tervola, W.D. O'Brien Jr., Spatial frequency domain technique: an approach for analyzing the scanning laser acoustic microscope interferogram images, IEEE Trans. Sonics Ultrason. 4 (1985) 544–554.

[13] S.A. Goss, W.D. O'Brien Jr., Direct ultrasonic velocity measurements of mammalian collagen threads, J. Acoust. Soc. Am. 65 (2) (1979) 507–511.

[14] F. Dunn, P.D. Edmonds, W.J. Fry, Absorption and dispersion of ultrasound in biological media, in: H.P. Schwan (Ed.), Biological Engineering, McGraw Hill, New York, 1969.

[15] B. Zeqiri, Reference liquid for ultrasonic attenuation, Ultrasonics 27 (1989) 314–315.

[16] Y.C. Fung, What principle governs the stress distribution in living organs? in: Y.C. Fung, E. Fukuda, W. Junjian (Ed.), Biomechanics in China, Japan and USA, Science, Beijing, 1983.

[17] R.N. Vaishnav, J. Vossoughi, Estimation of residual strain in aortic segments, in: C.W. Hall (Ed.), Biomedical Engineering. II. Recent Developments. Pergamon Press, New York, 1983, pp. 330–333.

[18] H. Gregersen, G.S. Kassab, Biomechanics of the gastrointestinal tract, Neurogastroent. Motil. 8 (1996) 277–297.

[19] H. Gregersen, G.S. Kassab, E. Pallencaoe, C. Lee, S. Chien, R. Skalak, Y.C. Fung, Morphometry and strain distribution in guinea pig duodenum with reference to the zero-stress state, Am. J. Physiol. 273 (1997) G865–G874.

[20] J.E. Assentoft, C.S. Jørgensen, H. Gregersen, L.L. Christensen, J.C. Djurhuus, W.D. O'Brien Jr., Characterizing biological tissue using scanning laser acoustic microscopy, IEEE Engng. Med. Biol. 15 (1996) 42–45.

[21] C.R. Hill (Ed.), Physical Principles of Medical Ultrasonics, Wiley, New York, 1986.

[22] C.A. Edwards, W.D. O'Brien Jr., Speed of sound in mammalian tendon threads using various reference media, IEEE Trans. Sonics Ultrason. SU32 (1985) 351–354.

[23] S. Fields, F. Dunn, Correlation of echographic visualization of tissue with biological composition and physiological state, J. Acoust. Soc. Am. 54 (1973) 809–812.

[24] N.B. Smith, Effect of myofibril length and tissue constituents on acoustic propagation properties of muscle, Ph.D. Thesis, University of Illinois at Urbana-Champaign, 1996.

# CHAPTER 14

# ULTRASONOGRAPHIC ALTERATIONS IN FUNCTIONAL DYSPEPSIA

ARNOLD BERSTAD AND ODD HELGE GILJA

A large proportion of patients undergoing upper gastrointestinal endoscopy have discomfort centred in the upper abdomen in the absence of oesophagitis, ulcer, cancer or other pathology which can explain their dyspepsia. Many of these cases are classified as having *functional dyspepsia*. The diagnosis does not imply that all examinations show completely normal results. For instance, the gastroscopy is often described as negative even though it may reveal minor mucosal abnormalities, like "erosive prepyloric changes" (1). These prepyloric fold formations with red spots, streaks or frank erosions on top of the folds are not due to *Helicobacter pylori*, intake of NSAIDs or other known exogenous or endogenous irritating substances. They are associated with and seem to be a manifestation of stress (2). Although they do not explain the dyspepsia, they may delineate a purer subgroup of patients with stress-induced, functional dyspepsia. The same thoughts may apply if we start to recognise "minor" stomach abnormalities seen on ultrasound.

## 1. What is Functional Dyspepsia?

Functional dyspepsia is a symptom complex including various meal-related sensations from the epigastrium, like unpleasant fullness, early satiety, bloating, nausea and belching. Although the symptoms resemble those in peptic ulcer disease, they cannot be satisfactorily explained by organic findings. The symptoms are, therefore, believed to arise due to motor or sensory disturbances of stomach function. The three abnormalities most regularly observed are prolonged gastric emptying, increased perception of discomfort in response to distension (gastric hypersensitivity), and impaired gastric accommodation (3). Each of these abnormalities might be related to particular symptom profiles, but the relationships are weak (4).

The condition is prevalent and a frequent cause for consulting a doctor both in general practice and in hospitals. The management of these patients continues to be a subject of dispute. Empirical treatment of undiagnosed dyspepsia is often recommended while others warn against misuse of drugs in a high proportion of the patients by doing so. When proton pump inhibitors are increasingly being used as antacids and antibiotics (against *Helicobacter pylori* infection) are given to patients without ulcer disease, the situation may be out of control.

## 2. Pathophysiology

Even in the absence of organic lesions, patients with functional dyspepsia may complain of severe symptoms and have a poor quality of life. They also often have a low estimate of own health and have complaints from several organ systems (i.e. somatization) (5, 6). Due to the complexity of the symptoms, both the central nervous system (stress, neuroticism etc.) and gastric (infectious or motor) disturbances are supposed to be involved, but their relative importance is controversial. Many of the patients who consult a doctor for dyspepsia have considerable psychological problems, and anxiety is often a major reason for consultation. Several studies have found that patients with functional dyspepsia as a group are more anxious and depressed, and have a higher level of neuroticism than controls (7). When patients with functional dyspepsia were asked to target their complaints, dyspepsia came only third place. Anxiety and family problems were more important (8). The fact that consultation is more often a consequence of anxiety than of abdominal discomfort is reasonable, but it seriously complicates the evaluation of the role of psychological factors in the pathophysiology of functional dyspepsia (9). While some think functional dyspepsia is mainly a psychological disorder, others think it is first and foremost a sensory-motor disorder of the stomach.

Anyhow, psychological factors are considered important in symptom generation. In a multifactorial way psychological factors and peripheral (gastric) mechanisms appear to be involved in symptom generation, implying an interaction between the central nervous and the enteric nervous systems. Our concept for the pathogenesis of functional dyspepsia is illustrated in Fig. 1.

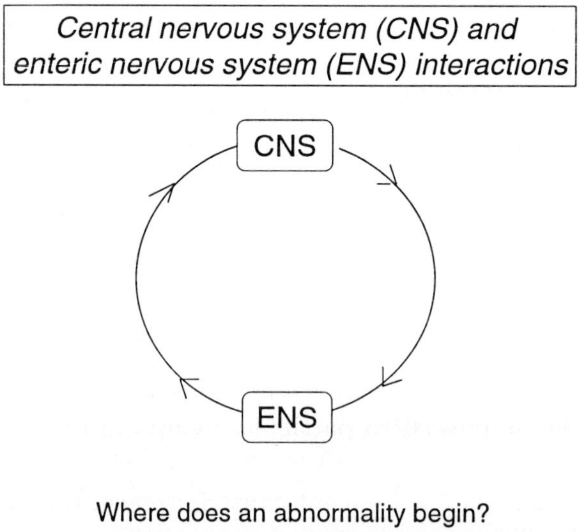


Fig. 1. Disturbances somewhere along the brain-gut axis are thought to be important in the pathogenesis of functional dyspepsia. Interactions between the central nervous system (CNS) and the enteric nervous system (ENS) involve both visceral efferent and afferent signals, some of which are mediated by the vagal nerve. Normally, efferent and afferent signals are balanced. When an imbalance is induced, as might be the case in functional dyspepsia, it is impossible to know where the disease begins or where it is located, centrally or peripherally.

We do not know where in the body functional gastrointestinal disorders begin. Consequently, we do not know where in the vicious circle to brake in for treatment. However, the good thing with a model like this is that it does not matter where the disease begins or where we apply the treatments. The pathogenetic mechanisms are all connected in a web of causation, which means that correcting one abnormality, central or peripheral, may break the vicious circle and generate a beneficial net result.

## 3. Conceptual Framework

A simple explanation of hypersensitivity to distension could be an abnormal firing of gastric mechanoreceptors coupled in series with smooth muscle cells. The response of the mechanoreceptors is then dependent on the contractile state of the smooth muscles, and distension of the stomach without prior proper adaptive relaxation of the muscles might be a key mechanism by which epigastric discomfort is elicited. Because functional dyspepsia patients often perceive considerable discomfort not only from the stomach, but from other organs as well, a central amplifying mechanism is thought to be involved. Whether visceral hypersensitivity merely is a combination of impaired gastric relaxation on one hand and "neuroticistic" amplification of afferent signals to the CNS on the other, we do not know.

Our working hypothesis for the pathogenesis of functional dyspepsia is illustrated in Fig. 2 (10). The association with psychological factors, like stress and neuroticism, is considered causal. The influence of stress on the stomach might be mediated by the vagus nerve, because we know that (acute) stress suppresses vagal tone, which is shown to be (chronically) low in these patients (11). A low vagal tone may impair vago-vagal reflexes regulating gastric emptying and accommodation and thus constitute an important mechanism by which the central nervous system modifies the function of the stomach (12).

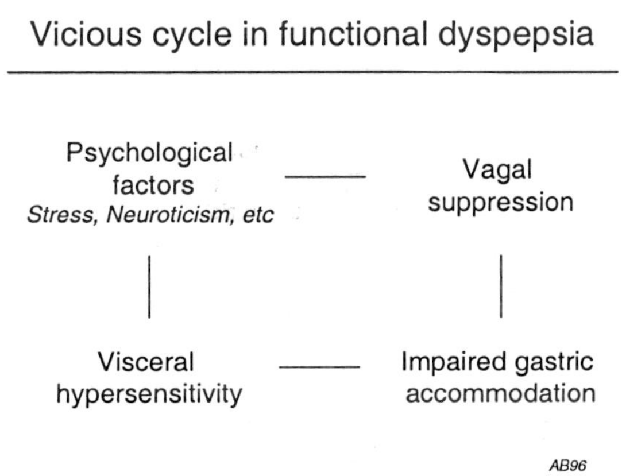


Fig. 2. A conceptual framework of functional dyspepsia:. When psychological factors like stress, neuroticism and depression are suppressing vagal activity, gastric relaxation in response to ingestion of food is impaired. This, in turn, impairs gastric accommodation and causes enhanced firing of tensoreceptors in the stomach wall in response to food intake. When the afferent signals are amplified centrally by a hypersensitive mind, visceral hypersensitivity and a vicious cycle may be created. The model implies that it does not matter where on the cycle we break in for treatment. Drugs acting centrally may work as well as those acting peripherally.

Impaired accommodation of the proximal stomach is shown by various techniques and by several research groups to be a characteristic feature of functional dyspepsia patients. The result is a relatively small proximal and a wide distal stomach in response to a meal (13). It appears as if the proximal stomach in functional dyspepsia patients is stiffer and allows less early postprandial accommodation of a meal as compared to healthy persons. Similar accommodation disturbances were seen after vagotomy and in patients with insulin dependent diabetes mellitus with vagal neuropathy. However, these patients complained of much less discomfort than patients with functional dyspepsia. The reason could be much less neuroticism among these patients or simply that the damaged vagal nerve allows less afferent signalling (14).

It is unlikely that symptom generation in functional dyspepsia is due to a wide range of gastric abnormalities. More likely the symptoms are caused by one single defect. Impaired receptive and adaptive gastric relaxation due to stress-induced suppression of vagal tone might be one such key mechanism by which several pathological findings (for instance, abnormal gastric accommodation) and symptoms (for instance, early satiety and epigastric fullness) in functional dyspepsia are generated. The model presented in Fig. 2 incorporates four established abnormalities in functional dyspepsia: increase in various psychological factors, low vagal tone, impaired gastric relaxation, and visceral hypersensitivity, in a logical interplay in one hypothetical pathophysiological mechanism.

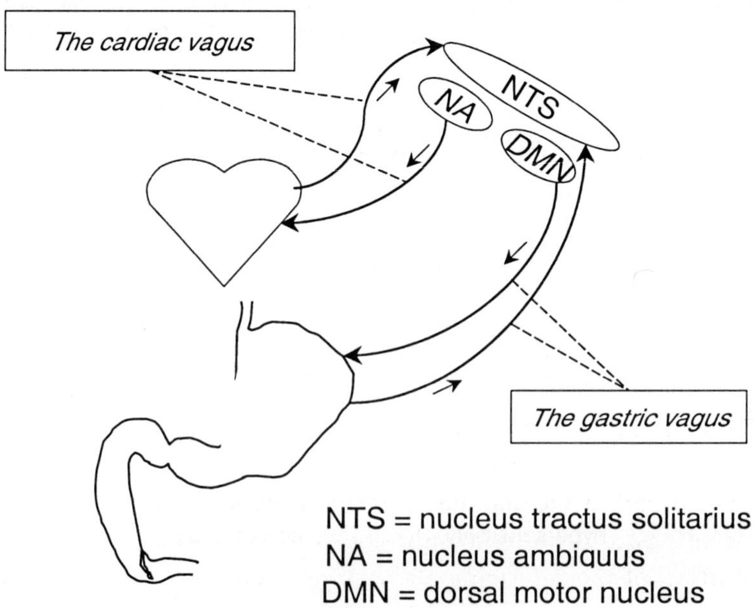


Fig. 3. Receptive and adaptive relaxation of the proximal stomach in response to ingestion of food is a vagally mediated and/or facilitated reflex allowing the proximal stomach to accommodate most of the meal without increase in intragastric pressure. Abdominal discomfort might be elicited when the stomach is distended by a meal without proper adaptive relaxation. Another possibility is that the afferent signals are triggered by hypersensitive mucosal chemoreceptors or by inflammation. Testing the activity in the gastric vagus nerve is impossible in man. For testing the cardiac vagal activity, respiratory sinus arrhythmia is used. The underlying assumption is that impairment of cardiac vagal activity also applies for the gastric activity.

## 4. Why Ultrasonography in Functional Dyspepsia

All kinds of acute stress, systemic or psychological, lead to the central release of corticotropin releasing factor (CRF), which in turn leads to the suppression of efferent vagal activity with various effects on secretion and motility in the upper gut, including delayed gastric emptying and presumably also impaired gastric accommodation (15). The latter is mediated by a vago-vagal reflex going to and from the vagal motor complex in the brainstem (Fig. 3). The reflex finely tunes the volume of the stomach to the size of the meal to avoid increase in intragastric pressure and perception of unpleasant fullness while eating. This reflex is most often studied by the gastric barostat, which is an air-filled balloon connected to a pump, which aspirates or installs air into the balloon to maintain a pre-set pressure within the stomach. By this technique, the normal accommodation to a meal is a volume increase (of the balloon) of around 400 ml. This impressive volume response tells that the reflex is important. In functional dyspepsia, this accommodation reflex is impaired in a large proportion of the patients.

Studying gastric accommodation with the barostat is a cumbersome, unpleasant and stressful procedure. Also, due to stress during the examination, the results might be poor measures of the normal gastric function of the patients.

Simply because functional dyspepsia is so strongly associated with psychological factors and stress, the examination should be performed in a quiet and relaxing atmosphere with a minimum of distress. Ultrasonography satisfies these criteria as it is non-invasive and does not by itself induce abnormal physiology in stress-responsive individuals. Hence, ultrasonography is a very attractive tool for investigating patients with functional disorders. Several studies from our group support the notion that ultrasonography may contribute a lot to the understanding of the pathophysiology of these conditions. Thus, gastric emptying, gastric distension, gastric accommodation, intragastric distribution and various motility indices can all be investigated using ultrasonography.

## 5. What Has Been Found in Functional Dyspepsia Using Ultrasound (Figs. 4–10)

### 5.1. *Wide gastric antrum*

Scintigraphic studies had indicated an abnormal intragastric distribution of liquid test meals within the stomach in patients with non-ulcer dyspepsia (16–18). However, scintigraphy exposes the subject to radiation and has relatively poor image resolution. Thus, we investigated whether ultrasonography, a radiation-free method, could be used to determine intragastric distribution of meals. Using the 2D ultrasonographic method of Bolondi *et al.* (19), Hausken *et al.* confirmed in several studies that a wide gastric antrum is a characteristic feature of patients with functional dyspepsia (13). In these patients, the antrum was wider 10 minutes after a liquid soup meal and also during fasting (11). Hveem *et al.* aspirated the content of the stomach during fasting and showed that the volume of the fasting content correlated with the width of the antrum (25).

Mean antral area was significantly wider in patients with non-ulcer dyspepsia (4.7 $cm^2$) than in controls (3.4 $cm^2$), and there was a significant correlation between width of the

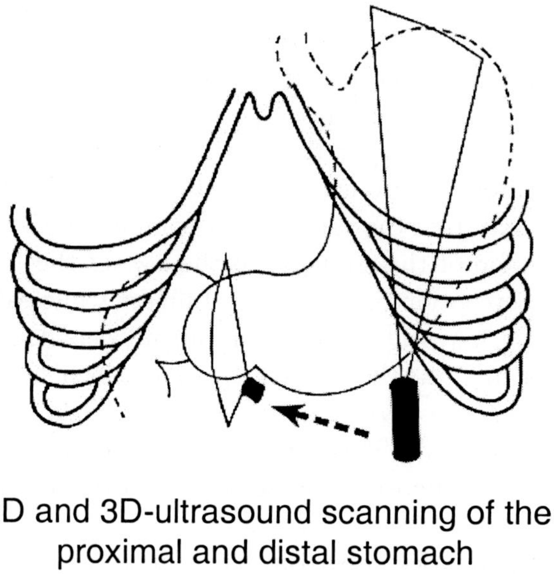


Fig. 4. Ultrasonography is an ideal tool for investigating patients with functional dyspepsia because it is non-invasive, radiation-free and allows repeated examinations without any discomfort to the patients. By new techniques both size, volume, and configuration of the proximal stomach, i.e. gastric accommodation, may be monitored. The figure indicates the position of the ultrasound probe used for two-dimensional (2D) and three-dimensional (3D) scanning of the proximal stomach.

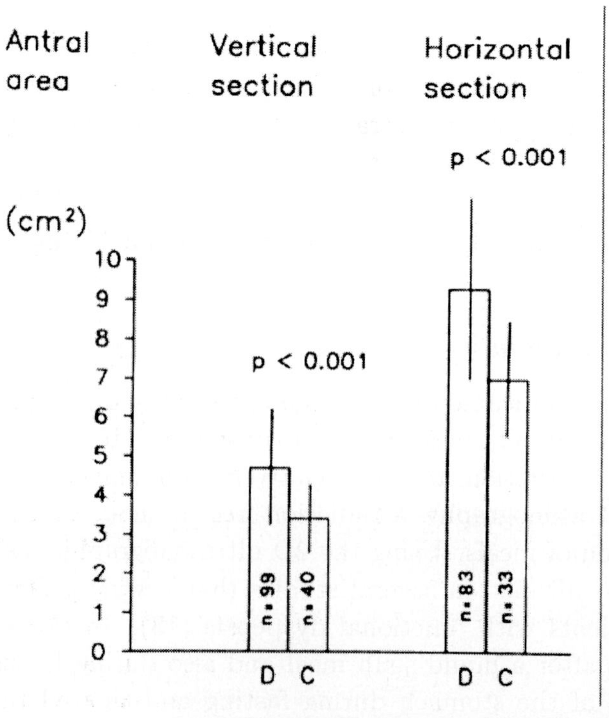


Fig. 5. Mean antral area in healthy control subjects (C) and in patients with non-ulcer dyspepsia and erosive prepyloric changes (D). (Vertical and horizontal sections).

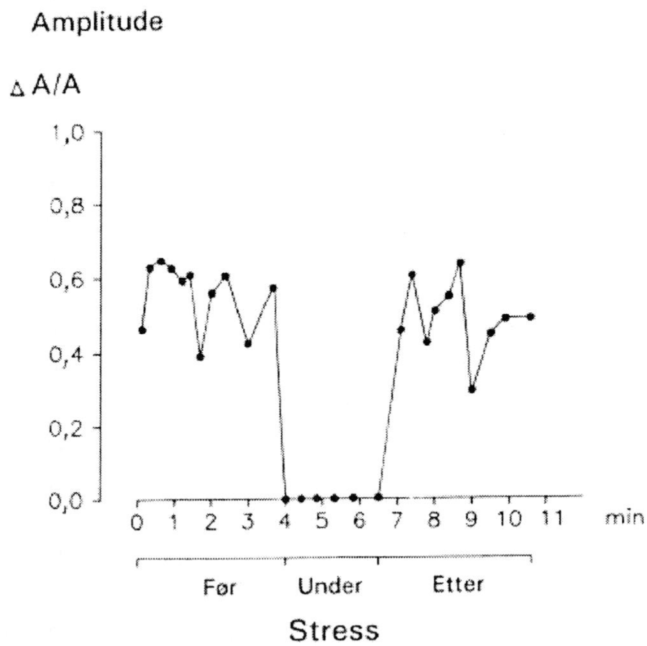


Fig. 6. Frequency and amplitudes of antral contractions can be monitored by external ultrasound. The figure shows amplitudes in a horizontal section of antral contractions before, during and after stress (by videoplay) in one healthy subject. Amplitudes are immediately decreased by stress. However, after cessation of stress, recovery is also quick.

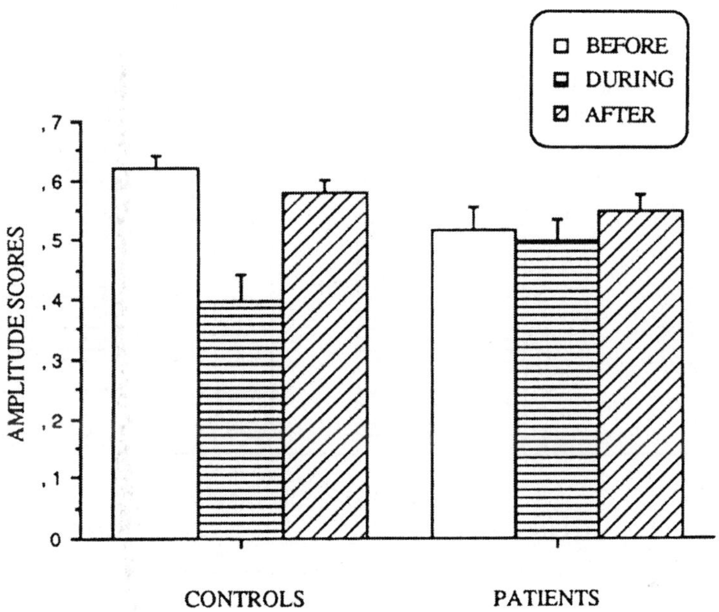


Fig. 7. Mean amplitude scores of antral contractions before, during, and after mental stress in healthy subjects (controls) and in patients with functional dyspepsia. The patients are less able to control antral activity than the controls.

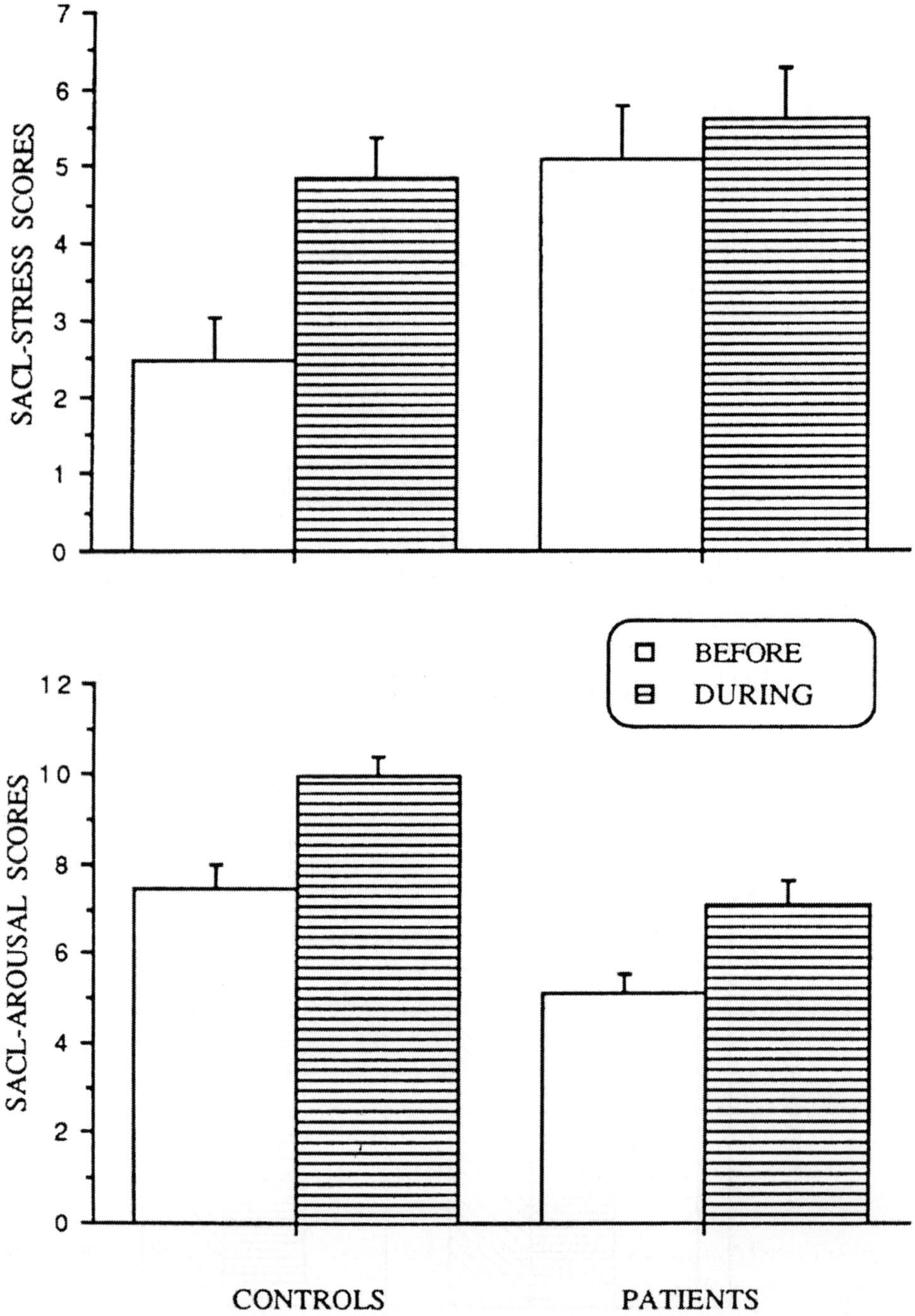


Fig. 8. In response to stress (during), healthy controls increase stress scores (upper panel) more than patients with functional dyspepsia. The patients are "stressed" already at baseline.

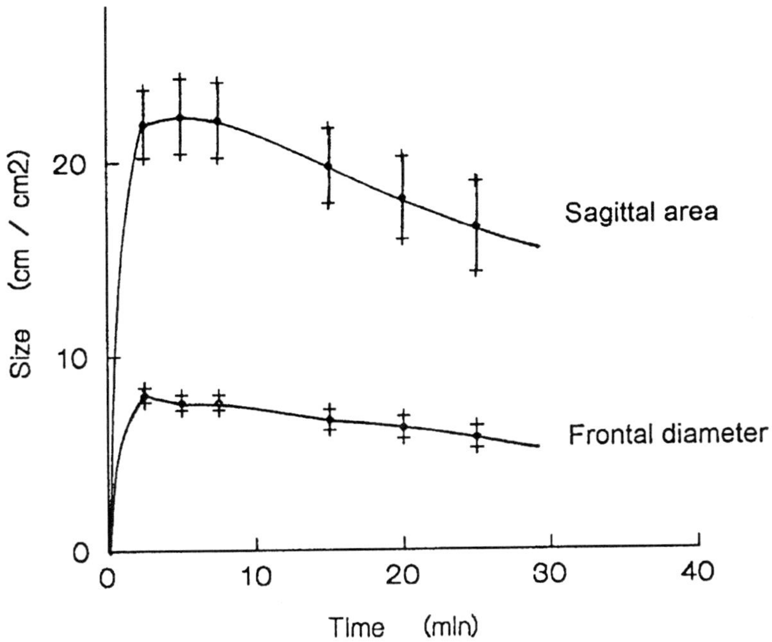


Fig. 9. Size of proximal stomach in response to food ingestion can be estimated by sagittal area and frontal diameter. (From Gilja *et al.* (32)).

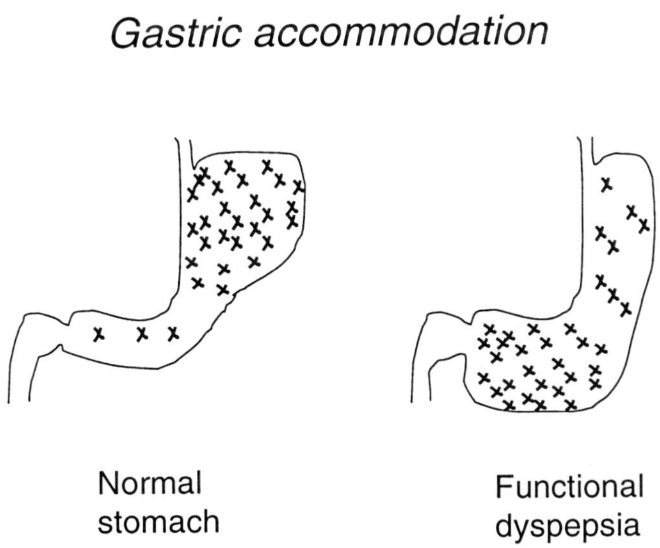


Fig. 10. Schematic drawing of gastric accommodation to a meal in functional dyspepsia. A wide gastric antrum and a small proximal stomach are typical. (From Berstad *et al.* (13)).

fasting gastric antrum and scores of abdominal bloating (20). Antral hypomotility (less than 5th percentile of controls) was seen in 32% and "wide" fasting antral area was seen in 35% of the patients. Treatment with cisapride reduced the enlarged antral area in non-ulcer dyspepsia patients. However, the symptomatic effect of cisapride was weak. Four weeks' treatment with cisapride 10 mg t.i.d. had a significant beneficial effect on the patients symptomatology only in 2, not in 4 weeks (21).

### 5.2. *Antral distension and postprandial fullness*

Hveem *et al.* showed that ingestion of both low and high nutrient drinks resulted in a decrease in hunger and in fullness. A direct relationship between fullness and the retention of the drink in the antrum was a novel observation consistent with the concept that fullness is related to antral distension. Both fullness and the magnitude of the increase in fullness after the drink were related to the increase in antral area and the scintigraphic content of the distal stomach. It was concluded that postprandial fullness, but not hunger, is closely related to antral distension (15, 22–27).

### 5.3. *Gastric emptying*

Two-dimensional (2D) ultrasonography is also utilized to assess gastric emptying. In the fasting state, the width of the antrum (in one single standardised section) reflects the amount of total fasting gastric juice. After a meal, gastric emptying can be monitored by repeated single 2D ultrasonic sections of the antrum. Hveem *et al.* found a good correlation between scintigraphic parameters of total stomach emptying and reduction of antral area as measured by ultrasound using both low (meat soup, 350 ml, 20 kcal) and high (dextrose, 350 ml, 300 kcal) nutrient liquids in healthy controls (24).

### 5.4. *Antral motility*

Frequency and amplitudes of antral contractions are the main ultrasonographic indexes of antral motility. Oral administration of the prostaglandin $E_2$ analogue enprostil in a single dose of 35 $\mu$g to 10 healthy volunteers reduced considerably antroduodenal co-ordination, frequency and amplitude of antral contractions, and size of antral area in response to ingestion of 500 ml of meat soup (28). The time during which the pylorus was wide open ($> 5$ mm) also increased after enprostil. The clinical effect of misoprostol, a prostaglandin $E_1$ analogue, was studied in 137 patients with non-ulcer dyspepsia and erosive prepyloric changes. Misoprostol had a significant worsening effect on epigastric pain, nausea, meteorism, lower abdominal pain, and diarrhoea, compared to placebo (29). Thus, opening the pylorus and facilitating gastric emptying by a prostaglandin analogue does not benefit these patients.

Patients with functional dyspepsia had smaller antral amplitudes in response to meat soup. In response to stress, however, patients with functional dyspepsia were unable to reduce postprandial amplitudes of antral contractions, as did healthy persons. Stress reduced mainly the amplitudes of antral contractions. Cisapride had no effect on these stress-induced responses (15).

Antral contractions and propagation were monitored simultaneously by concurrent manometry and ultrasound. Good concordance between the two methods was obtained with low inter-observer variability. Ultrasound was more sensitive than manometry in detecting wall motion and propagation of peristalsis (23).

### 5.5. *Transpyloric flow*

Soon after ingestion of meat soup, transpyloric flow commences without visible contractions of the gastroduodenal segment. Such emptying commenced significantly sooner in subjects without symptoms (24 sec) than in those with symptoms (70 sec) ($p = 0.02$). Duodenogastric reflux was not related to symptom profiles (30). In order to relate initial early transpyloric emptying and antral motility to early postprandial symptoms, twelve patients with functional dyspepsia were investigated with duplex sonography during 3 minutes of fasting, during 3 minutes of ingesting 500 ml of meat soup, and during the first 10 minutes postprandially (31). Gastric emptying commenced on an average of 52 seconds after the start of ingestion. Pendulating, transpyloric flow not generated by antral contractions appeared before contractile, peristaltic related flow, which commenced after an average of 116 seconds. Epigastric discomfort was experienced after the commencement of transpyloric flow by all patients, on average after 143 seconds. A negative correlation was found between intensity of fullness and duration of the time interval between commencement of transpyloric flow and commencement of symptoms. The occurrence of symptoms after the commencement of gastric emptying suggests that tasting of ingested material by duodenal chemo-receptors is involved in symptom generation. The inverse relationship between the duration of the tasting period, i.e. the period with pendulating, peristaltic-unrelated transpyloric flow, and intensity of fullness, suggests that the duration of the tasting period may have been too short in many of the dyspeptic patients. Possibly, proper gastric accommodation of a meal depends on duodenal tasting of the ingested material. If this tasting is inadequate and, as a consequence, reflex relaxation of the gastric musculature is impaired, the symptoms could be caused by undue stretching of the gastric mechanoreceptors coupled in series with the (still) contracted muscle cells.

### 5.6. *Small proximal stomach*

The proximal stomach had long been considered inaccessible for ultrasonic imaging because of its position behind the costal margins and the frequent presence of air pockets. However, by using the ultrasonographic area in a sagittal section and the maximal diameter in an oblique frontal section, Gilja *et al.* were able to monitor the postprandial size of the proximal stomach (32). By this technique they proved the existence of an impaired proximal gastric accommodation to a meal in patients with functional dyspepsia (33). Impaired proximal stomach accommodation was in fact a much more prevalent finding than a wide gastric antrum. The results suggest that in patients with functional dyspepsia, poor proximal accommodation may constitute the primary defect, the wide gastric antrum being a secondary consequence of a defect in the reservoir function of the proximal stomach.

Because NO is a key neurotransmitter in the reflex regulating adaptive relaxation, it was tempting to administer glyceryl trinitrate, an exogenous donor of NO, to patients with functional dyspepsia to examine if it would improve gastric accommodation and symptoms in response to a meal (34). In a double blind placebo-controlled cross-over study, Gilja *et al.* demonstrated that glyceryl trinitrate caused a concomitant improvement of proximal gastric accommodation and epigastric pain, nausea and total symptom scores in response to a meat soup meal (35).

### 5.7. *Stomach volume (3D-reconstruction)*

Volume estimation based on 2D sonograms is subject to significant errors because assumptions regarding configuration of the antrum have to be made prior to calculations. To overcome this limitation, we developed a method for volume estimation of organs based on 3D ultrasonography (36). This 3D ultrasound system demonstrated excellent accuracy *in vitro* both on phantoms and on animal organs, and intra- and interobserver variation was low also *in vivo* on human stomach (37). When validated *in vivo* against Magnetic Resonance Imaging, this 3D ultrasound system was in good agreement and presented in high precision (38).

A tilting device to acquire 3D ultrasound images was applied to explore whether antral volumes of patients with functional dyspepsia differed from healthy controls. In our first study, antral volumes were larger and postprandial antral filling was more pronounced in non-ulcer dyspepsia patients than in healthy controls. The soup meal induced dyspeptic symptoms in 15/17 of the patients and in only 2/18 of the controls. In another study, in 20 patients with functional dyspepsia and 20 healthy controls, we found no significant differences in antral volumes between dyspeptic patients and controls, neither fasting nor postprandially. The patients suffered more symptoms in response to the soup than controls ($p = 0.004$), but no significant correlation between antral volumes and symptoms was detected. Fasting antral volumes in *H. pylori* positive dyspeptics were smaller than in *H. pylori* negative patients ($p = 0.03$) (13).

Using 2D ultrasonography, Ahluwalia *et al.* found that the average values for postprandial antral width were similar in a group of functional dyspepsia patients compared to healthy controls, but the range of the values was significantly wider in patients than in controls (39). Thus, a wide gastric antrum may not be a consistent finding in functional dyspepsia. The divergent results might be due to a wide normal range of antral sizes and great overlap between the groups, making patient selection and group size important.

### 5.8. *Volume estimation with magnetic scanhead tracking*

In our previous ultrasonographic studies, only the most proximal and distal parts of the stomach are visualized for measurements, leaving a large portion of the stomach in between unseen. These shortcomings may be solved by recent developments in ultrasonography and data management.

Random or free-hand acquisition of 3D ultrasound data has been achieved using mechanical, acoustic and electromagnetic devices to locate the exact position and orientation of the transducer in space (36). Magnetic systems maintain the flexibility and smoothness of free-hand scanning, in contrast to mechanical tilting devices. The acoustic systems are limited by the fact that they do not tolerate physical interruptions of the acoustic wave without accuracy being compromised substantially. Accordingly, to enable scanning of a large organ like the fluid-filled stomach, a commercially available magnetometer-based position and orientation measurement (POM) device was interfaced. This system for magnetic scanhead tracking has been validated both with respect to its precision in locating specific points in space and to its accuracy in volume estimation. In these studies, the sensor system worked well in scanning human organs, and high precision and accuracy were revealed in point location and volume estimation (40).

This magnetic system was used to scan stomachs both *in vitro* and *in vivo*. It showed excellent *in vitro* accuracy, calculated gastric emptying rates more precisely than 2D ultrasound, and enabled estimation of intragastric distribution of a soup meal.

In a study on healthy subjects, the meal filled the stomach with a relatively high initial proximal/distal volume ratio, declining as the meal emptied. Interestingly, retrograde flow from the distal to the proximal stomach (assessed by proximal/distal volume shifts) occurred in 11% of measurement periods, and it was observed in half of the examinations. It is worth noting that there was a high intersubject variability in the proximal/distal ratio, a fact that questions the value of intragastric distribution being a useful parameter in diagnosis and work-up of patients. Nevertheless, further development of hardware and software for 3D ultrasonic image acquisition is in progress and may improve spatial and temporal resolution of this technique significantly, thus enabling a more precise and consistent division of the gastric compartments.

## 6. Similar Gastric Motor Abnormalities in Functional Dyspepsia, in Insulin-Dependent Diabetes Mellitus, and in Gallstone Disease

### 6.1. *Patients with diabetes mellitus*

Patients with insulin-dependent diabetes mellitus often display low heart rate variability indicating cardiac vagal neuropathy. Consistently, these patients also have slow gastric emptying, wide antral area and impaired accommodation of the proximal stomach in response to a meal, both when examined by barostat and by ultrasonography. The finding suggest that the disease damages not only the cardiac, but the gastric vagal nerves as well (14, 36, 41–43).

### 6.2. *Patients with gallstone disease*

Following cholecystectomy for uncomplicated gallstone disease some patients experience persistent symptoms suggesting an underlying functional disorder. We compared patients with symptomatic gallbladder stone disease with functional dyspepsia patients and healthy individuals with respect to putative pathogenetic mechanisms for dyspepsia (44). Gallbladder and gastric antrum volumes were estimated with three-dimensional (3D) ultrasonography before and ten minutes after ingestion of 500 ml of meat soup. Volume estimation was performed digitally after interactive manual tracing and organ reconstruction in three dimensions. Vagal tone was indexed by respiratory sinus arrhythmia. No significant differences were found between groups with respect to fasting gallbladder volume or gallbladder emptying. Antral volumes both fasting ($p < 0.05$) and postprandially ($p < 0.01$) were larger in gallbladder stone disease and in functional dyspepsia than in controls. The soup meal induced dyspeptic symptoms in 2/18 (11%) of controls, in 12/18 (67%) of patients with gallbladder stone disease and in 15/17 (88%) of patients with functional dyspepsia. Compared with controls, both gallbladder stone disease and functional dyspepsia patients had significantly decreased vagal tone ($p < 0.001$). There was no significant difference between gallbladde rstone disease and functional dyspepsia patients with respect to antral volume, vagal tone or symptoms. In conclusion, both gallbladder stone and functional dyspepsia patients are characterised by dyspeptic symptoms in response to ingestion of 500 ml meat soup, a wide gastric antrum, low vagal tone, but normal gallbladder size and emptying. Thus, patients with symptomatic, uncomplicated gallbladder stone disease and patients with functional dyspepsia have common pathogenetic mechanisms. Consequently, one may speculate whether gallbladder stone disease is, in fact, a serious complication of functional dyspepsia.

## 7. The Ultrasound Meal Accommodation Test

The Ultrasound Meal Accommodation Test (UMAT) was developed at Haukeland University Hospital on the basis of close interaction between scientific and clinical work in patients with dyspepsia. Before entering the protocol, the patients have been carefully worked-up with history, physical examination, blood tests, testing for *H. pylori*, and upper endoscopy. In some cases, additional examinations are performed to rule out organic causes for their symptoms. The protocol presented here is the mainstream *clinical* protocol. In scientific studies, other elements are often added.

### 7.1. *Test meal*

A 500 ml liquid meal of commercial meat soup (Toro® clear meat soup, Rieber & Søn A/S, Bergen, Norway) containing 1.8 g protein, 0.9 g bovine fat, and 1.1 g carbohydrate (20 kcal) is ingested over a period of 4 min. The soup is preheated and then cooled to 37°C to improve imaging quality by reducing the amount of air bubbles.

### 7.2. *Ultrasound scanning*

Patients are usually examined between 08:00 and 10:30 a.m. after overnight fasting. The individuals are scanned while sitting in a chair, leaning slightly backwards at an angle of 120°. Transducers in the range 2.5 to 5 MHz and both annular and curved arrays have been used for scanning. Two standardised sonographic image sections are chosen to measure the size of the proximal stomach (32). First, a sagittal section with the left renal pelvis in a longitudinal projection with the left lobe of the liver and the tail of the pancreas as internal landmarks, are recorded. Then the transducer is rotated 90° clockwise to obtain an oblique frontal section where the left hemidiaphragm, the top margin of the fundus and the liver parenchyma serve as landmarks. In the distal stomach, we apply a standard 2D sagittal section in which the aorta, the superior mesenteric vein, and the gastric antrum are visualized simultaneously (20, 45).

### 7.3. *Measurements*

An area of the proximal stomach in a sagittal section (SA) is outlined by tracing from the top margin of the fundus and 7 cm downward along the axis of the stomach. Then, the maximal diameter in an oblique frontal section (OFD), kept within 7 cm along the long axis of the proximal stomach is measured. In the distal stomach, an area is outlined by tracing the outer profile of the muscularis propria. In some cases, a 3D ultrasonographic examination is also performed (36).

### 7.4. *Evaluation of symptoms*

The patients are asked to evaluate their symptoms before and after the soup meal using visual analogue scales (VAS). The questionnaire often contains one VAS for pain, discomfort, nausea, fullness, bloating, feeling of hunger, as well as one VAS for total symptoms (37).

### 7.5. *Psychological assessment*

In order to characterize the patients regarding personality and possible psychopathology, they usually receive two self-rating instruments on the day of the examination. Eysenck Personality Questionnaire, Neuroticism scale (EPQ-N) is applied to indicate a general lifestyle of hyperresponsiveness or emotional overreactiveness. General Health Questionnaire (GHQ-28+) and Hospital Anxiety and Depression scale (HAD) are used to detect psychiatric morbidity in a somatic setting and to evaluate quality of life. In addition, other questionnaires are also used attempting to explore psychopathological mechanisms for their symptoms for further referral to a psychiatrist.

### 7.6. *Evaluation of vagal and sympathetic activity*

In som patients, we also apply measurement of vagal activity by Respiratory Sinus Arrythmia (RSA), as low vagal tone has been reported in functional dyspepsia (11, 12). Sympathetic activity is measured by skin conductance.

*Procedure*

(1) Ordinary ultrasound examination of the liver, gallbladder, biliary tract, spleen, pancreas, kidneys, and large vessels.

(2) Evaluation of fasting symptoms by VAS.

(3) Assessment of fasting motility pattern (phase I–III) by observing the pattern of contractility in the antrum.

(4) Measurement of fasting area of the distal stomach.

(5) Visualization of the proximal stomach to explore whether it is empty.

(6) 500 ml of preheated meat soup is ingested in 4 min at a constant speed.

(7) Postprandially the sagittal area (SA), the oblique frontal diameter (OFD), and·the antral area (AA) are measured.

(8) Postprandial symptom evaluation after 5 min.

(9) 10 min postprandially: SA, OFD, and AA measurement.

(10) 20 min postprandially: SA, OFD, and AA measurement.

(11) 30 min postprandially: SA, OFD, and AA measurement.

(12) Late postprandial symptom evaluation.

(13) AA is usually measured until fasting levels are reached for estimation of gastric emptying time.

In conjunction with the provocation test, psychometric tests are performed to improve our understanding of the symptoms and to tailor further work-up and treatment of the patient. Finally, the patient is informed about the findings and given appropriate advice and treatment.

## Conclusion

Claims that no findings are made in functional dyspepsia patients are not true. Both endoscopic and ultrasonographic imaging show changes (erosive prepyloric changes and accommodation abnormalities, respectively) in a high percentage of the patients. The diagnostic sensitivity and specificity of the changes are not yet known. The fact that they are also seen in several other conditions characterized by dyspepsia, for instance in gallstone disease, may indicate that they are linked to epigastric discomfort in general, and not to a specific dyspeptic condition. In our lab, we apply a meal provocation test (The Ultrasound Meal Accommodation Test) to study pathogenetic mechanisms and to tailor specific managements in these patients. For further understanding and treatment of dyspepsia, more attention should be paid to drugs improving gastric accommodation to a meal. In this context, ultrasonographic imaging may become an easily accessible, convenient, and reliable method for diagnosis and evaluation of the effects of treatment.

## References

1. Nesland, A. and Berstad, A., Erosive prepyloric changes in persons with and without dyspepsia. Scand J Gastroenterol 1985; 20: 222–228.
2. Nesland, A., Oktedalen, O., Opstad, P. K., Serck-Hanssen, A., Aase, S. and Berstad, A., Erosive prepyloric changes — A manifestation of stress? Scand J Gastroenterol 1989; 24: 522–528.
3. Tack, J., Piessevaux, H., Coulie, B., Caenepeel, P. and Janssens, J., Role of impaired gastric accommodation to a meal in functional dyspepsia. Gastroenterology 1998; 115: 1346–1352.
4. Tack, J., Caenepeel, P., Fischler, B., Piessevaux, H. and Janssens, J., Symptoms associated with hypersensitivity to gastric distention in functional dyspepsia. Gastroenterology 2001; 121: 526–535.
5. Wilhelmsen, I., Haug, T. T., Ursin, H. and Berstad, A., Discriminant analysis of factors distinguishing patients with functional dyspepsia from patients with duodenal ulcer. Significance of somatization. Dig Dis Sci 1995; 40: 1105–1111.
6. Wilhelmsen, I., Somatization, sensitization, and functional dyspepsia. Scand J Psychol 2002; 43, 177–180. Ref Type: Generic.
7. Haug, T. T., Svebak, S., Wilhelmsen, I., Berstad, A. and Ursin, H., Psychological factors and somatic symptoms in functional dyspepsia. A comparison with duodenal ulcer and healthy controls. J Psychosom Res 1994; 38: 281–291.
8. Haug, T. T., Wilhelmsen, I., Ursin, H. and Berstad, A., What are the real problems for patients with functional dyspepsia? Scand J Gastroenterol 1995; 30: 97–100.
9. Lydeard, S. and Jones, R., Factors affecting the decision to consult with dyspepsia: comparison of consulters and non-consulters. J R Coll Gen Pract 1989; 39: 495–498.
10. Berstad, A., Today's therapy of functional gastrointestinal disorders — Does it help? Eur J Surg Suppl 1998; 92–97.

11. Hausken, T., Svebak, S., Wilhelmsen, I., Haug, T. T., Olafsen, K., Pettersson, E., Hveem, K. and Berstad, A., Low vagal tone and antral dysmotility in patients with functional dyspepsia. Psychosom Med 1993; 55: 12–22.
12. Haug, T. T., Svebak, S., Hausken, T., Wilhelmsen, I., Berstad, A. and Ursin, H., Low vagal activity as mediating mechanism for the relationship between personality factors and gastric symptoms in functional dyspepsia. Psychosom Med 1994; 56: 181–186.
13. Berstad, A., Hausken, T., Gilja, O. H., Nesland, A. and Odegaard, S., Imaging studies in dyspepsia. Eur J Surg Suppl 1998; 42–49.
14. Undeland, K. A., Hausken, T., Gilja, O. H., Aanderud, S. and Berstad, A., Gastric meal accommodation and symptoms in diabetes. A placebo-controlled study of glyceryl trinitrate. Eur J Gastroenterol Hepatol 1998; 10: 677–681.
15. Hveem, K., Hausken, T., Svebak, S. and Berstad, A., Gastric antral motility in functional dyspepsia. Effect of mental stress and cisapride. Scand J Gastroenterol 1996; 31: 452–457.
16. Scott, A. M., Kellow, J. E., Shuter, B., Cowan, H., Corbett, A. M., Riley, J. W., Lunzer, M. R., Eckstein, R. P., Hoschl, R. and Lam, S. K., Intragastric distribution and gastric emptying of solids and liquids in functional dyspepsia. Lack of influence of symptom subgroups and H. pylori-associated gastritis. Dig Dis Sci 1993; 38: 2247–2254.
17. Troncon, L. E., Bennett, R. J., Ahluwalia, N. K. and Thompson, D. G., Abnormal intragastric distribution of food during gastric emptying in functional dyspepsia patients. Gut 1994; 35: 327–332.
18. Mangnall, Y., Houghton, L., Johnson, A. and Read, N. W., Abnormal distribution of a fatty liquid test meal within the stomach of patients with non-ulcer dyspepsia. Eur J Gastroenterol Hepatol 1994; 6: 323–327.
19. Bolondi, L., Bortolotti, M., Santi, V., Calletti, T., Gaiani, S. and Labo, G., Measurement of gastric emptying time by real-time ultrasonography. Gastroenterology 1985; 89: 752–759.
20. Hausken, T. and Berstad, A., Wide gastric antrum in patients with non-ulcer dyspepsia. Effect of cisapride. Scand J Gastroenterol 1992; 27: 427–432.
21. Hausken, T. and Berstad, A., Cisapride treatment of patients with non-ulcer dyspepsia and erosive prepyloric changes. A double-blind, placebo-controlled trial. Scand J Gastroenterol 1992; 27: 213–217.
22. Hveem, K., Svebak, S., Hausken, T. and Berstad, A., Effect of mental stress and cisapride on autonomic nerve functions in functional dyspepsia. Scand J Gastroenterol 1998; 33: 123–127.
23. Hveem, K., Sun, W. M., Hebbard, G., Horowitz, M., Doran, S. and Dent, J., Relationship between ultrasonically detected phasic antral contractions and antral pressure. Am J Physiol Gastrointest Liver Physiol 2001; 281: G95–101.
24. Hveem, K., Jones, K. L., Chatterton, B. E. and Horowitz, M., Scintigraphic measurement of gastric emptying and ultrasonographic assessment of antral area: relation to appetite. Gut 1996; 38: 816–821.
25. Hveem, K., Hausken, T. and Berstad, A., Ultrasonographic assessment of fasting liquid content in the human stomach. Scand J Gastroenterol 1994; 29: 786–789.
26. Hveem, K., Hausken, T. and Berstad, A., Ultrasonographic assessment of fasting liquid content in the human stomach. Scand J Gastroenterol 1994; 29: 786–789.
27. Jones, K. L., Doran, S. M., Hveem, K., Bartholomeusz, F. D., Morley, J. E., Sun, W. M., Chatterton, B. E. and Horowitz, M., Relation between postprandial satiation and antral area in normal subjects. Am J Clin Nutr 1997; 66: 127–132.
28. Hausken, T., Odegaard, S. and Berstad, A., Antroduodenal motility studied by real-time ultrasonography. Effect of enprostil. Gastroenterology 1991; 100: 59–63.

29. Hausken, T., Stene-Larsen, G., Lange, O., Aronsen, O., Nerdrum, T., Hegbom, F., Schulz, T. and Berstad, A., Misoprostol treatment exacerbates abdominal discomfort in patients with non-ulcer dyspepsia and erosive prepyloric changes. A double-blind, placebo-controlled, multicentre study. Scand J Gastroenterol 1990; 25: 1028–1033.
30. Hausken, T., Odegaard, S., Matre, K. and Berstad, A., Antroduodenal motility and movements of luminal contents studied by duplex sonography. Gastroenterology 1992; 102: 1583–1590.
31. Hausken, T., Gilja, O. H., Undeland, K. A. and Berstad, A., Timing of postprandial dyspeptic symptoms and transpyloric passage of gastric contents. Scand J Gastroenterol 1998; 33: 822–827.
32. Gilja, O. H., Hausken, T., Odegaard, S. and Berstad, A., Monitoring postprandial size of the proximal stomach by ultrasonography. J Ultrasound Med 1995; 14: 81–89.
33. Gilja, O. H., Hausken, T., Wilhelmsen, I. and Berstad, A., Impaired accommodation of proximal stomach to a meal in functional dyspepsia. Dig Dis Sci 1996; 41: 689–696.
34. Hausken, T. and Berstad, A., Effect of glyceryl trinitrate on antral motility and symptoms in patients with functional dyspepsia. Scand J Gastroenterol 1994; 29: 23–28.
35. Gilja, O. H., Hausken, T., Bang, C. J. and Berstad, A., Effect of glyceryl trinitrate on gastric accommodation and symptoms in functional dyspepsia. Dig Dis Sci 1997; 42: 2124–2131.
36. Gilja, O. H., Detmer, P. R., Jong, J. M., Leotta, D. F., Li, X. N., Beach, K. W., Martin, R. and Strandness, DE, Jr., Intragastric distribution and gastric emptying assessed by three-dimensional ultrasonography. Gastroenterology 1997; 113: 38–49.
37. Tefera, S., Gilja, O. H., Olafsdottir, E., Hausken, T., Hatlebakk, J. G. and Berstad, A., Intragastric maldistribution of a liquid meal in patients with reflux oesophagitis assessed by three dimensional ultrasonography. Gut 2002; 50: 153–158.
38. Gilja, O. H., Smievoll, A. I., Thune, N., Matre, K., Hausken, T., Odegaard, S. and Berstad, A., *In vivo* comparison of 3D ultrasonography and magnetic resonance imaging in volume estimation of human kidneys. Ultrasound Med Biol 1995; 21: 25–32.
39. Ahluwalia, N. K., Thompson, D. G., Mamtora, H. and Hindle, J., Evaluation of gastric antral motor performance in patients with dysmotility-like dyspepsia using real-time high-resolution ultrasound. Neurogastroenterol Motil 1996; 8: 333–338.
40. Gilja, O. H., Hausken, T., Olafsson, S., Matre, K. and Odegaard, S., *In vitro* evaluation of three-dimensional ultrasonography based on magnetic scanhead tracking. Ultrasound Med Biol 1998; 24: 1161–1167.
41. Undeland, K. A., Hausken, T., Gilja, O. H., Ropert, R., Galmiche, J. P. and Berstad, A., Gastric relaxation in response to a soup meal in healthy subjects. A study using a barostat in the proximal stomach. Scand J Gastroenterol 1995; 30: 1069–1076.
42. Undeland, K. A., Hausken, T., Aanderud, S. and Berstad, A., Lower postprandial gastric volume response in diabetic patients with vagal neuropathy. Neurogastroenterol Motil 1997; 9: 19–24.
43. Undeland, K. A., Hausken, T., Svebak, S., Aanderud, S. and Berstad, A., Wide gastric antrum and low vagal tone in patients with diabetes mellitus type 1 compared to patients with functional dyspepsia and healthy individuals. Dig Dis Sci 1996; 41: 9–16.
44. Hausken, T., Sondenaa, K., Svebak, S., Gilja, O. H., Olafsson, S., Odegaard, S., Soreide, O. and Berstad A., Common pathogenetic mechanisms in symptomatic, uncomplicated gallstone disease and functional dyspepsia: Volume measurement of gallbladder and antrum using three-dimensional ultrasonography. Dig Dis Sci 1997; 42: 2505–2512.
45. Hausken, T., Svebak, S., Wilhelmsen, I., Tangen Haug T., Olafsen, K., Pettersson, E., Hveem, K. and Berstad, A., Low vagal tone and antral dysmotility in patients with functional dyspepsia. Psychosom Med 1993; 55: 12–22.

Published with permission

*Digestive Diseases and Sciences, Vol. 41, No. 4 (April 1996), pp. 689–696*

# Impaired Accommodation of Proximal Stomach to a Meal in Functional Dyspepsia

O.H. GILJA, MD, T. HAUSKEN, MD, PhD, I. WILHELMSEN, MD, PhD, and A. BERSTAD, MD, PhD

In patients with functional dyspepsia, scanning by a novel ultrasonographic method was carried out to investigate postprandial accommodation of the proximal stomach. Twenty patients with functional dyspepsia and 20 controls were scanned fasting in a sitting position after drinking 500 ml meat soup. Images were recorded up to 25 min after the ingestion period using an ultrasound sector scanner with a 3.25-MHz transducer. The area in a sagittal section and the maximal diameter in an oblique frontal section were chosen as the main variables for calculating the emptying fraction of the proximal stomach, defined as: $(aV_{2.5min} - aV_{actual}/aV_{2.5min}$. All subjects were asked to score total symptoms (1–9) provoked by the meal. From 7.5 to 25 min after the ingestion period the patients exhibited both smaller area in the sagittal section ($P < 0.018$) and shorter diameter in the frontal section ($P < 0.046$) compared with healthy controls, and they suffered more symptoms in response to the meal ($P = 0.002$). Dyspeptic patients revealed higher emptying fractions ($P = 0.0005$, ANOVA), and *H. pylori* status did not influence the emptying fractions. Diagnostic sensitivity of the method at 20 min postprandially was 70% and the specificity was 65%. Patients with functional dyspepsia have impaired accommodation of the proximal stomach to a meal, temporarily related to symptom induction.

**KEY WORDS:** accommodation; adaptive relaxation; stomach; gastric emptying; ultrasonography; gastric physiology; functional dyspepsia.

Accommodation of the human stomach to a meal is a specialized motor function of the gastric corpus–fundus enabling high volume increase with minimal rise in intragastric pressure (1, 2). After an initial receptive relaxation of the proximal stomach induced by swallowing and bolus passage through the esophagus (3), an ongoing adaptive relaxation (4, 5) occurs providing the meal with a reservoir in the proximal stomach from which it is delivered to the antrum for grinding and final emptying through the pylorus.

The reservoir function of the proximal stomach has been studied both scintigraphically and by use of different balloon devices in patients with functional dyspepsia. Radionuclide methods have disclosed a delayed total gastric emptying (6) of both liquids (7) and solids (8, 9) in a subset of these patients. Furthermore, intragastric maldistribution of the meal, observed as a relatively higher portion of the meal residing in the antrum rather than in the proximal stomach, seems to be evident in these patients (10) and when total gastric emptying is normal (11).

Isobaric distension of the stomach (12) has shown that patients with functional dyspepsia exhibit a lower threshold to perception of visceral pain (13–15). These studies also advocate, although it has not been tested during meal ingestion, that the compliance of the proximal stomach is not altered in dyspeptic patients. The presence of an artificial balloon in the proximal stomach is known to influence the normal gastric physiology (16–18); thus a noninvasive

Manuscript received July 16, 1995; revised manuscript received December 19, 1995; accepted January 2, 1996.

From the Medical Department A and Department of Psychiatry, Haukeland Hospital, University of Bergen, Bergen, Norway.

Address for reprint requests: Dr. Odd Helge Gilja, Medical Department A, Haukeland Hospital, University of Bergen, N-5021 Bergen, Norway.



0163-2116/96/0400-0689$09.50/0 

Published with permission



TABLE 1. CHARACTERISTICS OF 20 PATIENTS WITH FUNCTIONAL DYSPEPSIA AND 20 HEALTHY CONTROLS AT ENTRY TO STUDY*

| | *Patients* | *Controls* |
|---|---|---|
| Male/female ratio | 6/14 | 6/14 |
| Median age (range), years | 38 (18–61) | 27 (22–50) |
| Mean weight ± SD, kg | 66 ± 7 | 64 ± 10 |
| Mean height ± SD, cm | 171 ± 8 | 171 ± 10 |
| Smokers | 8 | 5 |

*None of the differences between the groups are statistically significant.

method to evaluate the size of the proximal stomach during accommodation to a meal may yield significant information.

Transabdominal ultrasonography is a noninvasive and radiation-free method that has proven applicable in the study of antral motility in patients with functional dyspepsia (19, 20), partly due to the fact that it leaves gastric motility undisturbed. We have developed and evaluated a sonographic method to estimate postprandial size and emptying fraction of the proximal stomach (21). The objective of the present study was to investigate the accommodation of the proximal stomach and its relation to symptoms in patients with functional dyspepsia by using a soup meal, previously shown to induce symptoms in these patients (22, 23).

## MATERIALS AND METHODS

**Subjects.** Consecutive patients referred for upper gastrointestinal endoscopy were recruited to participate in the trial. A history of dyspeptic complaints for a minimum of three months and at least seven of the last 14 days were required to enter the study. All patients reported epigastric pain or discomfort as their main symptom, and one or more of the following symptoms were present: bloating, nausea, vomiting, early satiety, and postprandial fullness. Symptoms of irritable bowel syndrome could be present, but upper dyspepsia had to be the dominating complaint. No organic explanation for their symptoms was found during endoscopy or ultrasonography of the upper abdomen.

Twenty patients with functional dyspepsia, 6 men and 14 women, median age 38 years (range 18–61 years) were included in the study (Table 1). Six patients were *H. pylori* positive, as evaluated by rapid urease test or [$^{14}$C]urea breath test. Patients with functional dyspepsia had a mean symptom duration of 64 months, and the mean duration of symptoms in the 14 preceding days just prior to the investigation was 12.4 days. Twelve patients (60%) reported early satiety, 13 patients (65%) complained of nausea, and 14 (70%) patients stated that their symptoms were meal-related.

Criteria of exclusion from the study were serious systemic disease or possible malignant disease; clinical evidence of myalgia of the abdominal muscles; past surgery of the upper gastrointestinal tract; previous peptic ulcer disease; alcoholism; diseases of the liver, pancreas, or bile ducts; pregnancy or lactation; or drugs known to influence gastrointestinal motility.

Twenty healthy controls, 6 men and 14 women, median age 27 years (range 22–50 years) were recruited from medical students and staff at Haukeland Hospital (Table 1). The differences between patients and healthy controls with respect to age, height, weight, and smoking habits were not statistically significant.

**Psychological Assessment.** In order to characterize the patients and healthy controls regarding personality and possible psychopathology, both groups received two self-rating instruments on the day of examination. The Eysenck Personality Questionnaire, Neuroticism scale (EPQ-N), was applied to indicate a general life-style of hyperresponsiveness or emotional overreactiveness (24, 25). The General Health Questionnaire (GHQ-28+) was used to detect psychiatric morbidity in a somatic setting and to evaluate quality of life (26). Both test instruments were available in validated versions in Norwegian translation (27).

**Test Meal.** Five hundred milliliters of commercial meat soup (Toro clear meat soup, Rieber & Søn A/S, Bergen, Norway) containing 1.8 g protein, 0.9 g fat, and 1.1 g carbohydrate (20 kcal) was ingested during a period of 4 min. The soup was boiled and then cooled to 37°C, thus improving image quality by reducing the amount of air bubbles after ingestion. The pH of the soup varied between 5.4 and 5.7, and the osmolarity was 350 mosm/kg $H_2O$. Fat, protein, and carbohydrate were all soluble in water. In addition, the soup contained nonsoluble seasoning (0.4 g/liter). In previous studies, this soup meal induced antral contractions at a frequency of 3/min (fed state) in over 85% of patients and controls (20, 28). Fifteen grams of bovine fat (150 kcal) were added to the soup to increase the adaptive response of the stomach (29).

**Symptom Scores.** All participants were asked to evaluate their global dyspeptic symptoms both before and after the soup meal on a Likert scale from 0 to 9, also used in a previous study (23). Zero denotes absence of symptoms and 9 denotes excruciating symptoms.

**Experimental Procedure.** All participants were examined between 08:00 and 10:30 AM after an overnight fast. Smokers were not allowed to smoke on the morning of the examination. The individuals were scanned while sitting in a chair, leaning back slightly at an angle of 120°. The transducer was positioned in the epigastrium by the left subcostal margin and tilted cranially (Figure 1). Ultrasound images were obtained using a mechanical sector scanner (CFM 750, Vingmed Sound, Horten, Norway) with a 3.25-MHz annular array, enabling smooth rotation subcostally. The maximal angle of view (90°) obtained with this scanner was chosen to visualize as much of the proximal stomach as possible. The maximal depth of scanning in this study was 22 cm. Two standardized sonographic image sections were chosen to monitor the size of the proximal stomach. First, a sagittal section with the left renal pelvis in a longitudinal projection, the left lobe of the liver and the tail of the pancreas as internal landmarks, was recorded. Then the transducer was rotated 90° clockwise to obtain an oblique frontal section where the left hemidiaphragm, the top margin of the fundus, and the liver parenchyma served as landmarks. All selected ultrasound images were scanned at

Published with permission



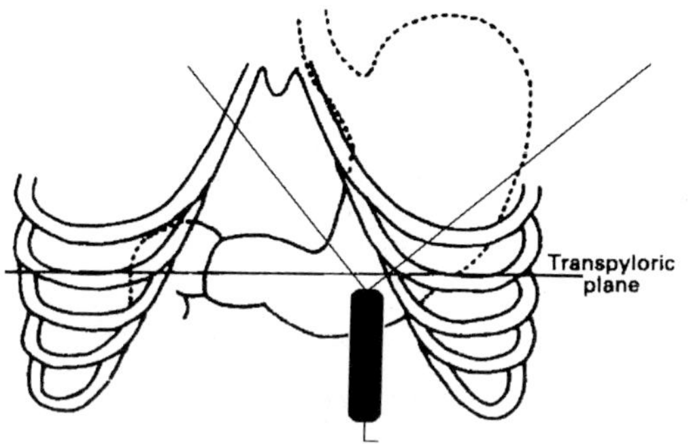


**Fig 1.** Drawing showing the position of the ultrasound transducer that enabled scanning of the proximal stomach in patients with functional dyspepsia and healthy controls.

the end of normal expiration and each standardized image was frozen before recording on a video tape.

**Measurements.** All measures of the size of the proximal stomach were obtained after replaying the tapes and by utilizing the manual tracing facilities on the CFM scanner. A proximal gastric area in a sagittal section (SA) was outlined by tracing from the top margin of the fundus and 7 cm downwards along the axis of the stomach (Figure 2). The maximal diameter in an oblique frontal section (OFD), kept within 7 cm along the long axis of the proximal stomach, was chosen as the second measure (Figure 3). By combining these two measures, an approximate volume (aV) of the proximal stomach was estimated ($aV = SA \times OFD$). The aV values were used to compute the individual's emptying fraction of the proximal stomach, defined as $(aV_{2.5\text{min}} - aV_{\text{actual}})/aV_{2.5\text{min}}$. Time zero was defined as the end of the ingestion period of 4 min. All measures were traced twice and the average results recorded. The ultrasound examinations and the measurements were performed by O.H.G., who was blinded with respect to diagnosis when measuring the scans.

**Definitions.** In order to address the problem of air pockets in the gastric fundus, the visible amount of air was graded from 0 to 3. Grade 0 denoted absence of visible air in the fundus, grade 1 small amounts of air, grade 2 moderate amounts, and grade 3 such great amounts of air that exclusion from the study was necessary.

**Ethical Approval.** The study was approved by the Regional Ethics Committee and was conducted in accordance with the revised Declaration of Helsinki. All participants gave a written, informed consent to participate in the trial.

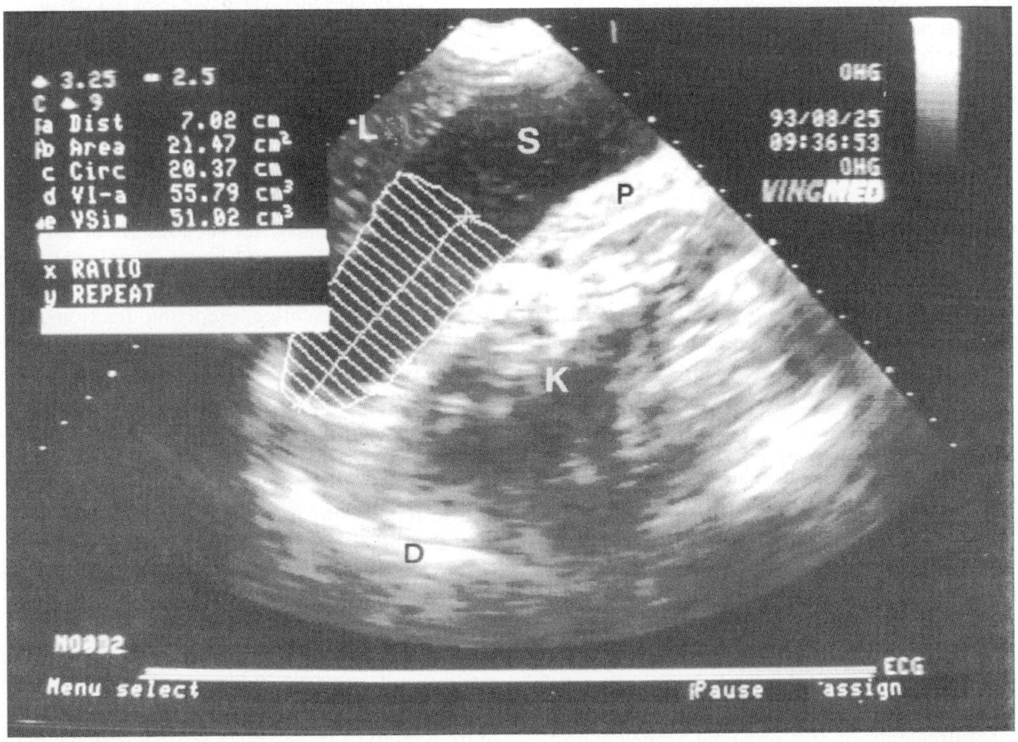


**Fig 2.** Ultrasonogram of the sagittal section applied for scanning of the proximal stomach with the area measurement denoted. The area was outlined by tracing from the top margin of the fundus and 7 cm downwards along the axis of the stomach. The right side of the image corresponds to the posterior part of the subject. S: stomach; L: liver; P: pancreas; K: kidney; D: diaphragm.

Published with permission



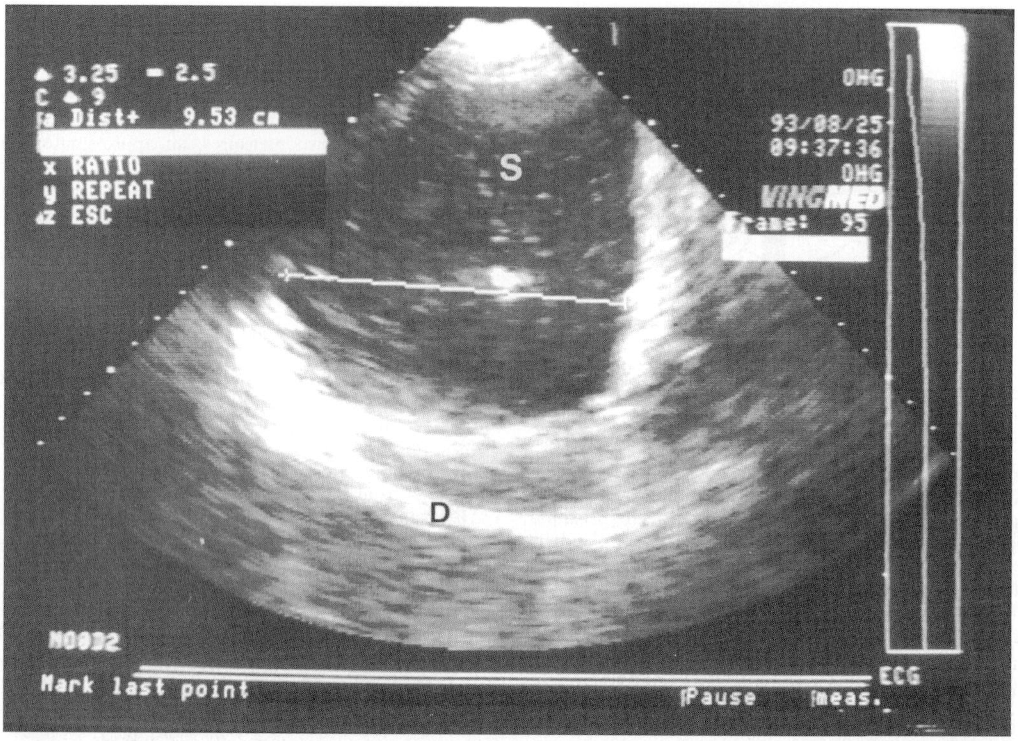


**Fig 3.** Ultrasonogram of the oblique frontal section applied for scanning of the proximal stomach including diameter measurement. The maximal diameter in this section, kept within 7 cm along the long axis of the proximal stomach, was traced. The right side of the image corresponds to the right side of the subject S: stomach; D: diaphragm.

**Statistical Analysis.** In the patient and control group mean values ± SD of variables are given, if not otherwise stated. The distribution of data was evaluated by inspecting a histogram and a probability plot and by utilising Kolmogorov-Smirnov test with Lillefors subanalysis. If the data were approximately normally distributed, Student's *t* test with two-sided probabilities was used to compare results between the groups. Separate variances were selected in the analysis, and $P < 0.05$ was chosen as the level of statistical significance. If the data did not follow an approximate normal distribution, the Mann-Whitney U test was applied to estimate group differences. Analysis of variance with repeated measurements was utilized to evaluate trends during the emptying time from the proximal stomach. All statistic calculations and graphic designs were performed using commercially available software (Systat, Systat Inc., Evanston, Illinois, USA).

## RESULTS

Patients with functional dyspepsia revealed smaller sagittal area measurements and shorter frontal diameter measurements of the proximal stomach postprandially than healthy controls. However, only 7.5, 15, 20, and 25 min after the ingestion period the differences in the sagittal sections ($P < 0.018$) and frontal sections ($P < 0.046$) were significantly different from healthy controls (Figures 4 and 5). Furthermore, when calculating emptying fractions of the proximal stomach and applying ANOVA, a highly significant difference ($P = 0.0005$; Greenhouse-Geisser: $P = 0.002$) between the two groups were detected (Figure 6).

Neither patients nor healthy controls had to be excluded from the study due to air (grade 3) in the gastric fundus impairing sonographic image quality. The number of subjects with grade 0 (absence of visible air) were 14 and 11, with grade 1 were 4 and 5, with grade 2 were 2 and 4, for patients with functional dyspepsia and healthy controls, respectively. None of these differences between the two groups were statistically significant ($P > 0.5$).

Patients with functional dyspepsia experienced more symptoms ($P = 0.002$), scored as global dyspepsia in response to the soup meal, than healthy controls (Figure 7). Sixteen of 20 patients (75%) experienced

Published with permission



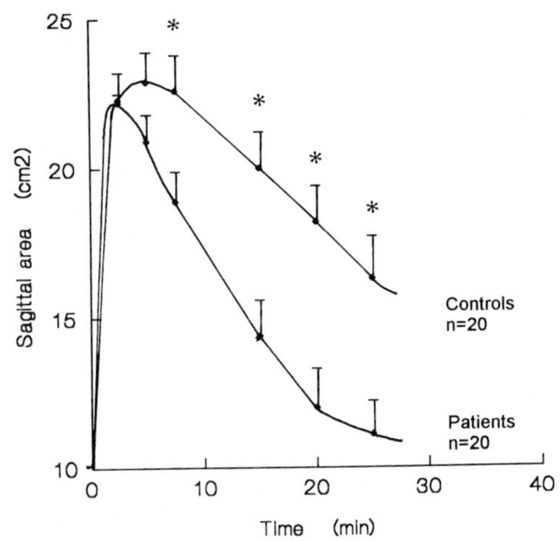


Fig 4. Graph showing the differences in area measurements in a sagittal section between patients with functional dyspepsia and healthy controls. SEM bars are shown. * $P < 0.05$.

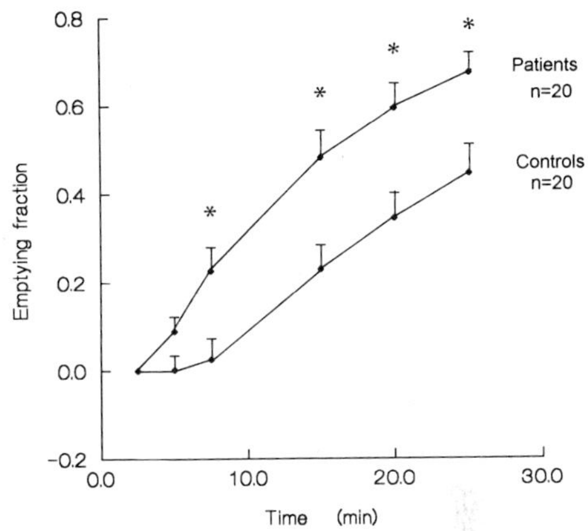


Fig 6. Plot revealing the differences in emptying fractions of the proximal stomach between healthy controls and patients with functional dyspepsia. Bars denoting SEM are drawn. * $P < 0.05$.

worsening of symptoms or induction of symptoms during or within 10 min after the ingestion of the meal. The emptying fractions were not correlated with symptoms induced by the soup. However, the duration of the disease was associated with the degree of symptom induction ($r = 0.58$, $P = 0.009$).

In the patient group, *H. pylori* status did not influence ($P = 0.44$, NS) the emptying fraction rate of the proximal stomach, nor did gender ($P = 0.23$, NS) or smoking habits ($P = 0.18$, NS). Patients with functional dyspepsia had higher scores on the GHQ-28+ registration ($P < 0.0005$), and neuroticism was a more dominant feature ($P < 0.0005$) compared with healthy controls (Figure 8).

With the present soup meal, the proximal gastric emptying fraction discriminating best between patients and healthy controls, was seen 20 min post-

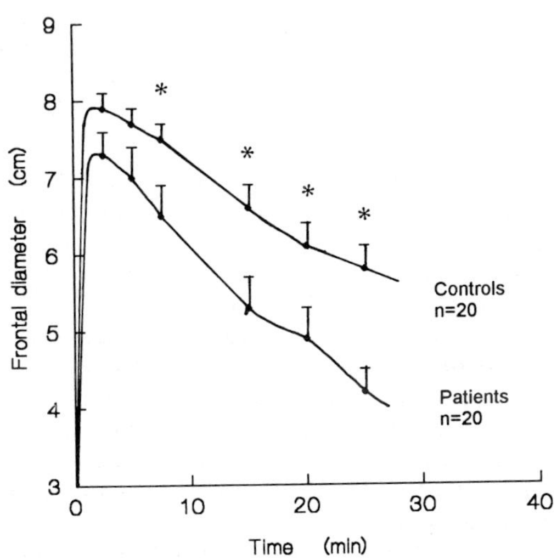


Fig 5. Graph demonstrating the differences in gastric diameter measured in an oblique frontal section between patients with functional dyspepsia and healthy controls. SEM bars are denoted. * $P < 0.05$.

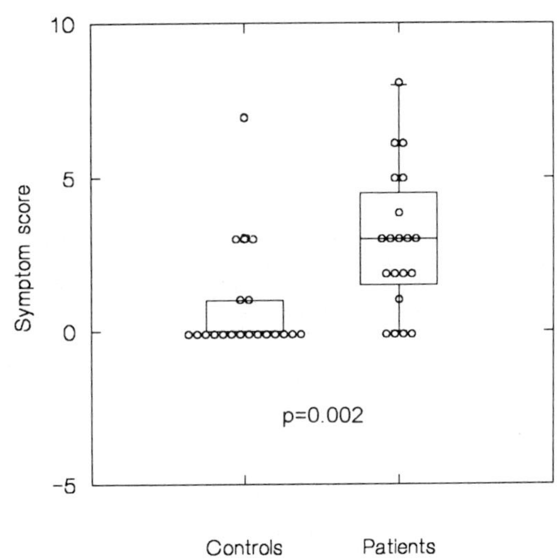


Fig 7. Combination of box and dot plot showing the differences in symptom scores between patients with functional dyspepsia and controls. The median of the batch is marked by the center horizontal line with a quartile on each side comprising the box.

Published with permission



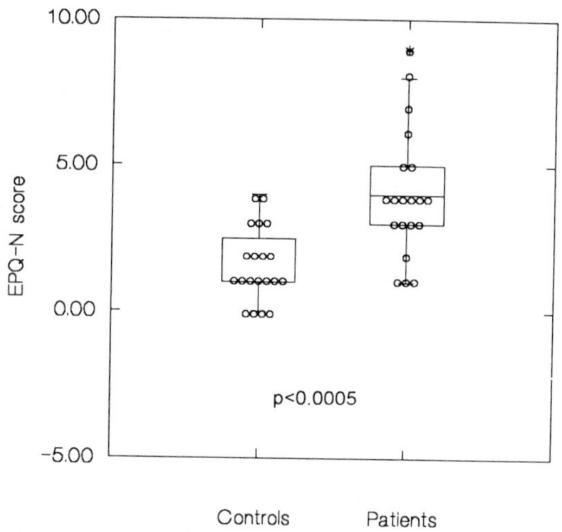


**Fig 8.** Combination of box and dot plot depicting the differences in EPQ-N score between functional dyspepsia patients and healthy controls. The median of the batch is marked by the center horizontal line with a quartile on each side embracing the box.

cibally. The diagnostic sensitivity of the method at 20 min postprandially was 70% and the specificity 65%. The positive predictive value using this method was 67%, and the negative predictive value was 68%.

## DISCUSSION

The present ultrasonographic method disclosed that patients with functional dyspepsia, in response to a soup meal, had smaller sizes and higher emptying fractions of the proximal stomach than healthy controls. This population of patients was also characterized by general hyperresponsiveness, lower quality of life, and higher susceptibility to psychiatric morbidity. Furthermore, ingestion of our soup meal induced significantly more symptoms in these patients than in healthy controls. Thus, this novel noninvasive method for measuring postprandial size and initial emptying fraction of the proximal stomach, previously shown to be applicable and to contribute to low intra- and interobserver error in healthy volunteers (21), seemed useful also in the evaluation of patients with functional dyspepsia.

Interestingly, there was no significant difference in the size of the proximal stomach between dyspeptics and controls immediately after the meal ingestion. This finding is consistent with other observations suggesting a normal compliance during pressure increments of the proximal stomach in fasting patients with functional dyspepsia (13, 15). Accordingly, in the time period before a substantial portion of the meal has reached the intestines, the proximal stomach seemed to relax adequately. However, after this initial, near-normal receptive relaxation, accommodation of the proximal stomach appeared to be impaired with abnormally high emptying fractions. It is documented that the proximal stomach receives reflex signals that induce gastric relaxation, both after volume expansion (30, 31) and nutrient infusion (32) into the duodenum. When the duodenum is properly exposed to nutrients or sufficiently dilated by the volume of the soup, feedback signals to the proximal stomach start to moderate the reservoir function of the corpus–fundus, interfering with normal adaptive relaxation. It is not possible from the present study to deduce which mechanism underlies the impaired accommodation in patients with functional dyspepsia, but our finding is supported by the previous detection of an impaired duodenogastric reflex in this patient group (33). Furthermore, intragastric maldistribution of a meal with a relatively lower proportion of the meal residing in the proximal stomach has been encountered in patients with functional dyspepsia (10, 11), substantiating our finding of impaired accommodation to a meal in these patients.

In patients with functional dyspepsia, it has been a constant challenge to establish valid associations between reported symptoms and actual physiological abnormalities. Evidence of altered gastric functions, like antral hypomotility (22, 34), delayed gastric emptying (6, 8, 9), and a wide antrum (20) have been found in subgroups of patients, but the diagnostic sensitivity and specificity of these findings are too low to allow conclusive diagnosis. We found a relatively high predictive value of the emptying fraction indicating that insufficient accommodation of the proximal stomach may constitute a significant sign in this patient population. Although no significant correlations between symptoms and emptying fraction were detected in this study, the patients experienced significantly more dyspepsia than controls following the meal at the same time as impaired adaptive relaxation of the proximal stomach was seen. Hence, as impaired accommodation and symptoms were temporarily related, a causal relationship is possible.

In accordance with previous studies (27, 35, 36), the present patients with functional dyspepsia were prone to a general lifestyle of hyperresponsiveness and emotional overreactiveness, as evaluated by EPQ-N score. In recent studies, a low vagal tone (22), and a significant negative correlation between EPQ-N score and vagal tone (37) was observed in patients with func-

Published with permission



tional dyspepsia. In fact, low vagal activity may constitute a mediating mechanism for the relationship between personal factors and gastric symptoms in functional dyspepsia (37). Both receptive and adaptive relaxation of the proximal stomach are facilitated by vagal nerves (38). In vagotomized patients, experiencing postcibal discomfort and fullness, increased intragastric pressure (16) and impairment of gastric adaptive relaxation (4, 39) have been discovered. Taken together with previous results, our study suggests a relation between impaired accommodation of the proximal stomach, low vagal tone, and induction of symptoms in patients with functional dyspepsia.

**Limitations of the Study.** In general, ultrasonographic methods require sonographic skills and a certain level of experience to fully decipher the information of the images. The present method is vulnerable with respect to the presence of gas pockets in the proximal stomach, and this problem was discussed in a previous paper (21). However, no patients or controls had to be excluded due to this phenomenon, and the amount of gas present was not statistically different in the two groups. In the validation study on healthy controls, we found a moderate day-to-day variation and low intra- and interobserver error of both the scanning procedure and the applied measurements.

The emptying fractions of the proximal stomach would be easier to interpret if total gastric emptying and intragastric distribution were known parameters. Unfortunately, it was practically impossible to measure gastric emptying by radionuclide methods in this study. Several studies have found that patients with functional dyspepsia exhibit delayed gastric emptying, including when ingesting liquid meals (6, 7, 40–42). Accordingly, it seems unlikely that our results are due to a rapid total gastric emptying in patients with functional dyspepsia. However, further studies are needed to elucidate the interplay and the coordination between the different parts of the stomach to facilitate accommodation of a meal.

The present ultrasonographic method is rather time consuming, but our results indicate that the ideal point of measurement, with respect to discriminating power, was at 20 min postprandially. Hence, to use this method in the clinical evaluation of patients with functional dyspepsia, it seems sufficient to measure postprandial sizes of the proximal stomach immediately after the meal and 20 min postprandially.

In conclusion, this novel noninvasive method to monitor the size and emptying fraction of the proximal stomach by ultrasonic scanning was also useful in evaluating the accommodation in a patient population. Patients with functional dyspepsia referred to a gastroenterologic unit for upper endoscopy exhibited greater symptom induction and impaired accommodation of the proximal stomach to a soup meal compared with healthy controls, suggesting a relationship between symptoms and impaired accommodation in these patients.

## ACKNOWLEDGMENTS

We want to express our thanks to Christen Bang, MD, PhD, for his kind support in recruiting patients to the study.

## REFERENCES

1. Grey EG: Observations on the postural activity of the stomach. Am J Physiol 45:272–285, 1918
2. Gianturco G: Some mechanical factors of gastric physiology. Am J Roentgenol 315:735–744, 1934
3. Cannon WB, Lieb CW: The receptive relaxation of the stomach. Am J Physiol 29:267–273, 1911
4. Jahnberg T, Abrahamsson H, Jansson G, Martinson J: Gastric relaxatory response to feeding before and after vagotomy. Scand J Gastroenterol 12(2):225–228, 1977
5. Hartley MN, Walker SJ, Mackie CR. Abnormal gastric adaptive relaxation in patients with gastrooesophageal reflux. Gut 31:500–503, 1990 (published erratum appears in Gut 31(7):799, 1990)
6. Jian R, Ducrot F, Piedeloup C, Mary JY, Najean Y, Bernier JJ: Measurement of gastric emptying in dyspeptic patients: Effect of a new gastrokinetic agent (cisapride). Gut 26:352–358, 1985
7. Jian R, Ducrot F, Ruskone A, Chaussade S, Rambaud JC, Modigliani R, Rain JD, Bernier JJ: Symptomatic, radionuclide and therapeutic assessment of chronic idiopathic dyspepsia. A double-blind placebo-controlled evaluation of cisapride. Dig Dis Sci 34:657–664, 1989
8. Tucci A, Corinaldesi R, Stanghellini V, Tosetti C, Di Febo G, Paparo GF, Varoli O, Paganelli GM, Labate AM, Masci C, et al: *Helicobacter pylori* infection and gastric function in patients with chronic idiopathic dyspepsia. Gastroenterology 103:768–774, 1992
9. Wegener M, Borsch G, Schaffstein J, Reuter C, Leverkus F: Frequency of idiopathic gastric stasis and intestinal transit disorders in essential dyspepsia. J Clin Gastroenterol 11:163–168, 1989
10. Scott AM, Kellow JE, Shuter B, Cowan H, Corbett AM, Riley JW, Lunzer MR, Eckstein RP, Hoschl R, Lam SK, Jones MP: Intragastric distribution and gastric emptying of solids and liquids in functional dyspepsia. Lack of influence of symptom subgroups and *H. pylori*-associated gastritis. Dig Dis Sci 38:2247–2254, 1993
11. Troncon LE, Bennett RJ, Ahluwalia NK, Thompson DG: Abnormal intragastric distribution of food during gastric emptying in functional dyspepsia patients. Gut 35:327–332, 1994
12. Azpiroz F, Malagelada JR: Physiological variations in canine gastric tone measured by an electronic barostat. Am J Physiol 248:G229–G237, 1985
13. Mearin F, Cucala M, Azpiroz F, Malagelada JR: The origin of

Published with permission



symptoms on the brain-gut axis in functional dyspepsia. Gastroenterology 101:999–1006, 1991
14. Bradette M, Pare P, Douville P, Morin A: Visceral perception in health and functional dyspepsia. Crossover study of gastric distension with placebo and domperidone. Dig Dis Sci 36:52–58, 1991
15. Lemann M, Dederding JP, Flourie B, Franchisseur C, Rambaud JC, Jian R: Abnormal perception of visceral pain in response to gastric distension in chronic idiopathic dyspepsia. The irritable stomach syndrome. Dig Dis Sci 36:1249–1254, 1991
16. Stadaas J, Aune S: Intragastric pressure-volume relationship before and after vagotomy. Acta Chir Scand 136:611–615, 1970
17. Moragas G, Azpiroz F, Pavia J, Malagelada JR: Relations among intragastric pressure, postcibal perception, and gastric emptying. Am J Physiol 264:G1112–G1117, 1993
18. Ropert A, des Varannes SB, Bizais Y, Roze C, Galmiche JP: Simultaneous assessment of liquid emptying and proximal gastric tone in humans. Gastroenterology 105:667–674, 1993
19. Bolondi L, Bortolotti M, Santi V, Calletti T, Gaiani S, Labo G: Measurement of gastric emptying time by real-time ultrasonography. Gastroenterology 89:752–759, 1985
20. Hausken T, Berstad A. Wide gastric antrum in patients with non-ulcer dyspepsia. Effect of cisapride. Scand J Gastroenterol 27:427–432, 1992
21. Gilja OH, Hausken T, Ødegaard S, Berstad A: Monitoring postprandial size of the proximal stomach by ultrasonography. J Ultrasound Med 14(2):81–89, 1995
22. Hausken T, Svebak S, Wilhelmsen I, Tangen Haug T, Olafsen K, Pettersson E, Hveem K, Berstad A: Low vagal tone and antral dysmotility in patients with functional dyspepsia. Psychosom Med 55:12–22, 1993
23. Hausken T, Berstad A: Effect of glyceryl trinitrate on antral motility and symptoms in patients with functional dyspepsia. Scand J Gastroenterol 29:23–28, 1994
24. Eysenck HJ: The Structure of Human Personality. London; Mitchum, 1953
25. Grayson DA: Latent trait analysis of the Eysenck Personality Questionnaire. J Psychiatr Res 20(3):217–235, 1986
26. Goldberg D: Identifying psychiatric illness among general medical patients. Br Med J 291:161–162, 1985
27. Tangen Haug T, Svebak S, Wilhelmsen I, Berstad A, Ursin H: Psychological factors and somatic symptoms in functional dyspepsia: A comparison with duodenal ulcer and healthy controls. J Psychosom Res 38(4):281–291, 1994
28. Hausken T, Ødegaard S, Matre K, Berstad A: Antroduodenal motility and movements of luminal contents studied by duplex sonography. Gastroenterology 102:1583–1590, 1992
29. Undeland KA, Hausken T, Gilja OH, Ropert A, Galmiche JP, Berstad A: Gastric relaxation in response to a soup meal in healthy subjects. A study using a barostat in the proximal stomach. Scand J Gastroenterol 30:1069–1076, 1995
30. Azpiroz F, Malagelada JR: Perception and reflex relaxation of the stomach in response to gut distention. Gastroenterology 98:1193–1198, 1990
31. Azpiroz F, Malagelada JR: Isobaric intestinal distension in humans: sensorial relay and reflex gastric relaxation. Am J Physiol 258:G202–G207, 1990
32. Ahluwalia NK, Thompson DG, Barlow J, Troncon LEA, Hollis S: Relaxation responses of the human proximal stomach to distension during fasting and after food. Am J Physiol 267:G166–G172, 1994
33. Coffin B, Azpiroz F, Guarner F, Malagelada JR: Selective gastric hypersensitivity and reflex hyporeactivity in functional dyspepsia. Gastroenterology 107:1345–1351, 1994
34. Stanghellini V, Ghidini C, Maccarini MR, Paparo GF, Corinaldesi R, Barbara L: Fasting and postprandial gastrointestinal motility in ulcer and non-ulcer dyspepsia. Gut 33:184–190, 1992
35. Talley NJ, Fung LH, Gilligan IJ, McNeil D, Piper DW: Association of anxiety, neuroticism, and depression with dyspepsia of unknown cause. A case–control study. Gastroenterology 90:886–892, 1986
36. Wilhelmsen I, Tangen Haug T, Ursin H, Berstad A: Discriminant analysis of factors distinguishing patients with functional dyspepsia from patients with duodenal ulcer. Significance of somatization. Dig Dis Sci 40(5):1105–1111, 1995
37. Tangen Haug T, Svebak S, Wilhelmsen I, Berstad A, Ursin H: Low vagal activity as mediating mechanism for the relationship between personality factors and gastric symptoms in functional dyspepsia. Psychosom Med 56:181–186, 1994
38. Kelly KA: Gastric motility after gastric operations. Surg Ann 6:103–123, 1980
39. Hartley MN, Mackie CR: Gastric adaptive relaxation and symptoms after vagotomy. Br J Surg 78:24–27, 1991
40. Ovartlarnporn B, Ratanalert S, Keowkarnkar W: Liquid meal emptying in non-ulcer dyspepsia: A study in 22 Thai patients. J Med Assoc Thai 75:236–239, 1992
41. Pfeiffer A, Aronbayev J, Schmidt T, Wendl B, Pehl C, Kaess H: Gastric emptying, esophageal 24-hour pH and gastric potential difference measurements in non-ulcer dyspepsia. Gastroenterol Clin Biol 16:395–400, 1992
42. Marzio L, DiFelice F, Laico MG, Imbimbo B, Lapenna D, Cuccurullo F: Gallbladder hypokinesia and normal gastric emptying of liquids in patients with dyspeptic symptoms. A double-blind placebo-controlled clinical trial with cisapride. Dig Dis Sci 37:262–267, 1992

CHAPTER 15

# ENDOSCOPIC ULTRASONOGRAPHY IN THE DIAGNOSIS OF GASTROINTESTINAL DISEASES WITH SPECIAL REFERENCE TO TUMOR STAGING

SVEIN ØDEGAARD AND LARS B. NESJE

Endosonography is the common denomination of ultrasound examinations using intracorporal transducers and was first described by Wild and Reid in 1956 (1). Endoscopic ultrasonography (EUS) is a method by which a high-frequency ultrasound probe is inserted into the gastrointestinal tract or similar luminal structures under endoscopic control. Thus, the visceral wall and adjacent structures can be imaged in detail (2–6). Acoustic coupling is usually achieved by filling water into the lumen or into a balloon around the ultrasound transducer. Alternatively, the ultrasound probe can be applied directly on the endoluminal surface. A water interface is usually preferred since it improves the ultrasound image by optimizing the focus and reducing acoustic artifacts.

EUS combines endoscopy with ultrasonography and may be regarded as a supplement to both modalities when detailed information is wanted from defined areas of the gastrointestinal system. The examiner need to be trained in endoscopy as well as in the interpretation of ultrasound images (7).

## 1. Endoluminal versus External Ultrasonography

EUS enables close vicinity between the ultrasound transducer and the target organ allowing high-frequency ultrasound, typically between 7.5 and 20 MHz, to be applied. Hence, improved image resolution can be accomplished. On the other hand, frequencies above 10 MHz have not been useful for transcutaneous ultrasound imaging of intra-abdominal structures due to limited ultrasound penetration. Skin, bone, and intestinal gas may attenuate a large proportion of the ultrasonic waves and further reduce their penetration (Fig. 1). The interpretation of ultrasound images is basically similar by external and endoluminal imaging. However, the echo texture may change with increasing frequency due to improved image resolution. Ultrasonographic examinations are usually guided by immediate interpretation of displayed images. This may be particularly important during EUS, since it may be difficult to define precisely the position of the intraluminal transducer as well as the angles of the acquired image planes.

Images of the GI wall as a structure with several layers can be obtained with both transcutaneous ultrasound and EUS. However, EUS can usually separate more wall layers and other details. The thickness of layers seen on ultrasound images differs from layers measured on histology. This is explained by interfaces occuring at the borders between tissue with different acoustical impedances. Kimmey *et al.* (8) have compared histology

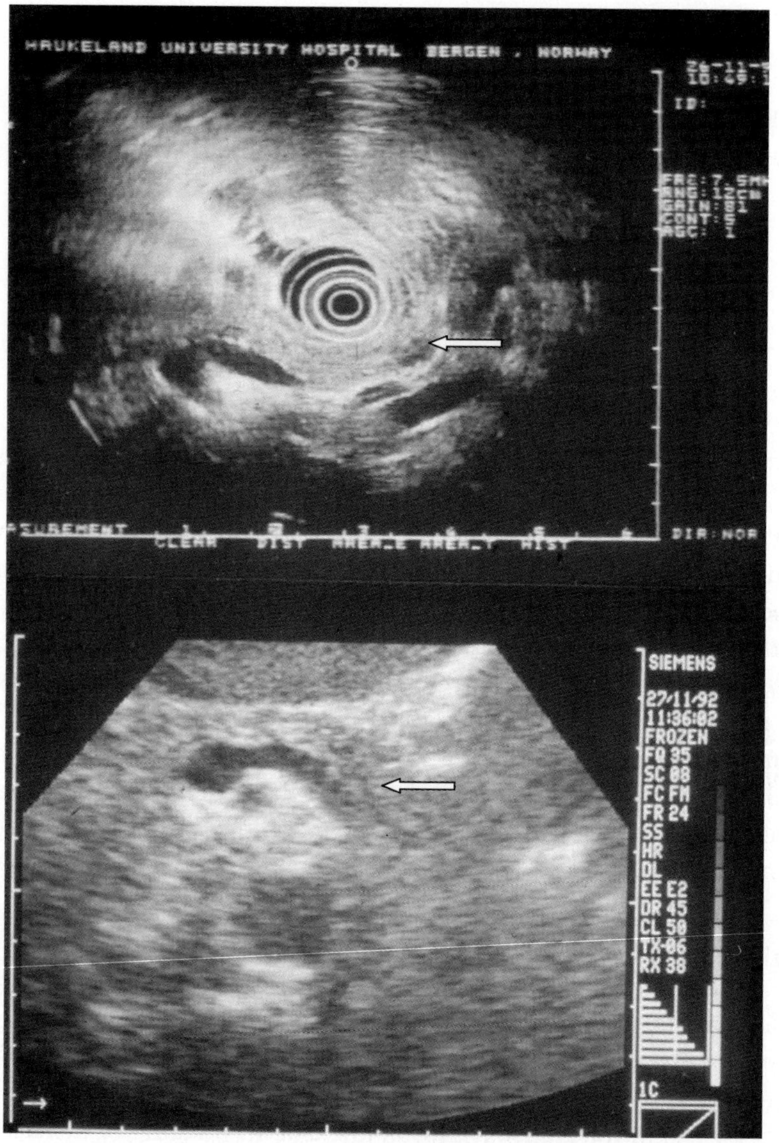


Fig. 1. Endoscopic ultrasound image (above) of a small tumor in the pancreatic tail (arrow). External ultrasound of the same pancreas (below). The pancreatic tail is not clearly seen.

and high-frequency ultrasound images of the GI tract and described the role of interface echoes between GI wall layers. Interface echoes are important in staging superficial GI cancer, because they represent a relatively major part of US images of the GI wall.

## 2. Endoscopic Ultrasonography versus Endoscopy

Endoscopy is a major tool for diagnosis and therapy of diseases in the digestive tract. However, the endoscopic investigation of visceral wall abnormalities is limited since only the superficial aspects can be evaluated (9). The depth of invasion of mucosal lesions like neoplasms or ulcers cannot be determined with endoscopy alone. Furthermore, although endoscopy may suggest the presence of a mass within or outside the gastrointestinal wall, it cannot further elucidate the location or character of the mass. EUS may thus extend the diagnostic ability and guide therapeutic endoscopic interventions. Using a miniature probe, EUS can be added to routine endoscopy without having to retract the endoscope. Otherwise, EUS must be performed as a separate procedure using a dedicated instrument.

## 3. Operator Dependence

EUS is a dynamic examination mode in which the result and the course of the procedure to a large degree depend on the examiner's skills and continuous assessments. The evaluation is based not only on the ultrasound image, which can be recorded on video and subsequently reviewed, but also on information from the endoscopic view, knowledge of the probe position, tissue displacement and deformation, provocation of symptoms during the examination, and technical performance of the instrument. Moreover, selection of target area may have to be reassessed during the procedure due to technical considerations or unexpected findings. Several authors have reported that the accuracy of their EUS examinations improved considerably with training and it is generally accepted that a rather long learning period is needed before the method is properly managed (10).

## 4. Endoscopic Ultrasound Instruments

Miniature ultrasound probes can be applied through the accessory channel of conventional endoscopes allowing EUS to be performed during routine endoscopy (11–13). On the other hand, dedicated ultrasound endoscopes with integrated ultrasound transducers can utilize lower ultrasound frequencies due to larger transducer size and may thus image larger areas along the gastrointestinal tract (14). Ultrasound endoscopes with a longitudinal image plane in the prolongation of the accessory channel can be applied for EUS-guided interventions (Fig. 2) (15–17).

Currently available ultrasound miniprobes are mechanical radial sector- , electronic phased array- or single crystal linear compound systems operating with frequencies between 12 MHz and 30 MHz (11–13, 18, 19). A system which combines linear scanning with mechanical radial sector scanning is also available making it possible to switch between these modalities (20). Some echoendoscopes have spectral-, colour- and power Doppler facilities and Doppler miniprobes have also been developed. Doppler technology gives important clinical information about vascular structures (21, 22).

A "push - back" probe with an ultrasound transducer with the size and frequency similar to that of an echoendoscope has been developed. The probe is inserted backwards through the working channel of a conventional endoscope allowing imaging of larger and deeper areas than what is possible with conventional transendoscopic miniprobes.

Other ultrasound systems designed for use within the GI tract do not have an optical system. Transrectal probes have been used for imaging the prostate, bladder, uterus, and rectum. These probes are either linear array or mechanical sector scanners with ultrasound frequencies of 3.5 to 7 MHz.

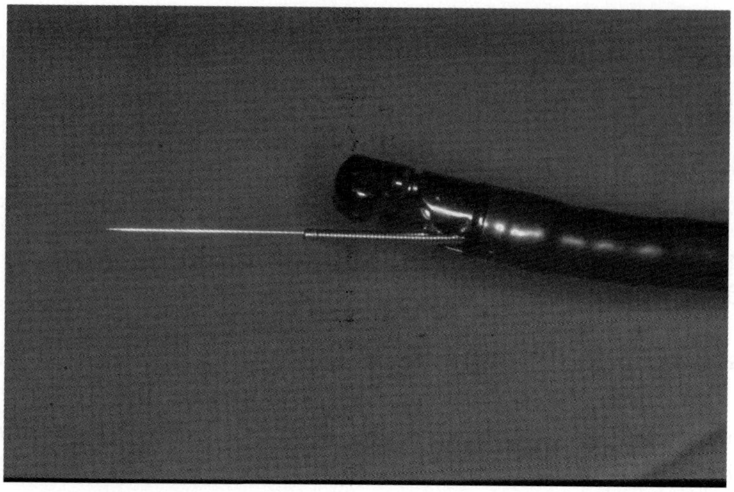

Fig. 2. Echoendoscope with curvilinear array transducer and biopsy needle.

## 5. Clinical Applications of Endoscopic Ultrasonography

Several benign and malignant gastrointestinal disorders may be investigated by EUS, both as a primary diagnostic procedure and in follow-up of patients with chronic diseases. From an endoscopist's point of view, EUS can be helpful in characterizing the intra- and extramural character of various lesions, such as polyps, ulcers, tumors, strictures, inflammation, suspected subepithelial lesions and abnormal vascular structures. The main application has so far been the assessment of tumor infiltration and regional lymph node metastasis in gastrointestinal cancer. Increased experience as well as technical improvements and specialization of the instruments have introduced new EUS applications, and the modality has evolved from a pure imaging method to an interventional tool for diagnostic sampling and endoscopic therapy. EUS has also been applied for diagnosis of diseases outside the gastrointestinal system, especially for the evaluation of mediastinal lymph nodes in different lung disorders (23–26).

## 6. Gastrointestinal Cancer Staging

EUS is an accurate method for $T$- and $N$-staging of carcinomas in the esophagus (14, 27–34), stomach (35–37), extrahepatic bile duct and pancreas (38–40). Reported accuracies of $T$-staging in these areas are usually between 70% and 85% and $N$-stage accuracy range between 60% and 80%. Similar figures apply for endosonographic staging of rectal cancer, for which a blind, rigid ultrasound probe is usually applied. A few studies have also been performed on EUS staging of colonic cancer, indicating a $T$-stage accuracy comparable to those mentioned above, but a less accurate $N$-staging. Lack of definite criteria for differentiating between metastatic and otherwise enlarged lymph nodes has been a problem in $N$-staging based on ultrasound imaging although malignant lymph nodes generally seem to be larger, rounder, more hypoechoic and homogeneous, sharply delineated, and closer to the primary tumor than those with benign lymphadenopathy (41–45).

In addition to the assessment of tumor infiltration depth, EUS can also be used for the evaluation of horizontal tumor growth and may indicate malignancy in deeper aspects of wall lesions despite negative biopsies, for instance in gastric linitis plastica. EUS-guided aspiration biopsies are valuable to confirm malignancy in deep visceral structures and enlarged lymph nodes (46–50). In some cases, it might be difficult to distinguish vessels from malignant lymph nodes because they are both echo poor. The use of Doppler probes are helpful in defining these structures.

## 7. Interventional Endosonography

EUS was initially developed as an imaging modality, but has subsequently been increasingly utilized to monitor interventional procedures. Specialized ultrasound endoscopes have been developed with longitudinal scanning planes in which biopsy needles introduced through the accessory channel of the instrument can be imaged in real time (15, 51). Thus, fine-needle biopsies of lymph nodes and other tumors can be performed under direct endosonographic surveillance. Therapeutic interventions, such as nerve blockades are also feasible (52–55). Recently, new instruments with larger channels have enabled new endosonography-guided therapeutic procedures like cyst drainages to be accomplished (55–57). It is also possible to perform other EUS guided therapies like endoscopic mucosal resection of early cancer and resection of submucosal tumors (58, 59).

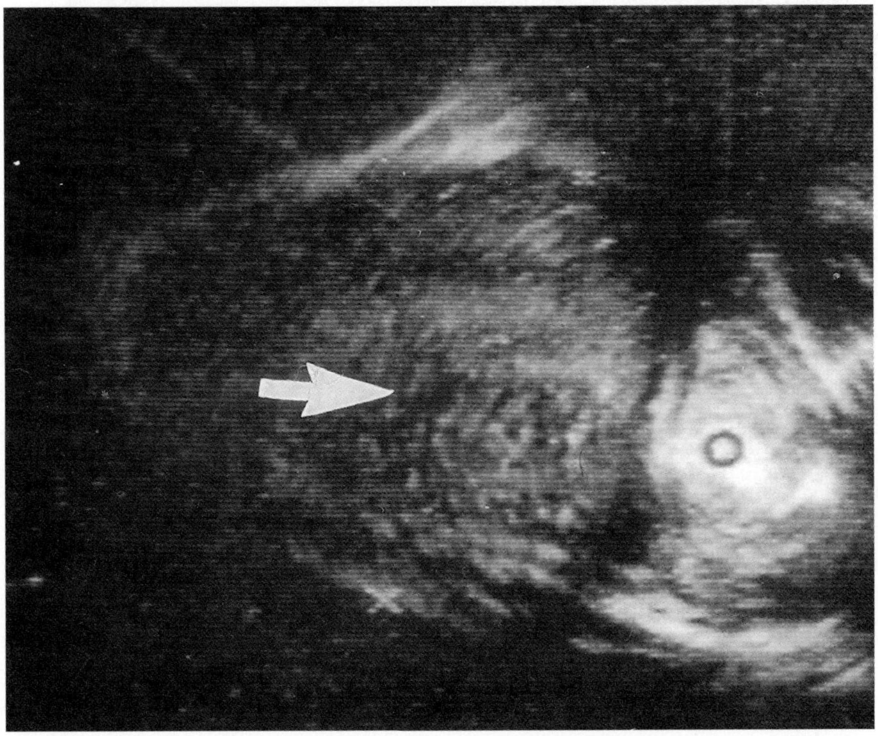

Fig. 3. An esophageal duplication cyst imaged with a miniprobe (arrow).

## 8. Esophageal Diseases

New options in esophageal cancer treatment have accentuated the need for pretherapeutic tumor staging. Important staging objectives may be to sort out early mucosal cancers which can be resected endoscopically, to identify irresectable tumors for which operation should be avoided or to predict whether a tumor can be subject to a curative or a palliative resection (20, 34, 59–65). EUS can visualize the esophageal wall and nearest surroundings in detail, but imaging of the mediastinum and adjacent organs may be limited, especially with frequencies above 15 MHz (Figs. 3 and 4).

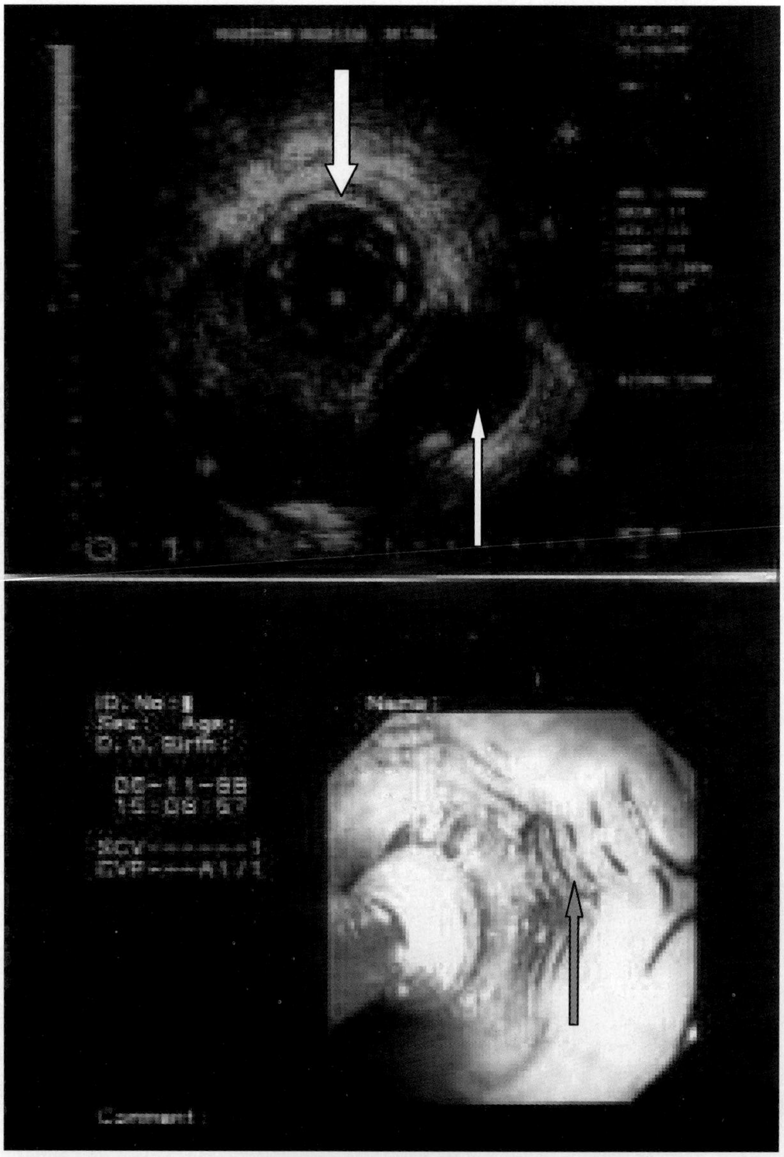


Fig. 4. Endoscopic ultrasound image (above) of an esophageal stent (thick arrow). Aorta (thin arrow). Endoscopic image (below) with stent (arrow).

The use of EUS for diagnosis and follow-up of precancerous conditions in the esophagus like Barrett's epithelium and squamous dysplasia is difficult because inflammatory changes cannot be reliably distinguished from dysplasia or tumor ingrowth (Fig. 5). Nevertheless, EUS may be helpful in the follow-up of individual patients with precancerous conditions in the esophagus and may help direct biopsies of suspected areas (65, 66). Reported $T$-staging accuracy of esophageal carcinomas using radial-scanning echo-endoscopes varies between 59–92%, and most series have obtained accuracy rates between 80–90% . Hasegawa *et al.* (14) compared an ultrasound miniprobe (15 MHz) with a radial echoendoscope in the staging of superficial esophageal carcinoma. The ultrasound probe was more accurate than conventional EUS in staging tumors localized to mucosa and submucosa (92 vs. 76%). However, the assessment of lymph node metastasis using this probe showed a sensitivity of only 25%, but a specificity of 80%.

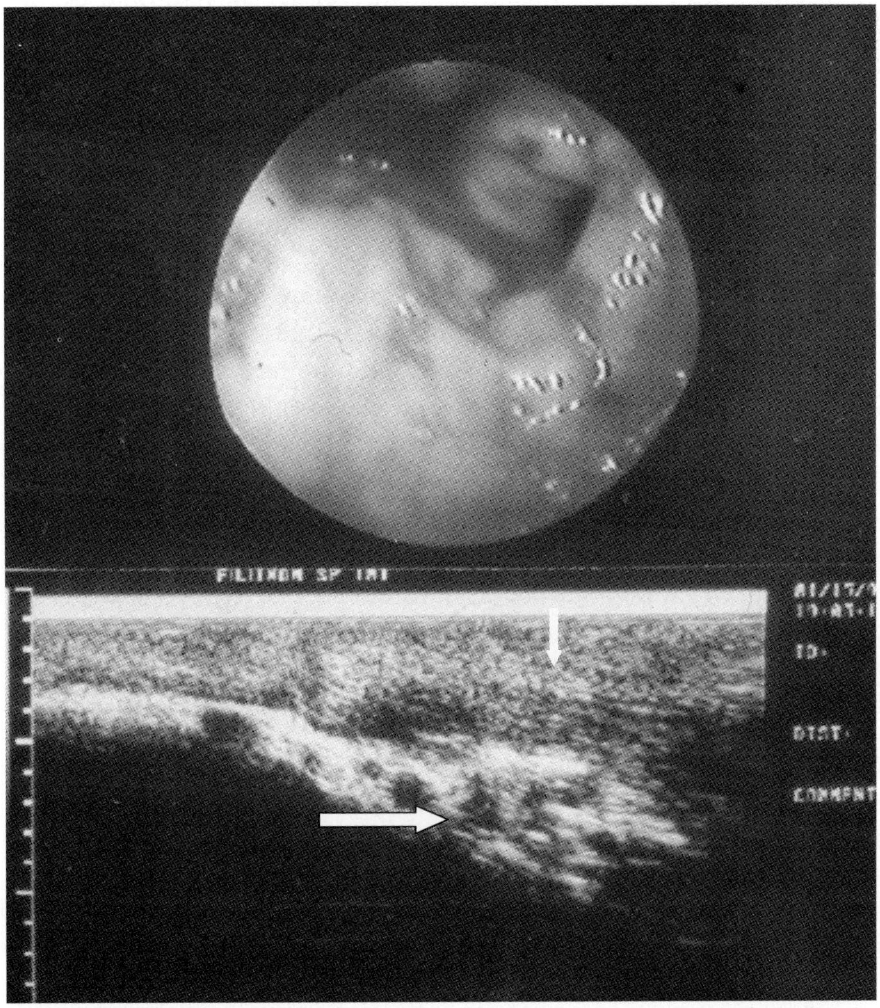


Fig. 5. Endoscopic image of inflammation in the distal esophageus (above). A linear ultrasound image shows thickening of the esophageal wall and loss of layer structure (thin arrow). Small periesophageal lymh nodes are seen (thick arrow).

Nesje *et al.* (61) compared a 20-MHz linear miniature ultrasound probe with a 7.5–/12–MHz radial-scanning ultrasound endoscope in preoperative $TN$-staging of esophageal cancers. The conclusions were that the two EUS systems had similar accuracy for assessing transmural tumor growth, but the ultrasound endoscope was superior in staging advanced transmural tumors and in predicting lymph node metastasis with traversable tumors.

EUS plays an important role not only in $TN$-staging of esophageal cancer but also in $M$-staging (67). Eloubeidi *et al.* (68) found that EUS imaging alone had a sensitivity of 77% and a specificity of 85% (overall accuracy 81%) in assessing celiac lymph nodes. When EUS-FNA was performed, the results were 98% and 100% respectively (overall accuracy 98%). Malignant celiac lymph nodes were found almost five times more often in patients with $T3$ and $T4$ tumors compared to $T1$ or $T2$ tumors. The importance of tissue diagnosis to guide therapy is pinpointed.

Helical CT has been regarded promising and superior to conventional CT in diagnosing celiac lymph nodes. Romagnuolo *et al.* (69) compared helical CT with EUS-FNA in 43 patients with esophageal cancer. Helical CT was inferior to EUS-FNA for $T$ and $N$ staging and was also poor at staging $T4$ tumors and in detecting celiac lymph nodes. EUS seems to be useful in the evaluation of conservative therapeutic strategies as demonstrated by Willis *et al.* (70) who studied 41 patients with esophageal cancer who received neoadjuvant treatment and radiotherapy. EUS was helpul in estimating the extent of the disease and in demonstrating tumor regression during therapy.

Murata *et al.* (59) stated recently that the five-year survival rate in patients with mucosal cancer ($m$ type) is much higher than that of patients with cancer invading the submucosa (sm type). Because the frequency of lymph node metastasis in $m$ type cancer is low, endoscopic mucosal resection (EMR) has been increasingly performed in these patients. The Japanese Society of Esophageal Diseases reviewed the histopathological findings in a group of 2,418 patients with superficial cancer, in which EMR was performed in 394 cases. The depth of superficial cancer was classified into 6 subgroups $m1$–$m3$ and $sm1$–$sm3$. The rate of lymph node metastasis in $m1$ and $m2$ was less than 5%, those of $m3$ and $sm1$ were 12–27%. Thus, $m1$ and $m2$ were regarded as suitable for EMR. EUS was performed in 145 cases using high frequency miniprobes and the esophageal wall could usually be delineated into nine layers. EUS findings were compared with histology of the lesions that had been removed either with EMR or surgery. EUS was correct in 81% of $m1$ and $m2$, in 60% of $m3$–$sm1$ and 87% of $sm2, 3$, respectively.

## 9. Endoscopic Ultrasonography in Gastroduodenal Diseases

Most EUS systems allow a good endoscopic view of the stomach making it possible to combine the endoscopic and ultrasonographic examination. It is generally accepted that EUS currently is better than other methods in evaluating gastric submucosal lesions, especially when impressions against the gastric wall is seen at endoscopy. Possible infiltration into the stomach wall from gastric polyps can be estimated and ultrasound imaging may also give important information about lesions before performing biopsies, punctions or polypectomies.

Gastric or duodenal ulcers typically exhibit an EUS pattern consisting of three separate elements: the ulcer crater, the echo-rich ulcer base, and the echo-poor inflammation zone, which can extend beyond the thickness of the wall and more widely than the endoscopic changes (71–73). It is usually not possible to separate malignant ulcers from benign ones on the basis of local infiltration pattern alone (Fig. 6). Enlarged vessels running into the ulcerated area can sometimes be demonstrated by EUS and may indicate an increased bleeding risk. EUS has the potential for evaluating the depth of invasion of gastric neoplasms

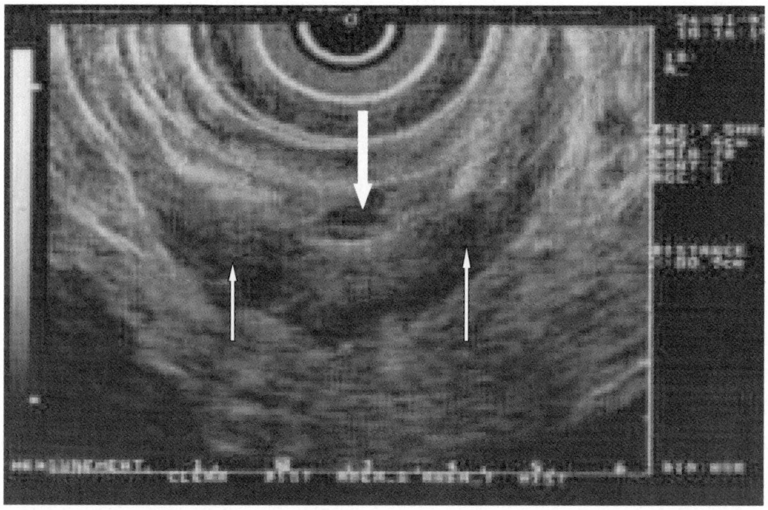

Fig. 6. Gastric ulcer crater (thick arrow). A hypoechoic mass is seen below and to both sides of the crater within the gastric wall (thin arrows). The ultrasound image can not differentiate between a benign and a malignant ulcer.

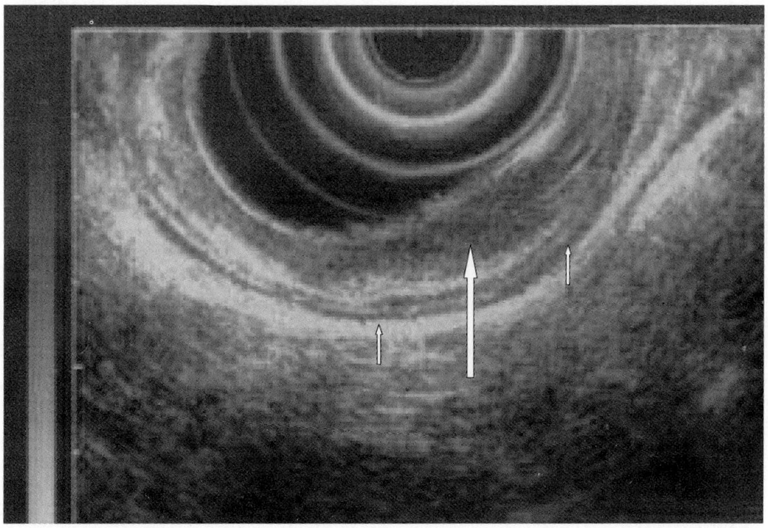

Fig. 7. A gastric tumor infiltrating mucosa and submucosa (thick arrow). Muscularis propria and serosa are intact (small arrows).

on the basis of layers seen on ultrasound images of the gastric wall (Fig. 7). Accuracy rates of approximately 90% are achieved in distinguishing early (confined to the mucosa or submucosa) from advanced (invasion of the muscularis propria or deeper) gastric cancer (74–77).

New treatment options for early gastric cancer make a precise diagnosis of this disease important. High-frequency EUS may distinguish a tumor located on the upper part of the mucosa from tumors invading through the muscularis mucosae and into the submucosa. Sometimes, the deeper part of the muscularis mucosae can be identified as an echopoor layer making it possible to demonstrate tumor penetration through this layer. If muscularis mucosae is not seen, tumors which seem to affect the superficial aspect of the echogenic third layer may still be in the muscularis mucosae (78).

Yanai *et al.* (79) assessed the depth of early gastric cancer invasion using a combined linear and radial 20 MHz ultrasound miniprobe system. They concluded that EUS was useful in combination with conventional endoscopy for staging such lesions. The malignant potensial of gastric submucosal stromal tumors (GIST) is difficult to identify by EUS (Fig. 8). Several authors have tried to define EUS criteria which might indicate malignancy in these tumors. However, this has so far been difficult (80–82). In this respect, EUS-FNA seems to be an important preoperative diagnostic procedure. Ando *et al.* (83) found an accuracy of EUS–FNA with histopathological examination in GIST to be 91% in diagnosing malignancy while the accuracy was only 78% with EUS alone.

Giant gastric folds can be caused by malignant disease such as lymphoma or linitis plastica or by benign disorders including varices, gastritis, or Menetrier's disease. EUS can demonstrate abnormalities in echogenicity and thickness of different wall layers and may help targeting biopsies for a definite diagnosis (47, 84, 85).

During endoscopy, it is often difficult to diagnose linitis plastica because this tumor at the early stage may have a nearly normal endoscopic appearance. If EUS is applied, the thickness and structure of the gastric wall can be evaluated. Increased wall thickness, especially in the third layer corresponding mainly to the submucosa and in the fourth layer mainly corresponding to the proper muscle is the most typical finding.

As stated by Songür *et al.* (84), EUS may distinguish between some malignant and benign diseases causing giant gastric folds. In Menetrier's disease, an isolated thickening of the second layer is usually found while in scirrhous carcinoma abnormalities are demonstrated in both the third and the fourth endosonographic layer.

Lymphomas involving the stomach can present either as an infiltrating or polypoid mass lesion or as a gastric ulcer. Endoscopic biopsy may reveal the diagnosis but biopsies may be non-diagnostic when the bulk of the tumor is subepithelial. EUS can detect the extent of lymphomatous involvement in infiltrating and ulcerative gastric lymphomas. Depth of wall invasion, involvement of surrounding organs such as the pancreas, and the presence of enlarged lymph nodes can be assessed with EUS. Reduction of tumor size following chemotherapy can also be demonstrated.

Primary low-grade malignant gastric lymphomas arising from the mucosa-associated lymphoid tissue (MALT) appear to have sequential development from gastritis through a phase of lymphoid hyperplasia. This sequence seems to be dependent on the presence of Helicobacter pylori (HP) and early stages of the lymphoma have been shown to regress after eradication of HP. Gastric lymphomas may have a rather typical appearance on EUS images exhibiting a selective thickening of the second and sometimes the third layer in the early, HP-dependent stages. Transmural tumor infiltration or lymph node metastasis seem to indicate HP-independent disease. EUS can be applied for staging of lymphomas and may thus influence directly on the choice of treatment strategy (86–90).

Levy *et al.* (89) characterized the endoscopic ultrasonographic aspects of low grade gastric MALT lymphomas and determined the value of this procedure in medical treatment assessment. Patients examined with EUS before treatment usually had increased gastric wall thickness, and the thickening was predominately of the mucosa alone and/or the submucosa, but never extended beyond the muscularis propria. The authors found that EUS could differentiate superficial from infiltrative types of gastric MALT lymphomas and confirm remission or persistence of the disease with medical treatment during follow-up.

Fusaroli *et al.* (91) evaluated in a multicenter study the interobserver agreement of EUS in MALT lymphoma. The aim of this study was to identify EUS characteristics for selecting correct therapy and for meaningful communication in patients with these lesions.They concluded that the agreement was suboptimal ranging from substantial to fair depending on the stage.

It is also possible to examine the duodenum with EUS. However, tumors in this area are mostly tumors of the papilla of Vater or tumor ingrowth from surrounding organs. Polyps

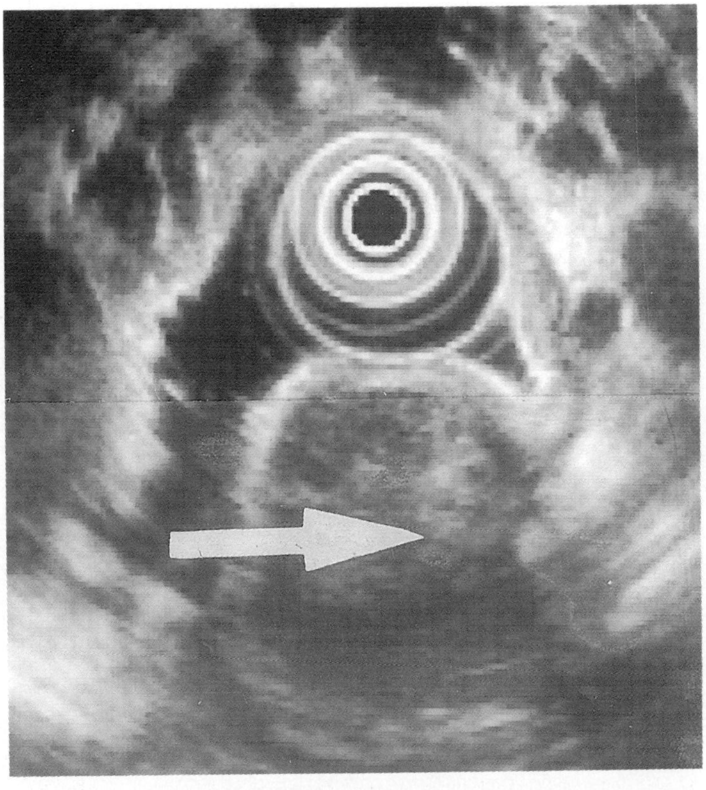

Fig. 8. A subepithelial hypoechoic tumor (arrow).

and cancers may occur in the duodenum and staging is then performed in the same manner as in other parts of the GI tract.

## 10. Subepithelial Masses

A subepithelial mass is often suspected by endoscopy when an elsewhere normal gastrointestinal wall is bulging into the lumen. Protrusion of the wall can be caused by intra- or extramural pathologic lesions as well as normal adjacent organs in some instances. EUS may demonstrate the location and echo features of subepithelial masses, which include malignant and benign tumors and also fluid-filled structures. When intramural tumors are imaged the layer of origin can usually be identified (80–82, 92–94).

Subepithelial masses are often serendipitous findings during endoscopy, but once identified they represent a managing challenge. Non-invasive imaging methods like transabdominal ultrasonography (US), computed tomography (CT) or magnetic resonance imaging (MRI) are often inadequate to characterize the cause of protrusion. The prevalence of suspected submucosal gastric lesions at routine endoscopy has been estimated to be about 0.5% (95).

Subepithelial tumors with large tumor size, ulceration, heterogeneous echo pattern (Fig. 9), cystic spaces and irregular tumor border have been associated with risk of malignancy (80, 81, 94). Serious symptoms like bleeding or obstruction and suspicion of malignancy usually prompt surgical therapy. However, lack of defined risk factors cannot exclude a malignant potential. EUS guided biopsy may be helpful in disclosing malignant tissue, but negative finding does not exclude malignancy. It may also be difficult to obtain adequate tissue samples from hard tumors and lesions within the GI wall (15, 49, 96).

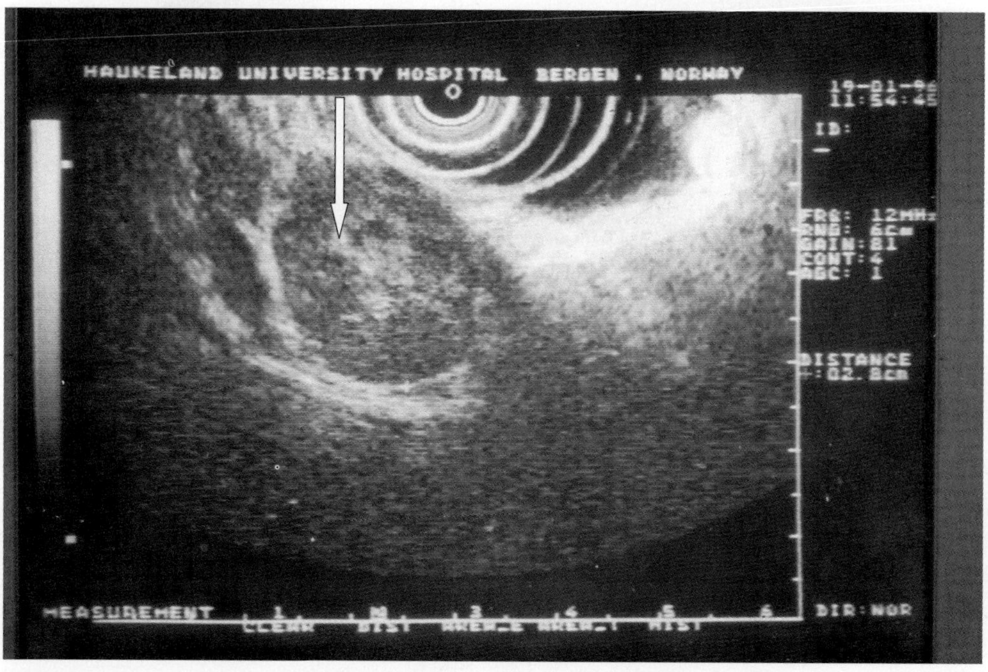


Fig. 9. Subepithelial gastric tumor with central echogenic structures (arrow).

A large proportion of submucosal tumors examined by endoscopic ultrasound appear to be gastrointestinal stromal tumors (GIST), demonstrated as a hypoechoic mass that is continuous with a myogenic layer of the normal gut wall. The majority of stromal tumors are benign, but up to 1/5 of them may be malignant. The clinical problem is to decide whether surgical resection should be performed or a follow-up would be sufficient. Chak *et al.* (80) demonstrated that tumor size (diameter $> 4$ cm), irregular extra luminal border, echogenic foci and cystic spaces were independently associated with malignancy in stromal cell tumors. Despite that it is difficult to separate malignant from benign lesions, EUS usually provides diagnostic information, which may help decide whether a lesion should be removed or followed up *in situ*. Future diagnosis of GIST may be improved if EUS is combined with other modalities like molecular marker detection in tissue samples and automatic texture analysis.

Nesje *et al.* (82) performed a study in fifty-four patients with suspected subepithelial lesions at endoscopy with the aim to diagnose and characterize subepithelial lesions of the gastrointestinal tract using EUS and search for markers of malignancy in stromal cell tumors. EUS disclosed 37 solid lesions and 10 fluid-filled structures. In 7 patients, including two with protrusion from a normal spleen, no pathology could be demonstrated. It was concluded that EUS can detect and characterize subepithelial masses in the gastrointestinal tract. Pathologic lesions of the overlying mucosa may indicate malignant development in stromal cell tumors, but valid markers of malignant potential are still lacking.

Lipomas are benign lesions, and can usually be seen as echo-rich well-defined structures located in the submucosa. In most cases, they are easy to diagnose with EUS, and they can usually be left *in situ*. Other tumors, like carcinoids, may however show a similar echogenicity (97).

Forceps biopsies from the mucosal surface are usually inconclusive for subepithelial masses and more aggressive biopsy techniques using snares or puncture may be hazardous when the cause of bulging is unknown. EUS-guided diagnostic and therapeutic procedures can improve safety and in some instances replace more extensive surgical procedures (58, 93). Doppler facilities may help distinguish vessels from other anechoic and hypoechoic structures. Contrast agents may also be used to assess vascularity and thus differentiate malignant and benign tumors. So far, however, the clinical usefulness of contrast agents in EUS examinations is still a matter of debate (98).

## 11. Other Gastrointestinal Diseases

Varices in the gastrointestinal wall, usually caused by portal hypertension, can be readily imaged by EUS as anechoic tubular structures, mainly located in the submucosa. Arterial abnormalities are less common but may cause severe, potentially life-threatening bleeding in the gastrointestinal tract. Due to a low number of cases, the role of EUS in the diagnosis and therapy of arterial malformations is not generally established. However, case reports have indicated that the method can be useful for investigation of severe gastric bleeding in the absence of gastric ulcer (21, 99).

Following sclerotherapy, submucosal varices may be obliterated but the effect on periesophageal collaterals is often uncertain (100). The sequence of acute variceal thrombosis and then organization of the thrombus following sclerotherapy has been shown with EUS. EUS may reveal recanalization of the varices indicating that further injection therapy is indicated. EUS can detect gastric varices and may be useful in distinguishing gastric varices from other causes of large rugal folds (Fig. 10). Extragastric venous collaterals in patients with portal hypertension can also be detected by EUS.

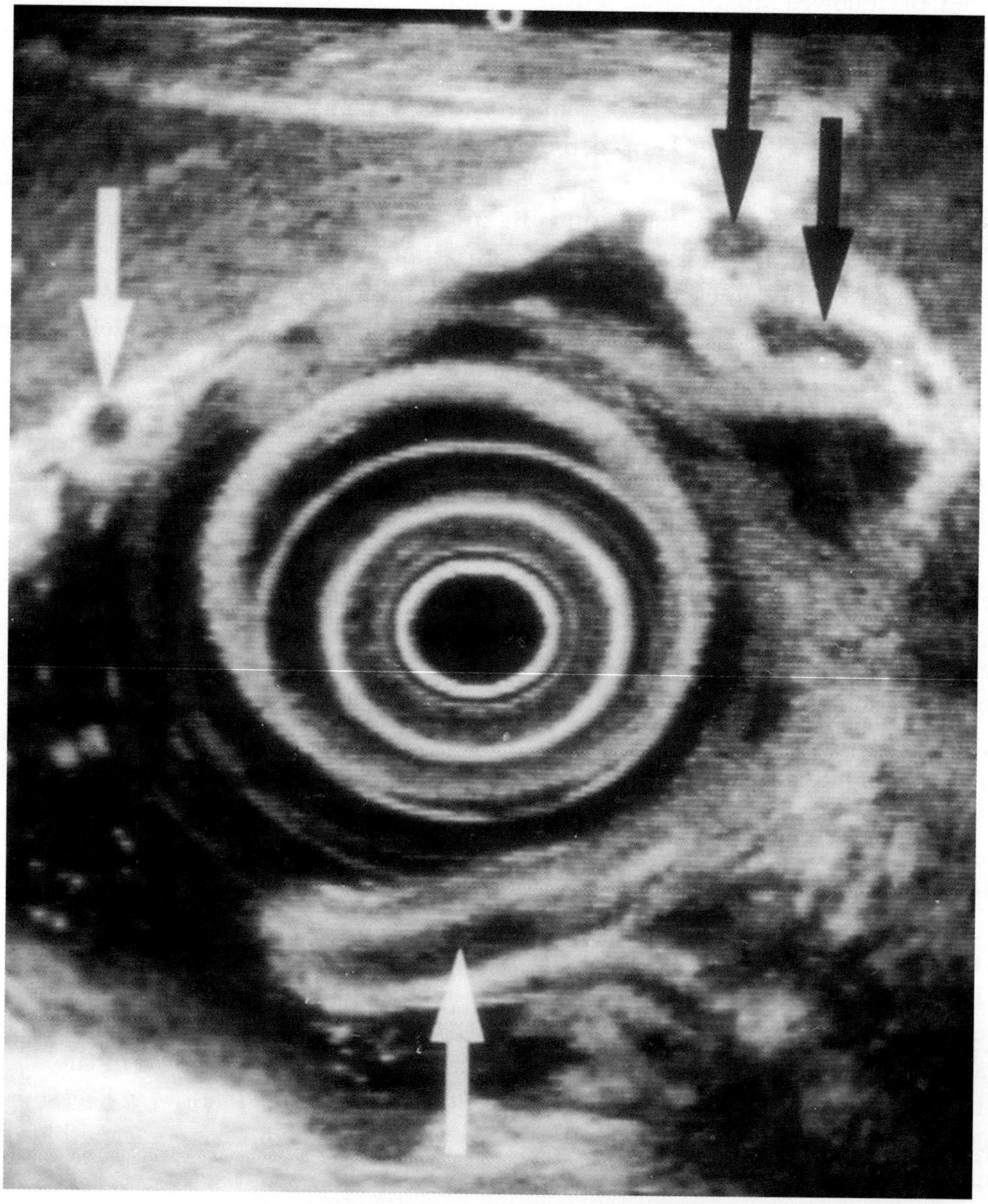

Fig. 10. Gastric varices (arrows) imaged with a 12 MHz rotating transducer.

Gastrointestinal polyps and adenomas can be evaluated by EUS with regard to their relationship to adjacent structures including blood vessels and the normal wall layers. Hence, EUS can predict whether an endoscopic resection is feasible and disclose possible risk factors. Signs of tumor infiltration can be visualized by EUS, but the method is usually not able to differentiate between benign and malignant mucosal tumors (99, 101).

Potentially premalignant diseases like Barrett's esophagus and ulcerative colitis have been subject to EUS investigations and EUS has also been applied to assess other inflammatory diseases of the gastrointestinal tract. EUS has demonstrated wall thickening, abscess formation and sometimes enlarged lymph nodes in cases of acute inflammation but has not been useful in order to disclose dysplastic changes or early malignancy in Barret's esophagus or ulcerative colitis (64, 102).

The carcinoid tumor is a unique neoplasm being neither completely malignant nor completely benign. It is thought to be an epithelial neoplasm and is known to originate in the mucosa. The tumor tends to penetrate the muscularis mucosa at an early stage, and to form a neoplastic nodule in the submucosa. Carcinoid tumors are therefore often diagnosed as submucosal tumors, and endoscopic biopsy specimen may reveal normal mucosa. Yasikane *et al.* (97) examined gastric, duodenal and rectal carcinoid tumors with endoscopic ultrasonography. The internal echo of these tumors was generally hypoechoic and homogeneous with clearly visualized borders. The tumors were mainly located in the third layer. A 20 MHz miniprobe allowed clearer imaging of the tumor margin in comparison with the conventional endosonography using an echoendoscope.

## 12. Liver, Bile Ducts, Gallbladder and Pancreas

The left liver lobe and parts of the right lobe can be visualized from the stomach and duodenum using echoendoscopes. Small tumors in the liver which cannot be seen on external ultrasound, CT scanning and MRI can thus sometimes be detected (Fig. 11). If transabdominal ultrasound guided FNA fails, EUS-FNA may be successful with regard to the diagnosis of malignant liver lesions (103). Examination of the pancreas, ampulla Vateri and the common bile duct have so far been important applications of EUS using rotating or curved array echoendoscopes. US images obtained with these instruments demonstrate the anatomy of these organs and the surrounding tissue better than what is possible with high-frequency miniprobes.

Most malignant tumours in the pancreas and bile duct can be localized using external ultrasound, CT and MRCP. However, small tumours may be difficult to see and EUS is regarded as a good imaging modality in detecting such tumours (104–112). Pancreatic endocrine tumors are rare with annual incidences below 10 per 1 million in the general population. Some of the tumors, particularly insulinomas and gastrinomas, can be small when causing severe symptoms. A major issue in the preoperative diagnostics may thus be to localize the tumor after clinical and biochemical verification. Non-invasive imaging methods tend to have insufficient sensitivity and the justification of applying invasive tests has been a matter of discussion in these cases. EUS has proved to be a sensitive modality for the imaging of pancreatic endocrine tumors, especially insulinomas (Fig. 12). EUS can demonstrate the size and the shape of the imaged tumors, as well as their relationship to adjacent structures like the pancreatic duct, bile duct, and large vessels. However, pedunculated and isoechoic tumors are usually difficult to identify by EUS (113).

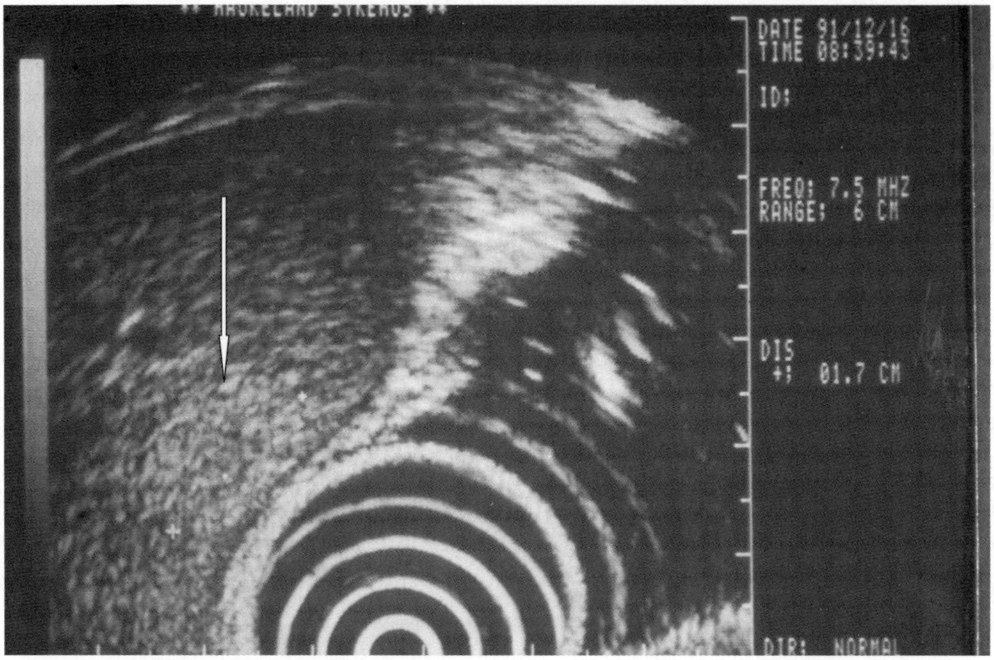


Fig. 11. Hyperechoic tumor (17 mm ×13 mm) in the liver (arrow).

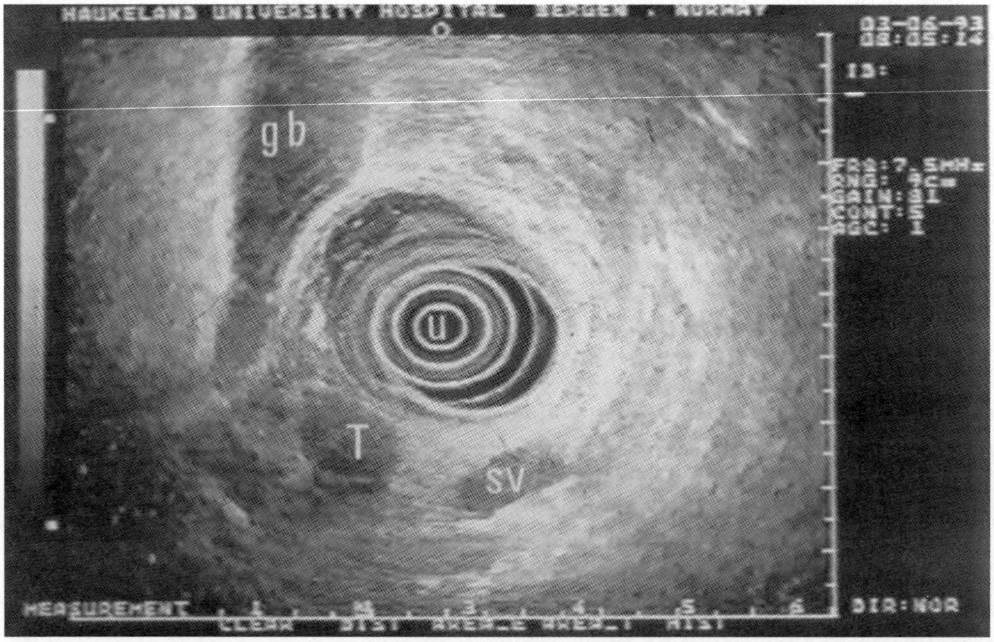


Fig. 12. Insulinoma in the head of pancreas (T). Splenic vein (sv), gall bladder (gb).

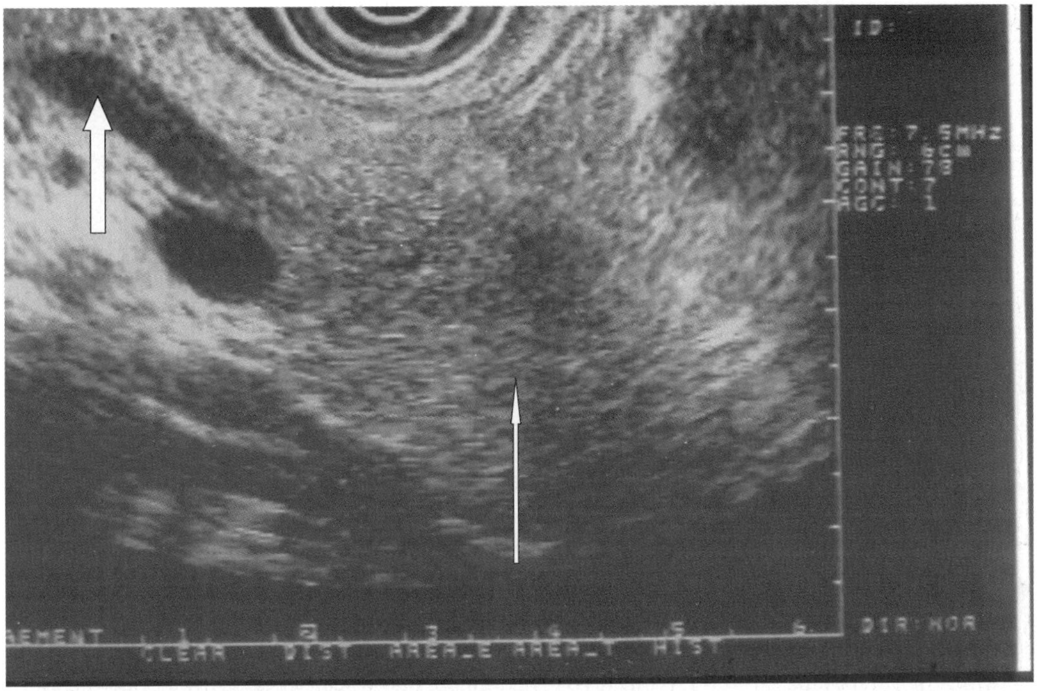

Fig. 13. Cancer in the pancreatic body and tail (thin arrow). Splenic vein (thick arrow).

Pancreatic cancer is mostly localized to the pancreatic head presenting with jaundice as the first symptom. However, most patients also have back pain at the time of diagnosis and tumors localized in the body and tail of the pancreas may present with only this symptom (Fig. 13). Early diagnosis and surgical treatment of pancreatic cancer is probably yet the only promising way to improve the treatment results of this cancer. Confirming the diagnosis of non-resectable pancreatic masses is important and EUS-FNA may influence on the therapeutic approach to such lesions.

Harewood and Wiersema (114) reported a sensitivity of EUS-FNA of 94% for malignant disease in 185 patients with inconclusive prior biopsies obtained by CT and ERCP. As demonstrated by Hahn and Faigel (115) mediastinal lymph nodes may be present in patients with pancreatic cancer. Thus, EUS, eventually EUS-FNA of the mediastinum should be performed for complete staging of pancreatic cancer.

Malignant cysts of the pancreas may be difficult to distinguish from benign cystic lesions. EUS-FNA of cystic and solid components may help making a correct diagnosis of such lesions (116). However, puncture procedures should generally be avoided in patients who are going to be operated anyway.

Carcinoma of the ampulla of Vater is infrequent compared to pancreatic cancer, but is important to recognize since patients often present with symptoms when the tumor is still resectable (Fig. 14). Five year survival after surgical resection of ampullary cancer can be expected in approximately 40% of patients. Studies indicate that EUS offers more than other imaging methoas in the preoperative staging of these tumors. Accurate staging of pancreatic and ampullary cancer is essential in choosing patients for radical resection

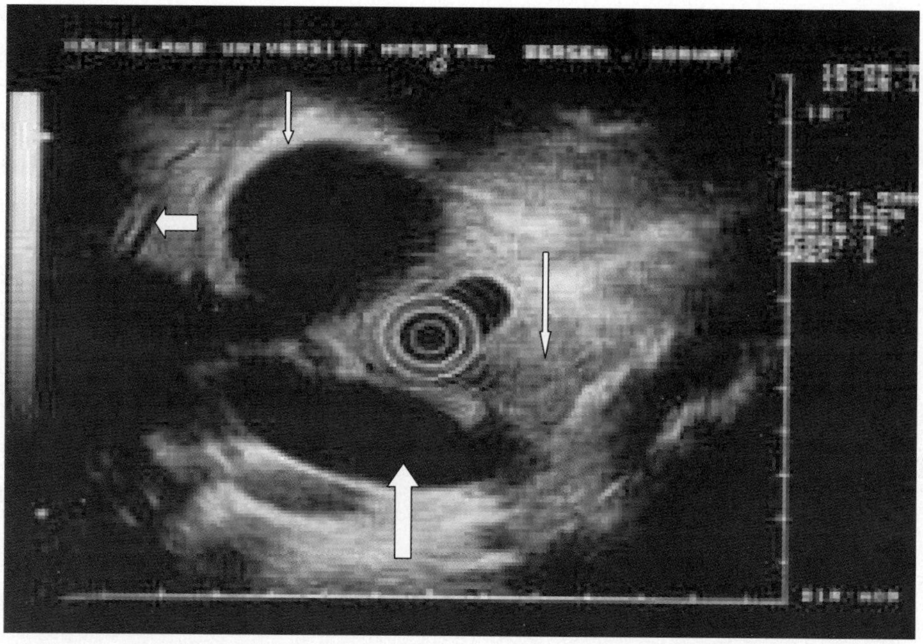

Fig. 14. Tumor of the papilla of Vater (thin arrow), common bile duct (thick arrow), gall bladder (small thin arrow), dilated intrahepatic bile ducts (small thick arrow).

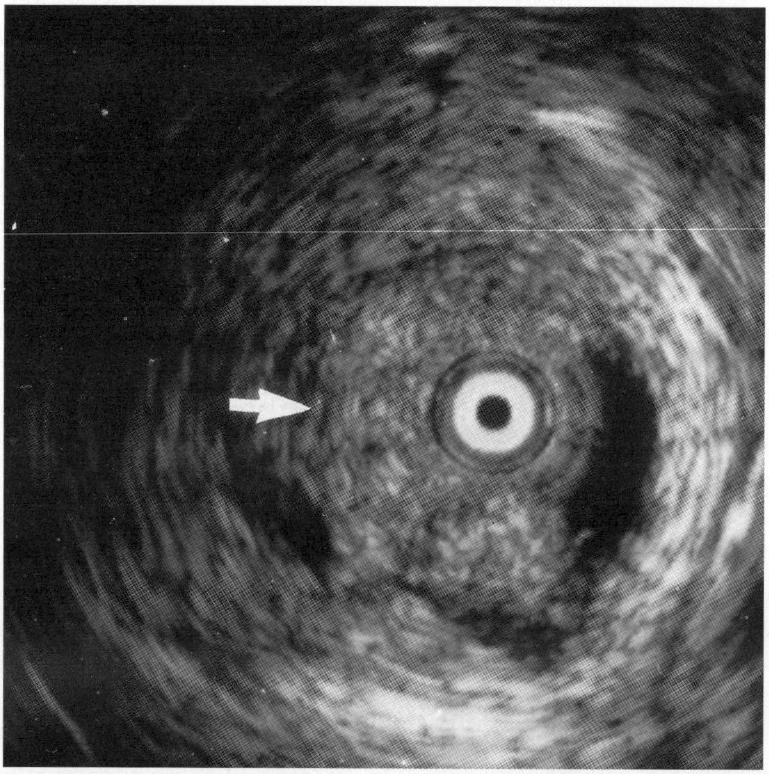

Fig. 15. Intraductal ultrasonography showing a bile duct tumor (arrow). Courtesy J. Menzel, Münster.

which until now has been the only possibility for curing patients with these diseases. EUS is a most accurate imaging method in detection and staging, and may help decide whether local resection can be sufficient or major surgery has to be performed (110, 112, 114, 117).

If cancer of the papilla of Vater is limited to the Oddi's muscle layer the prognosis is considered good. Recently, it has been shown possible to diagnose and stage even small tumors of the pancreas and bile ducts using intraductal miniprobe sonography (IDUS) (Fig. 15). This technique may be performed trans endoscopically or transcutaneously (117–120). The miniprobe can be inserted into the intrahepatic bile duct branches during ERCP or PTC. IDUS is not suitable for imaging distant metastases, but frequently the tumor and local metastases can be evaluated and tumor ingrowth into surrounding vessels my be seen indicating non-resectability. Itoh *et al.* (117) used a radial 20 MHz miniprobe for intraductal ultrasonography in diagnosing tumor extension of cancer of the papilla of Vater. In this study, IDUS was compared to EUS performed with a radial echoendoscope. The overall diagnostic accuracy rate was 87.5% in tumorstaging. IDUS was superior to EUS in detecting tumor infiltration into the bile and pancreatic ducts. Also Kuroiwa *et al.* (121) found a high accuracy rate (93%) in diagnosing tumor extension of bile duct cancer using IDUS and Menzel *et al.* (119) have recently demonstrated the potential of IDUS in the diagnosis of small insulinomas.

EUS has been proposed as a sensitive and specific imaging tool for the diagnosis of chronic pancreatitis. However, endosonographic features of chronic pancreatitis include a heterogeneous appearance of the pancreatic parenchyma with hypoechoic and echogenic areas. Focal pancreatitis may thus be difficult to separate from pancreatic cancer (Fig. 16). Ductal dilatation, strictures or stones may also be imaged with EUS, and small pseudocysts may be detected. (106, 107).

In many centers, EUS has replaced ERCP as the primary method for detection of bile duct stones (Fig. 17) since it is regarded as less invasive and has demonstrated a sensitivity similar to that of ERCP, which in some cases may cause serious pancreatitis (108, 109).

Enlargement of lymph nodes around the porta hepatis, aorta, celiac trunk, and splenic artery can be detected with EUS, and the presence of major vessel invasion by a pancreatic neoplasm precludes a curative resection. Unnecessary pancreaticoduodenectomies can be prevented in a significant number of patients if a reliable preoperative method of detecting vascular invasion is applied. EUS can detect portal vein and splenic vein involvement by pancreatic neoplasms. The presence or absence of portal vein involvement has been accurately predicted by EUS in over 90% of angiographically or histologically confirmed cases. The detection of splenic vein involvement is more difficult. Attenuation of the US beam by large tumor masses may hamper the evaluation of the splenic vein involvement in some cases.

## 13. Colon and Rectum

EUS using rectal probes is a well established method in the diagnosis and staging of rectal cancer, and EUS has also been increasingly used in some other abnormal conditions like fistula and anal disorders. Transrectal ultrasonography has been studied both for the preoperative staging and for the detection of postoperative recurrence of rectal cancer. The

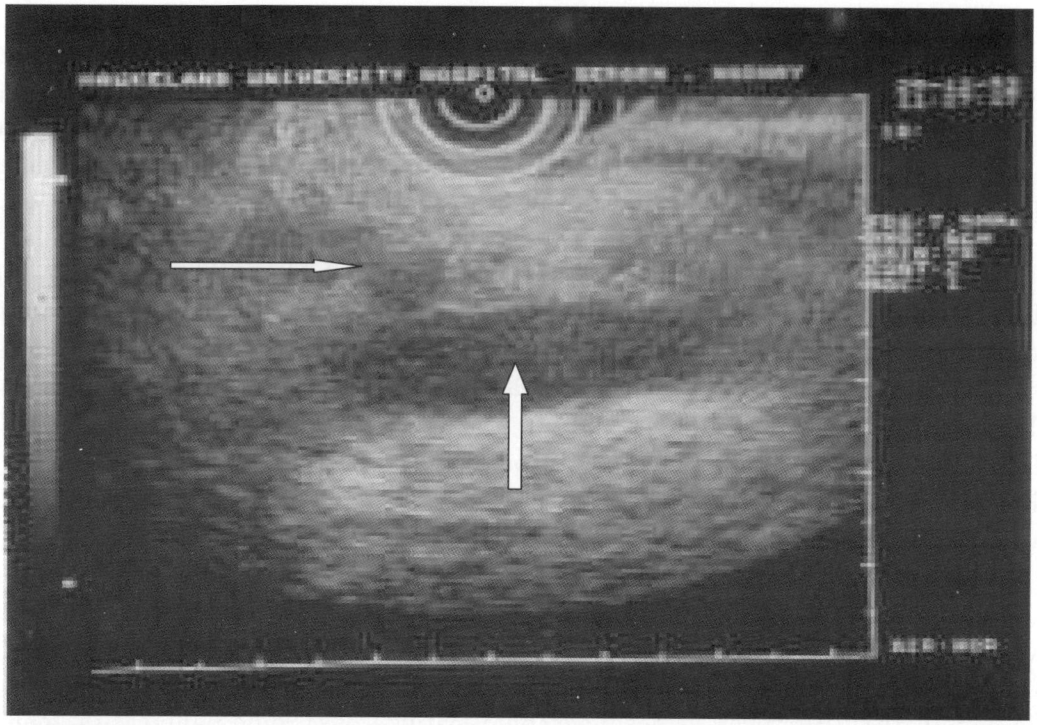

Fig. 16. Hypoechoic structure in the pancreas in a patient with pancreatitis after ERCP (thin arrow). Splenic vein (thick arrow).

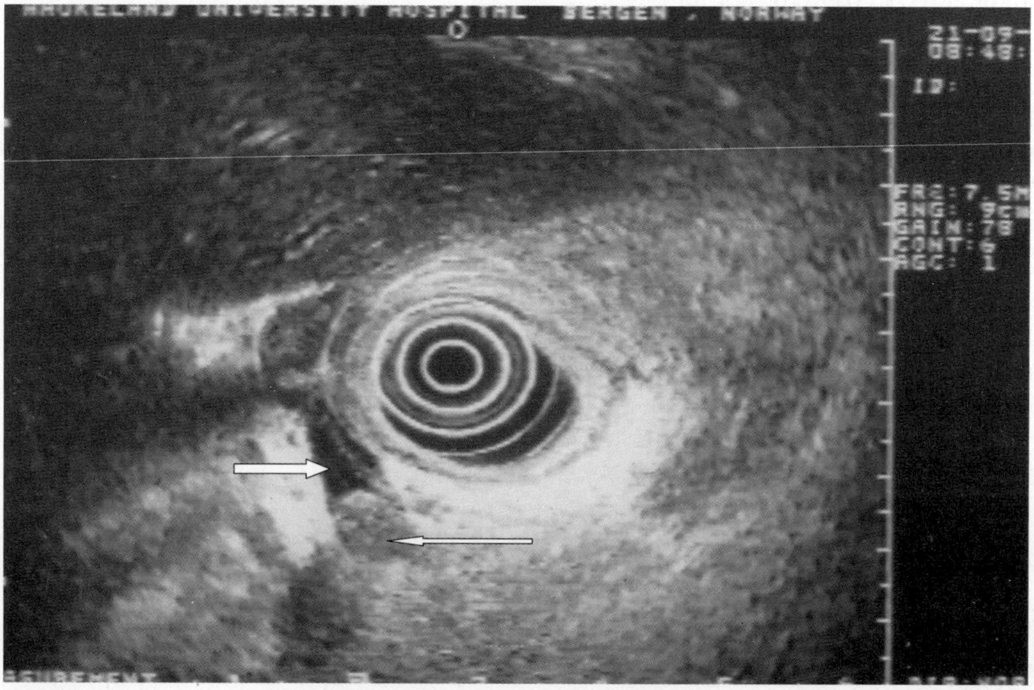


Fig. 17. Common bile duct (thick arrow) with a stone (thin arrow).

depth of cancer invasion in the rectal wall and surrounding tissue as well as the presence of malignant perirectal lymph nodes have been evaluated with transrectal ultrasound imaging. However, Marusch *et al.* (122) reported recently the results of a multicenter study including 1463 patients with rectal carcinoma. In approximately 1/3 of the patients comparison between EUS and histopathology was possible. The results were weaker than expected with an EUS diagnostic accuracy of 50.8%, 58.3%, 73.5% and 44.4% for $T1$, $T2$, $T3$ and $T4$, respectively. However, since 49 hospitals participated in the study, different experience with EUS may have influenced the results.

Dedicated echoendoscopes for use in the colon are available but have so far gained less application than those produced for use in the upper GI tract. Transendoscopic miniprobe EUS may be a practical method for EUS of the colon during conventional colonoscopy (Fig. 18) (92, 123, 124).

Evaluation of the GI wall in patients with precancerous disorders like long standing ulcerative colitis and in follow-up of patients treated for lymphomas is usually performed with colonoscopy and biopsies. EUS may be helpful in selecting areas where biopsies should be preferably obtained in these patients. Staging of cancer, evaluation of submucosal masses, polyps, wall thickening, and the surrounding area of the colon can be performed in the same way as mentioned for the upper GI tract. Watanabe *et al.* (123) stated a great need for accurate diagnosis of tumor invasion since endoscopic surgery is not indicated when a tumor has invaded beyond the middle of the submucosal layer. The combination of EUS using a miniprobe and injection of deaerated saline solution into the submucosa to elevate the tumor before ultrasonographic imaging (enhanced EUS) was helpful in staging such tumors. Recently, Kameyama *et al.* (92) evaluated several EUS systems in the diagnosis of submucosal lesions of the large intestine. Miniprobes were especially helpful for imaging lesions of the proximal colon since this part of the colon is difficult to reach with integrated echoendoscopes.

Waxman *et al.* (124) performed resection of submucosal tumors, including carcinoids, localized in the submucosa, using ultrasound miniprobe guidance. Resection was successful in 93% of the lesions.

## 14. Three-Dimensional EUS

3D-images are assumed to be easier to understand and communicate than the mental reconstruction of several 2D-images. 3D-techniques are currently under development for most imaging modalities and 3D-EUS may be applied for improved recognition of the GI anatomy and pathological lesions. 3D-EUS images can be obtained using images acquired by echoendoscopes or miniprobes (Fig. 19). Mostly, a pullback device is used to obtain parallel 2D images which are reconstructed to a 3D-image. Acquired ultrasound images can be stored and digitized using frame grabbing but direct digitizing of ultrasound raw data is being increasingly used in new scanners. Advanced software programs using different rendering or other reconstruction techniques are used for postprocessing and display of 3D ultrasound data, which can be studied using algorithms for anyplane slicing, segmentation, and volume calculation (125–129).

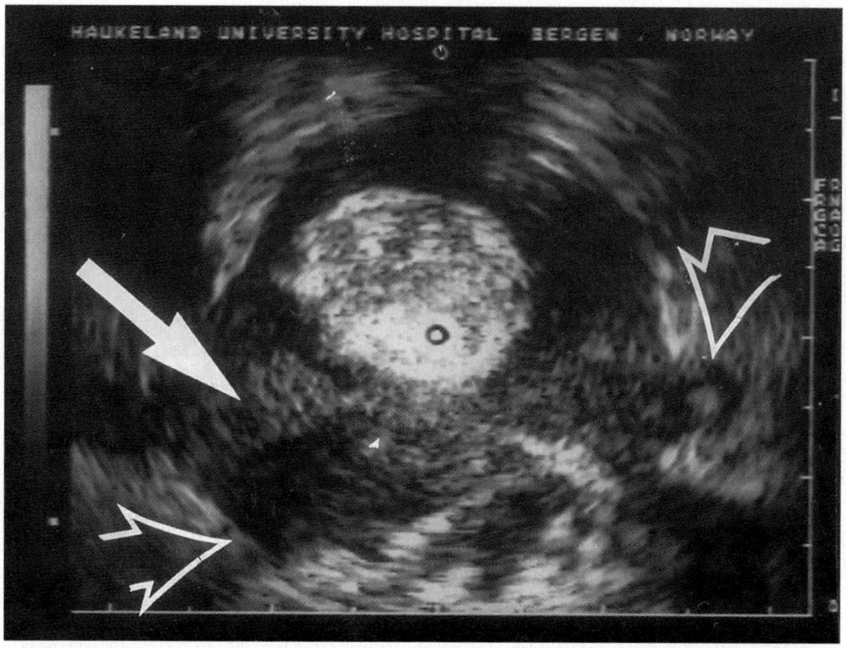


Fig. 18. A 12 MHz radial ultrasound image of a colonic cancer is shown. The hypoechoic tumor (closed arrow) is shown to infiltrate the pericolonic fatty tissue (open arrows).

## 15. EUS in Clinical Decision Making

The clinical implications of EUS have to be defined according to new medical and surgical treatment options which indicate the need for diagnostic tools capable of making a precise diagnosis, especially in selecting an appropriate treatment for cancer patients. In a prospective multicenter study, Nickl *et al.* (60) demonstrated that EUS changed the treatment plan in 74% of patients. In 31% the management changes were of major importance. The clinical impact of endoscopic ultrasound in gastrointestinal disease has also been evaluated by Jafri *et al.* (130) who concluded that endosonography is helpful in improving diagnostic certainty frequently leading to altered patient management.

## 16. Future Aspects

Lutz and Rösch (131) already performed a transgastroscopic EUS examination in 1976. EUS was initially developed as an imaging modality but has subsequently also become a tool for monitoring diagnostic and therapeutic interventions through the endoscope (132, 133). The number of different EUS instruments is increasing allowing the investigators to choose the most appropriate instruments for the separate tasks. The need for dedicated instruments and qualified investigators will probably limit the full utilization of EUS to larger centers. Miniature probes, which are less costly and easier to operate, will most likely be available in a majority of endoscopy units within a few years.

Systems for three-dimensional (3D) EUS have already been developed but need further refinement in order to allow true spatial reconstruction of imaged organs. Current systems

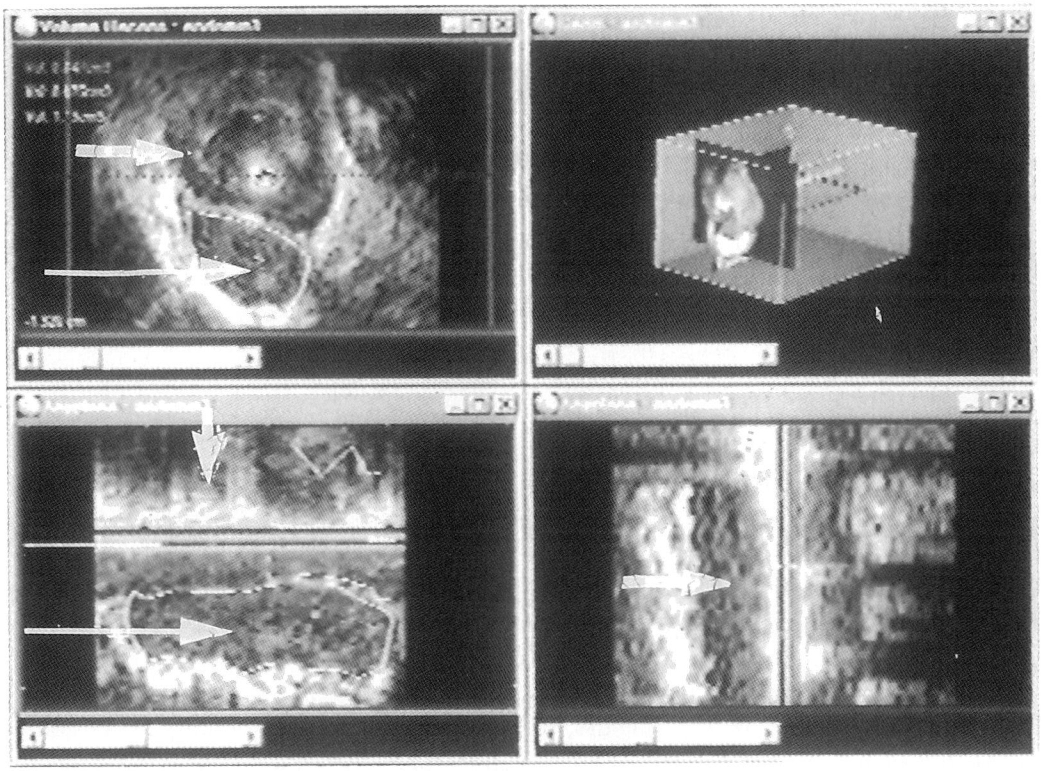

Fig. 19. 3D display (EchoPac 3D software) of esophageal cancer based on images aquired during pull-back of a radial-scanning ultrasound miniprobe. Original scan showing the esophageal wall (thick arrow) and a periesophageal lymph node (arrow) in the upper left window. The lower windows show two orthogonal reconstructed images with the lymph node (thin arrow) and a thickened esophageal wall (thick arrow). A geometric reconstruction is displayed in the upper right window. Manual outlining of structures in the reconstruction window (upper left) is automatically recorded in other windows.

are founded on linear pull-back of radial-scanning probes (129). In curved organs like the stomach, however, the lateral probe movement also has to be controlled. An electromagnetic position and orientation monitoring system will certainly be valuable for endoluminal probes (134, 135). Further improvement in electronic data processing systems may allow future 3D-EUS to be performed in real time, providing new possibilities for safe and accurate guiding of interventions.

If 3D-EUS reflects the true size, shape and relationship of visceral organs these 3D-images can be superimposed or combined with 3D-images from other modalities such as CT or MRI (136). Thus, the specific advantages of the different modalities can be utilized in common display systems allowing small details and overviews to be presented simultaneously.

Telemedicine is already established as a system for distant evaluation and assistance. High-capacity communication lines allow EUS examinations to be transferred in real-time (137). This may be important particulary in small centers with a few or single EUS investigators. 3D-EUS enables transfer of volumetric data sets in which a distant investigator at a later occasion can navigate and image virtual sections in any plane (138).

As various EUS systems technically develop, their role and impact in clinical practice has to be continously evaluated. Future studies on EUS will to a large degree have to be focused on its impact on management and clinical outcome of the patients.

## References

1. Wild, J. J. and Reid, J. M., Diagnostic use of ultrasound. Br J Phys Med 1956; 19: 248–57.
2. Tio, T. L., Endosonography in gastroenterology. Berlin, Springer-Verlag. 1988.
3. Kimmey, M. B. and Martin, R. W., Fundamentals of endosonography. Gastrointest Clin N Am 1992; 2: 557–73.
4. Rösch, T. and Classen, M., Gastroenterologic endosonography. Stuttgart, Georg Thieme Verlag. 1992.
5. Van Dam J. and Sivak, M. V., eds. Gastrointestinal endosonography. Philadelphia, W. B. Saunders Company, 1999.
6. Fukuda, M. and Hirata, K., Endoscopic ultrasonography in gastroenterology. Front Gastrointest Res 1997; 24: 182–202
7. Van Dam J., Brady, P. G., Freeman, M., Gress, F., Gross, G. W., Hassall, E., Hawes, R., Jacobsen, N. A., Liddle, R. A., Ligresti, R. J. *et al.*, Guidelines for training in endoscopic ultrasound: Guidelines for clinical application. From the ASGE. American Society for Gastrointestinal Endoscopy. Gastrointest Endosc 1999; 49: 829–33.
8. Kimmey, M. B., Martin, R. W., Haggitt, R. C., Wang, K. Y. and Franklin, D. W., Silverstein FE: Histological correlates of gastrointestinal endoscopic ultrasound images. Gastroenterology 1989; 96: 433–441.
9. Yanai, H., Noguchi, T., Mizumachi, S., Tokiyama, H., Nakamura, H., Tada, M. and Okita, K., A blind comparison of the effectiveness of endoscopic ultrasonography and endoscopy in staging early gastric cancer. Gut 1999; 44: 361–5.
10. Schlick, T., Heintz, A. and Junginger, T., The examiner's learning effect and its influence on the quality of endoscopic ultrasonography in carcinoma of the esophagus and gastric cardia. Surg Endosc 1999; 13: 894–8.
11. Kimmey, M. B., Martin, R. W. and Silverstein, F. E., Clinical application of linear ultrasound probes. Endoscopy 1992; 24(Suppl 1): 364–9.
12. Chak, A., Canto, M., Stevens, P. D., Lightdale, C. J., Van de Mierop, F., Cooper, G., Pollack, B. J. and Sivak, M. V. J., Clinical applications of a new through-the-scope ultrasound probe: Prospective comparison with an ultrasound endoscope. Gastrointest Endosc 1997; 45: 291–5.
13. Menzel, J. and Domschke, W., Gastrointestinal miniprobe sonography: The current status. Am J Gastroenterol 2000; 95: 605–16.
14. Hasegawa, N., Niwa, Y., Arisawa, T., Hase, S., Goto, H. and Hayakawa, T., Preoperative staging of superficial esophageal carcinoma: Comparison of an ultrasound probe and standard endoscopic ultrasonography. Gastrointest Endosc 1996; 44: 388–93.
15. Vilmann, P., Hancke, S., Henriksen, F. W. and Jacobsen, G. K., Endoscopic ultrasonography-guided fine-needle aspiration biopsy of lesions in the upper gastrointestinal tract. Gastrointest Endosc 1995; 41: 230–5.
16. Antillon, M. R. and Chang, K. J., Endoscopic and endosonography guided fine-needle aspiration. Gastrointest Endosc Clin N Am 2000; 10: 619–36.
17. Bhutani, M. S., Interventional endoscopic ultrasonography: State of the art at the new millenium. Endoscopy 2000; 32: 62–71.

18. Silverstein, F. E., Martin, R. W., Kimmey, M. B., Jiranek, G. C., Franklin, D. W. and Proctor, A., Experimental evaluation of an endoscopic ultrasound probe: *in vitro* and *in vivo* canine studies. Gastroenterology 1989; 96: 1058–1062.
19. Nesje, L. B., Ødegaard, S. and Kimmey, M. B., Transendoscopic ultrasonography during conventional upper gastrointestinal endoscopy. Scand J Gastroenterol 1997; 32: 500–508.
20. Yanai, H., Yoshida, T., Harada, T., Matsumoto, Y., Nishiaki, M., Shigemitsu, T. *et al.*, Endoscopic ultrasonography of superficial esophageal cancers using a thin ultrasound probe system equipped with switchable radial and linear scanning modes. Gastrointest Endosc 1996; 44: 578–82.
21. Matre, K., Ødegaard, S. and Hausken, T., Endoscopic ultrasound doppler probes for velocity measurements in vessels in the upper gastrointestinal tract using a multifrequency pulsed doppler meter. Endoscopy 1990; 22: 268–270.
22. Kohler, B. and Riemann, J. F., The role of endoscopic Doppler-sonography. Hepatogastroenterology 1999; 46: 732–6.
23. Panelli, F., Erickson, R. A. and Prasad, V. M., Evaluation of mediastinal masses by endoscopic ultrasound and endoscopic ultrasound-guided fine needle aspiration. Am J Gastroenterol 2001; 96: 401–8.
24. Pedersen, B. H., Vilmann, P., Folke, K., Jacobsen, G. K., Krasnik, M., Milman, N. and Hancke, S., Endoscopic ultrasonography and real-time guided fine-needle aspiration biopsy of solid lesions of the mediastinum suspected of malignancy. Chest 1996; 110: 539–44.
25. Aabakken, L., Silvestri, G. A., Hawes, R., Reed, C. E., Marsi, V. and Hoffman, B., Cost-efficacy of endoscopic ultrasonography with fine-needle aspiration vs. mediastinotomy in patients with lung cancer and suspected mediastinal adenopathy. Endoscopy 1999; 31: 707–11.
26. Fritscher-Ravens, A., Sriram, P. V., Bobrowski, C., Pforte, A., Topalidis, T., Krause, C., Jaeckle, S., Thonke, F. and Soehendra, N., Mediastinal lymphadenopathy in patients with or without previous malignancy: EUS-FNA-based differential cytodiagnosis in 153 patients. Am J Gastroenterol 2000; 95: 2278–84.
27. Brugge, W. R., Lee, M. J., Carey, R. W. and Mathisen, D. J., Endoscopic ultrasound staging criteria for esophageal cancer. Gastrointest Endosc 1997; 45: 147–52.
28. Menzel, J., Hoepffner, N., Nottberg, H., Schulz, C., Senninger, N. and Domschke, W., Preoperative staging of esophageal carcinoma: Miniprobe sonography versus conventional endoscopic ultrasound in a prospective histopathologically verified study. Endoscopy 1999; 31: 291–7.
29. Murata, Y., Suzuki, S., Mitsunaga, A., Iizuka, Y., Uchiyama, M., Uchida, K., Nakamura, S., Hayashi, K., Yoshida, K., Toki, F. and Ide, H., Endoscopic ultrasonography in diagnosis and mucosal resection for early esophageal cancer. Endoscopy 1998; 30(Suppl 1): A44–6.
30. Reed, C. E., Mishra, G., Sahai, A. V., Hoffman, B. J. and Hawes, R. H., Esophageal cancer staging: Improved accuracy by endoscopic ultrasound of celiac lymph nodes. Ann Thorac Surg 1999; 67: 319–21.
31. Rice, T. W., Clinical staging of esophageal carcinoma. CT, EUS, and PET. Chest Surg Clin N Am 2000; 10: 471–85.
32. Tio, T. L., Diagnosis and staging of esophageal carcinoma by endoscopic ultrasonography. Endoscopy 1998; 30(Suppl 1): A33–A40.
33. Heidemann, J., Schilling, M. K., Schmassmann, A., Maurer, C. A. and Buchler M. W., Accuracy of endoscopic ultrasonography in preoperative staging of esophageal carcinoma. Dig Surg 2000; 17: 219–24.
34. Fukuda, M., Hirata, K. and Natori, H., Endoscopic ultrasonography of the esophagus. World J Surg 2000; 24: 216–26.

35. Rosch, T., Endosonographic staging of gastric cancer: A review of literature results. Gastrointest Endosc Clin N Am 1995; 5: 549–57.
36. Willis, S., Truong, S., Gribnitz, S., Fass, J. and Schumpelick, V., Endoscopic ultrasonography in the preoperative staging of gastric cancer: Accuracy and impact on surgical therapy. Surg Endosc 2000; 14: 951–4.
37. Hunerbein, M., Ghadimi, B. M., Haensch, W. and Schlag, P. M., Transendoscopic ultrasound of esophageal and gastric cancer using miniaturized ultrasound catheter probes. Gastrointest Endosc 1998; 48: 371–5.
38. Tio, T. L., Cheng, J., Wijers, O. B., Sars, P. R. and Tytgat, G. N., Endosonographic TNM staging of extrahepatic bile duct cancer: Comparison with pathological staging. Gastroenterology 1991; 100: 1351–61.
39. Ahmad, N. A., Lewis, J. D., Ginsberg, G. G., Rosato, E. F., Morris, J. B. and Kochman, M. L., EUS in preoperative staging of pancreatic cancer. Gastrointest Endosc 2000; 52: 463–8.
40. Brugge, W. R., Pancreatic cancer staging. Endoscopic ultrasonography criteria for vascular invasion. Gastrointest Endosc Clin N Am 1995; 5: 741–53.
41. Hildebrandt, U., Schuder, G. and Feifel, G., Preoperative staging of rectal and colonic cancer. Endoscopy 1994; 26: 810–2.
42. Hunerbein, M., Totkas, S., Ghadimi, B. M. and Schlag, P. M., Preoperative evaluation of colorectal neoplasms by colonoscopic miniprobe ultrasonography. Ann Surg 2000; 232: 46–50.
43. Spinelli, P., Schiavo, M., Meroni, E., Di Felice, G., Andreola, S., Gallino, G., Belli, F. and Leo, E., Results of EUS in detecting perirectal lymph node metastases of rectal cancer: The pathologist makes the difference. Gastrointest Endosc 1999; 49: 754–8.
44. Faigel, D. O., EUS in patients with benign and malignant lymphadenopathy. Gastrointest Endosc 2001; 53: 593–8.
45. Bhutani, M. S., Hawes, R. H. and Hoffman, B. J., A comparison of the accuracy of echo features during endoscopic ultrasound (EUS) and EUS-guided fine-needle aspiration for diagnosis of malignant lymph node invasion. Gastrointest Endosc 1997; 45: 474–9.
46. Maruta, S., Tsukamoto, Y., Niwa, Y., Goto, H., Hase, S. and Yoshikane, H., Endoscopic ultrasonography for assessing the horizontal extent of invasive gastric carcinoma. Am J Gastroenterol 1993; 88: 555–9.
47. Tio, T. L., Large gastric folds evaluated by endoscopic ultrasonography. Gastrointest Endosc Clin N Am 1995; 5: 683–91.
48. Vilmann, P., Hancke, S., Henriksen, F. W. and Jacobsen, G. K., Endosonographically-guided fine needle aspiration biopsy of malignant lesions in the upper gastrointestinal tract. Endoscopy 1993; 25: 523–7.
49. Wiersema, M. J., Vilmann, P., Giovannini, M., Chang, K. J. and Wiersema, L. M., Endosonography-guided fine-needle aspiration biopsy: diagnostic accuracy and complication assessment. Gastroenterology 1997; 112: 1087–95.
50. Vazquez-Sequeiros, E., Norton, I. D., Clain, J. E., Wang, K. K., Affi, A., Allen, M., Deschamps, C., Miller, D., Salomao, D. and Wiersema, M. J., Impact of EUS-guided fine-needle aspiration on lymph node staging in patients with esophageal carcinoma. Gastrointest Endosc 2001; 53: 751–7.
51. Wiersema, M. J., Kochman, M. L., Cramer, H. M., Tao, L. C. and Wiersema, L. M., Endosonography-guided real-time fine-needle aspiration biopsy. Gastrointest Endosc 1994; 40: 700–7.
52. Gress, F., Schmitt, C., Sherman, S., Ikenberry, S. and Lehman, G., A prospective randomized comparison of endoscopic ultrasound- and computed tomography-guided celiac plexus block for managing chronic pancreatitis pain. Am J Gastroenterol 1999; 94: 900–5.

53. Abedi, M. and Zfass, A. M., Endoscopic ultrasound-guided (neurolytic) celiac plexus block. J Clin Gastroenterol 2001; 32: 390–3.
54. Gunaratnam, N. T., Sarma, A. V., Norton, I. D. *et al.*, A prospective study of EUS-guided celiac plexus neurolysis for pancreatic cancer pain. Gastrointest Endosc 2001; 54: 316–324.
55. Giovannini, M., Pesenti, C., Rolland, A. L. *et al.*, Endoscopic ultrasound-guided drainage of pancreatic pseudocysts or pancreatic abscesses using a therapeutic echoendoscope. Endoscopy 2001; 33: 473–477.
56. Vilmann, P., Hancke, S., Pless, T., Schell-Hincke, J. D. and Henriksen, F. W., One-step endosonography-guided drainage of a pancreatic pseudocyst: A new technique of stent delivery through the echo endoscope. Endoscopy 1998 Oct; 30(8): 730–3.
57. Seifert, H., Dietrich, C., Schmitt, T., Caspary, W. and Wehrmann, T., Endoscopic ultrasound-guided one-step transmural drainage of cystic abdominal lesions with a large-channel echo endoscope. Endoscopy. 2000 Mar; 32(3): 255–9.
58. Kawamoto, K., Yamada, Y., Furukawa, N., Utsunomiya, T., Haraguchi, Y., Mizuguchi, M., Oiwa, T., Takano, H. and Masuda, K., Endoscopic submucosal tumorectomy for gastrointestinal submucosal tumors restricted to the submucosa: A new form of endoscopic minimal surgery. Gastrointest Endosc 1997; 46: 311–7.
59. Murata, Y., Napoleon, B. and Odegaard, S., High-frequency endoscopic ultrasonography in the evaluation of superficial esophageal cancer. Endoscopy 2003; 35(5): 429–436.
60. Nickl, N. J., Bhutani, M. S., Catalano, M., Hoffman, B., Hawes, R., Chak, A., Roubein, L. D., Kimmey, M., Johnson, M., Affronti, J., Canto, M., Sivak, M., Boyce, H. W., Lightdale, C. J., Stevens, P. and Schmitt, C., Clinical implications of endoscopic ultrasound: The American Endosonography Club Study. Gastrointest Endosc 1996; 44: 371–7.
61. Nesje, L. B., Svanes, K., Viste, A., Lærum, O. D. and Ødegaard, S., Comparison of a linear miniature ultrasound probe and a radial scanning echoendoscope in TN staging of esophageal cancer. Scand J Gastroenterol 2000; 35: 997–1002.
62. Chak, A., Canto, M., Gerdes, H., Lightdale, C. J., Hawes, R. H., Wiersema, M. J., Kallimanis, G., Lok Tio, T., Rice, T. W., Boyce, H. W. and Sivak, M. V., Prognosis of esophageal cancers preoperatively staged to be locally invasive ($T4$) by endoscopic ultrasound (EUS): A multicenter retrospective cohort study. Gastrointest Endosc 1995; 42: 501–6.
63. Fockens, P., Manshanden, C. G., Lanschot, van J. B., Obertop, H. and Tytgat, G. N. J., Prospective study on the value of endosonographic follow-up after surgery for esophageal carcinoma. Gastrointest Endosc 1997; 46: 487–91.
64. Adrain, A. L., Ter, H. C., Cassidy, M. J., Schiano, T. D., Liu, J. B. and Miller, L. S., High-resolution endoluminal sonography is a sensitive modality for the identification of Barrett's metaplasia. Gastrointest Endosc 1997; 46: 147–51.
65. Fusaroli, P. and Caletti, G., Endoscopic ultrasonography. Endoscopy 2003; 35(2): 127–135.
66. Scotiniotis, I. A., Kochman, M. L., Lewis, J. D. *et al.*, Accuracy of EUS in the evaluation of Barrett's esophagus and high-grade dysplasia or intramucosal carcinoma. Gastrointest Endosc 2001; 54: 689–696.
67. Harewood, G. C. and Wiersema, M. J., A cost analysis of endoscopic ultrasound in the evaluation of esophageal cancer. Am J Gastroenterol 2002; 97: 452–458.
68. Eloubeidi, M. A., Wallace, M. B., Reed, C. E. *et al.*, The utility of EUS and EUS-guided fine-needle aspiration in detecting celiac lymph node metastasis in patients with esophageal cancer; a single-center experience. Gastrointest Endosc 2001; 54: 714–719.
69. Romagnuolo, J., Scott, J., Hawes, R. H. *et al.*, Helical CT versus EUS with fine-needle aspiration for celiac nodal assessment in patients with esophageal cancer. Gastrointest Endosc 2002; 55: 648–654.

70. Willis, J., Cooper, G. S., Isenberg, G. *et al.*, Correlation of EUS measurement with pathologic assessment of neoadjuvant therapy response in esophageal carcinoma. Gastrointest Endosc 2002; 55: 655–661.
71. Niwa, Y., Nakazawa, S., Tsukamoto, Y., Goto, H., Hase, S., Ohashi, S., Mizutani, K., Yoshikane, H., Yoshino, J., Nakamura, T. *et al.*, A new method for evaluating gastric ulcer healing by endoscopic ultrasonography. Scand J Gastroenterol 1991; 26: 457–64.
72. Tanaka, M., Maruoka, A., Chijiiwa, Y., Tanaka, M. and Nawata, H., Endoscopic ultrasonographic evaluation of gastric ulcer healing on treatment with proton pump inhibitors versus H2-receptor antagonists. Scand J Gastroenterol 1994; 29: 1140–1144.
73. Yoshikane, H., Tsukamoto, Y., Niwa, Y., Goto, H. and Hase, S., Sequential observation of gastric ulcer healing by endoscopic ultrasonography. Scand J Gastroenterol 1994; 29: 665–670.
74. Yanai, H., Tada, M., Karita, M. and Okita, K., Diagnostic utility of 20-megahertz linear endoscopic ultrasonography in early gastric cancer. Gastrointest Endosc 1996; 44: 29–33.
75. Yanai, H., Fujimura, H., Suzumi, M., Matsuura, S., Awaya, N., Noguchi, T., *et al.*, Delineation of the gastric muscularis mucosae and assessment of depth of invasion of early gastric cancer using a 20-megahertz endoscopic ultrasound probe. Gastrointest Endosc 1993; 39: 505–12.
76. Akahoshi, K., Chijiiwa, Y., Hamada, S., Sasaki, I., Maruoka, A., Kabemura, T. and Nawata, H., Endoscopic ultrasonography: A promising method for assessing the prospects of endoscopic mucosal resection in early gastric cancer. Endoscopy 1997; 29: 614–619.
77. Yasuda, K., Endoscopic ultrasonic probes and mucosectomy for early gastric carcinoma. Gastrointest Endosc 1996; 43: S29–S31.
78. Ødegaard, S. and Kimmey, M. B., Location of the muscularis mucosae on high frequency gastrointestinal ultrasound images. Eur J Ultrasound 1994; 1: 39–50.
79. Yanai, H., Matsumoto, M. D., Harada, T. *et al.*, Endoscopic ultrasonography and endoscopy for staging depth of invasion in early gastric cancer — A pilot study. Gastrointest Endosc 1997; 46: 212–216.
80. Chak, A., Canto, M. I., Rosch, T., Dittler, H. J., Hawes, R. H., Tio, T. L., Lightdale, C. J., Boyce, H. W., Scheiman, J., Carpenter, S. L., Van Dam J., Kochman, M. L. and Sivak, M. V. Jr., Endosonographic differentiation of benign and malignant stromal cell tumors. Gastrointest Endosc 1997; 45: 468–73.
81. Palazzo, L., Landi, B., Cellier, C., Cuillerier, E., Roseau, G. and Barbier, J. P., Endosonographic features predictive of benign and malignant gastrointestinal stromal cell tumours. Gut 2000; 46: 88–92.
82. Nesje, L. B., Laerum, O. D., Svanes, K., Ødegaard, S., Subepithelial masses of the gastrointestinal tract evaluated by endoscopic ultasonography. Eur J Ultrasound 2002; 15: 45–54.
83. Ando, N., Goto, H., Niwa, Y. *et al.*, The diagnosis of GI stromal tumors with EUS-guided fineneedle aspiration with immunohistochemical analysis. Gastrointest Endosc 2002; 55: 37–43.
84. Songür, Y., Okai, T., Watanabe, H. *et al.*, Endosonographic evaluation of giant gastric folds. Gastrointest endosc 41; 1995: 468–74.
85. Caletti, G., Fusaroli, P., Togliani, T., Bocus, P. and Roda, E., Endosonography in gastric lymphoma and large gastric folds. Eur J Ultrasound 2000; 11: 31–40
86. Fischbach, W., Dragosics, B., Kolve-Goebeler, M. E., Ohmann, C., Greiner, A., Yang, Q., Bohm, S., Verreet, P., Horstmann, O., Busch, M., Duhmke, E., Muller-Hermelink, H. K. and Wilms, K., Primary gastric B-cell lymphoma: Results of a prospective multicenter study. The German-Austrian Gastrointestinal Lymphoma Study Group. Gastroenterology 2000; 119: 1191–202.

87. Sackmann, M., Morgner, A., Rudolph, B., Neubauer, A., Thiede, C. *et al.*, Regression of gastric malt lymphoma after eradication of helicobacter pylori is predicted by endosonographic staging. Gastroenterology 1997; 113: 1087–1090.
88. Van Dam J., The role of endoscopic ultrasonography in monitoring treatment: Response to chemotherapy in lymphoma. Endoscopy 1994; 26: 772–773.
89. Levy, M., Hammel, P., Lamarque, D., Marty, O., Chaumette, M.-T., Haioun, C., Blazquez, M. and Delchier, J.-C., Endoscopic ultrasonography for the initial staging and follow-up in patients with low-grade gastric lymphoma of mucosa-associated lymphoid tissue treated medically. Gastrointest Endosc 1997; 46: 328–33.
90. Lugering, N., Menzel, J., Kucharzik, T. *et al.*, Impact of miniprobes compared to conventional endosonography in the staging of low-grade gastric MALT lymphoma. Endoscopy 2001; 33: 832–837.
91. Fusaroli, P., Buscarini, E., Peyre, S. *et al.*, Interobserver agreement in staging gastric malt lymphoma by EUS. Gastrointest Endosc 2002; 55: 662–668.
92. Kameyama, H., Niwa, Y., Arisawa, T., Goto, H. and Hayakawa, T., Endoscopic ultrasonography in the diagnosis of submucosal lesions of the large intestine. Gastrointest Endosc 1997; 46: 406–411
93. Hizawa, K., Matsumoto, T., Kouzuki, T., Suekane, H., Esaki, M., Fujishima, M., Cystic submucosal tumors in the gastrointestinal tract: Endosonographic findings and endoscopic removal. Endoscopy 2000; 32: 712–4.
94. Sun, S., Wang, M. and Sun, S., Use of endoscopic ultrasound-guided injection in endoscopic resection of solid submucosal tumors. Endoscopy 2002; 34: 82–85.
95. Hedenbro, J. L., Ekelund, M. and Wetterberg, P., Endoscopic diagnosis of submucosal gastric lesions. The results after routine endoscopy. Surg Endosc 1991; 5: 20–3.
96. Gress, F. G., Hawes, R. H., Savides, T. J., Ikenberry, S. O. and Lehman, G. A., Endoscopic ultrasound-guided fine-needle aspiration biopsy using linear array and radial scanning endosonography. Gastrointest Endosc 1997; 45: 243–250.
97. Yoshikane, H., Tsukamoto, Y., Niwa, Y., Goto, H., Hase, S., Mizutani, K. and Nakamura, T., Carcinoid tumors of the gastrointestinal tract: evaluation with endoscopic ultrasonography. Gastrointest Endosc 1993; 39: 375–83.
98. Bhutani, M. S., Hoffman, B. J., van Velse, A. and Hawes, R. H., Contrast-enhanced endoscopic ultrasonography with galactose microparticles: SHU508A (Levovist). Endoscopy 1997; 29: 635–639.
99. Nesje, L. B., Skarstein, A., Matre, K., Myking, A. O. and Ødegaard, S., Dieulafoy's vascular malformation: Role of endoscopic ultrasonography in therapeutic decision-making. Scand J Gastroenterol 1998; 33: 104–108.
100. Helmy, A. and Hayes, P. C., Current endoscopic therapeutic options in the management of variceal bleeding. Aliment Pharmacol Ther 2001; 15: 575–94.
101. Hunerbein, M., Totkas, S., Ghadimi, B. M. and Schlag, P. M., Preoperative evaluation of colorectal neoplasms by colonoscopic miniprobe ultrasonography. Ann Surg 2000; 232: 46–50.
102. Gast, P. and Belaiche, J., Rectal endosonography in inflammatory bowel disease: Differential diagnosis and prediction of remission. Endoscopy 1999; 31: 158–66.
103. TenBerge, J., Hoffman, B. J., Hawes, R. H. *et al.*, EUS-guided fine-needle aspiration of the liver; indications, yield, and safety based on an international survey of 167 cases. Gastrointest Endosc 2002; 55: 859–862.
104. Anderson, M. A., Carpenter, S., Thompson, N. W., Nostrant, T. T., Elta, G. H. and Scheiman, J. M., Endoscopic ultrasound is highly accurate and directs management in patients with neuroendocrine tumors of the pancreas. Am J Gastroenterol 2000; 95: 2271–7.

105. De Angelis, C., Carucci, P., Repici, A. and Rizzetto, M., Endosonography in decision making and management of gastrointestinal endocrine tumors. Eur J Ultrasound 1999; 10: 139–50.
106. Wallace, M. B., Hawes, R. H., Durkalski, V., Chak, A., Mallery, S., Catalano, M. F., Wiersema, M. J., Bhutani, M. S., Ciaccia, D., Kochman, M. L., Gress, F. G., Van Velse, A. and Hoffman, B. J., The reliability of EUS for the diagnosis of chronic pancreatitis: Interobserver agreement among experienced endosonographers. Gastrointest Endosc 2001; 53: 294–9.
107. Brand, B., Pfaff, T., Binmoeller, K. F., Sriram, P. V., Fritscher-Ravens, A., Knofel, W. T., Jackle, S. and Soehendra, N., Endoscopic ultrasound for differential diagnosis of focal pancreatic lesions, confirmed by surgery. Scand J Gastroenterol 2000; 35: 1221–8.
108. Buscarini, E. and Buscarini, L., The role of endosonography in the diagnosis of choledocholithiasis. Eur J Ultrasound 1999; 10: 117–25.
109. Canto, M. I., Chak, A., Stellato, T. and Sivak, M. V. Jr., Endoscopic ultrasonography versus cholangiography for the diagnosis of choledocholithiasis. Gastrointest Endosc 1998; 47: 439–48.
110. Quirk, D. M., Rattner, D. W., Fernandez-del, Castillo. C., Warshaw, A. L. and Brugge, W. R., The use of endoscopic ultrasonography to reduce cost of treating ampullary tumors. Gastrointest Endosc 1997; 46: 334–7.
111. Ueno, N., Tomiyama, T., Tano, S., Wada, S., Aizawa, T. and Kimura, K., Utility of endoscopic ultrasonography with color doppler function for the diagnosis of islet cell tumor. Am J Gastroenterol 1996; 91(4): 772–776.
112. Tio, T. L., Hoei Sie, L., Kallimanis, G., Luiken, G. J. H. M., Nicola Kimmings, A., Huibregtse, K. and Tytgat, G. N. J., Staging of ampullary and pancreatic carcinoma: Comparison between endosonography and surgery. Gastrointest Endosc 1996; 44: 706–13.
113. Nesje, L. B., Varhaug, J. E., Husebye, E. S. and Ødegaard, S., Endoscopic ultrasonography for preoperative diagnosis and localization of Insulinomas. Scand J Gastroenterol 2002; 37: 732–737.
114. Harewood, G. C. and Wiersema, M. J., Endosonography-guided fine-needle aspiration biopsy in the evaluation of pancreatic masses. Am J Gasroenterol 2002; 97: 1386–1391.
115. Hahn, M. and Faigel, D. O., Frequency of mediastinal lymph node metastases in patients undergoing EUS evaluation of pancreaticobiliary masses. Gastrointest Endosc 2001; 54: 331–335.
116. Ahmad, N. A., Kochman, M. L., Lewis, J. D. *et al.*, Can EUS alone differentiate between malignant and benign cystic lesions of the pancreas? Am J Gastroenterol 2001; 96: 3295–3300.
117. Itoh, A., Goto, H., Naitoh, Y., Hirooka, Y., Furukawa, T. and Hayakawa, T., Intraductal ultrasonography in diagnosing tumor extension of cancer of the papilla of Vater. Gastrointest Endosc 1997; 45: 251–60.
118. Engström, C.-F. and Wiechel, K.-L., Endoluminal ultrasound of the bile ducts. Surg Endosc 1990; 4: 187–190.
119. Menzel, J. and Domschke, W., Intraductal ultrasonography (IDUS) may localize islet cell tumours negative on endoscopic ultrasound. Scand J Gastroenterol 1998; 33: 109–112.
120. Taki, T., Goto, H., Naitoh, Y., Hirooka, Y., Furukawa, T. and Hayakawa, T., Diagnosis of mucin-producing tumor of the pancreas with an intraductal ultrasonographic system. J Ultrasound Med 1997; 16: 1–6.
121. Kuroiwa, M., Tsukamoto, Y., Naitohm, Y. *et al.*, New technique using intraductal ultrasonography for the diagnosis of bile duct cancer. J Ultrasound Med 1994; 13: 189–95.
122. Marusch, F., Koch, A., Schmidt, U. *et al.*, Routine use of transrectal ultrasound in rectal carcinoma: results of a prospective multicenter study. Endoscopy 2002; 34: 385–390.

123. Watanabe, H., Miwa, H., Terai, T., Imai, Y., Ogihara, T. and Sato, N., Endoscopic ultrasonography for colorectal cancer using submucosal saline solution injection. Gastrointest Endosc 1997; 45: 508–511.
124. Waxman, I., Saitoh, Y., Raju, G. S. *et al.*, High-frequency probe EUS-assisted endoscopic mucosal resection: A therapeutic strategy for submucosal tumors of the GI tract. Gastrointest Endosc 2002; 55: 44–49.
125. Nishimura, K., Niwa, Y., Goto, H., Hase, S., Arisawa, T. and Hayakawa, T., Three-dimensional endoscopic ultrasonography of gastrointestinal lesions using an ultrasound probe. Scand J Gastroenterol 1997; 32: 862–868.
126. Kanemaki, N., Nakazawa, S., Inui, K., Yoshino, J., Yamao, K. and Okushima, K., Three-dimensional intraductal ultrasonography: Preliminary results of a new technique for the diagnosis of diseases of the pancreatobiliary system. Endoscopy 1997; 29: 726–731.
127. Loehnert, M., Doniec, J. M., Kovacs, G., Schroeder, J. and Dohrmann, P., New method of radiotheraphy for anal cancer with three-dimensional tumor reconstruction based on endoanal ultrasound and ultrasound — Guided afterloading therapy. Dis Colon rectum 1998; 41: 169–176.
128. Hunerbein, M., Gretschel, S., Ghadimi, B. M. and Schlag, P. M., Three-dimensional endoscopic ultrasound of the esophagus. Surg Endosc 1997; 11: 991–994.
129. Molin, S. O., Nesje, L. B., Gilja, O. H., Hausken, T., Martens, D. and Odegaard, S., 3D-endosonography in gastroenterology: methodology and clinical applications. Eur J Ultrasound 1999; 10: 171–7.
130. Jafri, I. H., Saltzman, J. R., Colby, J. M. *et al.*, Evaluation of the clinical impact of endoscopic ultrasonography in gastrointestinal disease. Gastrointest Endosc 1996; 44: 367–70.
131. Lutz, H. and Rosch, W., Transgastroscopic ultrasonography. Endoscopy 1976; 8: 203–5.
132. Mortensen, M. B., The role of gastrointestinal endosonography in diagnostic and therapeutic interventional procedures. Eur J Ultrasound 1999; 10: 93–104.
133. Mallery, S. and Van Dam J., Interventional endoscopic ultrasonography: Current status and future direction. J Clin Gastroenterol 1999; 29: 297–305.
134. Detmer, P. R., Bashein, G., Hodges, T., Beach, K. W., Filer, E. P., Burns, D. H. and Strandness, DE Jr., 3D ultrasonic image feature localization based on magnetic scanhead tracking: *in vitro* calibration and validation. Ultrasound Med Biol 1994; 20: 923–36.
135. Matre, K., Stokke, E. M., Martens, D. and Gilja, O. H., *In vitro* volume estimation of kidneys using three-dimensional ultrasonography and a position sensor. Eur J Ultrasound 1999; 10: 65–73.
136. Krivonos, O., Gebhard, F., Keppler, P., Kinzl, L., Hesser, J. and Manner, R., Computer assisted treatment of pelvis fractures. Stud Health Technol Inform 2001; 81: 242–6.
137. Burgul, R., Gilbert, F. J. and Undrill, P. E., Methods of measurement of image quality in teleultrasound. Br J Radiol 2000; 73: 1306–12.
138. Kratochwil, A., Lee, A. and Schoisswohl, A., Networking of three dimensional sonography volume data. Ultrasound Obstet Gynecol 2000; 16: 335–40.

Published with permission

ORIGINAL ARTICLE

# Comparison of a Linear Miniature Ultrasound Probe and a Radial-scanning Echoendoscope in TN Staging of Esophageal Cancer

**L. B. Nesje, K. Svanes, A. Viste, O. D. Lærum & S. Ødegaard**
Institutes of Internal Medicine and Surgery, and The Gade Institute, Dept. of Pathology, Haukeland University Hospital, University of Bergen, Bergen, Norway

Nesje LB, Svanes K, Viste A, Lærum OD, Ødegaard S. Comparison of a linear miniature ultrasound probe and a radial-scanning echoendoscope in TN staging of esophageal cancer. Scand J Gastroenterol 2000;35:997–1002.

**Background:** Endoscopic ultrasonography is a precise method for TN staging of esophageal cancer. We explored the staging properties of a linear miniprobe as compared with a radial-scanning echoendoscope. **Methods:** Sixty-eight patients with esophageal cancer underwent preoperative TN staging using a 20-MHz linear miniprobe and a 7.5/12-MHz radial-scanning echoendoscope. Tumor stage was verified by surgery and/or histology. **Results:** T and N stages were verified in 53 and 54 patients, respectively. T-staging accuracy using the echoendoscope was 70%. The high-frequency miniprobe could not differentiate between T3 and T4 tumors, but both systems had an accuracy of 87% in discriminating between T1, T2, and T3/4 stages. With traversable tumors, the accuracy of N staging was significantly better with the echoendoscope than with the miniprobe (90% vs. 48%, $P = 0.008$). **Conclusions:** The two endosonographic systems had similar accuracy for assessing transmural tumor growth, but the echoendoscope was superior in staging advanced transmural tumors and in predicting lymph node metastasis with traversable tumors.

**Key words:** Endosonography; esophageal neoplasm; instrumentation; neoplasm staging; ultrasound methods

*Lars Birger Nesje, M.D., Dept. of Medicine, Haukeland University Hospital, N-5021 Bergen, Norway (fax: +47 55 97 29 50)*

Several studies have demonstrated that endoscopic ultrasonography (EUS) is currently the most accurate method for preoperative staging of esophageal cancer (1–8). Most EUS studies have been performed using dedicated endoscopes with integrated ultrasound (US) transducers, and conventional endoscopy is usually performed prior to EUS of the esophagus. During recent years, miniature ultrasound probes (MUP) have been developed allowing EUS to be performed through the accessory channel of conventional endoscopes.

In our hospital, we first got access to a prototype linear MUP system, which produced static compound scans when the transducer was moved over the area of interest (9–11). However, different probes with rotating transducers providing real-time radial scans have subsequently been introduced onto the market and improved (12–14) and recently, probes with switchable radial and linear modalities have also been developed (15). The role of different MUP systems as compared to integrated echoendoscopes (EE) is still not completely established.

Use of the linear MUP system seems to have been limited to a few centers (9–11, 16, 17). Despite technical limitations due to small transducer size, high US frequency and static US images, it has been reported that linear MUP may add clinically valuable information to that obtained by endoscopy alone (10). The present study was performed with the aim to compare a 20-MHz linear MUP to a 7.5/12-MHz radial-scanning EE in TN staging of esophageal cancers.

## Material and Methods

During the 5-year period from 1991 to 1996, we prospectively registered 68 consecutive patients (56 men, 12 women, median age 66 years, range 39–83 years) with esophageal carcinoma who were referred for preoperative endosonographic staging at our hospital. Forty-three patients had tumor locations restricted to the esophagus, while in 25 patients, the tumor also involved the cardia region of the stomach. Tumor histology showed adenocarcinoma in 45 patients (66%), squamous cell carcinoma in 20 patients (29%), and combined adeno-squamous cell type in 3 patients (4%). In 36 patients (53%), the tumor was traversable with EE, while 32 patients (47%) had non-traversable esophageal stenosis.

All patients underwent initial endoscopy, during which

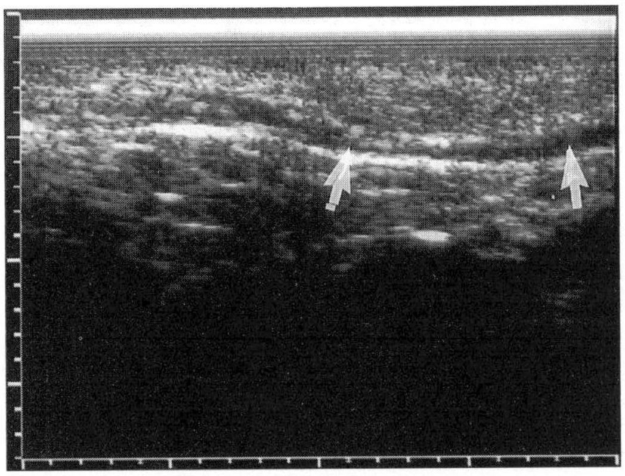

Fig. 1. Tumor stage T1 imaged with a linear 20-MHz miniature ultrasound probe applied on the luminal surface (top of image). The tumor is seen as an echo-poor wall thickening involving the superficial wall layers. The muscularis propria layer (arrows) is seen unaffected below the tumor.

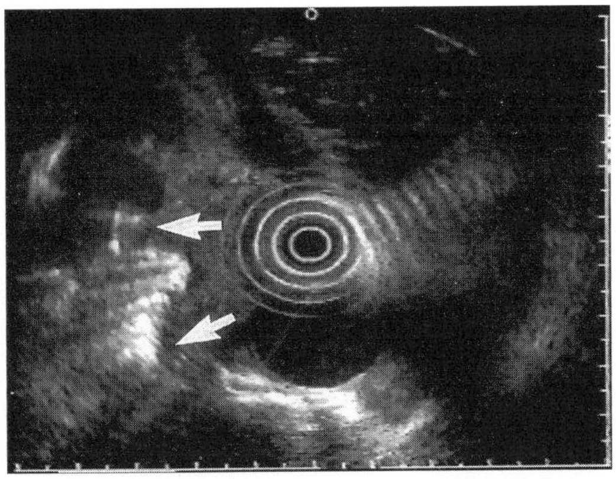

Fig. 3. T4 stage tumor imaged with the radial-scanning echoendoscope using a 7.5-MHz transducer located in the esophageal lumen. The tumor is seen as an echo-poor mass infiltrating through the esophageal wall and into the right pleura (arrows).

EUS was performed with the linear 20-MHz MUP (Fujinon Sonoprobe SP-101, Fujinon Co., Omiya, Japan). Subsequently, an examination with a 7.5/12-MHz radial-scanning EE (Olympus EU-M3 or EU-M20, Olympus Optical Co., Tokyo, Japan) was carried out. Both EUS examinations were performed by one or two gastroenterologists with several years of training in endoscopy and transabdominal ultrasonography. However, one of the examiners had less than 1 year of training in endosonography when the study started. T and N stage, as determined by MUP, was noted before proceeding to EE examination. Due to the limited number of trained examiners in the hospital, the two EUS procedures usually had to be performed by the same person. Most patients also had a preoperative computed tomography (CT) examination, but the CT results were not known when performing EUS.

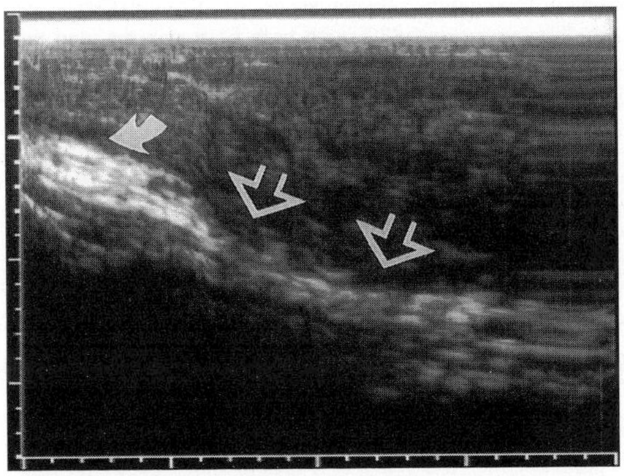

Fig. 2. T3 stage cancer imaged with a linear 20-MHz miniature ultrasound probe. The tumor appears as a diffuse, echo-poor wall thickening obscuring all layers of the esophageal wall and extending beyond the outer wall delineation (open arrows). Curved arrow indicates muscularis propria layer.

The tumors were usually imaged as an echo-poor expansion of the gastrointestinal (GI) wall. A tumor was staged T1 if it was limited to the area superficial to the muscularis propria layer, with a visible interface echo between the tumor and the muscle layer (Fig. 1). If the tumor was continuous with the echo-poor muscularis propria layer, it was staged T2 as long as the outer wall delineation remained smooth without extensions into the surrounding tissue. An irregular outer border (Fig. 2) was regarded as an indicator of transmural wall infiltration (T3), and when the tumor extended across the limitation of adjacent organs (pericard, pleura, vessels, bronchi, or diaphragm) with a loss of interface echo, it was staged T4 (Fig. 3). When comparing the two EUS systems T3 and T4 stages were merged into a T3/4-stage category, because of the MUP's limited ability to separate T4 from T3 stage tumors.

Hypoechoic lymph nodes with a short axis diameter of at least 5 mm, sharp delineation, and a rounded shape on EUS were generally regarded to be metastatic, constituting nodal stage N1. Stage N0 was denoted when no indication of regional lymph node metastasis was demonstrated by EUS, including cases where the evaluation was hampered by stenosis or technical limitations. If possible, celiac, perigastric, and mediastinal lymph nodes up to the level of the right recurrent nerve were evaluated.

Surgery was performed after a mean of 8 days following EUS. Nineteen patients were operated the subsequent day, while three patients waited for more than 3 weeks to be operated. Endosonographic TN stages, as determined by MUP and EE, were compared to surgical and/or histopathologic staging when available after surgery. Operation was

Published with permission



undertaken unless preoperative examinations showed definite signs of irresectability or disseminated disease. When curative surgery was regarded as possible, a radical resection of regional lymph nodes in the abdomen and the mediastinum was attempted. Lymph nodes from different locations were sampled in separate containers. Histology of resected specimens was performed according to standard procedures, including examination of all available lymph nodes. The tissue was fixed in 4% formaldehyde solution, embedded in paraffin and cut into 5-μm thick sections before staining with hematoxylin and eosin. Transmural tumors that were macroscopically resectable at surgery, but histologically showed infiltration of small vessels in the periesophageal fat, were staged T3. Only histologically evaluated lymph nodes were used as a reference for endosonographic N staging.

The kappa statistic (18) was applied to describe agreement between the two EUS methods in determining T and N stage categories. The kappa ($\kappa$) value has a maximum of 1.00 when the agreement is perfect, and 0.00 indicates no agreement better than chance. Strength of agreement is usually classified as poor ($\kappa < 0.20$), fair ($\kappa = 0.21$–$0.40$), moderate ($\kappa = 0.41$–$0.60$), good ($\kappa = 0.61$–$0.80$), or very good ($\kappa = 0.81$–$1.00$). Staging accuracy was defined as the number of cases with a correct staging as a percentage of all evaluated cases. Proportions of correct N staging with the two methods were compared using the Fisher exact test.

## Results

Resective surgery with histologic examination of resected specimen was performed in 46 patients; 25 patients had a transthoracic resection, while transhiatal resection was performed in 21 patients. In one of these cases, T stage of a resected tumor could not be histologically determined due to tissue violation. In patients undergoing explorative laparotomy or thoracotomy, T stage could be reliably determined by the surgeon in 8 cases and N stage in 8 cases. Thus, T stage was verified by surgery and/or histology in 53 patients (78%), as was N stage in 54 patients (79%), and these groups of patients were subject to the evaluation of preoperative endosonographic tumor staging.

In 15 patients (22%), the depth of tumor infiltration could not be histologically or surgically verified. Seven of these patients were not operated on due to preoperative signs of advanced disease, while six patients underwent limited surgical exploration with disclosure of previously unrecognized distant metastases in the liver and/or the peritoneum. One patient died before operation and no autopsy was performed, and one resected specimen could not be evaluated by histology, as mentioned above. All patients with non-confirmed T stage had signs of transmural tumor growth on both EUS modalities (Table I), and signs of lymph node metastases were found in all but one patient on EUS.

Among patients in whom surgical and pathologic staging information was available, 4 T1 stage (8%), 7 T2 stage (13%), 32 T3 stage (60%), and 10 T4 stage tumors (19%) were found. Regional lymph node metastases were demonstrated in 46 (85%) out of 54 patients. In patients undergoing transhiatal esophageal resection leaving unevaluated lymph nodes of the upper mediastinum, lymph node metastases were demonstrated in 17 out of 21. Twenty-nine patients (55%) with confirmed T stage and 31 patients (57%) with confirmed N stage had tumors that could be traversed with both endoscope systems.

The overall accuracy in T staging with EE was 70% in patients with confirmed tumor stage (Table I), and in the subgroup of patients with traversable tumors, the accuracy was 69% (Table II). Both EUS systems had an accuracy of 91% in assessing whether the tumor infiltrated through the wall. All evaluated patients with non-traversable stenoses had transmural tumor infiltration, as was correctly demonstrated in 23 cases (96%) with MUP and in all 24 cases with EE. The 20-MHz MUP system could not reliably distinguish between T3 and T4 stage tumors due to limited US penetration depth. When differentiating between stages T1, T2, and T3/T4, the overall accuracy was 87% with both EUS systems, and the corresponding accuracy figures in patients with traversable tumors were 79% with MUP and 76% with EE. Three non-

Table I. Endosonographic T staging of esophageal cancers (traversable and non-traversable) using a miniature ultrasound probe (MUP) and a radial-scanning echoendoscope (EE), presented as number of cases per category

| Surgical/histologic T stage | T stage with MUP | T stage with EE |
|---|---|---|
| T1 ($n = 4$) | 2 T1 | 2 T1 |
| | 2 T2 | 2 T2 |
| T2 ($n = 7$) | 3 T2 | 3 T2 |
| | 4 T3 | 4 T3 |
| T3 ($n = 32$) | 1 T2 | 1 T2 |
| | 17 T3 | 28 T3 |
| | 14 at least T3 | 3 T4 |
| T4 ($n = 10$) | 3 T3 | 6 T3 |
| | 7 at least T3 | 4 T4 |
| T stage not confirmed | 4 T3 | 9 T3 |
| ($n = 15$) | 11 at least T3 | 6 T4 |

Table II. Endosonographic T staging of traversable esophageal cancers using a miniature ultrasound probe (MUP) and a radial-scanning echoendoscope (EE), presented as number of tumors per category

| Surgical/histologic T stage | T stage with MUP | T stage with EE |
|---|---|---|
| T1 ($n = 4$) | 2 T1 | 2 T1 |
| | 2 T2 | 2 T2 |
| T2 ($n = 7$) | 3 T2 | 3 T2 |
| | 4 T3 | 4 T3 |
| T3 ($n = 16$) | 12 T3 | 1 T2 |
| | 4 at least T3 | 14 T3 |
| | | 1 T4 |
| T4 ($n = 2$) | 2 at least T3 | 1 T3 |
| | | 1 T4 |
| T stage not confirmed ($n = 7$) | 1 T3 | 3 T3 |
| | 6 at least T3 | 4 T4 |

Published with permission



Table III. Endosonographic N staging of esophageal cancers (traversable and non-traversable) using a miniature ultrasound probe (MUP) and a radial-scanning echoendoscope (EE), presented as number of patients per category

| Surgical/histologic N stage | N stage with MUP | N stage with EE |
|---|---|---|
| N0 ($n = 8$) | 8 N0 | 6 N0 |
| | | 2 N1 |
| N1 ($n = 46$) | 21 N0 | 10 N0 |
| | 25 N1 | 36 N1 |
| N stage not confirmed | 5 N0 | 1 N0 |
| ($n = 14$) | 9 N1 | 13 N1 |

Table V. Agreement data of the miniature ultrasound probe (MUP) and the radial-scanning echoendoscope (EE) in T staging of esophageal cancer, presented as number of examinations per category

| | T stage with EE | | | | |
|---|---|---|---|---|---|
| T stage with MUP | T1 | T2 | T3 | T4 | Total |
| T1 | 2 | | | | 2 |
| T2 | | 4 | 2 | | 6 |
| T3 | | 2 | 23 | 3 | 28 |
| At least T3 | | | 22 | 10 | 32 |
| Total | 2 | 6 | 47 | 13 | 68 |

traversable T4 stage tumors infiltrating the pleura ($n = 2$) and the large pulmonary vessels ($n = 1$) were correctly staged with EE, as was one traversable tumor with pancreatic infiltration. Five non-traversable T4 cancers infiltrating the pleura ($n = 2$), pulmonary vessels, diaphragm, or posterior abdominal wall were understaged T3 with EE, as was one traversable tumor infiltrating the posterior abdominal wall.

N stage of evaluated patients was correctly assessed in 61% of cases using the MUP and in 78% with the EE ($P = 0.09$, Table III). In patients with traversable tumors, the N staging accuracy was 58% with MUP and 90% with EE ($P = 0.008$, Table IV), while the corresponding accuracy figures with non-traversable tumors were 65% and 61%, respectively ($P = 1.0$).

The agreement between the two EUS systems was good when assessing transmural tumor infiltration or not ($\kappa = 0.72$), and in the differentiation between T1, T2, and T3/T4 stages ($\kappa = 0.72$) (Table V). In the group of patients with confirmed T stage, there was also good agreement, with kappa values of 0.71 and 0.72, respectively, in the evaluations described above.

By N staging with MUP and EE, the overall agreement in detecting regional lymph node metastases was fair with a kappa value of 0.26 (Table VI), varying from 0.17 (poor) in patients with non-traversable tumors to 0.34 (fair) in the traversable group. In evaluating patients with confirmed N stage, the corresponding kappa values were 0.25 (fair), 0.16 (poor), and 0.32 (fair), respectively.

## Discussion

New options in esophageal cancer treatment have accentuated the need for pretherapeutic tumor staging. Important staging objectives include: to sort out early mucosal cancers which can be resected endoscopically (19–21), to identify irresectable tumors for which operation should be avoided (22), and to predict whether a tumor can be subject to a curative or a palliative resection (4, 23).

The present study included all patients referred for preoperative staging of esophageal cancer at our hospital during a 5-year period. For the evaluation of T and N stages, 22% and 21%, respectively, of the patients were excluded, primarily due to advanced disease which precluded surgical exploration. Among the evaluated patients, more than 40% had non-traversable esophageal stenosis leading to an incomplete endosonographic examination, especially with regard to lymph node evaluation. The accuracy figures of the linear MUP and EE systems were comparable in classifying T1, T2, and T3/4 stage cancers of the esophagus including the cardia. The agreement in assessing tumor penetration through the GI wall was also good. However, the EE was more accurate in assessing regional lymph node metastasis, due to its better visualization of the mediastinum when the tumor was traversable by endoscopy.

In previously published reports, T staging accuracy of esophageal carcinomas using the radial-scanning EE varies between 59%–92% (3, 5), and most series have obtained accuracy rates between 80%–90% (24). In the present study, the accuracy of T staging was 70%. Interestingly, the

Table IV. Endosonographic N staging of traversable esophageal cancers using a miniature ultrasound probe (MUP) and a radial-scanning echoendoscope (EE), presented as number of patients per category

| Surgical/histologic N stage | N stage with MUP | N stage with EE |
|---|---|---|
| N0 ($n = 7$) | 7 N0 | 6 N0 |
| | | 1 N1 |
| N1 ($n = 24$) | 13 N0 | 2 N0 |
| | 11 N1 | 22 N1 |
| N stage not confirmed ($n = 5$) | 1 N0 | 5 N1 |
| | 4 N1 | |

Table VI. Agreement data of the miniature ultrasound probe (MUP) and the radial-scanning echoendoscope (EE) in N staging of esophageal cancers, presented as number of examinations per category

| | N stage with EE | | |
|---|---|---|---|
| N stage with MUP | N0 | N1 | Total |
| N0 | 13 | 21 | 34 |
| N1 | 4 | 30 | 34 |
| Total | 17 | 51 | 68 |

Published with permission



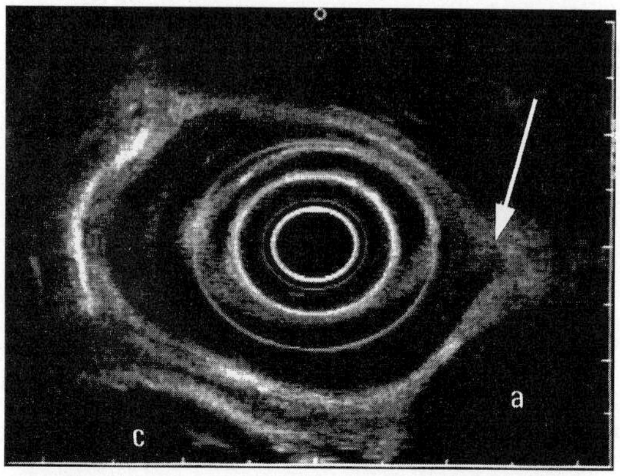


Fig. 4. T2 stage tumor overstaged as T3 by EUS. Irregular wall delineation (arrow) was misinterpreted as tumor extension. Image produced with radial-scanning echoendoscope in the esophagus, US frequency 12 MHz. a = descending aorta, c = columna.

accuracy was not better in patients with traversable tumors. This may in part be explained by the fact that all non-traversable tumors were stages T3 or T4, making overstaging, which was the dominating error on EUS, less likely. The most evident staging error was overstaging of T1 and T2 stage tumors. However, the number of tumors in these categories was low, and the accuracy figures should therefore be interpreted with care.

Understaging of T4 tumors occurred especially in patients where the level of maximal infiltration depth could not be reached by the instrument due to non-traversable esophageal stenosis. In these cases, the risk of understaging is evident and should always be taken into consideration when interpreting the examination results. In contrast to some other reports (25, 26), we found that all non-traversable tumors had transmural infiltration constituting stage T3 or T4.

An intriguing psychological bias, sometimes referred to as the 'T3 syndrome', may occur based on the knowledge that most esophageal cancers show transmural growth at the time of diagnosis (27). Although T3 is over-represented in our EUS staging, it is not possible to assess the role of this bias separately. Some tumors showed infiltration through a major part of the muscularis propria layer, but had no signs of extramural extension on histologic examination. In these cases, the number and position of histologic slides are crucial for assessing EUS accuracy, since the slice distance in routine histologic examinations may vary. In our study, all specimens with borderline or poorly defined infiltration depth at histology were reevaluated by an experienced pathologist.

Several advanced tumors were excluded from evaluation since they were not operated on, and many of these tumors had obvious signs of irresectability on EUS. Exclusion of the most advanced tumors may thus have influenced the staging accuracy in the study. Another point is that the present material also includes our early experience in endosonographic tumor staging, and staging accuracy has in other studies been shown to improve with number of examinations performed (28, 29). Interpretation of EE images may to a certain degree have been biased in those cases where the examiner knew the results of the previous MUP examination, and theoretically, this would tend to diminish the differences between the two systems.

The imaging capacity of MUP systems has generally been limited by the small size of the transducers and reduced penetration due to increased US frequency. Some studies, however, have indicated an advantage of high-frequency MUP in staging early cancers of the upper GI tract, mainly due to increased image resolution and avoidance of influence from the EE's balloon embedding the transducer (14, 30–32). MUP can also be applied in some areas not accessible with EE, for example, in stenotic lesions, and can be used as an accessory to routine endoscopy. Generally, MUP systems are less expensive and easier to use than EE systems.

We were not able to demonstrate differences between linear MUP and radial-scanning EE in terms of categorization into T1, T2, and T3/T4 stages. However, in patients with traversable tumors, the acquired information about tumor localization and relationship to adjacent tissue was generally better with the radial-scanning, real-time system. In many cases, a more detailed description of infiltration pattern and extramural tumor masses will constitute a valuable supplement to the T stage information in choosing the appropriate cancer therapy. Furthermore, the echoendoscope was superior in the assessment of regional lymph node metastases. Hence, our experience does not indicate that linear MUP can replace radial-scanning EE in cancer staging. On the other hand, although the linear MUP system seems to be incomplete as a stand-alone staging modality, additional tumor information may be obtained when longitudinal image planes are applied. We therefore believe that the combined linear and radial-scanning MUP systems may be adopted as a valuable tool while waiting for improved three-dimensional endosonographic systems allowing any-plane slicing in high-quality spatial US images.

## Acknowledgements

This work was financially supported by Haukeland University Hospital Strategic Research Program, Bergen, Norway and by grants from Norwegian Cancer Society, Oslo, Norway and Rebekka Ege Hegermann's Foundation, Bergen, Norway.

## References

1. Murata Y, Suzuki S, Hashimoto H. Endoscopic ultrasonography of the upper gastrointestinal tract. Surg Endosc 1988;2:180–3.
2. Tio TL, Coene PP, den Hartog Jager FC, Tytgat GN. Preoperative TNM classification of esophageal carcinoma by endosonography. Hepatogastroenterology 1990;37:376–81.
3. Botet JF, Lightdale CJ, Zauber AG, Gerdes H, Urmacher C,

Published with permission



Brennan MF. Preoperative staging of esophageal cancer: comparison of endoscopic US and dynamic CT. Radiology 1991;181:419–25.
4. Rosch T, Lorenz R, Zenker K, von Wichert A, Dancygier H, Hofler H, et al. Local staging and assessment of resectability in carcinoma of the esophagus, stomach, and duodenum by endoscopic ultrasonography. Gastrointest Endosc 1992;38: 460–7.
5. Rice TW, Boyce GA, Sivak MV. Esophageal ultrasound and the preoperative staging of carcinoma of the esophagus. J Thorac Cardiovasc Surg 1991;101:536–43.
6. Dittler HJ, Siewert JR. Role of endoscopic ultrasonography in esophageal carcinoma. Endoscopy 1993;25:156–61.
7. Grimm H, Binmoeller KF, Hamper K, Koch J, Henne BD, Soehendra N. Endosonography for preoperative locoregional staging of esophageal and gastric cancer. Endoscopy 1993;25: 224–30.
8. Souquet JC, Napoleon B, Pujol B, Keriven O, Ponchon T, Descos F, et al. Endoscopic ultrasonography in the preoperative staging of esophageal cancer. Endoscopy 1994;26:764–6.
9. Martin RW, Silverstein FE, Kimmey MB. A 20-MHz ultrasound system for imaging the intestinal wall. Ultrasound Med Biol 1989;15:273–80.
10. Nesje LB, Ødegaard S, Kimmey MB. Transendoscopic ultrasonography during conventional upper gastrointestinal endoscopy. Clinical evaluation of a linear 20-MHz probe system. Scand J Gastroenterol 1997;32:500–8.
11. Kimmey MB, Ødegaard S. High-resolution endoluminal sonography of the upper gastrointestinal tract: the linear scanning ultrasound probe. In: Van Dam J, Sivak MV, editors. Gastrointestinal endosonography. Philadelphia: Saunders; 1999. p. 67–79.
12. Rosch T, Classen M. A new ultrasonic probe for endosonographic imaging of the upper GI tract. Preliminary observations. Endoscopy 1990;22:41–6.
13. Yasuda K. Development and clinical use of ultrasonic probes. Endoscopy 1994;26:816–7.
14. Chak A, Canto M, Stevens PD, Lightdale CJ, Van de Mierop F, Cooper G, et al. Clinical applications of a new through-the-scope ultrasound probe: prospective comparison with an ultrasound endoscope. Gastrointest Endosc 1997;45:291–5.
15. Yanai H, Yoshida T, Harada T, Matsumoto Y, Nishiaki M, Shigemitsu T, et al. Endoscopic ultrasonography of superficial esophageal cancers using a thin ultrasound probe system equipped with switchable radial and linear scanning modes. Gastrointest Endosc 1996;44:578–82.
16. Kimmey MB, Martin RW, Silverstein FE. Clinical application of linear ultrasound probes. Endoscopy 1992;24 Suppl 1:364–9.
17. Yanai H, Tada M, Karita M, Okita K. Diagnostic utility of 20-megahertz linear endoscopic ultrasonography in early gastric cancer. Gastrointest Endosc 1996;44:29–33.
18. Altman DG. Practical statistics for medical research. London: Chapman & Hall; 1991. p. 403–9.
19. Murata Y, Suzuki S, Mitsunaga A, Iizuka Y, Uchiyama M, Uchida K, et al. Endoscopic ultrasonography in diagnosis and mucosal resection for early esophageal cancer. Endoscopy 1998;30 Suppl 1:A44–6.
20. Soehendra N, Binmoeller KF, Bohnacker S, Seitz U, Brand B, Thonke F, et al. Endoscopic snare mucosectomy in the esophagus without any additional equipment: a simple technique for resection of flat early cancer. Endoscopy 1997;29:380–3.
21. Toh Y, Baba K, Ikebe M, Adachi Y, Kuwano H, Sugimachi K. Endoscopic ultrasonography in the diagnosis of an early esophageal carcinoma. Hepatogastroenterology 1993;40:212–6.
22. Mortensen MB, Scheel HJ, Madsen MR, Qvist N, Hovendal C. Combined endoscopic ultrasonography and laparoscopic ultrasonography in the pretherapeutic assessment of resectability in patients with upper gastrointestinal malignancies. Scand J Gastroenterol 1996;31:1115–9.
23. Peters JH, Hoeft SF, Heimbucher J, Bremner RM, DeMeester TR, Bremner CG, et al. Selection of patients for curative or palliative resection of esophageal cancer based on preoperative endoscopic ultrasonography. Arch Surg 1994;129:534–9.
24. Rosch T, Classen M. Staging esophageal cancer: the Munich experience. In: Van Dam J, Sivak MV, editors. Gastrointestinal endosonography. Philadelphia: Saunders; 1999. p. 139–45.
25. Van Dam J, Rice TW, Catalano MF, Sivak Jr MV. High-grade malignant stricture is predictive of esophageal tumor stage. Risks of endosonographic evaluation. Cancer 1993;71:2910–7.
26. Binmoeller KF, Seifert H, Seitz U, Izbicki JR, Kida M, Soehendra N. Ultrasonic esophagoprobe for TNM staging of highly stenosing esophageal carcinoma. Gastrointest Endosc 1995;41:547–52.
27. Bolton JS, Fuhrman GM, Richardson WS. Esophageal resection for cancer. Surg Clin North Am 1998;78:773–94.
28. Fockens P, Van den Brande JH, van Dullemen HM, van Lanschot JJ, Tytgat GN. Endosonographic T staging of esophageal carcinoma: a learning curve. Gastrointest Endosc 1996;44:58–62.
29. Rice TW, Zuccaro G. Staging esophageal cancer: the Cleveland experience. In: Van Dam J, Sivak MV, editors. Gastrointestinal endosonography. Philadelphia: Saunders; 1999. p. 131–8.
30. Hasegawa N, Niwa Y, Arisawa T, Hase S, Goto H, Hayakawa T. Preoperative staging of superficial esophageal carcinoma: comparison of an ultrasound probe and standard endoscopic ultrasonography. Gastrointest Endosc 1996;44:388–93.
31. Menzel J, Hoepffner N, Nottberg H, Schulz C, Senninger N, Domschke W. Preoperative staging of esophageal carcinoma: miniprobe sonography versus conventional endoscopic ultrasound in a prospective histopathologically verified study. Endoscopy 1999;31:291–7.
32. Ødegaard S, Kimmey MB, Martin RW, Yee HC, Cheung AGS, Silverstein FE. The effects of applied pressure on the thickness, layers, and echogenicity of gastrointestinal wall ultrasound images. Gastrointest Endosc 1992;38:351–6.

Received 12 July 1999
Accepted 7 March 2000

# CHAPTER 16

# ULTRASOUND IN PATIENTS WITH GASTROESOPHAGEAL REFLUX DISEASE

SOLOMON TEFERA AND JAN GUNNAR HATLEBAKK

## 1. Gastroesophageal Reflux Disease

The term gastroesophageal reflux disease (GERD) refers to the presence of esophageal mucosal breaks or to the occurrence of symptoms induced by abnormal exposure of the esophagus to gastric and duodenal contents. Symptomatic GERD should be diagnosed only if symptoms are severe enough to impair the quality of life (1). This is a common condition with a variety of clinical manifestations and if untreated may lead to complications such as reflux esophagitis, peptic stricture of the esophagus, or Barrett's esophagus which is a premalignant condition and a precursor for adenocarcinoma of the esophagus (2, 3). Gastroesophageal reflux in itself is not necessarily pathological: indeed, moderate amounts of reflux can be demonstrated in most subjects. Such episodes most often occur after meals, do not usually cause symptoms and are of short duration (4–6). Physiological reflux often accompanies eructation. Generally, GERD is accompanied by typical clinical symptoms such as heartburn, acid regurgitation or dysphagia (7, 8). However, atypical symptoms such as unexplained chest pain, hoarseness, asthma/chronic cough, laryngitis, hiccups and loss of dental enamel are also seen (9), but the role of acid reflux in these conditions are not always recognized.

## 2. Pathogenesis of GERD

GERD is a multifactorial disease (10–12). Although it is primarily a motility disorder, several other disturbances can interfere and contribute to determine the severity of symptoms and the degree of lesions. The multiple factors that may contribute to GERD are the barrier to reflux provided by the LES (13, 14), the ability of the esophagus to clear refluxed material (15, 16), the potential of refluxed material to damage the esophagus (17–19), the role of the stomach in terms of gastric secretion, distention, and emptying (20–30), the intrinsic resistance of the esophageal mucosa to damage (19, 31–34), and a hiatal hernia, which is found in up to 80% of the patients (35–40). In normal subjects, as in patients with abnormal reflux, nearly all the episodes of reflux result from one of the following three general mechanisms:

(1) Gastroesophageal reflux associated with transient LES relaxation (TLESR) (14, 41).
(2) Stress reflux resulting from transient increases in intra-abdominal pressure caused by abdominal muscle contraction (42–44).
(3) Spontaneous free reflux across an atonic sphincter (5, 6).

The TLESR is the dominating reflux mechanism in healthy subjects and in patients with endoscopy-negative GERD or mild reflux esophagitis, whereas the other mechanisms assume more importance in patients with severe and complicated reflux disease (5, 6, 14).

## 3. Diagnosis of GERD

There has been proposed many different tests for the evaluation of acid reflux disease, but it has become more and more clear that there is no single gold standard for the diagnosis of GERD. Endoscopy is the diagnostic method most frequently used and best suited to document esophageal mucosal injury (erosions or ulcerations). Twenty-four-hour ambulatory esophageal pH monitoring is frequently considered to be a gold standard in the diagnosis and quantification of acid reflux, and particularly useful in endoscopy-negative patients (45, 46). Symptom evaluation is a useful diagnostic approach and when the association of symptoms with reflux episodes is evaluated as part of the pH monitoring study, the gains in sensitivity and specificity are of great practical value (47). The use of a 1- to 2-week course of high-dose proton pump inhibitor (PPI) therapy has been suggested as a useful, cost-effective diagnostic approach for GERD (48). Recent studies have shown high sensitivity, but insufficient specificity of this diagnostic approach to the disease (49).

## 4. Challenges in the Diagnosis of GERD

The evaluation of symptoms in patients with upper gastrointestinal disorders is difficult. Heartburn as a predominant symptom is relatively specific for GERD, as confirmed by other methods (46), but the sensitivity of individual symptoms as a diagnostic tool of reflux disease is only around 50%. Attempts at developing disease-specific questionnaires to better recognize patterns of symptoms have been moderately successful (50).

Even though endoscopy is the diagnostic approach most frequently used to investigate esophageal mucosal injury in GERD, abnormal findings are absent in more than 50% of individuals who have had heartburn two or more times a week for six months (45, 51–53). If only the cumulative acid exposure time from 24-hour pH-monitoring is used for the diagnosis of GERD, a minority of patients with definite, even severe reflux esophagitis, will have a false-negative result. Cumulative esophageal acid exposure values are abnormal in between half and two thirds of endoscopy-negative patients with symptomatic GERD (45). In these patients, repeat testing gives diagnostically inconsistent findings in a significant minority (54). More complex scoring systems integrating more variables extracted from the pH-recording, such as the DeMeester score, does not alleviate this problem. The inclusion of a variable evaluating the temporal relationship between individual symptom episodes and reflux episodes, such as the Symptom Index (SI) (55) and the Symptom Association Probability (SAP) (56) has however increased the sensitivity of a 24-hour pH-metry significantly, which is of great importance in low-grade GERD.

Barium upper gastrointestinal series has limited diagnostic value, except in the case of peptic strictures, hiatal herniation and ulcerations. The diagnosis of abnormal reflux is particularly difficult and not very reproducible. The result is dependent on the state of competence of the antireflux mechanism at a particular moment. Radiographic reflux has been demonstrated in as few as 60% of severely symptomatic patients or in as many as 25% of patients having no reflux symptoms. It has therefore both poor specificity and sensitivity (13, 57).

The abovementioned diagnostic tools for reflux disease are supplementary to one another. However, most of these tools are invasive and unpleasant for the patient. Furthermore, from time to time we deal with pediatric and elderly patients who have difficulties in cooperating for such examinations. Therefore, the diagnostic tests for GERD should be categorized and selected according to the specific questions being asked, to reduce patient discomfort and optimize resource utilization.

## 5. The Potential of Ultrasonographic Methods in GERD

The non-invasive transabdominal sonographic methods have been available for some time. These techniques have not achieved extensive clinical use in the investigation of esophageal pathology or disease mechanisms, because other imaging modalities have seemed to present advantages over ultrasonography in the thoracic region. Indirectly, ultrasound has still contributed to our insights in the pathogenesis of certain esophageal diseases.

Ultrasound is a valuable method to assess certain aspects of gastric function — gastric size, volume, intragastric distribution and emptying of a test meal, as well as contractile activity of the wall of the distal stomach. However, when assessing the cardia, this method is not so accurate, especially in adult patients, due to the position of the gastroesophageal junction behind the costal margins and sternum (Fig. 1). Although several studies investigating gastro-esophageal reflux with conventional transcutaneous ultrasound have been reported, they have focused mostly on pediatric patients (58–66), in whom the proximal stomach is more easily accessible with a transcutaneous approach. Pathogenetic

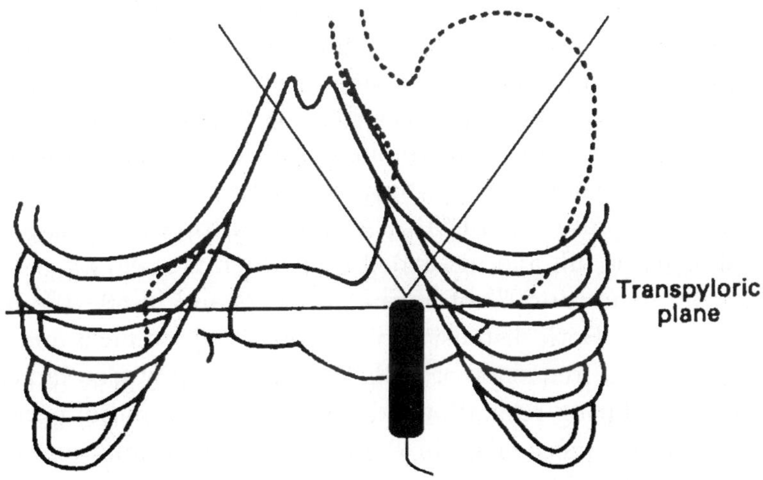


Fig. 1. The figure shows the position of the transducer for scanning the proximal stomach with 2D and 3D ultrasound (adapted from Gilja *et al.*, *J. Ultrasound. Med.* **14**(2), 81–89 (1995).) With transabdominal ultrasonography, there are technical limitations for assessing esophageal disease including GERD in adult patients due to the position of the gastroesophageal junction behind the costal margins and lower sternum.

mechanisms of gastroesophageal reflux disease in young children may however differ from those common in adults, except for incompetence of LES function.

There are therefore technical limitations when using transabdominal sonography in the area of the distal esophagus and upper portion of the stomach, due to the sternum, costal margins, lung and gas in the stomach. Recent advances in ultrasound technology, such as the application of color Doppler technology (67–70), and the high-frequency intraluminal ultrasound probe (71–74) have increased the potential use of ultrasound as diagnostic tools for the detection of upper gastrointestinal tract pathology, especially so in the study of esophageal disorders. Endosonography has facilitated the understanding of esophageal wall motility and pathogenetic mechanisms of GERD development.

Ultrasound can be applied for studies of several aspects of upper gastrointestinal function which are relevant for GERD or other esophageal disease, employing either transcutaneous or endosonograhic approaches:

(1) Gastric accommodation and emptying in GERD patients (20, 21, 75, 76).
(2) Esophageal mucosal abnormalities (before and after treatment of GERD), distension or wall thickness in case of motility disturbances (in GERD patients) (71–74, 77).
(3) Gastric and duodenogastric reflux to the esophagus (59–70, 78, 79).
(4) Presence of a hiatal hernia, when a non-invasive method is required (67, 80, 81).

### 5.1. *Gastric accommodation and emptying in GERD patients*

Gastric accommodation is a complex process, which describes how the proximal gastric compartment changes in response to a meal. Abnormal gastric accommodation and emptying is one of the multiple factors that may contribute to GERD.

In healthy subjects, as well as in the great majority of patients with GERD, most reflux episodes occur during transient lower esophageal sphincter relaxation TLESRs. TLESR is a prolonged relaxation of the lower esophageal sphincter not associated with swallowing (82). Stimulation of tensoreceptors, especially in the subcardial area, caused by the distension of the proximal stomach, is supposed to be a major factor that increases the frequency of TLESR (82–84). On the other hand, gastric volume is mainly determined by the rate of gastric emptying, basal acid secretory rate, duodenogastric reflux, and the degree of gastric distension. Increased gastric volume not only provides more gastric contents available for reflux but also increases the rate of TLESRs. Acid reflux to the esophagus is more likely to occur when the stomach is full and distended than when it is empty. TLESR is accompanied by acid reflux in about 40–50% of normal subjects and in 60–70% of patients with reflux disease (5, 14, 85–87). Both distension of the proximal stomach and delayed gastric emptying can cause increased frequency of TLESRs and possibly also increased frequency of gastroesophageal reflux during relaxations, during the postprandial period (14, 83, 84). It is the major pathogenethic mechanism in the development of mild and moderate reflux disease in children and adults alike. However, none of the commonly employed diagnostic techniques in GERD allows studying the gastric accommodation to meals.

Scintigraphy, the gold standard for the study of gastric emptying, is applicable for studying intragastric distribution of a meal. However, this method does not allow determination of intragastric volumes. It involves a radiation hazard and can be performed only with certain kinds of meals. Volume visualization methods such as MRI, computed tomography, single-photon emission computed tomography, and position emission tomography have all been available for some time (88), but these techniques have not achieved extensive clinical use, partly due to high costs and the time required to obtain and process high-resolution image data.

Gastric accommodation in GERD patients has previously been studied with a barostat. The barostat measures gastric wall relaxation and from that one can infer about gastric tone. However, introducing the barostat balloon into the gastric lumen may influence the gastric motility patterns (89, 90). Furthermore, the examination is invasive and unpleasant. Neither the barostat nor scintigraphy allows for estimation of the size of the proximal stomach.

Gastric emptying both in normal children and pediatric GERD patients have been evaluated by LiVoti *et al.* (75), using 2 dimensional transcutaneous ultrasound. They found three different patterns of gastric emptying: (a) normal in 20%; (b) clearly delayed in 15%; and (c) intermediate in 65% of cases in which the plateau curve was abnormal (slow emptying) but the end time of gastric emptying was normal. The estimate of frequency in patients with GERD is similar to the reported data of the literature. Rico *et al.* (76) studied gastric emptying and the degree of antral dilation using real-time ultrasound in 25 healthy children and 25 children with gastroesophageal reflux. They found that patients with gastroesophageal reflux had significantly longer gastric emptying time when compared with the healthy subjects and showed a dilated antrum for longer periods after ingestion of a test meal. Carroccio *et al.* (91) evaluated gastric emptying in 12 children with gastroesophageal reflux and 12 normal control children by means of real-time ultrasonography before and after treatment with cisapride. They found that the patients had a significantly greater antral area than the controls (postprandialy double) and the gastric emptying time was significantly greater in the patients than in the controls before treatment. After 8 weeks of treatment with cisapride ultrasonography showed a decreased antral area with no significant difference between patients and controls. The gastric emptying time was also significantly lower than before treatment. The technique used to measure gastric emptying by these authors (75, 76) was the one described by Bolondi et al. based on measuring the changes in either antral cross-sectional area or diameter (92). It was, however, uncertain how the rate of gastric emptying of liquids could be related to changes in antral area.

Using two-dimensional ultrasonography, we evaluated gastric accommodation to a meal in 20 adult patients with reflux esophagitis and 20 healthy subjects, by investigating not the whole but only the uppermost part of the proximal stomach (7 cm from the top margin of the fundus downward along the axis of the stomach, see Fig. 2) and the antral area or diameter (20). The position of the transducer used for scanning the stomach is shown in Fig. 1. Reflux esophagitis patients revealed significantly larger sagittal area of the proximal stomach at 5 min and 15 min postprandially and experienced more epigastric fullness after the meal (Fig. 3). We found no significant difference in the antral area and gastric emptying fraction between patients and healthy controls. In GERD patients, postprandial fullness and sagittal area of the proximal stomach correlated significantly. The finding of postprandial distention of the proximal stomach may be a significant pathogenetic factor in patients with reflux esophagitis, by inducing more often TLESRs or by keeping a larger reservoir for

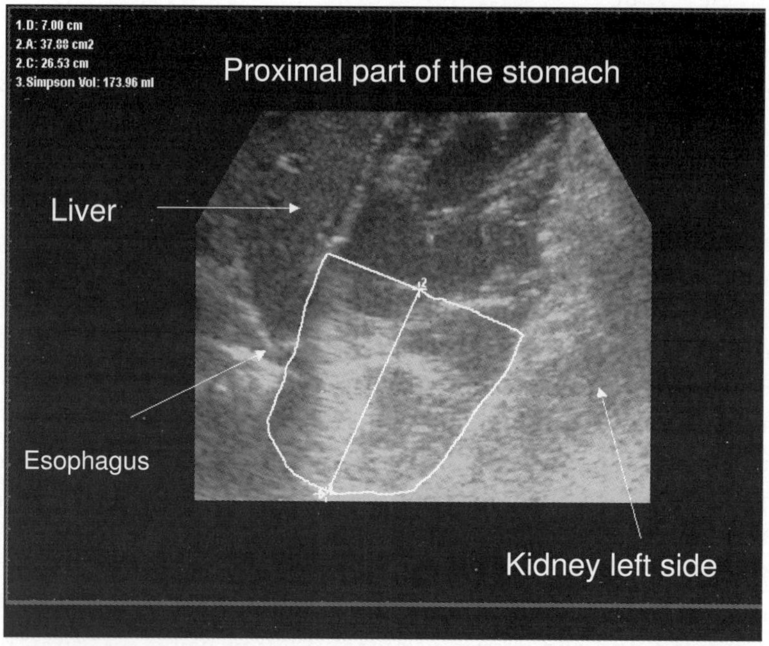


Fig. 2. Using two-dimensional ultrasonography, we evaluated gastric accommodation to a soup meal in patients with reflux esophagitis and healthy subjects, by investigating only the uppermost part of the proximal stomach (7 cm from the top margin of the fundus downward along the axis of the stomach). The left lobe of the liver, the left renal pelvis, and the tail of the pancreas served as internal landmarks to obtain the sagittal section of the proximal stomach. Unfortunately the pancreas is not included in this picture due to lack of space. In this picture one can easily identify the esophagus (but cannot be identified in all images).

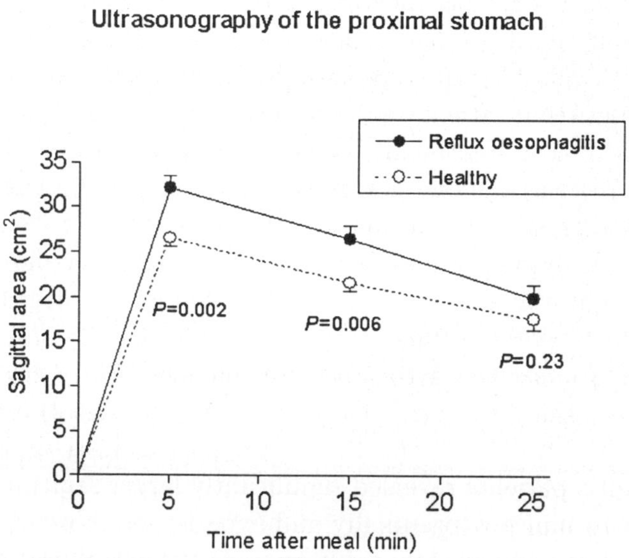


Fig. 3. Changes in sagittal area of the proximal stomach following a 500 mL soup meal as studied with 2D ultrasonography. Bars denoting SEM are depicted. Patients with reflux esophagitis grade I or II had a significantly larger sagittal area of the proximal stomach at 5 min. and at 15 min. postprandially compared with healthy subjects.

gastroesophageal reflux. This method did not allow a simultaneous imaging of the entire stomach.

Using a position sensor based on magnetic scanhead tracking for the acquisition of three-dimensional images, we evaluated gastric accommodation to a meal in 20 patients with reflux esophagitis and 20 healthy subjects by investigating not only the uppermost part of the proximal stomach but in principle the whole stomach (Fig. 4) (21). *In vivo* accuracy of this 3D ultrasonography method was evaluated by scanning a soup-filled barostat bag positioned in the proximal stomach of six healthy subjects. The 3D ultrasound system showed excellent agreement with the true volumes and a low interobserver variation. In patients with reflux esophagitis, after ingestion of a 500 ml meat soup meal, we measured a larger volume of the total and proximal stomach ultrasonographically at 2 min and 10 min, and an increased proximal/distal intragastric volume ratio at 10 min (Fig. 5). The patients also experienced more epigastric fullness than the controls.

The findings with both 2D and 3D ultrasound methods in GERD patients is consistent with the results of other recently published studies (23–25). Zerbib *et al.* found a more pronounced relaxation of the proximal stomach in GERD patients using a barostat, and

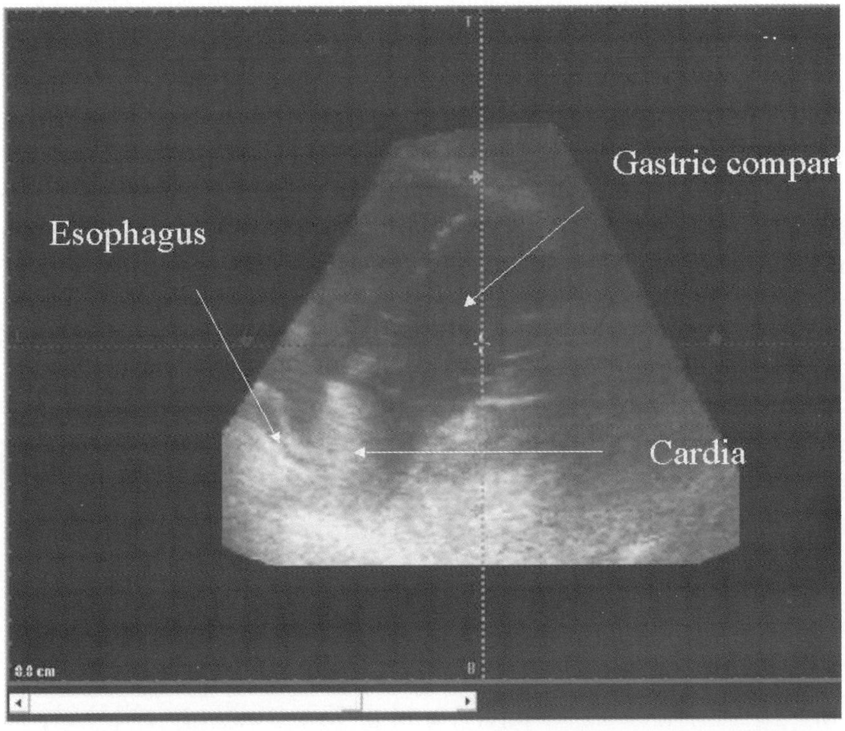


Fig. 4. Using three-dimensional ultrasonography, we evaluated gastric volume and intragastric distribution of a liquid meal in patients with reflux esophagitis and healthy subjects, by investigating the entire stomach. The stomach was scanned starting in the proximal end where the transducer was positioned by the left subcostal margin and then moved distally to the gastroduodenal junction. For each scan approximately 60–70 ultrasound images were stored (a frame rate of 10 per second and a scan typically lasting 6–7 seconds). The above figure represents one of the middle frames which shows the whole stomach. Here one can easily identify the esophagus, which is however not always visible.

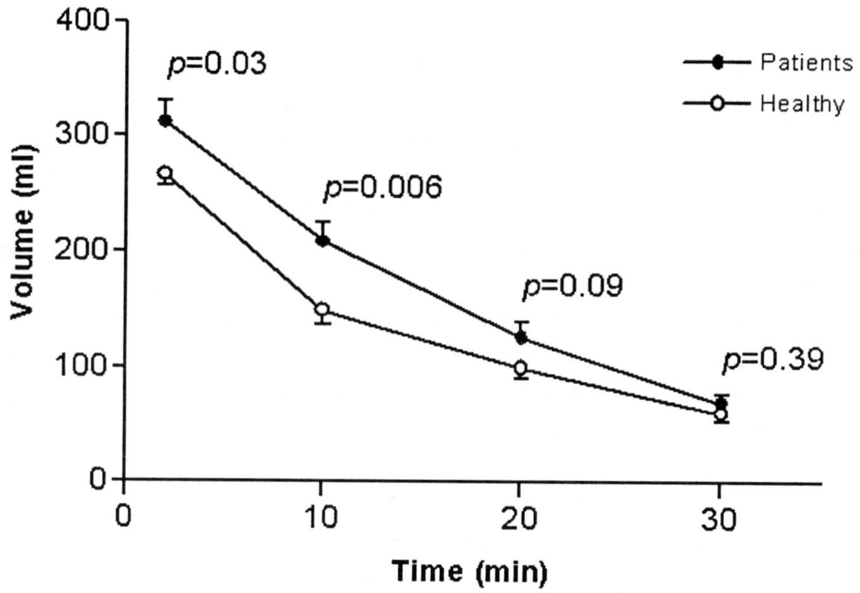


Fig. 5. Proximal gastric volume estimated with 3D ultrasonography in 20 healthy controls and 20 patients with mild or moderate reflux oesophagitis, following ingestion of a 500 mL soup meal. Patients with reflux esophagitis revealed a larger volume of the proximal stomach at 2 min and 10 min postprandially compared with healthy controls. Bars denoting SEM are drawn.

observed an inverse correlation between maximal postprandial relaxation and severity of the disease (23). Penagini *et al.* found delayed recovery of proximal gastric tone after intake of a combined solid and liquid meal in GERD patients (24). Recently, Vu *et al.* found that postprandial gastric relaxation was significantly prolonged in patients with GERD compared to GERD patients who had undergone Nissen fundoplication or controls (25). The technique used by these authors for the evaluation of gastric accommodation in GERD was barostat and scintigraphy. Taken together, these studies show that there are significant abnormalities in proximal gastric motor function in patients with GERD. Therefore, if TLESRs result from distension, or if distension is the major stimulus to TLESRs as suggested previously (14, 83, 84), then the non-invasive methods such as the ultrasound technique used in our laboratory could be a useful tool for investigating gastric accommodation, with clear advantages compared to invasive methods.

### 5.1.1. *Two-dimensional versus three-dimensional ultrasonography of the stomach*

Both the 2D and 3D ultrasound techniques used in this study are relatively new and have certain limitations. These methods are subject to the same limitations as ultrasonography in general, demanding a certain level of sonographic skills and experience to interpret the images. Measurement of gastric accommodation using this method is dependent on the amount of a food residing in the stomach. A high body mass index in GERD patients could presumably create difficulties, but none of our patients or the healthy volunteers in our study (20, 21) had to be excluded because of impaired image quality.

Using a 2D ultrasound scanner, one can obtain a real-time ultrasound image. It is a method that is available in almost every hospital and is easy to use, if not necessarily to interpret. Using 2D ultrasound one can only investigate the uppermost or distal part of the proximal stomach at a time. 3D ultrasound exploits the real-time capability of two-dimensional ultrasound to build a volume of the organ. But 3D ultrasonography cannot be accomplished in real time for larger volumes of hollow organs. The process of creating 3D images based on ultrasonography is time consuming and needs professional expertise. Using 3D ultrasound one can investigate in principle the whole stomach (21). We believe that 2D ultrasound is not more accurate than a position sensor based scanning for acquisition of 3D images in the assessment of gastric emptying time. Preparation, data acquisition and volume estimation with 2D or 3D ultrasound systems for the study of gastric accommodation is very similar when performed in other patient groups.

#### 5.1.2. *Concerns about the volume estimation using 3-dimensional ultrasound technique in GERD patients*

The volume estimation cannot be carried out by continuous recordings. It is very difficult to ensure that the frames obtained during this study truly represent the dynamic nature of gastric volume distribution postprandially in GERD patients. As indicated in the article (21), we found a significantly increased proximal to distal intragastric volume ratio at 10 min, but not at 2 min postprandially. This redistribution of the meal from the distal to the proximal stomach might as likely happen at any time over the eight minutes time window between recordings. We have no exact data on the reliability of the method due to great difficulties in doing simultaneous comparison with other imaging modalities. Nevertheless, we believe that using this low caloric liquid meal (93–96), which has an average half emptying time of $21.2 \pm 9.9$ min in healthy controls, gives us a good impression of the dynamic nature of gastric volume distribution (and redistribution) postprandially.

Using our ultrasound technique, it is impossible to discriminate between the amount of gastric juice produced during the examination period and the amount of the ingested test meal in GERD patients. Hirschowitz (17) found no difference in basal and maximal outputs of acid and pepsin between patients with or without oesophagitis. Meal stimulated gastric secretion is dependent on the caloric content and composition of the meal. Using meat soup as a test meal (calorie content 48 kcal/mL), Frislid *et al* (97) found that the amount of gastric secretion was no more than 3 ml/min. In our study, with a low caloric (20 kcal/mL) liquid meal, we speculate that the amount of acid and other secretion in the stomach was significantly lower than what Frislid *et al.* found, and it should therefore not affect the results significantly.

The presence of air pockets in the gastric fundus is a natural enemy of ultrasonography. However, the amount of postprandial gas varies greatly between individuals. This problem can be reduced by leaning the individuals slightly backwards. The gas is seldom visible in the oblique frontal sections. Preparation of the test meal according to their recommendations should minimize this particular problem (98). We have no exact data on how reliable the measurements of the sagittal area of the proximal stomach in GERD patients is in cases of fundic gas accumulation, due to the great difficulties in doing simultaneous comparison with other imaging modalities. In our studies (20, 21), we found that using the common landmarks (liver, kidney and pancreas) as a starting point and tracing the outer border of the air pocket, is more reliable than blind tracing of the inner echogenic layer. We have also carefully evaluated the amount of visible gas in the sagittal section in the 2 study groups (20) to establish if there are group differences with regard to gas. In this study, we found no differences, and that makes the ultrasound examination of the proximal stomach in GERD patients clinically valid.

Ultrasound examination of the gastric compartment in GERD patient with large hiatus hernia may also create difficulties because the exact fundic margins are difficult to delineate. In our study (20, 21) patients with hiatus hernia with an axial length longer than 5 cm were excluded. There were only 10 patients who had hiatus hernia and the mean length of the hiatus hernia was 2.9 cm. We believe that the volume of a liquid test meal retained in the 2.9 cm hernia is not more than what the patients produce and swallow (saliva) during the examination period. Outlining of the proximal stomach started from the top margin of the fundus, and not from the top of the hiatus hernia. The presence of hiatus hernia is a potential confounder, still should not significantly relate to the results presented in this study.

The barostat and ultrasound methods measure different aspects of gastric motor function. The barostat measures gastric muscular relaxation and from that one can infer about gastric tone, whereas ultrasound measures the gastric size and from that one can infer about gastric accommodation. In the late postprandial period, most of the liquid meal has been emptied from the stomach, and the proximal stomach is collapsed, which makes it difficult for ultrasound to detect the gastric wall. In that sense, ultrasound may be less sensitive than the barostat in detecting the effect of small volumes on proximal gastric stomach function. However, the ultrasound technique is non-invasive, comfortable to the patient and does not disturb the normal gastric motility. Gastroesophageal reflux is mainly a postprandial phenomenon, and any motility events during this period may imaginably contribute to it.

During ultrasound examination, errors may be introduced when the transducer is rotated 90°, when the image is frozen in expiration and when finding the maximal diameter of the frontal section in case of image scanning with 2D ultrasound. In case of 3D image scanning, the slightest rotation of the transducer might create poor image visualization, and difficulties in upgrading of the intermediate frames, due to crossing of manually traced organ contours. In spite of subjective errors like these, which are also frequently encountered with other sonographic methods (99–102), we found no differences in the applicability of the present 2D and 3D method in GERD patients.

### 5.1.3. *The value of ultrasound in studying gastric accommodation in GERD*

We have demonstrated that in adult patients with reflux disease postprandial ultrasonic imaging of the stomach was informative and achievable using either a 2D or a 3D ultrasound system. The ultrasonographic method offers advantages over established methods for the study of gastric accommodation in GERD patients, such as barostat and scintigraphy because it is non-invasive and safe.

Abnormal gastric accommodation and gastric emptying can be found in other gastrointestinal disorders as well. This ultrasonographic finding is therefore not diagnostic for GERD, but can be supplementary to the well-established methods such as endoscopy and 24-h ambulatory esophageal pH monitoring, and will add information on pathogenetic mechanisms. Since the ultrasonographic studies of the stomach are time consuming, this technique is likely to be used mainly for research purposes.

Our findings with this method in GERD patients may not be unconditionally applicable to all other centers. Currently, we are the only center which uses three-dimensional ultrasound with a magnetic scanhead tracking system for the evaluation of gastric accommodation in this group of patients. We still feel that certain aspects of the method are inadequately developed; therefore warranting further research on the gastric volume estimation using 3D ultrasound in GERD patients, as well as other patient groups.

## 5.2. *Esophageal mucosal injury, motility disturbances and distension in GERD patients*

Endoscopy is important for evaluating mucosal changes in patients with GERD, including metaplasia, and for grading reflux esophagitis. High-resolution endoscopy can detect minor signs of reflux-induced injury, both proximal to and distal to the *z*-line. Except for full-thickness biopsies, none of the available diagnostic techniques allows us to study the esophageal wall (measure the thickness of individual wall layers) or the mucosal injury in depth. Both the inner circular muscle layer and outer longitudinal muscles of the esophagus participate in peristalsis, and various measurement techniques have yielded conflicting information as to the temporal relationship between contraction in the two individual muscle layers. Contractions in the longitudinal layer have been hypothesized to contribute to the development of a hiatal hernia or *brachyoesophagus*, imaginably as a response to repeated esophageal acid exposure (36, 103).

Several motility abnormalities are found in patients with GERD. A low resting pressure and/or shortened lower esophageal sphincter is found in an important subgroup of patients with moderate to severe GERD. Abnormal esophageal acid exposure is thought to underlie the hypertensive peristalsis of "nutcracker esophagus" in at least 50%. Conversely, ineffective esophageal motility, defined as distal esophageal contraction amplitude below 30 mmHg, is probably the most common finding at manometry of the esophageal body in patients with chronic GERD. Acid reflux has variably been considered both cause of and result from motility disturbances. Experimental distension of the esophagus can cause heartburn and chest pain in healthy subjects as well as patients with GERD and other esophageal disease (104–107). Endoscopic ultrasonography (EUS), especially high-frequency endoscopic ultrasound, has a potential to elucidate certain clinical problems in esophagology that have not been solved by traditional diagnostic methods.

### 5.2.1. *Endoscopic ultrasonography*

Endoscopic ultrasonography (EUS) is the only technique that allows detailed in vivo study of the wall of each organ and to some extent, the closest neighboring organs (108, 109). It is a clinically useful technique currently indicated for staging GI cancers, assessment of submucosal tumors, and diagnosis of intestinal wall infiltrative diseases, common bile duct stones, and gut neuroendocrine tumors (110) (see chapter 15).

In a recent publication of a randomized, double-blind clinical trial by Mine *et al.*, EUS gave a very useful evaluation of submucosal injury in GERD patients (77). Using the miniature EUS probe (UM-3R, 20 MHz, Olympus, Tokyo, Japan), they evaluated 25 patients with reflux complaints before treatment, finding a variable degree of wall thickening in the lower esophagus as compared with 20 normal subjects. 6 weeks of therapy with lansoprazole reduced the thickening of the esophageal wall significantly when compared to patients treated with a standard-dose H2-receptor antagonist. The endosonographic finding strongly suggests that inflammatory damage to the submucosal and muscle layers of the lower esophagus might contribute to heartburn and associated symptoms such as dysphagia in patients with endoscopy-negative reflux disease.

In GERD patients, EUS allows not only the localization of damaged esophageal mucosa or diffuse thickening of the esophageal wall, but also characterization of the exact anatomic layers involved in these pathological processes (111). Episodes of noncardiac chest pain (NCCP) are often difficult to diagnose. Recent prospective double-blind studies have shown that about 44% of these patients with NCCP may have underlying GERD (112). EUS examination has shown that a subgroup of patients with no evidence for abnormal reflux or motility abnormalities in the esophagus still had sustained muscular contractions with a mean duration of 68 seconds immediately preceding episodes of chest pain (112). These contractions were secondary to isometric contraction of the circular muscle, which did not cause luminal constriction nor were related to contraction of the longitudinal muscle layer. EUS can be an alternative diagnostic tool for patients with NCCP who do not have classic motility abnormalities such as diffuse esophageal spasm, or respond to high-dose PPIs. The role of EUS in the assessment of patients with atypical GERD or other esophageal disease, is the subject of intense evaluation.

The potential of EUS in the detection of Barrett's esophagus and high-grade dysplasia or intramucosal carcinoma was compared with surgical/histopathologic evaluation (113). EUS detected unsuspected submucosal invasion and lymph node involvement in several cases. Sensitivity, specificity, and negative predictive values of preoperative EUS for submucosal invasion of carcinoma were 100%, 94%, and 100%, respectively, and for lymph node involvement were 100%, 81%, and 100%, respectively.

EUS has also been used recently for detecting the position and integrity of bulking materials employed to increase the competency of the cardia region to limit gastroesophageal reflux in our laboratory. This includes polymeric compounds implanted in case of the Gatekeeper® method (Fig. 6) or injected with the Enteryx® protocol in GERD patients.

### 5.2.2. *High-frequency intraluminal ultrasound (HFIUS)*

Using high-frequency intraluminal ultrasound (HFIUS), Yamamoto *et al.*, investigated the temporal correlation between contraction of the circular and longitudinal muscle layers during ascending excitatory and descending inhibitory reflexes in 10 normal healthy subjects. Their data indicate that the two muscle layers contract and relax in a coordinated manner during distension-related peristaltic reflexes in the esophagus (71). Using the same technique Balaban *et al.* studied the changes in esophageal muscle thickness in 10 healthy subjects and in 10 patients with chest pain unexplained by cardiological workup, manometry or 24-hour pH-metry (72). In this study, sustained esophageal contractions, found to have

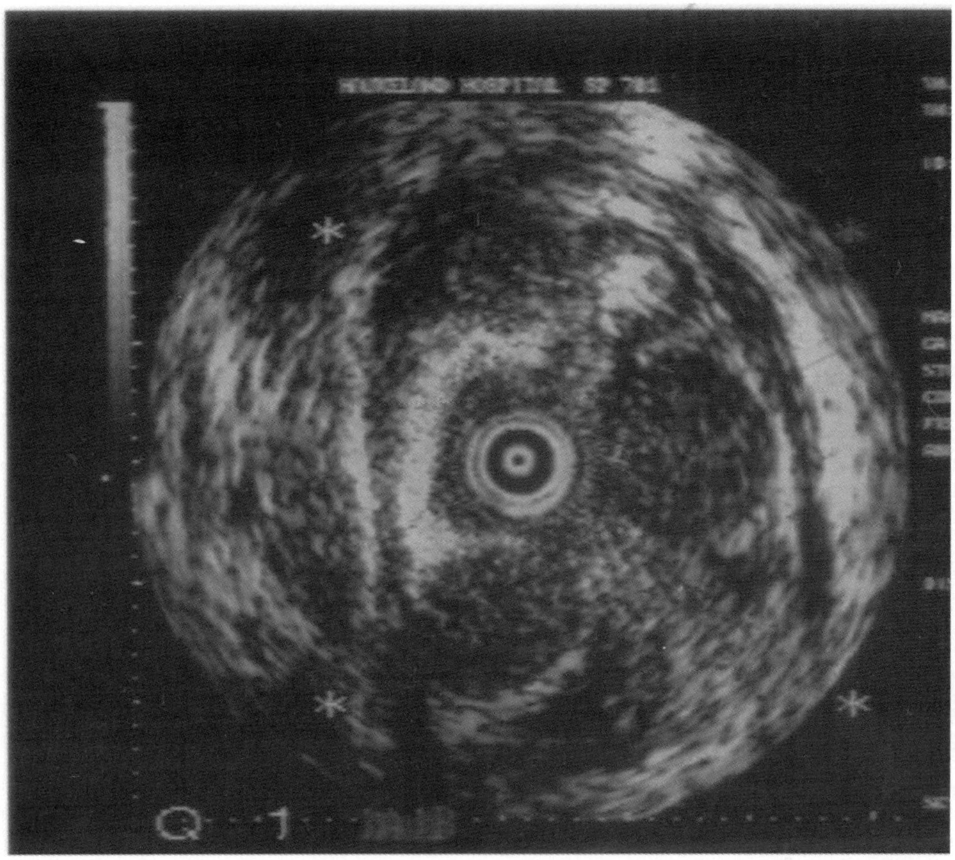

Fig. 6. Endosonographic image of submucosal implants employed in the Gatekeeper(r) method for reducing gastroesophageal reflux. The prostheses have a diameter of 2 mm when implanted, but expand to a diameter of about 7–9 mm over 24 hours. The figure shows the implants after 4 weeks and they can be seen to be safely located in the submucosa, to be intact and not to have induced inflammatory changes in the surrounding tissues.

a mean duration of 68 sec, were not detected in normal subjects, but in the patient group 18 of 24 spontaneous chest pain episodes were preceded by such contractions on ultrasonography. Pehlivanov *et al.* studied the relationship between the baseline (relaxed) and peak (contracted) muscle thickness and the manometrically defined contraction amplitude during swallow-induced contractions along the length of the esophagus in 15 normal subjects (73). They found that in the resting state, muscle thickness was significantly higher in the LES compared with the rest of the esophagus. Baseline muscle thickness was also significantly higher 2 cm as compared to 10 cm above the LES. A typical image from the distal esophagus in a patient with dysphagia and chest pain is shown in Fig. 7. Recently, Rhee *et al.* evaluated the technique of HFIUS to measure the esophageal cross-sectional area in 7 healthy subjects during swallowing of defined and increasing volumes of liquids. They furthermore observed episodes of gastroesophageal reflux and found HFIUS to be a valid technique to measure configurational changes of the esophagus *in vivo* during gastroesophageal reflux (74).

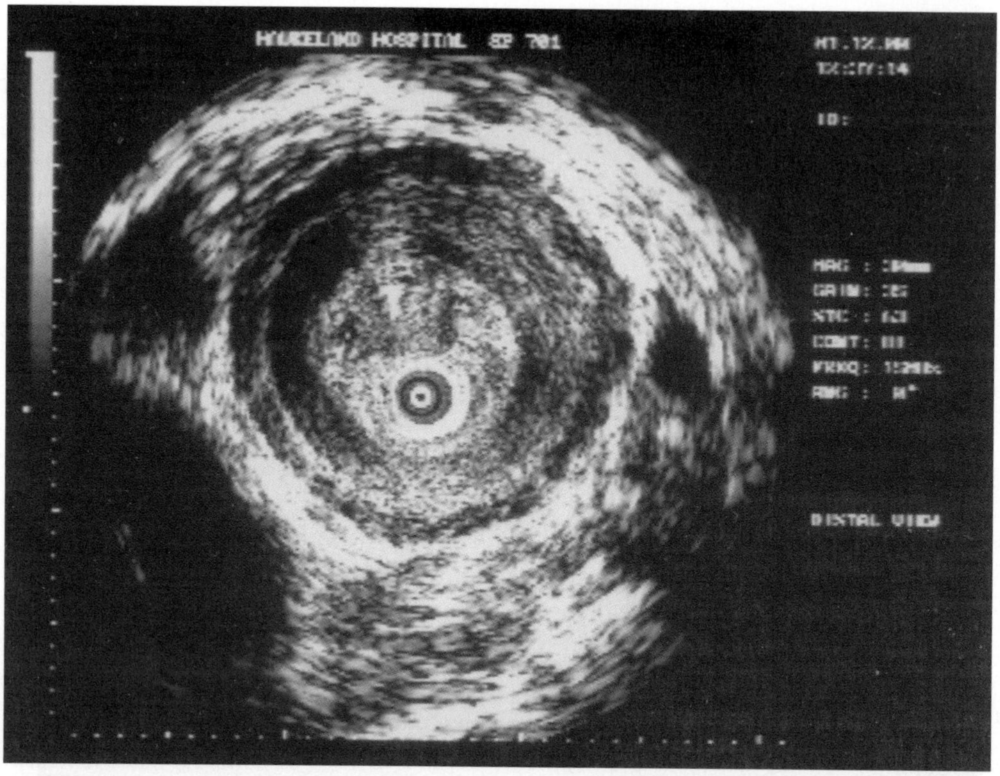

Fig. 7. Ultrasonographic image obtained from the distal esophagus with a 15 MHz miniprobe in a patient with dysphagia and chest pain. One can readily see how several layers of the esophageal wall can be discerned, including the two sublayers of the muscularis propria: the inner circular layer which broadens distally to form the lower esophageal sphincter, and the outer longitudinal layer.

HFIUS is a novel and unique technique to detect contraction of the individual longitudinal and circular muscle layers of the esophagus. It is, however, invasive and time consuming for analysis. Furthermore, it can be very difficult to detect the esophageal distension with reflux, since the volumes of refluxed material can be relatively small. This may reduce the sensitivity of the method as compared to a 24-hour pH-monitoring, which is likely to detect even small volumes of reflux. It is well known, however, that pH-metry is unable to identify all reflux episodes since two pH-electrodes at the same level do not measure identical pH-curves. This technique might be useful in the evaluation of achalasia and for the investigation of other esophageal motility disorders than those related to GERD.

### 5.3. *Evaluation of gastroesophageal reflux episodes*

In children, it is almost always possible to visualize the cardia region by transcutaneous ultrasound and passage of ingested fluids and refluxed material can be observed. Imaginably, this could be used as a simple method to diagnose abnormal reflux tendency. Comparison between ultrasonography (B-mode) and 24 hour esophageal pH-monitoring by Milocco *et al.* in 40 infants with suspected gastroesophageal reflux (GER) showed that ultrasonography could not be considered a faithful diagnostic tool in screening for GERD in infants. In this study, the positive and negative predictive value of sonography versus the result of continuous 24 hour pH-monitoring was 80% and 50% respectively (59).

Hirsch *et al.* performed a comparative study of ultrasonography (abnormal reflux or physiological reflux) with and without the use of color Doppler versus 24 hour esophageal pH measurements in eighty-four high-risk children for suspected gastroesophageal reflux (67, 69). He found abnormal reflux in 60.7% by pH-metry, in 51.2% by B-mode ultrasonography and in 59.5% by color Doppler ultrasonography. There was agreement between pH-metry and B-mode ultrasonography in 87% of patients as compared to 94% between pH-metry and color Doppler ultrasonography, and increased sensitivity of reflux detection from 84.4% to 98% when color Doppler was added to B-mode ultrasonography. This improvement was thought to be due to the higher sensitivity of CD for rapid and small quantities of reflux. The small number of discrepancies between pH-metry and CD US is probably due to the inability of the former to detect neutral reflux of contents or short duration ($< 30$ s), while CD US may miss some cases of acid reflux due to the short time of the examination (10 min). The addition of CD increased the sensitivity of US for detecting reflux. This rapid, easy and reliable method can be used to screen high-risk populations when reflux is suspected of being the cause of respiratory symptoms.

Jang *et al.* (68) compared color Doppler sonography and 24 hour esophageal pH monitoring in 54 children ranging in age from 2 months to 10 years (mean, 3 years) with suspected gastroesophageal reflux (GER). The study showed that Color Doppler sonography was highly sensitive and was thought to be easier to use and more acceptable to the child than pH monitoring. In this study, the two tests showed 81.5% agreement in the detection of GER. These two different tests were not performed simultaneously; therefore it is difficult to give definite criteria for evaluating the severity of GER on color Doppler imaging. Nevertheless, this modality may be clinically useful in screening children for GER.

Color Doppler ultrasonography is an easy and reliable method. It increases the sensitivity of ultrasonography for detecting reflux, because it is sensitive for rapid and small quantities of reflux. However, color Doppler ultrasonography is unable to detect reflux of a short duration. Nevertheless, it can be used to screen high-risk populations when reflux is thought to be the cause as in patients with respiratory symptoms or in case of children with suspected reflux disease.

### 5.4. *Hiatal hernia*

A hiatal hernia represents the migration of the esophago-gastric junction and later the stomach through the esophageal hiatus of the diaphragm into the posterior mediastinum (35). In our laboratory hiatal hernia is defined as gastric folds seen at least 2 cm above the diaphragm in adult patients. Little is known about the cause of hiatal hernia. Factors such as age (typical age of onset is in the fifth decade of life), with loss of elasticity, pregnancy and overweight (114), may play a role. Hiatal hernia may also be a consequence rather than a cause of GERD, because of spasms and shortening secondary to reflux or esophagitis (36, 103). The role of hiatal hernia in GERD is controversial. Hiatal hernia is not always associated with GERD, only one in three patients with a hiatal hernia have esophagitis and, on the other hand, endoscopic and radiographic studies suggest that 50–94% of patients with reflux disease have a hiatal hernia (17, 37–40, 115–118). It is believed that a hiatal hernia increases the chance of LES dysfunction and may worsen the symptoms of reflux disease. It acts as a fluid trap that promotes gastroesophageal reflux during swallowing-induced LES relaxation in supine patients (119).

Endoscopy and radiographic examinations are the established tools for identification of a hiatal hernia. However, there are patients who are not suitable for the above-mentioned examination namely infants and some elderly patients. In those cases ultrasound could be an alternative method for identifying hiatal hernia, even though it has low sensitivity and specificity. Westra and coworkers have defined the principal ultrasonographic findings associated with abnormal gastroesophageal reflux associated with hiatal herniation of the distal esophagus in infants and young children (65). These include an intra-abdominal esophagus measuring less than 2 cm, rounding of the gastroesophageal angle and the presence of a beak at the esophagogastric junction.

The best approach to diagnose a hiatal hernia with ultrasound in patients is the same as the standard ultrasonographic image section to measure the size of the proximal stomach (20, 21). In infant patients, the ultrasound probe must be placed in the midline under the xiphisternum and the distal esophagus. The transducer is then rotated and repositioned to obtain a longitudinal section through the intra-abdominal part of the distal esophagus. In adults the finding is dependent on a certain size of the hiatal hernia (in our experience a hernia larger than 3 cm in axial length). For visualization of the hiatal hernia the patients must swallow a liquid meal or water during the ultrasound examination to locate the encroachment of the liquid prior to the gastroesophageal junction. This process must be repeated until the suspected hiatus is demonstrated (at least 100 ml of water). Increased swallowing of the liquid may however also lead to the presence of air pockets in the gastric fundus, which distorts the image.

## 6. Ultrasound in the Clinical Setting of GERD/Summary

Ultrasound has limited diagnostic value in reflux disease, especially in adult GERD patients due to the position of the gastroesophageal junction behind the costal margins and xiphoid process. Potential uses in GERD in adults are partly the study of gastric accommodation using a transcutaneous approach, partly, by endosonography, to study motility changes and reflux events. In children, ultrasound has gained the widest routine use. The appropriate role for ultrasonography as a replacement for the upper gastrointestinal series in vomiting infants remains undefined. However, whenever reflux persists despite medical treatment, ultrasound can be useful to look for a hiatus hernia and gastric stasis. Although its role in the evaluation of patients with Barrett's esophagus and various strictures of the esophagus appears promising, its clinical use in evaluating GERD patients remains largely unproven.

The result of ultrasonograhic examinations is dependent on the state of competence of the antireflux mechanisms at a particular moment. It is also dependent on the experience of the performer with the method and the patient's cooperation. Transcutaneous ultrasound of the stomach is unable to differentiate between the different pathologic entities and may not always contribute to the diagnosis of GERD. The intraluminal approach is invasive. Endoluminal ultrasound gives a detailed study of the anatomy and dynamics of the esophagus and stomach, but such studies have no value as a first-line examination. It has poor specificity and sensitivity for uncomplicated reflux esophagitis (69, 79). Therefore, we do not recommend routine ultrasound examinations of the upper gastrointestinal tract in clinically obvious GERD.

## References

1. Dent, J., Brun, J., Fendrick, A. M. *et al.*, An evidence-based appraisal of reflux disease management — The Genval Workshop Report. Gut 1999; 44(Suppl 2): S1–S16.
2. Winters, C., Spurling, T. J. and Chobanian, S. J., Barrett's esophagus. A prevalent occult complication of gastroesophageal reflux disease. Gastroenterology 1987; 92: 118.
3. Sampliner, R. E., Barrett's esophagus, a complication of GERD. Curr. Treat. Options. Gastroenterol. 2002; 5: 45–50.
4. Dent, J., Dodds, W. J., Friedman, R. H. *et al.*, Mechanism of gastroesophageal reflux in recumbent asymptomatic human subjects. J. Clin. Invest. 1980; 65: 256–267.
5. Dodds, W. J., Dent, J., Hogan, W. J. *et al.*, Mechanisms of gastroesophageal reflux in patients with reflux esophagitis. N. Engl. J. Med. 1982; 307(25): 1547–1552.
6. Dent, J., Holloway, R. H., Toouli, J. *et al.*, Mechanisms of lower esophageal sphincter incompetence in patients with symptomatic gastroesophageal reflux. Gut 1988; 29: 1020–1028.
7. Klauser, A. G., Schindlbeck, N. E. and Muller-Lissner, S. A., Symptoms in gastro-oesophageal reflux disease. Lancet 1990; 335(8683): 205–208.
8. Berstad, A., Overview of ranitidine in reflux oesophagitis. Its effect on symptoms, endoscopic appearances and histology. In: The clinical use of ranitidine. Eds. Misiewicz, J. J., Wormsley, K. G., International Symposium. Med. Int. 1982.
9. Katz, P. O., Gastroesophageal reflux disease — State of the art. Rev. Gastroenterol. Disord. (2001); 1(3): 128-138.
10. Holloway, R. H. and Dent, J., Pathophysiology of gastroesophageal reflux. Lower esophageal sphincter dysfunction in gastroesophageal reflux disease. Gastroenterol. Clin. North. Am. 1990; 19(3): 517–535.
11. Altorki, N. k. and Skinner, D. B., Pathophysiology of gastroesophageal reflux. Am. J. Med. 1989; 86: 685–689.
12. Timmer, R., Breumelhof, R., Nadorp, J. H. S. M. *et al.*, Recent advances in the pathophysiology of gastro-oesophageal reflux disease. Eur. J. Gastroenterol. Hepatol. 1993; 5: 485–491.
13. Richter, J. E. and Castell, D. O., Gastroesophageal reflux. Pathogenesis, diagnosis, and therapy. Ann. Intern. Med. 1982; 97: 93–103.
14. Mittal, R. K. and McCallum, R. W., Characteristics and frequency of transient relaxation of the lower oesophageal sphincter on patients with reflux oesophagitis. Gastroenterology (1988); 95: 593–599.
15. Helm, J. F., Dodds, W. J., Pelc, L. R. *et al.*, Effect of esophageal emptying and saliva on clearance of acid from the esophagus. New. Engl. J. Med. 1984; 310: 84–288.
16. Kahrilas, P. J., Doods, W. J. and Hogan, W. J., Effect of peristalitic dysfunction on esophageal volume clearance. Gastroenterology 1988; 94: 73–80.
17. Hirschowitz, B. I., A critical analysis, with appropriate controls, of gastric acid and pepsin secretion in clinical esophagitis. Gastroenterology 1991; 101: 1149–1158.
18. Zhu, H., Pace, F., Sangaletti, O. *et al.*, Gastric acid secreation and pattern of gastroesophageal reflux in patients with esophagitis and concomitant duodenal ulcer. Scand. J. Gastroenterol. 1993; 28: 387–392.

19. Lillemoe, K. D., Johnson, L. F. and Harmon. J. W., Alkaline esophagitis: A comparison of the ability of components of gastroduodenal contents to injure the rabbit esophagus. Gastroenterology 1983; 85(3): 621–628.
20. Tefera, S., Gilja, O. H., Hatlebakk, J. G. and Berstad, A., Gastric accommodation studied by ultrasonography in patients with reflux esophagitis. Dig. Dis. Sci. 2001; 46(3): 618–625.
21. Tefera, S., Gilja, O. H., Olafsdottir, E., Hausken, T., Hatlebakk, J. G. and Berstad, A., Intragastric maldistribution of a liquid meal in patients with reflux esophagitis assessed by three-dimensional ultrasonography. Gut 2002; 2: 153–158.
22. Hartley, M. N., Walker, S. J. and Mackie, C. R., Abnormal gastric adaptive relaxation in patients with gastrooesophageal reflux. Gut 1990; 31: 500–503.
23. Zerbib, F., des Varannes, S. B., Ropert, A. *et al.*, Proximal gastric tone in gastro- oesophageal reflux disease. Eur. J. Gastroenterol. Hepatol. 1999; 11: 511–515.
24. Penagini, R., Hebbard, G., Horowitz, M. *et al.*, Motor function of the proximal stomach and visceral perception in gastro-oesophageal reflux disease. Gut 1998; 42: 251–257.
25. Vu, M. K., Straathof, J. W. A., vd Schaar, P. J. *et al.*, Motor and sensory function of the proximal stomach in reflux disease and after laparoscopic Nissen fundoplication. Am. J. Gastroenterol. 1999; 94: 1481–1489.
26. McCallum, R. W., Berkowitz, D. M. and Lerner. E., Gastric emptying in patient with gastroesophageal reflux. Gastroenterology 1981; 80: 285–291.
27. Shay, S., Eggli, D., McDonald, C. *et al.*, Gastric emptying of solid food in a patients with gastroesophageal reflux. Gastroenterology 1987; 92: 459–465.
28. Myers, J. C., Collins, P. J., Dehn, T. C. B. *et al.*, Which part of the stomach is responsible for delay in gastric emptying of solids in patients with gastro-oesophageal reflux disease. J. Gastroenterol. Hepatol. 1988; 3: 988.
29. Collins, B. J., McFarland, R. J., O'Hare, M. M. T. *et al.*, Gastric emptying of solid-liquid meal and gastroentestinal hormone responses in patients with erosive esophagitis. Digestion 1986; 33: 61-68.
30. Maddern, G. J., Chatterton, B. E., Collins, P. J. *et al.*, Solid and liquid gastric emptying in patients with gastro-oesophageal reflux. Br. J. Surg. 1985; 72(5): 44–347.
31. Orlando, R. C., Esophageal epithelial resistance. J. Clin. Gastro. 1986; 1: 12–16.
32. Orlando, R. C., Esophageal epithelial defense against acid injury. J. Clin. Gastroenterol. 1991; 13(Suppl 2): S1–S5.
33. Bor, S., Caymaz-Bor, C., Tobey, N. A. *et al.*, Effect of ethanol on the structure and function of rabbit esophageal epithelium. Am. J. Physiol. 1998; 274: G819–G826
34. Salo, J. A. and Kivilaakso, E., Role of luminal $H^+$ in the pathogenesis of experimental esophagitis. Surgery 1982; 92: 61–68.
35. Santos, G. H., Is hiatus hernia responsible for reflux? Chest 1983; 84: 242–244.
36. Bremner, R. M., Crokkes, P. F., Costantini, M. *et al.*, The relationship of esophageal length to hiatal hernia in gastroesophageal reflux disease (GERD). Gastroenterology 1992; 102: A45.
37. Petersen, H., The clinical significance of hiatus hernia. Scand. J. Gastroenterol. 1995; 211 Suppl: 19–20.
38. Berstad, A., Weberg, R., Froyshov, L. I. *et al.*, Relationship of hiatus hernia to reflux oesophagitis. A prospective study of coincidence, using endoscopy. Scand. J. Gastroenterol. 1986; 21(1): 55–58.
39. Kahrilas, P. J., Hiatus hernia causes reflux: Fact or fiction? Gullet 1993; 3(Suppl): 21.
40. Kahrilas, P. J., Wu, S., Ponderoix, P. *et al.*, Attenuation of esophageal shortning during peristalisis with hiatus hernia. Gastroenterology 1995; 109: 1818–25

41. Dodds, W. J., Kahrilas, P. J., Dent, J. *et al.*, Analysis of spontaneous gastroesophageal reflux and esophageal acid clearance in patients with reflux esophagitis. J. Gastrointest. Motil. 1990; 2: 79–89.
42. Dent, J., Wylie, J., Dodds, J. *et al.*, Interdigestive phasic contractions of the human lower esophageal sphincter. Gastroenterology 1983; 84: 453.
43. Holloway, R. H., Blank, E., Takahashi, I. *et al.*, Variability of lower esophageal Sphincter pressure in the fasted unanesthetized opossum. Am. J. Physiol. 1985; 248 (4 Pt 1): G398–406.
44. Holloway, R. H., Blank, E., Takahashi, I. *et al.*, Motilin: A mechanism incorporating the opossum lower esophageal sphincter into the migrating motor complex. Gastroenterology 1985; 89(3): 507–515.
45. Lind, T., Havelund, T., Carlsson, R. *et al.*, Heartburn without oesophagitis: efficacy of omeprazole therapy and features determining therapeutic response. Scand. J. Gastroenterol. 1997; 32: 974–979.
46. Hatlebakk, J. G., Hyggen, A., Madsen, P. H., Walle, P. O., Schulz, T., Mowinckel, P., Bernklev, T. and Berstad, A., Heartburn treatment in primary care: randomised, double blind study for 8 weeks. BMJ 1999; 319(7209): 550–553.
47. Smout, A. J. P. M., Evaluation and significance of reflux from the duodenum and stomach. Aliment. Pharmacol. Ther. 1997; 11(Suppl 2): 27–32.
48. Bate, C. M., Riley, S. A., Chapman, R. W., Durnin, A. T. and Taylor, M. D., Evaluation of omeprazole as a cost-effective diagnostic test for gastro-oesophageal reflux disease. Aliment. Pharmacol. Ther. 1999; 13(1): 59–66.
49. Johnsson, F., Hatlebakk, J. G., Klintenberg, A.-C., Román, J., Toth, E., Stubberöd, A., Falk, A. and Edin, R., One-week esomeprazole treatment: an effective confirmatory test in patients with suspected gastroesophageal reflux disease. Scand J Gastroenterol 2003; 38: 354–359.
50. Manterola, C., Munoz, S., Grande, L. and Bustos, L., Initial validation of a questionnaire for detecting gastroesophageal reflux disease in epidemiological settings. J. Clin. Epidemiol. 2002; 55(10): 1041–1045.
51. Venables, T., Newland, R., Oatel, A. C. *et al.*, Omeprazole 10 milligrams once daily, omeprazole 20 milligrams once daily, or ranitidine 150 milligrams twice daily, evaluated as initial therapy for the relief of symptoms of gastro-oesophageal reflux disease in general practice. Scand. J. Gastroenterol. 1997; 32: 965–973.
52. Carlsson, R., Dent, J., Watts, R. *et al.*, Gastro-oesophageal reflux disease (GORD) in primary care: An international study of different treatment strategies with omeprazole. Eur. J. Gastroenterol. Hepatol. 1998; 10: 119–124.
53. Galmiche, J, P., Barthelemy, P. and Hamelin, B., Treating the symptoms of gastro-oesophageal reflux disease: A double-blind comparison of omeprazole and cisapride. Aliment. Pharmacol. Ther. 1997; 11: 765–773.
54. Johnsson, F. and Joelsson, B., Reproducibility of ambulatory oesophageal pH monitoring. Gut 1988; 29: 886–889.
55. Wienere, G. J., Richter, J. E., Copper, J. B., Wu, W. C. and Castell, D. O., The symptom index: A clinically important parameter, of ambulatory 24-hour esophageal pH monitoring. Am. J. Gastroenterol. 1988; 83: 358–361.
56. Weusten, B. L., Roelofs, J. M., Akkermans, L. M., van Berge, Henegouwon. G. P. and Smout, A. J., The symptom association probability: an improved method for symptom analysis of 24-hour esophageal pH data. Gastroenterology 1994; 107: 1741–1745.
57. Johnston, B. T., Troshinsky, M. B., Castell, J. A. *et al.*, Comparison of barium radiography with esophageal pH monitoring in the diagnosis of gastroesopageal reflux disease. Am. J. Gastroenterol. 1996; 91(6): 1181–1185.

58. Wynchank, S., Mann, M. D., Fisher, R. *et al.*, Ultrasound as a screening study for gastro-oesophageal reflux in children. Ann. Trop. Paediatr. 1997; 17(4): 343–348.
59. Milocco, C., Salvatore, C. M., Torre, G. *et al.*, Sonography versus continuous 24 hours oesophageal pH-monitoring in the diagnosis of infant gastroesophageal reflux. Peadiatr. Med. Chir. 1997; 19(4): 245–246.
60. Di Mario, M., Bergami, G., Fariello, G. *et al.*, Diagnosis of gastroesophageal reflux in childhood. Comparison of ultrasonography and barium swallow. Radiol. Med. (Torino) 1995; 89(1–2): 76–81.
61. Gomes, H., Gastroesophageal reflux in infants: ultrasonographic reading of pHmetry. Arch. Pediatr. 1994; 1(7): 639–645.
62. Le Dosseur, P., Moutounet, L., Eurin, D. *et al.*, Ultrasonography of the esophagus in children. Ann. Radiol. (Paris) 1994; 37(7–8): 494–499.
63. Tani, G., Sciutti, R., Teglia, F. *et al.*, Diagnosis of gastro-esophageal reflux in children. Ultrasonography versus pH monitoring. Radiol. Med. (Torino) 1993; 86(5): 626–629.
64. Vogt, S., Schramm, D., Frenzel, J. *et al.*, Sonographic diagnosis of gastroesophageal reflux in infancy. Kinderarztl. Prax. 1990; 58(7): 349–53.
65. Westra, S. J., Wolf, B. H. and Staalman, C. R., Ultrasound diagnosis of gastroesophageal reflux and hiatal hernia in infants and young children. J. Clin. Ultrasound. 1990; 18(6): 477–485.
66. Naik, D. R., Bolia, A. and Moore, D. J., Comparison of barium swallow and ultrasound in diagnosis of gastro-oesophageal reflux in children. Br. Med. J. (Clin. Res. Ed.) 1985; 290(6486): 1943–1945.
67. Hirsch, W., Kedar, R. and Preiss, U., Color doppler in the diagnosis of the gastroesophageal reflux in children: Comparison with pH measurements and B-mode ultrasound. Pediatr. Radiol. 1996; 26(3): 232–235.
68. Jang, H. S., Lee, J. S., Lim, G. Y. *et al.*, Correlation of color Doppler sonographic findings with pH measurements in gastroesophageal reflux in children. J. Clin. Ultrasound. 2001; 29(4): 212–217.
69. Hirsch, W., Preiss, U. and Kedar, R., Color coded Doppler ultrasound in diagnosis of gastroesophageal reflux. Klin. Padiatr. 1997; 209(1): 6–10.
70. Yamada, M., Kobayashi, I., Kawamura, N. *et al.*, Color Doppler ultrasonography for evaluation of gastroesophageal reflux in a sick child. Acta. Paediatr. 1998; 87(2): 229–230.
71. Yamamoto, Y., Liu, J., Smith, T. K. *et al.*, Distension-related responses in circular and longitudinal muscle of the human esophagus: an ultrasonographic study. Am. J. Physiol. 1998; 275: G805–G811.
72. Balaban, D. H., Yamamoto, Y., Liu, J. *et al.*, Sustained esophageal contraction: A marker of esophageal chest pain identified by intraluminal ultrasonography. Gastroenterology 1999; 116(1): 29–37.
73. Pehlivanov, N., Liu, J., Kassab, G. S. *et al.*, Relationship between esophageal muscle thickness and intraluminal pressure in patients with esophageal spasm. Am. J. Physiol. Gastrointest. Liver. Physiol. 2001; 280: G1093–G1098.
74. Rhee, P. L., Liu, J., Puckett, J. L. *et al.*, Measuring esophageal distension by high-frequency intraluminal ultrasound probe. Am. J. Physiol. Gastrointest. Liver. Physiol. 2002; 283(4): G886–G892.
75. LiVoti, G., Tulone, V., Bruno, R. *et al.*, Ultrasonography and gastric emptying: Evaluation in infants with gastroesophageal reflux. J. Pediatr. Gastroenterol. Nutr. 1992; 14(4): 397–399.
76. Rico, M. E., Codoner, F. P., Molla, O. E. *et al.*, Gastric emptying in children with gastroesophageal reflux. Evaluation by real time ultrasonography of the pyloric antrum. An. Esp. Pediatr. 1999; 51: 33–38.

77. Mine, S., Fujisaki, T., Tabata, T. *et al.*, Ultrasonographic evaluation of lansoprazole-induced improvement of submucosal injury in patients with gastroesophageal reflux. Am. J. Gastroenterol. 2000; 95(2): 381–386.
78. Westra, S. J., Derkx, H. H. and Taminiau, J. A., Symptomatic gastroesophageal reflux: Diagnosis with ultrasound. J. Pediatr. Gastroenterol. Nutr. 1994; 19(1): 58–64.
79. Lazzari, L. R., Collina, A., Pession, A., Corvaglia, L. *et al.*, The diagnosis of gastroesophageal reflux in childhood: A comparison between echography and pH measurement. Pediatr. Med. Chir. 1991; 13(6): 617–619.
80. Aliotta, A., Rapaccini, G. L., Pompili, M. *et al.*, Ultrasonographic signs of sliding gastric hiatal hernia and their prospective evaluation. J. Ultrasound. Med. 1995; 14(6): 457–61.
81. Zaragosi, E. A., Cabanas, A. M. D., Garre, S. M. C. *et al.*, Ultrasonography-hiatal hernia and gastro-esophageal reflux disease. Rev. Esp. Enferm. Dig. 1998; 90(3): 198–199.
82. Mittal, R. K., Holloway, R. H., Penagini, R., Blackshaw, L. A. and Dent, J., Transient lower esophageal sphincter relaxation. Gastroenterology 1995; 109: 601–610.
83. Holloway, R. H., Hongo, M., Berger, K. *et al.*, Gastric distention: a mechanism for postprandial gastroesophageal reflux. Gastroenterology 1985; 89: 779–784.
84. Franzi, S. J., Martin, C. J., Cox, M. R. *et al.*, Response of canine lower esophageal sphincted to gastric distention. Am. J. Physiol. 1990; 259: G380–G385.
85. Schoeman, M. N., Tippett, M. D., Akkermans, L. M. A. *et al.*, Mechanisms of gastroesophageal reflux in ambulant healthy human subjects. Gastroenterology 1995; 108: 83–91.
86. Holloway, R. H., Kocyan, P. and Dent, J., Provocation of transient lower esophageal sphincter relaxations by meals in patients with symptomatic gastroesophageal reflux. Dig. Dis. Sci. 1991; 36: 1034–1039.
87. Penagini, R., Schoeman, M. N., Holloway, R. H. *et al.*, Mechanisms of gastroesophageal reflux in ambulant patients with reflux esophagitis (abstr). Gastroenterology 1994; 106: A159.
88. Fishman, E. K., Magid, D., Ney, D. R. *et al.*, Three-dimensional imaging. Radiology 1991; 181: 321–337.
89. Moragas, G. M., Azpiroz, F., Pavia, J. *et al.*, Relation among intragastric pressure postcibal percebtion, and gastric emptying. Am. J. Physiol. 1993; 264: G1112–1117.
90. Ropert, A., des Varannes, S. B., Bizais, Y. *et al.*, Simultaneous assessment of liquid emptying and proximal gastric tone in humans. Gastroenterology 1993; 105: 667–674.
91. Carroccio, A., Iacono, G., Li Voti, G., Montalto, G., Cavataio, F., Tulone, V., Lorello, D., Kazmierska, I., Acierno, C. and Notarbartolo, A., Gastric emptying in infants with gastroesophageal reflux. Ultrasound evaluation before and after cisapride administration. Scand. J. Gastroenterol. 1992; 27(9): 799–804.
92. Bolondi, L., Bortolotti, M., Santi, V. *et al.*, Measurement of gastric emptying time by real-time ultrasonography. Gastroenterology 1985; 89(4): 752–759.
93. Hausken, T. and Berstad, A., Wide gastric antrum in patients with non-ulcer dyspepsia. Effect of cisapride. Scand. J. Gastroenterol. 1992; 27: 427–432.
94. Hausken, T., Ødegaard, S., Matre, K. *et al.*, Antroduodenal motility and movements of luminal contents studied by duplex sonography. Gastroenterology 1992; 102: 1583–1590.
95. Hveem, K., Jones, K., Chatterton, B. E. *et ala.*, Scintigraphic and ultrasonographic measurment of the antral area — Relationship to appetite. Gut 1996; 38: 816–821.
96. Gilja, OH., Detmer, P. R., Jong, J. M. *et al.*, Intragastric distribution and gastric emptying assessed by three-dimensional ultrasonography. Gastroenterology 1997; 113: 38–49.

97. Frislid, K., Berstad, A. and Guldvog, I., Simulated meal test. A new method for estimation of parietal and non-parietal secretion in response to food. Scand. J. Gastroenterol. 1985; 20(1): 115–122.
98. Gilja, O. H., Hausken, T., Odegaard, S. *et al.*, Monitoring postprandial size of the proximal stomach by ultrasonography. J. Ultrasound. Med. 1995; 14(2): 81–9.
99. Szebeni, A. and Beleznay, E., New simple method for thyroid volume determination by ultrasonography. J. Clin. Ultrasound. 1992; 20(5): 329–337.
100. Terris, M. K. and Stamey, T. A., Determination of prostate volume by transrectal ultrasound. J. Urol. 1991; 145(5): 984–987.
101. Jones, T. B., Riddick, L. R., Harpen, M. D. *et al.*, Ultrasonographic determination of renal mass and renal volume. J. Ultrasound. Med. 1983; 2(4): 151–154.
102. Everson, G. T., Braverman, D. Z., Johnson, M. L. *et al.*, A critical evaluation of real-time ultrasonography for the study of gallbladder volume and contraction. Gastroenterology 1980; 79(1): 40–46.
103. Clouse, R. E., Eckert, T. C. and Staiano, A., Hiatus hernia and esophageal contraction abnormalities. Am. J. Med. 1986; 81: 447–450.
104. Barish, C. F., Castell, D. O. and Richter, J. F., Graded esophageal ballon distension: A new provocative test for non-cardiac chest pain. Dig. Dis. Sci. 1986; 31: 1292–1298.
105. De Caestecker, J. S., Pryde, A. and Heading, R. C., Site and mechanism of pain Perception with oesophageal ballon distension and intravenous edrophonium in patients with oesophageal chest pain. Gut 1992; 33: 580–586.
106. Richter, J. F., Barish, C. F. and Castell, D. O., Abnormal sensory perception in patients with esophageal chest pain. Gastroenterology 1986; 91: 845–852.
107. Takeda, T., Liu, J., Gui, A. *et al.*, The relationship between esophageal sensation and biomechanical properties of the wall of the esophagus (Abstract). Gastroenterology 2001; 120(Suppl 1): A631.
108. Caletti, G. C., Bolondi, L., Zani, L. *et al.*, Technique of endoscopic ultrasonography investigation: Esophagus, stomach and duodenum. Scand. J. Gastroenterol. 1986; 21(Suppl 123): 1–5.
109. Tsukamoto, Y., Goto, H., Hase, S. *et al.*, Endosonographic evaluation of the quality of ulcer healing induced by proton pump inhibitors. J. Clin. Gastroenterol. 1995; 20(Suppl 2): S40–S43.
110. Caletti, G. C., Fusaroli, P. and Bocus, P., Endoscopic ultrasonography. Digestion 1998; 59: 509–529.
111. Caletti, G. C., Ferrari, A., Mattioli, S. *et al.*, Endoscopy versus endoscopic ultrasonography in staging reflux esophagitis. Endoscopy 1994; 26: 794–797.
112. Shrestha, S. and Pasricha, P. J., Update on noncardiac chest pain. Dig. Dis. 2000; 18(3): 138–146.
113. Scotiniotis, I. A., Kochman, M. L., Lewis, J. D., Furth, E. E., Rosato, E. F. and Ginsberg, G. G., Accuracy of EUS in the evaluation of Barrett's esophagus and high-grade dysplasia or intramucosal carcinoma. Gastrointest. Endosc. 2001; 54(6): 689–96.
114. Stene-Larsen, G., Weberg, R., Frøyshov, L. I. *et al.*, Relationship of overweight to hiatus hernia and reflux oesophagitis. Scand. J. Gastroenterol. 1988; 23: 427–432.
115. Johannessen, T., Petersen, H., Kleveland, P. M. *et al.*, The predictive value of history in dyspepsia. Scand. J. Gastroenterol. 1990; 25: 689–697.
116. Kaul, B., Petersen, H., Myrvold, H. E. *et al.*, Hiatus hernia in gastroesophageal reflux disease. Scand. J. Gastroenterol. 1986; 21(1): 31–34.

117. Ott, D. J., Gelfand, D. W., Chen, Y. M. *et al.*, Predictive relationship of hiatal hernia to reflux esophagitis. Gastrointest. Radiol. 1985; 10(4): 317–320.
118. Wright, R. A. and Hurwitz, A. L., Relationship of hiatal hernia to endoscopically proved reflux esophagitis. Dig. Dis. Sci. 1979; 24(4): 311–313.
119. Mittal, R, K., Lange, R. C. and McCallum, R. W., Identification and mechanism of delayed esophageal acid clearance in subjects with hiatus hernia. Gastroenterology (1987); 92: 130–135.

Published with permission

*Digestive Diseases and Sciences, Vol. 46, No. 3 (March 2001), pp. 618–625*

# Gastric Accommodation Studied by Ultrasonography in Patients with Reflux Esophagitis

S. TEFERA, MD, O.H. GILJA, MD, PhD, J.G. HATLEBAKK, MD, PhD, and A. BERSTAD, MD, PhD

The aim of this study was to investigate gastric accommodation to a meal in patients with reflux esophagitis using ultrasonography. Twenty consecutive patients with reflux esophagitis of grade I (14) or II (6) and 20 healthy subjects underwent ultrasonographic measurements of the stomach before and after ingestion of a 500 ml soup meal. Reflux esophagitis patients revealed a significantly larger sagittal area of the proximal stomach at 5 min ($P = 0.002$) and 15 min ($P = 0.007$) postprandially and experienced more epigastric fullness after the meal ($P = 0.0006$). Postprandial fullness and sagittal area of the proximal stomach correlated significantly ($r = 0.69$; $P = 0.0007$). We conclude that patients with mild or moderate reflux esophagitis have a larger sagittal area of the proximal stomach and more postprandial fullness in response to a soup meal than healthy subjects. Postprandial distension of the proximal stomach may be a pathogenetic factor in reflux esophagitis.

**KEY WORDS:** gastric accommodation; gastroesophageal reflux disease; postprandial fullness; proximal part of the stomach; transient lower esophageal sphincter relaxation; ultrasonography

Following a meal the proximal stomach relaxes and acts as a reservoir. This gastric accommodation to a meal involves both receptive relaxation of the corpus–fundus region of the stomach starting when food enters the pharynx and esophagus and adaptive relaxation in response to small increases in intragastric pressure as food builds up in the stomach. The responses are mediated by vagal reflexes (1–4), which, under physiological conditions, enable the proximal part of the stomach to maintain a low balanced pressure and adapt its volume to the size of the ingested meal.

Using scintigraphy, McCallum et al found normal gastric emptying of liquids but delayed emptying of solids in 41% of patients with reflux esophagitis (5), whereas Maddern et al found delayed emptying of both liquid and solid meals (6). Using an electronic barostat, Zerbib et al found a more pronounced reduction of gastric tone in patients with gastroesophageal reflux disease (GERD) than in dyspeptic patients or healthy subjects (7). However, the barostat balloon may influence the normal gastric motility pattern (8, 9), and neither the barostat nor scintigraphy allow estimation of the size of the proximal stomach. Gilja et al recently developed a method by which the size of the proximal stomach in response to a liquid meal can be measured using noninvasive, transcutaneous ultrasound (10). By this method, patients with functional dyspepsia, patients with diabetes, and children with recurrent abdominal pain have been studied (11–14).

The purpose of this study was to investigate gastric accommodation to a liquid meal in patients with mild or moderate reflux esophagitis using transcutaneous ultrasound.

Manuscript received December 29, 1999; revised manuscript received May 1, 2000; accepted September 30, 2000.

From the Division of Gastroenterology, Department of Medicine, Haukeland Hospital, University of Bergen, Norway.

Address for reprint requests: Dr. Solomon Tefera, Medical Department, Haukeland Hospital, University of Bergen, N-5021 Bergen, Norway.

Published with permission



TABLE 1. DEMOGRAPHIC DATA FOR HEALTHY SUBJECTS AND PATIENTS WITH REFLUX ESOPHAGITIS GRADE I OR II

| | *Healthy* | *Patients* | P |
|---|---|---|---|
| Patients (*N*) | 20 | 20 | NS |
| Male/female ratio | 7/13 | 7/13 | NS |
| Age (range), years | 43 (27–62) | 42 (25–57) | NS |
| Weight, kg | 69.90 ± 12.34 | 83.15 ± 8.85 | 0.0004 |
| Height, cm | 171.8 ± 9.97 | 176.2 ± 9.38 | NS |
| Esophagitis grade I/II | NA | 14/6 | NA |
| Hiatal hernia, no. of patients | NA | 10 | NA |
| Mean length of hiatal hernia, cm | NA | 2.9 | NA |
| Body mass index (range) | 23 (19–28) | 27 (20–38) | 0.003 |

## MATERIALS AND METHODS

**Subjects.** Between October 1997 and March 1999, twenty consecutive untreated patients of both genders and between 25 and 57 years old, with chronic heartburn and/or acid regurgitation and reflux esophagitis confirmed at endoscopy, were recruited for the study. Twenty randomly selected healthy subjects of both genders and between 27 and 62 years old with no history of dyspepsia or reflux symptoms served as the control group (Table 1).

**Exclusion Criteria.** Hiatial hernia larger than 5 cm and diseases other than reflux esophagitis grade I or II, eg, scleroderma, peptic stricture, serious systemic or suspected malignant disease, previous gastric surgery, previous peptic ulcer disease, *Helicobacter pylori* infection, alcoholism, disease of the liver, pancreas, or bile ducts, pregnant or lactating women, or patients on drug therapy that may influence gastric motor function were excluded.

**Endoscopy.** The endoscopic examination was performed by one of the authors. The severity of macroscopic esophagitis were graded as: 0 = normal; I = red streaks or spots along the ridge of the mucosal folds, with or without fibrinous exudate: II = broded lesions, each involving the entire width of a fold or coalescing into fields of erythaema, with or without fibrinous exudate; III = stricture or endoscopically visible ulcer in the distal esophagus (15). Evaluation of *H. pylori* status was made by rapid urease test which was read after 24 hr (16). Hiatial hernia was defined as gastric folds seen at least 2 cm above the diaphragmatic incisura.

**Study Protocol.** Patients returned for ultrasound scanning within seven days after endoscopy. Smoking was not allowed before the examination, which was done between 8:00 AM and 10:00 AM after an overnight fast. The participants were scanned while sitting in a wooden chair, leaning slightly backwards at an angle of 120°. Sonographic images were obtained using an ultrasound scanner (System Five, GE Vingmed Sound, Horten, Norway) with a 3.5-MHz broadband curvilinear transducer. Before ingestion of the test meal, the occurrence of antral contractions was observed for at least 2 min to evaluate whether the subject's interdigestive migrating motor complex was in phase III (regular contractions with a frequency of 3/min). If phase III was observed, ingestion of test meal was postponed until phase I (quiescence) was observed. Scanning was performed in the fasting state, and 5, 15, 25, and 35 min postprandially right after a 4-min ingestion of the test meal. The maximal angel of view was 90°, and the maximal depth of the scanning was 22 cm for sagittal and oblique frontal sections of the proximal part of the stomach and 15 cm for the antral section. Two standardized sonographic image sections were chosen to monitor the size of the proximal stomach. First a sagittal section, with the left renal pelvis in a longitudinal projection, the left lobe of the liver and the tail of the pancreas as internal landmarks, was recorded. Then the transducer was rotated 90° clockwise to obtain an oblique frontal section where the left hemidiaphragm, the top margin of the fundus, and the liver parenchyma served as landmarks. To obtain the sagittal antral area, the aorta, the superior mesenteric vein, and the left lobe of the liver were used as landmarks. All selected ultrasound images were scanned at the end of normal expiration. The time required for scanning each part was < 1 min. One investigator (S.T.) was able to perform all the scans and operate the image workstation.

**Measurements.** Each standardized image was frozen before being recorded on videotape and stored on System Five ultrasound scanner. At the end of the examination, the stored images were transferred to a 1.3-GB magneto optical (MO) disk (Sony Corp., Recording and Energy Company, Shinagawa-Ku, Tokyo). Data processing was done on a Windows-NT version 4.0 workstation (Compac Proline, 100-MHz Pentium, San Jose, California, USA equipped with 48 MB RAM.

All measures were traced twice after replaying the videotapes by utilizing the manual tracing facilities on the scanner. The ultrasonograms also were traced once from the MO disk using a newly developed software package with rendering and volume estimation capabilities (EchoPAC-3D, GE Vingmed Sound, Horten, Norway).

In order to assess the problem of air pockets in the gastric fundus, the visible amount of air in the proximal stomach was graded from 0 to 3. Grade 0 denoted absence of visible air in the fundus, grade 1 small amounts of air, grade 2 moderate amounts, and grade 3 amounts of air so great that exclusion from the study was necessary.

A proximal gastric area in a sagittal section (SA) was outlined by tracing from the top margin of the fundus 7 cm downward along the axis of the stomach. The maximal diameter in an oblique frontal section (FD), kept within 7 cm along axis of the proximal stomach, was chosen as the second measure. Within 7 cm along the axis of the outlined sagittal section of the proximal stomach, the maximal diameter was chosen as sagittal diameter. The sagittal section of the antral area was measured by tracing the outer profile of the muscularis propria of the gastric wall. The inner echogenic layer corresponding to the interface between the soup and the mucosa of the gastric wall was outlined (17). In those cases in which air pockets were present in the selected sonographic section, the outer border of the air pocket was traced. Blinded to the values first obtained, the same investigator repeated the workstation procedure after four months.

**Test Meal.** Five hundred milliliters of commercially available meat soup (Toro clear meat soup, Rieber & Son A/S, Bergen, Norway) containing 1.8 g protein, 0.9 g fat, and 1.1 carbohydrate (20 kcal) at the temperature of 37°C was ingested over a period of 4 min (during ultrasound scanning). The pH of the soup was between 5.4 and 5.7 and the osmolarity was 350 mosm/kg $H_2O$. This low-calorie soup meal has been extensively investigated in our laboratory in patients with dyspepsia, where it has important advantages: it gives an excellent ultrasonographic view and it provokes symptoms in the majority of patients. The meal has a mean half emptying time of 22.1 ± 3.8 min (18), and it induces fed-state antral contractions at a rate of 3/min in over 85% of patients with functional dyspepsia and healthy controls (19, 20).

**Symptom Scores.** All participants were asked to score their abdominal symptoms (pain, nausea, fullness, abdominal discomfort, and hunger or satiety) 1 min before and 5 min after the test meal using a visual analog scale from 0 (no symptom) to 10 (intolerable symptom).

**Statistics Analysis.** All calculations and graphic designs were done using commercially available computer software (Graphpad Prism, GraphPad Software Inc, San Diego, California, USA). The measurements are given as means ±SD, if not otherwise stated. The distribution of data was evaluated by inspecting a probability plot and by using the Kolmogorov-Smirnov test with Lilliefors subanalysis. If the data appeared normally distributed, Student's $t$ test with two-sided probabilities was used to evaluate the statistical significance of differences between means. If not normally distributed, a **Mann-Whitney nonparametric test** was applied. The association between postprandial fullness and sagittal area of the proximal stomach was assessed by Pearson's correlation coefficient. $P < 0.05$ was chosen as the level of statistical significance.

## RESULTS

None of the patients or healthy subjects had to be excluded due to air pockets in the gastric fundus, technical difficulties, or symptoms after the ingestion of the test meal. Air pockets were graded 0 in 15 and 14, grade 1 in 4 and 3, and 2 in 1 and 3 patients and controls, respectively ($P > 0.5$). Prior to soup ingestion, the proximal stomach was empty both in the patients and healthy subjects. We found no difference in the application of internal landmarks between patients and healthy subjects. The data presented in the results are the averaged values.

Patients with reflux esophagitis had a significantly larger sagittal area of the proximal stomach at 5 min (32.1 ± 6.1 vs 26.5 ± 4.1 $cm^2$, $P = 0.002$) and at 15 min (26.5 ± 6.3 vs 21.6 ± 4.2 $cm^2$, $P = 0.007$) postprandially compared with healthy subjects (Figure 1). The corresponding differences in the sagittal diameter were 5.3 ± 1.0 vs 4.7 ± 0.9 cm ($P = 0.04$) after 5 min and 4.4 ± 1.2 vs 3.9 ± 0.8 cm, ($P = 0.09$) after 15 min (Table 2). In the fasting state the antral area tended to be larger in patients than in healthy subjects (4.9 ± 3.2 vs 3.4 ± 1.1 $cm^2$; $P = 0.05$) (Table 3). Postprandially, there were no significant difference in either oblique frontal diameter of the proximal stomach, antral area, or ratio of proximal to distal stomach area between patients and healthy subjects (Tables 2 and 3). The degree of esophagitis or the presence of a hiatus hernia did not influence the results.

Pain and discomfort were significantly greater in patients before ingestion of the meal (0.72 ± 1.08 vs 0.14 ± 0.19 cm, $P = 0.02$ and 1.16 ± 1.83 vs 0.44 ± 0.91 cm, $P = 0.005$, respectively (Table 4). In the postprandial period both groups experienced fullness, but patients with reflux esophagitis experienced significantly more postprandial fullness than the healthy subjects (3.76 ± 2.20 vs 1.16 ± 1.08 cm, $P = 0.0004$) (Figure 2). In the patient group there was a significant correlation between postprandial sagittal area of the proximal stomach and postprandial fullness at 5 min ($r = 0.69$; $P = 0.0007$) (Figure 3) and at 15 min ($r = 0.51$; $P = 0.02$), but not in the control group. In this study we did not find any significant correlation between postprandial epigastric fullness and size of antral area neither in patients nor in healthy subjects.

Patients with reflux esophagitis had greater body mass index ($P = 0.003$) (Table 1), but there was no significant correlation between body mass index and postprandial sagittal area of the proximal stomach ($r = 0.01$; $P = 0.6$), or postprandial fullness ($r = 0.03$; $P = 0.9$). The degree of esophagitis or the presence of a hiatial hernia did not significantly influence to the above results.

## DISCUSSION

This is the first study to employ ultrasonography to investigate gastric accommodation in patients with mild or moderate reflux esophagitis. The finding of an enlarged sagittal area of the proximal stomach soon after intake of a liquid meal is the opposite of what we previously found using the same ultrasonographic method in patients with functional dyspepsia (11, 19). Functional dyspepsia patients as a group were found to have a significantly smaller sagittal area of the proximal stomach and a wider gastric antrum in re-

Published with permission



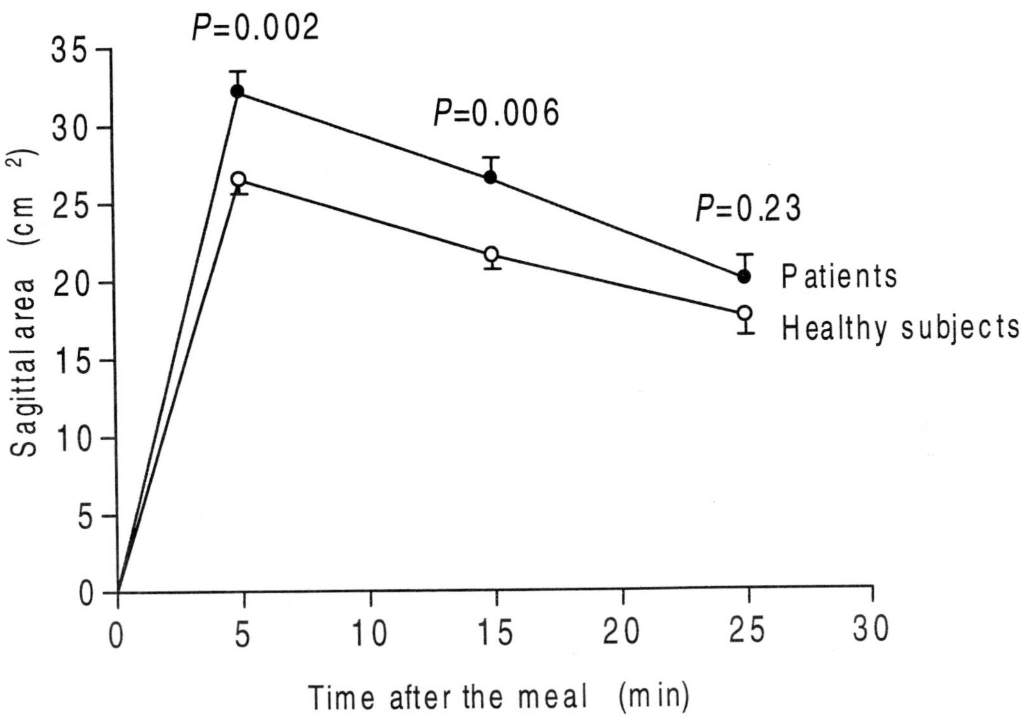


**Fig 1.** Changes in sagittal area of the proximal stomach following a 500-ml soup meal studied by ultrasonography. Bars denoting SEM are depicted. Patients with reflux esophagitis grade I or II revealed a significant larger sagittal area of the proximal stomach at 5 and 15 min postprandially compared with healthy subjects.

sponse to the meal than healthy subjects (11, 19). One might have expected similar findings in patients with functional dyspepsia and patients with GERD because there is a considerable overlap in symptoms between the two patient groups. Many patients with reflux disease complain of upper abdominal discomfort (21–23). Thus, in the present study, the most pronounced early postprandial symptom in patients with reflux esophagitis was postprandial fullness, which is a symptom also often seen in patients with functional dyspepsia. Nevertheless, our ultrasonographic findings support the view that functional dyspepsia and GERD are two separate disorders.

Both the early symptom generation and the significant correlation between postprandial fullness and sagittal proximal stomach area suggest that postprandial fullness is causally related to gastric distension. In a review of 670 upper gastrointestinal endoscopies,

Table 2. Postprandial Sagittal and Oblique Frontal Diameter of Proximal Stomach*

| *Postprandial time (min)* | *Healthy (cm)* | *Patients (cm)* | P |
|---|---|---|---|
| Sagittal diameter | | | |
| 5 min | 4.74 ± 0.87 (4.58) | 5.35 ± 0.96 (5.35) | 0.04 |
| 15 min | 3.89 ± 0.84 (3.95) | 4.45 ± 1.21 (4.21) | 0.09 (NS) |
| 25 min | 3.15 ± 0.80 (3.16) | 3.51 ± 1.18 (3.52) | 0.27 (NS) |
| Oblique frontal diameter | | | |
| 5 min | 7.38 ± 1.05 (7.59) | 7.68 ± 1.01 (7.85) | 0.36 (NS) |
| 15 min | 6.02 ± 1.12 (6.11) | 6.43 ± 1.19 (6.43) | 0.27 (NS) |
| 25 min | 5.07 ± 1.27 (4.81) | 5.50 ± 1.18 (5.86) | 0.28 (NS) |

*In 20 healthy subjects and 20 patients with reflux esophagitis obtained by ultrasonographic scanning. Mean ± SD (median) values.

Published with permission



TABLE 3. ANTRAL AREA AND RATIO OF PROXIMAL TO DISTAL SAGITTAL AREA*

| *Postprandial time (min)* | *Healthy* | *Patients* | P |
|---|---|---|---|
| Antral area ($cm^2$) | | | |
| Fasting | 3.36 ± 1.12 (3.19) | 4.89 ± 3.21 (4.50) | 0.052 (NS) |
| 5 min | 15.92 ± 6.67 (16.44) | 14.77 ± 5.10 (12.78) | 0.54 (NS) |
| 15 min | 12.73 ± 6.89 (12.24) | 11.98 ± 5.79 (12.16) | 0.71 (NS) |
| 25 min | 9.94 ± 6.41 (9.20) | 9.89 ± 5.30 (9.69) | 0.98 (NS) |
| 35 min | 7.86 ± 5.02 (7.45) | 8.17 ± 4.92 (7.75) | 0.83 (NS) |
| Ratio of proximal to distal | | | |
| 5 min | 2.17 ± 1.38 (1.42) | 2.38 ± 0.80 (2.33) | 0.56 (NS) |
| 15 min | 2.07 ± 1.02 (1.67) | 3.31 ± 3.40 (2.38) | 0.13 (NS) |
| 25 min | 2.37 ± 1.21 (2.17) | 2.64 ± 1.72 (2.00) | 0.58 (NS) |

*In 20 healthy subjects and 20 patients with reflux esophagitis studied by ultrasound. Mean ± SD (median) values.

patients with grade I or II reflux esophagitis were significantly more likely to be overweight (24). Consistent with this prior finding, the present patients as a group had greater body mass indexes than healthy subjects, but the severity of postprandial fullness and sagittal proximal stomach area were unrelated to

TABLE 4. SYMPTOM SCORES ASSESSED ON A VISUAL ANALOG SCALE BEFORE AND AFTER TEST MEAL*

| | *Fasting* | | | *Postprandial* | | |
|---|---|---|---|---|---|---|
| *Symptoms* | *Controls* | *Patients* | P | *Controls* | *Patients* | P |
| Pain | 0.14 ± 0.19 | 0.72 ± 1.08 | 0.02 | 0.16 ± 0.17 | 0.73 ± 1.36 | NS |
| Nausea | 0.34 ± 0.96 | 0.63 ± 0.94 | NS | 0.86 ± 1.71 | 1.02 ± 1.75 | NS |
| Fullness | 0.34 ± 0.70 | 1.16 ± 1.83 | 0.07 | 1.57 ± 1.44 | 3.76 ± 2.20 | 0.0006 |
| Discomfort | 0.44 ± 0.91 | 1.67 ± 1.62 | 0.005 | 0.93 ± 1.36 | 1.67 ± 1.80 | NS |
| Hunger/satiety | 2.71 ± 2.07 | 3.01 ± 2.33 | NS | 5.40 ± 2.32 | 5.52 ± 2.37 | NS |

*In 20 healthy subjects and in 20 patients with reflux esophagitis. Mean ± SD values. Scores are in centimeters based on a 10-cm scale

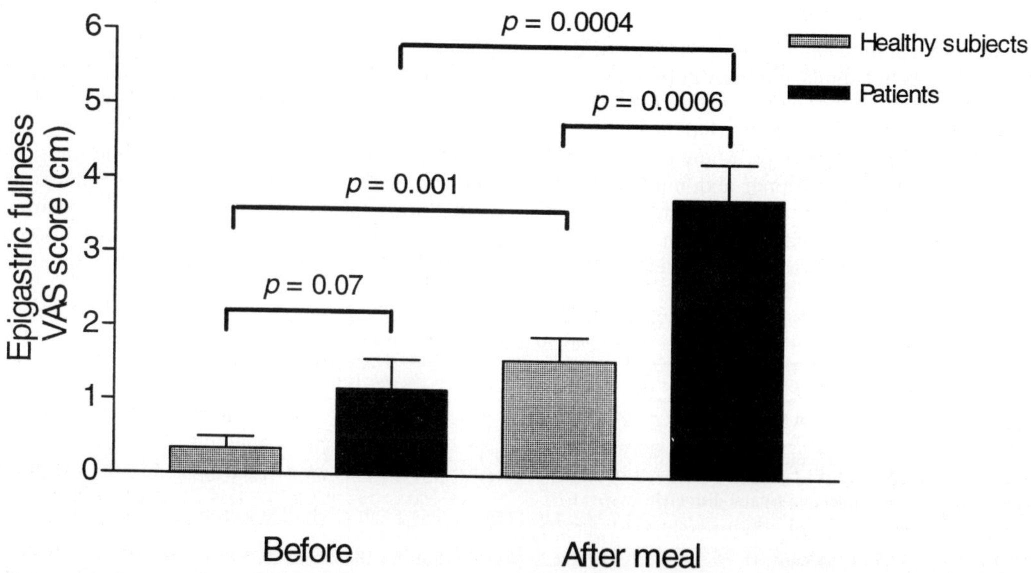


**Fig 2.** Pre- and postprandial epigastric fullness in 20 healthy subjects and 20 patients with reflux esophagitis grade I or II. Mean values with SEM.

Published with permission



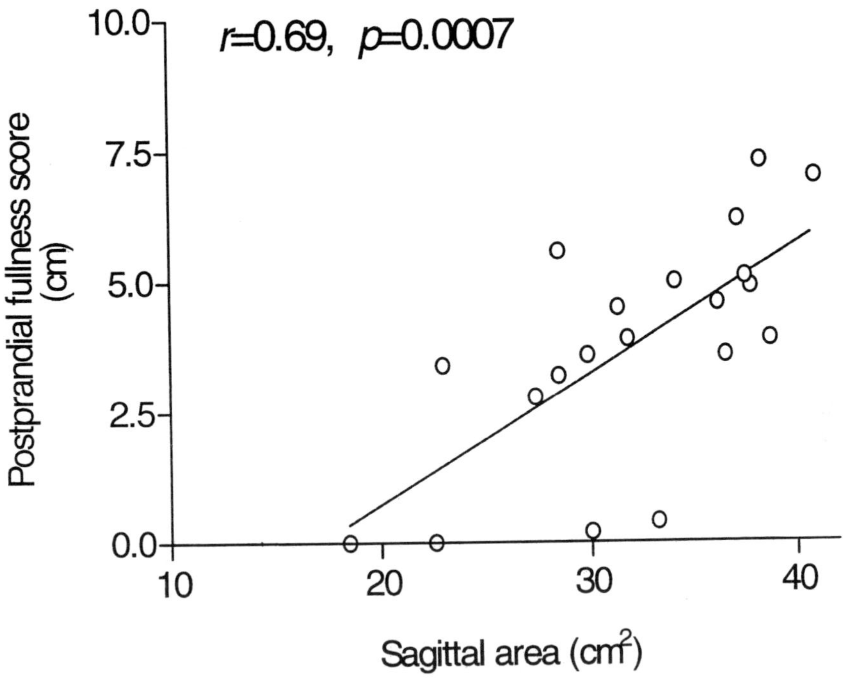


**Fig 3.** Correlation between postprandial fullness and 5-min postprandial sagittal area of the proximal stomach in 20 healthy subjects and 20 patients with reflux esophagitis grade I or II. There was a comparable correlation at 15 min postprandially ($r$ = 0.51; $P$ = 0.02).

body mass index, suggesting that a high body mass index can explain neither the postprandial fullness nor the increased stomach area in these patients.

In patients with GERD the majority of reflux episodes are preceded by a transient lower esophageal sphincter relaxation (TLESR), which is a prolonged relaxation of the lower esophageal sphincter not associated with swallowing (25–27). Stimulation of tensoreceptors, especially in the subcardial area, caused by distension of the proximal stomach, is supposed to be a major factor that increases the frequency of TLESR (28–30). TLESR is accompanied by acid reflux in about 40–50% of normal subjects and in 60–70% of patients with reflux disease (25, 31–34). Acid reflux is more likely to occur when the stomach is full and distended than when it is empty. Enhanced postprandial gastric distension may provide a potent stimulus for triggering TLESRs and facilitate gastroesophageal reflux. Hence, the abnormally wide proximal stomach, as observed in the present study, might contribute to the main event in GERD.

Gastric relaxation in patients with reflux esophagitis has previously been studied by barostat. The barostat can measure gastric tone and from that one can make inferences about gastric accommodation. Penagini et al found delayed recovery of proximal gastric tone after intake of a combined solid and liquid meal (35). Zerbib et al found postprandial gastric relaxation to be more pronounced in GERD patients than in normal controls or patients with dyspepsia (7), while Hartley et al found that the gastric pressure response to distension was reduced in fasting patients with GERD (36). Recently, Vu et al found that postprandial gastric relaxation was significantly prolonged in patients with GERD compared to GERD patients who had undergone Nissen fundoplication or controls (37). Taken together, these studies show that there are significant abnormalities in proximal gastric motor function in patients with GERD. We have documented abnormal gastric accommodation as soon as the first 15 min postprandially. Together with the delayed postprandial recovery of gastric tone, as shown by Penagini et al (35), our results suggest an impairment of vagal reflexes in patients with reflux esophagitis as previously noted by Ogilvie et al (38). Vagal nerve dysfunction might also

Published with permission



be important in the etiology of other motility disturbances commonly found in patients with GERD, such as delayed esophageal transit, abnormal peristalsis, and LES dysfunction (30, 39).

Using a computerized gastric tensostat, Distrutti et al (40) showed that gastric wall tension determines the perception of distension. We did not measure intragastric pressure, and we are therefore unable to calculate wall tension. Our findings of an increased proximal sagittal area and unchanged oblique frontal diameter suggest an increased proximal stomach volume. Because this volume increase might be causally related to the perception of postprandial fullness/distension, we are inclined to suppose that even though the volume of the proximal stomach increased more than in controls, the increase might be too small to balance a change in intragastric pressure and thus avoid the perception of distension during the first 15 min after the meal.

The present ultrasonographic method offers advantages over established methods for the study of gastric accommodation, such as the gastric barostat, because it is noninvasive, safe, comfortable, and does not disturb normal gastrointestinal motility. Our ultrasonographic measurements indicate an abnormal postprandial distension of the proximal stomach in GERD patients, which might constitute a major underlying mechanism for impaired lower esophageal sphincter function and abnormal gastroesophageal reflux.

## REFERENCES

1. Desai KM, Sessa WC, Vane JR: Involvment of nitric oxide in the reflaxation of the stomach to accommodate food or fluid. Nature 351:477–479, 1991
2. Desai KM, Zembowicz A, Sessa WC, Vane JR: Nitroxergic nerves mediate vagally induced relaxation in the isolated stomach of the guinea pig. Proc Natl Acid Sci USA 88:11490–11494, 1991
3. Uno H, Arakawa T, Fukuda T, Higuchi K, Kobayashi K: Involvment of capsaicin-sensitive sensory nerves in gastric adaptive relaxation in isolated guinea-pig stomachs. Digestion 58:232–239, 1997
4. Jahnberg T, Abrahamsson H, Jansson G, Martinson J: Gastric relaxatory response to feeding before and after vagotomy. Scand J gastroenterol 12(2):225–228, 1977
5. McCallum RW, Berkowitz DM, Lerner E: Gastric emptying in patient with gastroesophageal reflux. Gastroenterology 80:285–291, 1981
6. Maddern GJ, Chatterton BE, Collins PJ, Horowitz M, Shearman DJC, Jamieson GG: Solid and liquid gastric emptying in patients with gastro-oesophageal reflux. Br J Surg 72:344–347, 1985
7. Zerbib F, des Varannes SB, Ropert A, Lamouliatte H, Quinton A, Galmiche JP: Proximal gastric tone in gastro-oesophageal reflux disease. Eur J Gastroenterol Hepatol 11:511–515, 1999
8. Moragas GM, Azpiroz F, Pavia J, Malagelada J-R: Relation among intragastric pressure postcibal percebtion, and gastric emptying. Am J Physiol 264:G1112–G1117, 1993
9. Ropert A, des Varannes SB, Bizais Y, Roze C, Galmiche JP: Simultaneous assessment of liquid emptying and proximal gastric tone in humans. Gastroenterology 105:667–674, 1993
10. Gilja OH, Hausken T, Odegaard S, Berstad A: Monitoring postprandial size of the proximal stomach by ultrasonography. J Ultrasound Med 14(2):81–89, 1995
11. Gilja OH, Hausken T, Wilhelmsen I, Berstad A: Impaired accommodation of proximal stomach to a meal in functional dyspepsia. Dig Dis Sci 41(4):689–696, 1996
12. Gilja OH, Hausken T, Bang CJ, Berstad A: Effect of glyceryl trinitrate on gastric accommodation and symptoms in functional dyspepsia. Dig Dis Sci 42(10):2124–2131, 1997
13. Undeland KA, Hausken T, Gilja OH, Aanderud S, Berstad A: Gastric meal accommodation studied by ultrasound in diabetes. Relation to vagal tone. Scand J Gastroenterol 33(3):236–241, 1998
14. Olafsdottir E, Gilja OH, Aslaksen A, Berstad A, Fluge G: Impaired accommodation of the proximal stomach in childeren with recurrent abdominal pain. J Pediatr Gastroenterol 1999 (in press)
15. Hatlebakk JG, Berstad A, Carling L, et al: Lansoprazole versus omeprazole in short-term treatment of reflux oesophagitis. Scand J Gastroenterol 28:224–228, 1993
16. Berstad A, Olafsson S, Tefera S, et al: A review of five years experience at a university hospital in Norway. J Physiol Pharmacol 47:31–49, 1996
17. Kimmey MB, Martin RW, Haggitt RC, Wang KY, Franklin DW, Silverstein FE: Histologic correlated of gastrointestinal ultrasound images. Gastroenterology 96:433–441, 1989
18. Gilja OH, Detmer PR, Jong JM, Leotta DF, Li XN, Beach KW, Martin R, Strandness E: Intragastric distribution and gastric emptying assessed by three-dimensional ultrasonography. Gastroenterology 113:38–49, 1997
19. Hausken T, Berstad A: Wide gastric antrum in patients with non-ulcer dyspepsia. Effect of cisapride. Scand J Gastroenterol 27:427–432, 1992
20. Hausken T, Odegaard S, Matre K, Bersatd A: Antroduodenal motility and movements of luminal contents studied by duplex sonography. Gastroenterology 102:1583–1590, 1992
21. Talley NJ, Colin-Jones D, Koch KL, Koch M, Nyren O, Stanghellini V: Functional dyspepsia: a classification with guidelines for diagnosis and management. Gastroenterol Int 4:145–160, 1991
22. Klauser A, Schindlbeck N, Muller-Lissner S: Symptoms in gastro-oesophageal reflux disease. Lancet 335:205–208, 1990
23. Shi G, Bruley des Varannes S, Scarpignato C, Le Rhun M, Galmiche JP: Reflux related symptoms in patients with normal oesophageal exposure to acid. Gut 37:457–464, 1995
24. Berstad A, Weberg R, Froyshov Larsen I, Hoel B, Hauer-Jensen M: Relationship of hiatus hernia to reflux oesophagitis. A prospective study of coincidence, using endoscopy. Scand J Gastroenterol 21(1):55–58, 1986
25. Dodds WJ, Dent J, Hogan WJ, Helm JF, Hauser RG, Patel GW, Egide M: Mechanisms of gastrooesophageal reflux in patient with reflux oesophagitis. N Engl J Med 307:1547–1552, 1982
26. Dent J, Holloway RH, Toouli J, Dodds WJ: Mechanisms of

# INDEX

## M

**R**

**T**